Skin Cancer

Recognition and Management

Second Edition

Robert A. Schwartz, MD, MPH, FACP, FAAD
Professor and Head, Dermatology
Professor of Pathology
Professor of Medicine
Professor of Pediatrics
Professor of Preventive Medicine and Community Health
New Jersey Medical School
Newark, New Jersey
USA

Blackwell
Publishing

© 2008 by Blackwell Publishing
Blackwell Publishing, Inc., 350 Main Street, Malden, Massachusetts 02148-5020, USA
Blackwell Publishing Ltd, 9600 Garsington Road, Oxford OX4 2DQ, UK
Blackwell Publishing Asia Pty Ltd, 550 Swanston Street, Carlton, Victoria 3053, Australia

The right of the Author to be identified as the Author of this Work has been asserted in accordance with the Copyright, Designs and Patents Act 1988.

First published 2008

1   2008

Library of Congress Cataloging-in-Publication Data

Skin cancer : recognition and management / [edited by] Robert Schwartz. – 2nd ed.
    p. ; cm.
   Includes bibliographical references.
   ISBN 978-1-4051-5961-6 (alk. paper)
1. Skin–Cancer.   I. Schwartz, Robert A., 1947–
   [DNLM: 1. Skin Neoplasms–diagnosis.   2. Skin Neoplasms–therapy. WR 500
S628 2007]

RC280.S5S58 2007
616.99′477–dc22

                    2007010197

ISBN: 978-1-4051-5961-6

A catalogue record for this title is available from the British Library

Set in Meridien 9pt/12pt by Aptara Inc., New Delhi, India
Printed and bound in Singapore by Fabulous Printers Pte Ltd

Commissioning Editor: Martin Sugden
Editorial Assistant: Jennifer Seward
Development Editors: Adam Gilbert, Fiona Pattison
Production Controller: Debbie Wyer

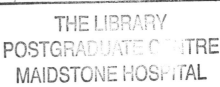

For further information on Blackwell Publishing, visit our website:
http://www.blackwellpublishing.com

The publisher's policy is to use permanent paper from mills that operate a sustainable forestry policy, and which has been manufactured from pulp processed using acid-free and elementary chlorine-free practices. Furthermore, the publisher ensures that the text paper and cover board used have met acceptable environmental accreditation standards.

Designations used by companies to distinguish their products are often claimed as trademarks. All brand names and product names used in this book are trade names, service marks, trademarks or registered trademarks of their respective owners. The Publisher is not associated with any product or vendor mentioned in this book.

The contents of this work are intended to further general scientific research, understanding, and discussion only and are not intended and should not be relied upon as recommending or promoting a specific method, diagnosis, or treatment by physicians for any particular patient. The publisher and the author make no representations or warranties with respect to the accuracy or completeness of the contents of this work and specifically disclaim all warranties, including without limitation any implied warranties of fitness for a particular purpose. In view of ongoing research, equipment modifications, changes in governmental regulations, and the constant flow of information relating to the use of medicines, equipment, and devices, the reader is urged to review and evaluate the information provided in the package insert or instructions for each medicine, equipment, or device for, among other things, any changes in the instructions or indication of usage and for added warnings and precautions. Readers should consult with a specialist where appropriate. The fact that an organization or Website is referred to in this work as a citation and/or a potential source of further information does not mean that the author or the publisher endorses the information the organization or Website may provide or recommendations it may make. Further, readers should be aware that Internet Websites listed in this work may have changed or disappeared between when this work was written and when it is read. No warranty may be created or extended by any promotional statements for this work. Neither the publisher nor the author shall be liable for any damages arising herefrom.

Contents

Contributors

Mary S. Brady, MD
Assistant Professor, Surgery
Joan and Sanford I. Weill College
    of Medicine of Cornell University
Memorial Sloan-Kettering Cancer Center
New York, New York, USA

Günter Burg, MD
Professor and Chairman Emeritus
Dermatology
Universität Zürich
Zürich, Switzerland

Eds Chua, MD
Visiting Procedural Dermatology Fellow
Skin Laser and Surgery Specialists of
    New York and New Jersey
New York, New York, USA

Philip J. Cohen, MD
Chief of Dermatology
VA New Jersey Health Care System
East Orange, New Jersey, USA

Denis K. Dudley, MD, FRCS (C)
Executive Director, Laserderm
Ottawa, Canada

Reinhard Dummer, MD
Professor of Dermatology
Universität Zürich
Zürich, Switzerland

Jeffrey I. Ellis, MD
Dermatology, SUNY Downstate
    School of Medicine
Director, Dermatologic Surgery

North Shore University Hospital and
    Long Island Jewish Medical Center
New Hyde Park, New York, USA

David J. Goldberg, MD, JD
Clinical Professor of Dermatology
Mt. Sinai School of Medicine
Clinical Professor of Dermatology
New Jersey Medical School
Adjunct Professor of Law
Fordham Law School
Director, Skin Laser and Surgery Specialists of
    New York and New Jersey
New York, New York, USA

Klaus Helm, MD
Professor of Dermatology and Pathology
Director, Dermatopathology
Pennsylvania State University
    College of Medicine
Milton S. Hershey Medical Center
Hershey, Pennsylvania, USA

Thomas N. Helm, MD
Clinical Associate Professor of Dermatology and
    Pathology
State University of New York at Buffalo
Buffalo, New York, USA

Ulrich R. Hengge, MD
Professor of Dermatology
Heinrich-Heine-University
Düsseldorf, Germany

Maja A. Hofmann, MD
Department of Dermatology and Allergy
Skin Cancer Center

Charité - Universitätsmedizin
Berlin, Germany

Werner Kempf, MD
Lecturer and Consultant Physician
Department of Dermatology
Universität Zürich
Co-Director
Kempf und Pfaltz
Histologische Diagnostik
Zürich, Switzerland

Emanuel G. Kuflik, MD
Clinical Professor of Dermatology
New Jersey Medical School
Newark, New Jersey, USA

Francesco Lacarrubba, MD
Assistant Professor, Dermatology
University of Catania
Catania, Italy

W. Clark Lambert, MD, PhD
Professor and Associate Head, Dermatology
Professor of Pathology
Chief, Dermatopathology
New Jersey Medical School
Newark, New Jersey, USA

Sharyn A. Laughlin, MD, FRCS (C)
Assistant Professor of Dermatology
University of Ottawa Faculty of Medicine
Ottawa, Ontario, Canada

Arthur Mashberg, DDS
Professor of Surgery, Emeritus
New Jersey Medical School
Newark, New Jersey, USA

Giuseppe Micali, MD
Professor and Chair, Dermatology
University of Catania
Catania, Italy

Beatrice Nardone, MD
Resident in Dermatology
University of Catania
Catania, Italy

Robert A. Schwartz, MD, MPH, FACP, FAAD
Professor and Head, Dermatology
Professor of Pathology
Professor of Medicine
Professor of Pediatrics
Professor of Preventive Medicine and
    Community Health
New Jersey Medical School
Newark, New Jersey, USA

Kyu H. Shin, MD
Professor of Radiation Oncology
State University of New York at Buffalo
Director, CCS Oncology Center
Buffalo, New York, USA

Daniel M. Siegel, MD, MS
Clinical Professor of Dermatology
Director, Procedural Dermatology
    Fellowship
State University of New York Downstate
    Medical Center
Brooklyn, New York, USA

Christopher J. Steen, MD
Staff Physician
Department of Dermatology
New Jersey Medical School
Newark, New Jersey, USA

Wolfram Sterry, MD
Professor and Head
Department of Dermatology
University of Medical Faculty Charite
Berlin, Germany

James R. Trimble, MD
Private practice
Jacksonville, Florida, USA

James W. Trimble, MD
Private practice
Jacksonville, Florida, USA

Mark R. Wick, MD
Professor and Associate Director,
    Surgical Pathology
University of Virginia School of Medicine
Charlottesville, Virginia, USA

Preface

The skin, uniquely positioned at the interface between the human body and the external world, plays a multifaceted role in the expression of cancer. Primary skin cancer is the most common cancer afflicting mankind and is rising in incidence, despite the fact that it is often preventable. Besides primary cancer, the skin may show direct and indirect evidence of internal cancer, thus serving as a window to the body for both laymen and physicians alike. In addition, the accessibility of the skin is useful for the study of carcinogenesis as well as cancer treatment options.

I owe much of my interest in skin cancer to Leon Goldman, the father of dermatologic laser surgery, and to Edmund Klein, the father of modern immunotherapy. I am also grateful to Peter J. Lynch for recruiting me as an early faculty member in the dermatology program he had founded at the University of Arizona. Their support and guidance has proven invaluable in preparing me for academia, as I complete my 25th year as professor and founding head of dermatology at this the New Jersey Medical School. I am grateful to Dr. Stewart Taylor, formerly Publisher, Medical Division, Blackwell Publishing in Oxford, United Kingdom, for encouraging and gaining approval for this 2nd edition, and to his successor, Martin Sugden, working alongside Adam Gilbert (Development Editor), for facilitating its fruition. I thank my talented and loyal administrative staff person, Mrs. Linda D. Hesselbirg. My dermatologist wife, Camila, and I are also thankful for the encouragement of our mentor, Professor Stefania Jabłońska, and our distinguished colleagues, including in alphabetical order: Professors Julian Ambrus (Buffalo), Gerimanta Balévičiene (Vilnius), Eugeniusz Baran (Wrocław), Jerzy Bowszyc (Poznań), Walter H. C. Burgdorf (Munich), Stefano Calvieri (Rome), Luiz G. Martins Castro (São Paolo), Olegas Čeburkov (Kaunas), Enrico Ceccolini (Bologna), Hong-Duo Chen (Shenyang), Bożena Chodynicka (Białystok), William P. Coleman III (New Orleans), Vincent A. De Leo (New York), Richard L. Dobson (Charleston), Peter M. Elias (San Francisco), Michael D. Fox (Mill Valley), Pere Gascón (Barcelona), Alberto Giannetti (Modena), Lawrence E. Gibson (Rochester), Harald Gollnick (Magdeburg), Vladimír Hegyi (Bratislava), Jana Hercogová (Prague), Karl Holubar (Vienna), Chull-Wan Ihm (Chonju), Daniele Innocenzi (Rome), Aleksej Kansky (Ljubljana), Djordjije Karadaglic (Podgorica), Helmut Kerl (Graz), Neena Khanna (New Delhi), Uday Khopkar (Mumbai), Cezary Kowalewski (Warsaw), Alicja Kurnatowska (Łódź), Piotr Kurnatowski (Łódź), Jonas Lelas (Vilnius), Jasna Lipozenčič (Zagreb), Torello M. Lotti (Florence), Sławomir Majewski (Warsaw), Romuald Maleszka (Szczecin), Jon G. Meine (Cleveland), Giuseppi Micali (Catania), Felix Milgrom (Buffalo), Halina Milgrom (Buffalo), Anastazy Omulecki (Łódź), Joseph L. Pace (Valletta), Lawrence C. Parish (Philadelphia), Zofia Piela (Rzeszów), Mario Pippione (Torin), Waldemar Placek (Bydgoszcz), Murlidhar Rajagopalan (Chennai), Jadwiga

Roszkiewicz (Gdańsk), Andris Y. Rubins (Riga), Vincenzo Ruocco (Naples), Zbigniew Ruszczak (Berlin), Thomas Ruzicka (Munich), Stuart J. Salasche (Tucson), D.V. Siva Sankar (Westbury), Jean-Hilaire Saurat (Geneva), Wojciech Silny (Poznań), Jay Siwek (Washington DC), Georg Stingl (Vienna), Anna Sysa-Jędrzejowska (Łódź), Henryk Szarmach (Gdańsk), Jacek C. Szepietowski (Wrocław), James S. Taylor (Cleveland), Aurora Tedeschi (Catania), Wally J. Temple (Calgary), Kenneth J. Tomecki (Cleveland), Barbara Toruniowa (Lublin), Takuo Tsuji (Nagoya), Skaidra Valiukevičíene (Kaunas), František Vosmík (Prague), and Alexander Zajczenko (Lviv). Helping anchor Camila and me on a nonmedical front is our mother, Lusia Krysicka (a hero of the Warsaw Resurrection); 102-year-old uncle, Robert Upright, back home in San Francisco; and aunt Dolly Schwartz in Oakland, California.

We are fortunate in this work to have some of the world's foremost authorities in their areas of expertise as contributors, in alphabetical order: Professors Mary Sue Brady, Günter Burg, David J. Goldberg, Ulrich R. Hengge, Emanuel G. Kuflik, W. Clark Lambert, Arthur Mashberg, Giuseppe Micali, Daniel M. Siegel, Wolfram Sterry, and Mark R. Wick. I am also blessed with the strong support and encouragement of my colleagues at this New York City metropolitan area medical school (founded in 1954 as Seton Hall College of Medicine; New Jersey College of Medicine 1965 to 1970; New Jersey Medical School, since 1970).

I have been honored to serve in multiple roles at the New Jersey Medical School, including as the first tenured head of dermatology in the history of the state of New Jersey, being able with Professors W. Clark Lambert, Roger H. Brodkin, Tamotsu Imaeda, and George Kihiczak to establish the first dermatology residency training program in New Jersey. From this medical school faculty I also thank Michael P. Bagley, Soly Baredes, Santiago A. Centurión, Stanley Cohen, Manuel A. Cruz, Hugh E. Evans, Lawrence P. Frohman, Bunyad Haider, George J. Hill, Robert L. Johnson, Mark Jordan, Rajendra Kapila, Julianne H. Kuflik, John Kwittken, Carroll Moton Leevy, Ruy V. Lourenço, Judit Nyirady, Jerry Rothenberg, Christopher W. Scialis, Kenneth G. Swan, Isabelle Thomas, and Jeffrey M. Whitworth. Dermatology has become an important part of our academic community, allowing me to serve as Faculty President, Alpha Omega Alpha National Honor Medical Society Chapter Councilor, and as Sigma Xi Chapter President. I am gratified that one of my first dermatology residents, Philip J. Cohen, has coauthored two chapters in this book as he continues his thriving academic career after years with Professor Stephen I. Katz at the National Institutes of Health, returning to his alma mater as chief of dermatology at our New Jersey Veterans Administrations Medical Center in East Orange. It is satisfying to have one of my loftiest chief residents, Christopher J. Steen, as a coauthor of a chapter. I am appreciative of my talented current residents—Christopher J. Steen, Robyn D. Siperstein, Lenis M. González, George G. Kihiczak, Smeeta Sinha, Stephen J. Nervi, Justin Brown, Anjali K. Butani, Mordechai M. Tarlow, and Geover Fernández—as well as our dermatopathology residents Wen Chen, Rajit Malliah, and Wanda M. Patterson—with particular thanks to Lenis González, George G. Kihiczak, Sharon E. Hwang, and Wen Chen with regard to this book.

I am fortunate for many reasons. It is inspiring to have the friendship of Theodore Cardinal E. McCarrick, PhD. Munificent colleagues have facilitated my election as an honorary member of the national dermatology societies of Italy, Czech Republic, Korea, Poland, Slovenia, Slovakia, Latvia, Lithuania, Ukraine, and Yugoslavia. I am indebted to Institute of Immunology and Experimental Therapeutics Director Jacek Szepietowski, rector and the academic senate for the Academia Medica Wratislasiensis Medal, awarded in June 2007 by the University Rector Magnificus, Medical University of Wrocław (Breslau). Special thanks goes to Professor Wiesław Gliński, Chairman, Dermatology, Medical University of Warsaw, for his timely assistance and to Katie Greczylo for her superb efforts as project manager.

CHAPTER 1
Introduction

Robert A. Schwartz

Skin cancer, the most common cancer worldwide, has an incidence doubling every 15 to 20 years! The principle factor inducing most of the primary skin cancers discussed in this book is ultraviolet light–induced carcinogenesis. However, as we will stress, other parts of the electromagnetic spectrum, such as x-rays and infrared rays (heat), may also be carcinogenic (Table 1.1). In addition, viral and chemical carcinogenesis may be very important. Details of ultraviolet light–induced carcinogenesis are delineated within the respective chapters on basal cell carcinoma, squamous cell carcinoma, actinic keratosis, melanoma, and the deadliest of all skin cancers: Merkel cell carcinoma [1]. The increased risks for five additional cancer types (prostate, breast, and colon cancers, non-Hodgkin's lymphoma, and multiple myeloma) in first-degree relatives of melanoma cases suggest that individuals with a family history of melanoma should strictly adhere to recommended screenings for all cancers [2].

There are two major challenges in dealing with cancer, the first being prevention. The use of sunscreens has been emphasized and needs to be stressed. Actual skin protection chiefly depends on the way sunscreens are used and the quantity applied [3]. Skin cancer prevention is facilitated by explicit labeling and free provision of sunscreen. Prevention should begin early in childhood [4]. Proper young ladies and men should be seen with bonnets or hats and long sleeves, not photoaging themselves unnecessarily. Certainly, the structural and functional changes of normal cutaneous aging include decreased growth of the epidermis, hair, and nails; delayed wound healing; and impaired cutaneous immune responses. Photoaging,

however, is a different process [5]. Evidence suggests that topical retinoids not only may decelerate the photoaging process but also are capable of repairing photoaged skin at both the clinical and biochemical levels and may prevent photoaging [6]. In addition, topical retinoids could be beneficial in the treatment of intrinsically aged skin. Antioxidants may also be employed, particularly in combination, to reduce and neutralize free radicals [7]. Importantly, for every light-complexioned individual (Fig. 1.1), protection from the premature and unsightly effects of sun exposure is mandatory (Table 1.2). As both melanocytic nevi and sunburn are risk factors for the development of melanoma, we should target fair-skinned transplant recipients with melanocytic nevi for sun avoidance education [8]. The goal should be the prevention of both photoaging and photocarcinogensis [9]. Risk assessment is a good idea [10].

A secondary challenge is detection, because most cancers are curable if caught early. This point is emphasized by the "developing epidemic of melanoma" in Hispanic men in California [11]. A statistically significant 1.8% per year increase in incidence of invasive melanomas among Hispanic males has been observed between 1988 and 2001. Among them, melanomas thicker than 1.5 mm at presentation increased at 11.6% per year. This increase in melanoma in Hispanics, confined to thicker tumors with a poor prognosis, emphasizes the need for both prevention and early detection.

The worldwide scourge of AIDS, beginning for us in Europe and America in the early 1980s, is an epidemic that is not abating [12–16]. Kaposi's sarcoma has been an intrinsic part of this epidemic, as delineated in the Kaposi's sarcoma chapter. Since the

Table 1.1 Electromagnetic spectrum

Type of Radiation	Wavelength
Gamma rays, x-rays, Grenz rays	Below 1 nm (10 angstroms)
Ultraviolet light (UV)	
UV "C" range	1–290 nm
UV B	290–320 nm (through ozone layer)
UV A	320–400 nm (through window glass)
Visible light	400–700 nm
Infrared radiation (heat)	700–1,000,000 nm
Radio waves	1,000,000 nm and above

Table 1.2 Preventing skin cancers and premature aging (photoaging)

Avoid sun exposure
Use sunscreen preparations and cover body with clothing
Consider topical retinoid use

first edition of this book was published, the etiologic agent of Kaposi's sarcoma has been identified [17]. Although the incidence of Kaposi's sarcoma has declined dramatically in areas with access to highly active antiretroviral therapy, it remains the most common AIDS-associated malignancy in the developed world and is one of the most common malignancies in developing nations. Current treatment options are ineffective, unavailable, or toxic to many affected persons. A growing body of basic science, preclinical, and observational data suggests that antiviral medications may play an important role in the prevention and treatment of Kaposi's sarcoma–associated herpesvirus, providing hope for the future [18]. The skin may serve as an important organ for study in these patients and often manifests the first signs of AIDS.

Some cutaneous tumors remain an enigma. A good example, one even better than melanoma, is perhaps the deadliest of all skin cancers—Merkel cell carcinoma—which appears to have tripled in incidence from 1986 to 2001 in the United States and Canada [1]. Often appearing as an asymptomatic nodule on sun-exposed skin, it may resemble a basal cell carcinoma, a common misdiagnosis both clinically and histologically that may have fatal consequences. Its origin from the normal epidermal Merkel cell remains controversial, because this neoplasm originates in the dermis and only rarely

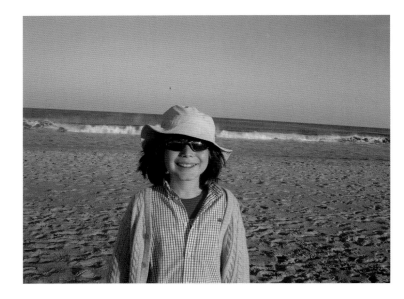

Fig. 1.1 The author's light-complexioned 10-year-old son, Edmund, exhibiting evidence of skin cancer prevention at a New Jersey beach.

Table 1.3 Cancers mimicking dermatitis

Erythroplasia of Queyrat and other sites
Paget's disease of the breast
Extramammary Paget's disease
Inflammatory metastatic carcinoma
Bowen's disease
Amelanotic lentigo maligna melanoma
Scar carcinoma

demonstrates epidermal involvement. It may be de-rived from the haarscheibe or hair disc (touch cor-puscles), composed predominantly of Merkel cells. Advances in our understanding of it are moving for-ward [19].

Viral oncogenesis has taken large leaps ahead through exciting technologic advances that have al-lowed the typing of human papillomaviruses and have linked them with a variety of skin cancers [20]. In the chapters that follow, some of the probable as-sociations of human papillomavirus infections and cancer are discussed. Through the study of model diseases, such as epidermodysplasia verruciformis and xeroderma pigmentosum, much has been and will continue to be learned about skin cancer. The topical application of the bacterial DNA repair en-zyme T4 endonuclease V to sun-damaged skin of patients with xeroderma pigmentosum has promise in lowering the rate of development of actinic ker-atoses and basal cell carcinoma [21,22].

As the chapters on recognition of skin cancer note, diagnosing skin cancers may at times be dif-ficult. It is amazing how often skin cancer may mimic dermatitis (eczema; Table 1.3). Conversely, worrisome skin tumors may represent benign cu-taneous processes or cutaneous infections, espe-cially in immunocompromised persons. The ability to immunosuppress transplant recipients and the AIDS epidemic bring dermatology to the forefront of medicine.

Modern molecular biology has led to much progress. There are important genetic changes con-tributing to the development of melanoma, basal cell carcinoma and squamous cell carcinoma, and other less common skin cancers [23]. Although our understanding of oncogenes and tumor suppressor genes involved in the development and progres-sion of skin tumors remains fragmentary, recent advances have shown alterations affecting con-served signaling pathways that control cellular pro-liferation and viability. The *BRAF* oncogene is a good example [24,25]. There have been more than 30 distinct *BRAF* mutations in melanomas described, varying in biological activity. Some may be predic-tive of clinically relevant tumor differences. *BRAF* somatic mutations are often found in primary and metastatic melanomas and melanocytic nevi. *BRAF*-mutant melanomas appear to be linked with host phenotype, tumor location, and pigmentation, with this somatic mutation sometimes associated with a germline one [26].

All of our modern advancements are of particular advantage in studying patients with genetic cancer syndromes, such as the dysplastic nevus syndrome, the basal cell nevus syndrome, xeroderma pigmen-tosum, and the Muir-Torre syndrome—all of which are also covered in the chapters to follow.

References

1 Schwartz RA, Lambert WC. The Merkel cell carcinoma: a 50-year retrospect. J Surg Oncol 2005;89:5.

2 Larson AA, Leachman SA, Eliason MJ, et al. Population-based assessment of non-melanoma can-cer risk in relatives of cutaneous melanoma probands. J Invest Dermatol 2007;127:183–8.

3 Nicol I, Gaudy C, Gouvernet J, et al. Skin protection by sunscreens is improved by explicit labeling and provid-ing free sunscreen. J Invest Dermatol 2007;127:41–8.

4 Azfar RS, Schwartz RA, Berwick M. Primary melanoma prevention in children. G Ital Dermatol Venereol 2004;139:267–72.

5 Rabe JH, Mamelak AJ, McElgunn PJ, et al. Photoag-ing: mechanisms and repair. J Am Acad Dermatol 2006;55:1–19.

6 Singh M, Griffiths CE. The use of retinoids in the treat-ment of photoaging. Dermatol Ther 2006;19:297–305.

7 Baumann L. Skin ageing and its treatment. J Pathol 2007;211:241–51.

8 Thomson MA, Suggett NR, Nightingale PG, et al. Skin surveillance of a U.K. paediatric transplant population. Br J Dermatol 2007;156:45–50.

9 Afaq F, Mukhtar H. Botanical antioxidants in the pre-vention of photocarcinogenesis and photoaging. Exp Dermatol 2006;15:678–84.

10 Schwartz RA. Cutaneous malignant melanoma risk assessment. G Ital Dermatol Venereol 2005;140:315–6.

11 Cockburn MG, Zadnick J, Deapen D. Developing epidemic of melanoma in the Hispanic population of California. Cancer 2006;106:1162–8.

12 Dourmishev LA, Dourmishev AL, Palmeri D, et al. Molecular genetics of Kaposi's sarcoma–associated herpesvirus (human herpesvirus-8) epidemiology and pathogenesis. Microbiol Mol Biol Rev 2003;67:175–212.

13 Hengge UR, Ruzicka T, Tyring SK, et al. Update on Kaposi's sarcoma and other HHV8 associated diseases. Part 1: epidemiology, environmental predispositions, clinical manifestations, and therapy. Lancet Infect Dis 2002;2:281–92.

14 Hengge UR, Ruzicka T, Tyring SK, et al. Update on Kaposi's sarcoma and other HHV8 associated diseases. Part 2: pathogenesis, Castleman's disease, and pleural effusion lymphoma. Lancet Infect Dis 2002;2:344–52.

15 Schwartz RA. Kaposi's sarcoma: an update. J Surg Oncol 2004;87:146–51.

16 Borkovic SP, Schwartz RA. Kaposi's sarcoma presenting in the homosexual man—a new and striking phenomenon! Ariz Med 1981;38:902–4.

17 Moore PS, Chang Y. Kaposi's sarcoma (KS), KS-associated herpesvirus, and the criteria for causality in the age of molecular biology. Am J Epidemiol 1998;147:217–21.

18 Casper C, Wald A. The use of antiviral drugs in the prevention and treatment of Kaposi sarcoma, multicentric Castleman disease and primary effusion lymphoma. Curr Top Microbiol Immunol 2007;312:289–307.

19 Fernandez-Figueras MT, Puig L, Musulen E, et al. Expression profiles associated with aggressive behavior in Merkel cell carcinoma. Mod Pathol 2007;20:90–101.

20 Majewski S, Jablonska S. Current views on the role of human papillomaviruses in cutaneous oncogenesis. Int J Dermatol 2006;45:192–6.

21 Wright TI, Spencer JM, Flowers FP. Chemoprevention of nonmelanoma skin cancer. J Am Acad Dermatol 2006;54:933–46; quiz 947–50.

22 Yarosh D, Klein J, O'Connor A, et al. Effect of topically applied T4 endonuclease V in liposomes on skin cancer in xeroderma pigmentosum: a randomised study. Xeroderma Pigmentosum Study Group. Lancet 2001;357:926–9.

23 Pons M, Quintanilla M. Molecular biology of malignant melanoma and other cutaneous tumors. Clin Transl Oncol 2006;8:466–74.

24 Thomas NE. BRAF somatic mutations in malignant melanoma and melanocytic naevi. Melanoma Res 2006;16:97–103.

25 Liu W, Kelly JW, Trivett M, et al. Distinct clinical and pathological features are associated with the BRAF(T1799A(V600E)) mutation in primary melanoma. J Invest Dermatol 2006;127:900–5.

26 Landi MT, Bauer J, Pfeiffer RM, et al. MC1R germline variants confer risk for BRAF-mutant melanoma. Science 2006;313:521–2.

CHAPTER 2
Actinic keratosis

Robert A. Schwartz

Actinic (or solar) keratoses (AKs) are common. Almost all elderly light-complexioned people have one or more of them. They represent a cutaneous dysplasia, akin to those of the uterine cervix, which may progress to full thickness in situ and then invasive squamous cell carcinoma (SCC). However, a good case can also be made that an AK is from inception an SCC [1,2]. There are approximately 5.2 million visits annually in America for AKs, with an estimated cost of at least $920 million [3]. The prevalence in the white population of northwest England in people over 40 years of age was 15.4% in men and 5.9% in women [4]. As the recreational habits of recent times have encouraged large amounts of sun exposure, one identifies more and more AKs on younger and younger people. The sites on which one most commonly sees AKs are the face (especially the forehead) and dorsal hands. Often the AK can better be palpated as a roughened spot than visualized. AKs may gradually enlarge to form plaques, which may be skin colored, slightly erythematous, or at times brownish or grayish yellow. The essentials of diagnosis are delineated in Table 2.1.

In the individual with AKs, one tends to also find obvious evidence of chronic solar exposure. Dilated capillaries may be evident around the nose. The skin may appear thickened or yellowish and elastotic. In regions with year-round solar exposure, one sees relatively young people with these chronic degenerative changes. I usually mention to my patients that our grandparents never deliberately exposed themselves to chronic destructive sun exposure. It is unfortunate that the tan, which was once equated with common laborers, remains fashionable.

The development of AK and SCC is likely an example of multistage carcinogenesis resulting from a complex sequence of events initiated by exposure to ultraviolet (UV) light [5,6]. Initial damage takes place in the DNA. Mutations in the tumor suppressor gene *p53* are common in AK and SCC.

History

Although Dubreuilh is credited with describing the typical AK in 1904 [7], it took another two decades to separate it from seborrheic keratosis and verruca vulgaris in the medical literature. The careful work of Montgomery [8] and MacKee and Cipollaro [9] helped clarify any residual confusion in the United States, as did more recent work [10].

As it was easily linked with sun exposure, the term *solar keratosis* became fashionable, followed more recently by *actinic keratosis*, the preferred term today. The term *senile keratosis*, which has also been employed, is misleading, as its development appears to be a function of sun exposure rather than age per se.

Clinical features

The AK usually appears on sun-exposed areas in light-complexioned people as a minute skin-colored to yellowish-brown macule or papule, often with a dry adherent scale (Fig. 2.1). It may be considerably larger, up to several centimeters in diameter. It is characterized by a roughened quality on palpation, which is often considerably more striking than its visual qualities. The AK is often without symptoms. Sometimes a patient will notice a mildly irritating quality to the AKs and on occasion gently rub them. If induration, erythema, or erosion is observed, the physician should suspect

Table 2.1 The actinic keratosis: essentials of diagnosis

Roughened papule (often ill defined)
Light-skinned individual
Sun-exposed site
Size: pinhead to 1 cm
Skin colored or reddish, sometimes reddish brown or
    yellowish black
Evidence of associated sun damage of skin
    Telangiectasias
    Solar elastosis
    Freckling

Table 2.2 Clinical types of actinic keratosis

Palpable papular AK
Hypertrophic AK
Actinic cheilitis
Superficial pigmented AK
Atrophic AK
Lichenoid AK
Actinic conjunctivitis

possible evolution into an SCC. Clinical parameters indicating AKs with an increased risk of malignancy have been emphasized by the pneumonic IDRBEU: I (Induration/Inflammation), D (Diameter > 1 cm), R (Rapid Enlargement), B (Bleeding), E (Erythema), and U (Ulceration) [11]. Occasionally an AK exhibits proliferative characteristics both histologically and clinically, in which case it may be resistant to standard therapies because of deep migration of abnormal cells along hair follicles and sweat ducts. This type may have an increased risk of becoming an infiltrative SCC and has been labeled a distinctive AK variant: the proliferative AK [12].

One technique that can be employed to better visualize AKs is the application of topical 5-fluorouracil (5-FU), which produces intense lesional inflammation 2 weeks later and often delineates otherwise unobserved early AKs. However, topical chemotherapy is best advised for the treatment rather than the diagnosis of AKs.

There are a number of types of AKs (Table 2.2). These variations and their differential diagnoses follow (Table 2.3). The subtleties of distinguishing the common AK from other entities, such as disseminated superficial actinic porokeratosis, may require clinical experience [13] (Fig. 2.2). The clinical diagnosis of nonpigmented facial AK may be enhanced by dermatoscopy, which may show a peculiar "strawberry" appearance [14].

The hypertrophic actinic keratosis
The AK may become hyperkeratotic. This phenomenon is often observed on the dorsal hands

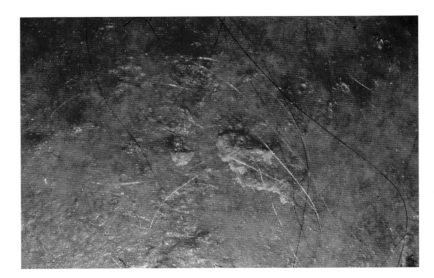

Fig. 2.1 Roughened papules on bald scalp are better palpated than visualized. (Reprinted with permission from Schwartz RA. Actinic keratoses. J Am Acad Dermatol 1984;11(6):27A, 30A.)

Table 2.3 Differential diagnosis of actinic keratosis

Discoid lupus erythematous (small papule)
  Salmon colored, atrophy, carpet-tacking
  This photo-induced lesion may require biopsy to
    distinguish
Seborrheic keratosis
  Under magnification, lesion shows pits and furrows
Solitary cutaneous papulonodule of coccidioidomycosis
  History of travel to or residence in endemic areas
Disseminated superficial actinic porokeratosis
  Small keratotic ridge on border of each lesion
Large cell acanthoma
  Slightly pigmented and keratotic 5–10 mm nondescript
    plaque

and face. Sometimes the exophytic growth may be so impressive that a "cutaneous horn" is formed. This term is purely morphologic; however, the overwhelming majority of cutaneous horns in light-complexioned adults are actually exuberantly prolific AKs. The full range of cutaneous horns is discussed in a separate chapter. The trauma of chronic rubbing may produce the hyperkeratosis. A hypertrophic AK may be so hyperkeratotic as to resemble the horn of an animal. This cutaneous horn, or cornu cutaneum, appears as a solid, dry, conical protuberance of variable coloration and angulation, which varies in size from minute to huge. Most appear 2 to 8 mm in diameter, projecting up to 3 cm (Fig. 2.3), as covered in Chapter 3.

The lichenoid actinic keratosis

In 1967, Hirsh and Marmelzat [15] employed the term *lichenoid actinic keratosis* to describe five patients with a specific localized skin lesion on sun-exposed areas. Each patient was a white woman with a single lesion situated on the upper anterior chest. Clinically, the lesions resembled lichen planus, lichenoid drug eruption, lichenoid polymorphous light eruption, lichenoid contact dermatitis, and lichen actinicus. However, microscopically, the salient features were epidermal dysplasia and a lichenoid infiltrate.

Other descriptions, both preceding and since the above account, called it solitary lichen planus-like keratosis [16], solitary lichen planus [17], and benign lichenoid keratosis [18,19]. The histologic features, however, are not those of AK, lacking evidence of cellular atypia or anaplasia. Melanocytic nevi with lichenoid regression may resemble a benign lichenoid keratosis histologically [20]. The clinicopathologic spectrum of benign lichenoid keratosis is broad, encompassing several unrelated entities [21]. It has been proposed to classify lichenoid keratosis into the following lichenoid entities: seborrheic keratosis, solar lentigo, AK, and idiopathic

Fig. 2.2 Roughened papule in solar exposure distribution disseminated superficial actinic porokeratosis.

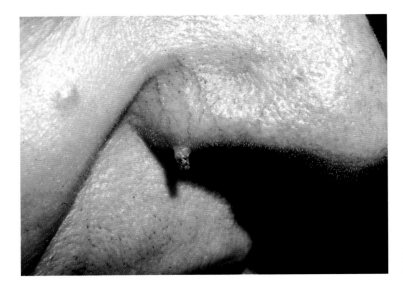

Fig. 2.3 Hypertrophic AK on a nose; a cutaneous horn.

lichen planus [22]. I have observed lichenoid AKs, as have James and colleagues [23]; it is my impression that most solitary lichenoid keratoses are not lichenoid AKs. The James group noted pigmentation in lichenoid AKs, the pigment being located in upper dermal macrophages.

Spreading pigmented actinic keratoses

In 1978, James, Wells, and Whimster [23] described 10 patients with asymptomatic pigmented plaques of the face between 1.5 and 4.0 cm in diameter. Although six had been diagnosed clinically as a lentigo maligna (Hutchinson's freckle), all were microscopically found to be pigmented AKs. Most AKs exhibit little tendency for centrifugal growth over 1 cm. The surface of the spreading pigmented AK is variably pigmented and either smooth, slightly warty, or scaly. Spreading pigmented AK and melanoma may exhibit overlapping clinical features; dermoscopy may facilitate diagnosis [24]. Clinical features of spreading pigmented AK may suggest seborrheic keratosis, senile lentigo, and melanocytic nevus as well as early melanoma [25].

Their histology is similar to that of the typical AK, although epidermal and melanophage pigmentation is more prominent. James and associates [23] found that melanocytes appeared normal in size, number, and morphology. The hyperpigmentation is the result of enhanced melanosome formation and distribution and not a melanocyte–keratinocyte melanosome transfer block [26].

The evolution of the superficial pigmented AK is unknown, although one suspects the same behavior as with typical AKs. Whether they evolve into pigmented Bowen's disease is an unanswered question at present.

Actinic cheilitis

The most important type of AK is that located on the lip, the actinic cheilitis (AC). This incipient form of actinically induced SCC of the lower lip is of great concern, as SCC of the lip has a high malignant potential [27] (see "Lip Squamous Cell Carcinoma" in Chapter 5). The AC invariably occurs on the lower rather than the upper lip, because the carcinogenic agent is solar radiation. ACs are similar morphologically to AKs on cutaneous surfaces, although a more prominent atrophic quality may be noted on the lip (Fig. 2.4). One series divided AC into three clinical forms: white nonulcerated lesions (29%), erosions or ulcers of the lip (48%), and mixed white and erosive (23%) [28]. A recent study of 20 patients with AC analyzed the entire lip vermilion searching for microscopic areas of progression; foci of invasive SCC were found in four (20%) of them [29]. Patients with AC having poorly demarcated lesions may have severe histopathologic changes irregularly distributed along the vermilion. An intense

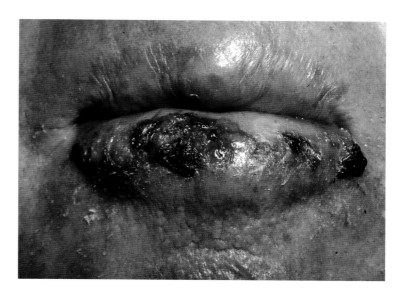

Fig. 2.4 Roughened papule, lip, AK (actinic cheilitis).

inflammatory infiltrate was found to be predictive of an adjacent invasive SCC [30]. In this study of 70 cases of chronic AC, the p53 protein immunoreactivity was not a marker of malignant transformation. Differential diagnostic considerations are noted in Table 2.4.

Actinic conjunctivitis

Ultraviolet light produces conjunctival alterations classified clinically as a pinguecula or pterygium. It appears as a wedge-shaped opaque plaque near the limbus. Actinic conjunctivitis may progress to SCC of the conjunctiva [31,32].

Histopathology

The AK is a cutaneous dysplasia of the epidermis [2,10]. Thus, alterations of cellular polarity, dysplasia, and nuclear atypia are evident and characteristic. Epidermal cells appear abnormal, less basophilic than normal keratinocytes, and variable

Table 2.4 Differential diagnosis of actinic cheilitis

Necrotizing sialometaplasia
Factitial lip crusting
Lupus erythematosus
Cheilitis granulomatosis

in size and shape. Often one can observe a few nuclei that are enlarged and contain prominent nucleoli. Some cells may be multinucleated; others may display mitotic figures. Individual cell keratinization is present sometimes. The overlying epidermis is slightly to markedly hyperkeratotic, with some stratum corneum appearing either loose or compact. Orthokeratotic hyperkeratosis and parakeratosis may alternate, with the normal hyperkeratosis appearing above the adnexal structures. The acanthosis is irregular; often small buds extend downward. Dyskeratosis may be prominent. Spaces in the epidermis with partially keratinized cells called *corps rounds and grains* may be seen [8].

The dermis often shows basophilic degeneration with a mild inflammatory infiltrate and edema of the upper dermis. Hair follicles, sebaceous glands, apocrine and eccrine sweat glands, and ducts appear unaltered.

Acantholytic changes were noted consistently in 18 of 402 cases of AK (4.4%) and involved both the epidermis and appendageal epithelia [33]. Suprabasal clefting with acantholytic cells portends no special clinical or prognostic distinction; however, it is this type of AK that probably evolves into the so-called adenoid SCC [34]. The AK may occasionally show the changes of epidermolytic hyperkeratosis along the entire epidermis (except adnexa) [35].

Table 2.5 Histologic types of actinic keratoses

Typical (SCC grade 1/2)
Bowenoid (full-thickness epidermal change)
Hypertrophic
Acantholytic
Pigmented
Lichenoid
Proliferative

Of the previously mentioned 402 skin biopsy specimens, 49.7% were labeled atrophic-type AKs, 38% were of the hypertrophic type, and 7.7% of the bowenoid type [33]. A breakdown of histologic types of AKs is given in Table 2.5. When AKs extend to the biopsy specimen margins, about half recur within 3 years [36].

Although the AK is most closely linked with SCC, occasionally a basal cell carcinoma [37] and rarely a sebaceous carcinoma may arise on or from an AK [38].

Histologic differential diagnosis

The characteristic AK involves focal dysplasia sparing dermal appendages. Atypical vacuolated cells may resemble mammary and extramammary Paget's disease [39]. However, the presence of desmosomes and keratinocyte dyskeratosis usually allows distinction.

At times, AKs may show hypergranulosis, atrophy, and basal cell layer liquefactive degeneration, prompting confusion with lupus erythematosus, lichen planus, and other lichenoid eruptions. Columns of parakeratosis may resemble the coronoid lamella of the porokeratoses and be difficult to distinguish from disseminated superficial actinic porokeratosis. Unusual findings occasionally occur, such as a primary cutaneous extraskeletal osteosarcoma under a previous electrodessicated actinic keratosis [40].

Prognosis

It is generally accepted that, except on the lip, AKs are of low-grade malignant potential [2]. One study of 560 individuals from Wales found that 21% of AKs resolved spontaneously over a 12-month period and none progressed into SCC [41]. An Australian analysis of 1140 aged 40 years and over found 616 (59.2%) with solar keratoses, 224 (36.4%) of whom had spontaneous remission of at least one of their solar keratoses within 1 year [42]. A total of 485 lesions (25.9%) underwent spontaneous remission out of the 1873 AKs evident at the first examination of these 224 people. The incidence rate of SCC occurring in those with solar keratoses was 0.24% for each solar keratosis evident at the original examination. In up to 20% to 25% of patients with AKs, one or more of the AKs display evidence of SCC, either in situ or invasive [8]. Another analysis found 7.7% of AKs displayed bowenoid change [33]. Graham and Helwig [34] reviewed data on patients with AKs and found that about 13% showed actual change of SCC. Bendl and Graham [43] studied the data from 156 patients with 163 AKs having evidence of dermal invasion, which they labeled "solar keratosis with squamous cell carcinoma," and found the metastatic potential nonexistent or infinitesimally low.

Histologic evidence of a contiguous AK was found in eight of 18 patients (44%) with SCC that had metastasized from skin [44]. If sampling errors are considered, this figure may be even higher. Increased tumor thickness and depth of invasion were the most consistent histologic features linked with these metastasizing SCCs. Such SCCs may be locally aggressive but do not commonly metastasize. Although some AKs may become clinically inapparent, possibly either because of immune rejection or simply because their external surface unknowingly has been scraped off, an untreated AK represents a potentially curable fatal cancer.

Treatment

The therapeutic options for treating AKs are multiple (Table 2.6). Treatment includes cryosurgery, curettage and excisional surgery, dermabrasion, chemical peels, laser resurfacing, 5-FU, imiquimod, diclofenac, and tretinoin [45]. I prefer liquid nitrogen cryosurgery for individual AKs and 5-FU for field therapy. Field cancerization is particularly important with AC, as one must evaluate and, if

Table 2.6 Therapeutic options for actinic keratoses

Liquid nitrogen cryosurgery
Topical 5-FU
Imiquimod
Diclofenac
Curettage and electrodessication
Photodynamic therapy
Dermabrasion
Topical retinoids
Chemical peel
T4 endonuclease V (T4N5) liposome lotion
Systemic retinoids

need be, treat the entire lip vermilion, searching for microscopic areas of invasive SCC. Liquid nitrogen cryotherapy has a cure rate approaching 100% [46,47]. Moreover, it and topical 5-FU can be employed in combination. A 1-week course of topical 0.5% fluorouracil before cryosurgery was significantly more effective in reducing AKs 6 months after treatment than cryosurgery alone [48].

Topical 5-FU has been effectively used since it was pioneered by Edmund Klein in the early 1960s [49–53]. It is an excellent option, particularly for AKs occurring on the face [54], but many patients experience considerable discomfort for weeks. Several formulations and concentrations of topical fluorouracil are Food and Drug Administration approved for the treatment of AK and AC, with the most commonly employed being the 5% and 0.5% creams [55]. They eradicate AKs, often with application site irritation, erythema, and burning. Comparative data suggest that the fluorouracil 0.5% cream is more cost-effective and may be safer, more tolerable than, and as efficacious as fluorouracil 5% cream. I sometimes use a moderately potent topical steroid after the 5-FU to reduce irritation. In AKs of the forearms and hands, 5-FU alone has been relatively ineffective whereas the combination of 5% 5-FU cream twice daily followed by nightly application of 0.05% tretinoin cream may be efficacious [56,57]. The efficacy and tolerability of 5% 5-FU cream and imiquimod cream were compared in 36 patients with four or more AKs who were randomly assigned to receive 5% 5-FU cream twice daily for 2 to 4 weeks or 5% imiquimod cream twice weekly

for 16 weeks [58]. 5-FU was more effective than imiquimod in exposing presumed subclinical AKs, reducing the final AK count (total AK count declined during the 24-week study by 94% vs. 66%), achieving complete clearance (incidence of 84% vs. 24% by week 24), and achieving clearance rapidly. Tolerability was similar, although erythema was initially significantly higher with 5-FU than with imiquimod but resolved rapidly and was significantly lower than with imiquimod by week 16. This study concluded that 5% 5-FU remains the gold standard field therapy for AKs.

Some favor imiquimod as having a higher efficacy than 5-FU for AK lesions located on the face and scalp [59–62]. Local adverse events with imiquimod in one study were erythema (27%), scabbing or crusting (21%), flaking (9%), erosion (6%), edema (4%), and weeping (3%) [63]. Aphthous stomatitis may also become evident when using imiquimod to treat AC [64]. Imiquimod 5% cream used three times weekly for 16 weeks is effective in the treatment of AK [65]. It stimulates a cutaneous immune response characterized by increases in activated dendritic cells and CD4$^+$ and CD8$^+$ T cells [66]. It also encourages keratinocytes to secrete cytokines and chemokines, attracting inflammatory cells, resulting in immune cell–mediated destruction of AKs [62].

The relationship between a key mediator in the proinflammatory cascade, cyclooxygenase, and carcinogenesis has provided a rationale for the use of topical nonsteroidal anti-inflammatory drugs for the treatment of AK, with 3% diclofenac coming to the forefront [61]. It has shown moderate efficacy with low morbidity in mild AKs. Treatment has been well tolerated; side effects were mainly pruritus, dry skin, and application site reactions. Assessing clinically meaningful end points in managing AKs with diclofenac 3% gel may be challenging [67].

Other approaches are noteworthy. In areas of widespread involvement, such as the bald scalp, dermabrasion may be a useful option and, moreover, may have a long-term prophylactic effect [68,69]. Patients who have undergone both topical 5-FU and dermabrasion appear to find dermabrasion more tolerable [47]. Photodynamic therapy (PDT) is also an effective and safe treatment of nonhypertrophic

Table 2.7 Dangers and opportunities posed by actinic keratoses

May evolve into metastatic SCC
  Rare except on lip
Educate physician and patient about other skin-induced
  cancers
  Examine entire skin surface, especially for melanoma
  Reexamine every 6 months
Warn physician and patient about skin cancer prevention
In young patients, consider rare genetic syndrome:
  xeroderma pigmentosum
If patient is immunocompromised, watch carefully for
  other skin cancers and aggressive AKs

Table 2.8 Curiosities about actinic keratoses

DNA repair deficiency in lymphocytes in patients with AK
Cutaneous vitamin A level may be low in AK
DNA repair after UV light exposure in skin fibroblasts of
  patients with AKs may be defective
Topical retinoids appear to moderate or reduce skin
  photoaging with elimination of dysplasia and atypia,
  but whether their use becomes popular remains to be
  seen

AKs of the scalp and face. PDT is good for multiple AKs and AC, without the adverse effects of 5-FU or imiquimod [70,71]. Blue light PDT is being explored for treating AKs [72]. Blue light patch may be a safe, effective, and alternative method for light delivery and topical aminolevulinic acid activation during PDT [73]. Tretinoin cream, a topical retinoid, may moderate or reverse photoaging [74].

Topical or systemic retinoids may ultimately prove useful in the chemoprevention of AKs, but preliminary evidence is contradictory [57,75]. People with moderately severe AKs using daily vitamin A have experienced a 32% risk reduction in cutaneous SCCs. The vitamin A doses of 50,000 and 75,000 IU/day for 1 year have proven safe and efficacious and have been recommended for future skin cancer chemoprevention studies [76]. Intralesional α_2-interferon has demonstrated efficacy in inducing complete regression of AKs but requires multiple injections and is less practical [77]. In patients with xeroderma pigmentosum, T4 endonuclease V (T4N5) liposome lotion applied for 1 year reduced the rates of AK and skin cancer compared with placebo. Thus, T4 endonuclease V, an enzyme that repairs damaged bacterial DNA, apparently reduces DNA damage and/or increases the rate of DNA repair in these patients [78].

An overview

Actinic keratosis tags the patient with a marker of excessive sun exposure. In selected model diseases, such as xeroderma pigmentosum and oculocutaneous albinism, the solar limits are lower than for the rest of the population. In recent years, it has become apparent that immunocompromised patients should also be considered at increased risk of AKs with progression to SCC. The dangers of AKs and opportunities posed by their detection are listed in Table 2.7.

Actinic keratosis also represents an opportunity as a model for carcinogenesis and cancer therapy. It is not surprising that DNA repair deficiencies have been found in lymphocytes [79] and fibroblasts of patients with AKs. Other curious findings are listed in Table 2.8 [57,74,76,77,79–81].

Much of the challenge of AKs lies in prevention by public education [82]. Avoidance of sun exposure and the use of protective agents and garments if solar radiation is mandatory are difficult concepts for a public that craves deep tans. The use of sunscreens and sun blocks, such as zinc oxide ointment, is recommended.

References

1 Ackerman AB, Mones JM. Solar (actinic) keratosis is squamous cell carcinoma. Br J Dermatol 2006;155:9–22.

2 Schwartz RA. The actinic keratosis. A perspective and update. Dermatol Surg 1997;23:1009–19; quiz 1020–1.

3 Warino L, Tusa M, Camacho F, et al. Frequency and cost of actinic keratosis treatment. Dermatol Surg 2006;32:1045–9.

4 Memon AA, Tomenson JA, Bothwell J, et al. Prevalence of solar damage and actinic keratosis in a Merseyside population. Br J Dermatol 2000;142:1154–9.

5 Ortonne JP. From actinic keratosis to squamous cell carcinoma. Br J Dermatol 2002;146 Suppl 61: 20–3.

6 Person JR. An actinic keratosis is neither malignant nor premalignant: it is an initiated tumor. J Am Acad Dermatol 2003;48:637–8.

7 Bloch B. Cancers and precancerous afflictions from the dermatological viewpoint. Cancer Review 1932;7:65–98.

8 Montgomery H. Precancerous dermatosis and epithelioma in situ. Arch Dermatol Syphilol 1939;39:387–408.

9 MacKee GM, Cipollaro AC. Cutaneous cancer and precancer: a practical monograph. New York: The American Journal of Cancer; 1937. p. 1–222.

10 Schwartz RA, Stoll HL Jr. Epithelial neoplasms and precancerous lesions. In: Freedberg IM, Eisen AZ, Wolff K, Austen KF, Goldsmith LA, Katz SI, Fitzpatrick TB, editors. Fitzpatrick's dermatology in general medicine. 5th ed. New York: McGraw-Hill; 1999. p. 823–39.

11 Quaedvlieg PJ, Tirsi E, Thissen MR, et al. Actinic keratosis: how to differentiate the good from the bad ones? Eur J Dermatol 2006;16:335–9.

12 Goldberg LH, Chang JR, Baer SC, et al. Proliferative actinic keratosis: three representative cases. Dermatol Surg 2000;26:65–9.

13 Wiltz H, Schwartz RA, Lambert WC. Disseminated superficial actinic porokeratosis: appearance after suntan parlor exposure. Photodermatology 1987;4:47–8.

14 Zalaudek I, Giacomel J, Argenziano G, et al. Dermoscopy of facial nonpigmented actinic keratosis. Br J Dermatol 2006;155:951–6.

15 Hirsch P, Marmelzat WL. Lichenoid actinic keratosis. Dermatol Int 1967;6:101–3.

16 Shapiro L, Ackerman AB. Solitary lichen planus-like keratosis. Dermatologica 1966;132:386–92.

17 Lumpkin LR, Helwig EB. Solitary lichen planus. Arch Dermatol 1966;93:54–5.

18 Barranco VP. Multiple benign lichenoid keratoses simulating photodermatoses: evolution from senile lentigines and their spontaneous regression. J Am Acad Dermatol 1985;13:201–6.

19 Goette DK. Benign lichenoid keratosis. Arch Dermatol 1980;116:780–2.

20 Dalton SR, Fillman EP, Altman CE, et al. Atypical junctional melanocytic proliferations in benign lichenoid keratosis. Hum Pathol 2003;34:706–9.

21 Morgan MB, Stevens GL, Switlyk S. Benign lichenoid keratosis: a clinical and pathologic reappraisal of 1040 cases. Am J Dermatopathol 2005;27:387–92.

22 Glaun RS, Dutta B, Helm KF. A proposed new classification system for lichenoid keratosis. J Am Acad Dermatol 1996;35:772–4.

23 James MP, Wells GC, Whimster IW. Spreading pigmented actinic keratoses. Br J Dermatol 1978;98:373–9.

24 Zalaudek I, Ferrara G, Leinweber B, et al. Pitfalls in the clinical and dermoscopic diagnosis of pigmented actinic keratosis. J Am Acad Dermatol 2005;53:1071–4.

25 Subrt P, Jorizzo JL, Apisarnthanarax P, et al. Spreading pigmented actinic keratosis. J Am Acad Dermatol 1983;8:63–7.

26 Dinehart SM, Sanchez RL. Spreading pigmented actinic keratosis. An electron microscopic study. Arch Dermatol 1988;124:680–3.

27 Boddie AW Jr, Fischer EP, Byers RM. Squamous carcinoma of the lower lip in patients under 40 years of age. South Med J 1977;70:711–2, 5.

28 Markopoulos A, Albanidou-Farmaki E, Kayavis I. Actinic cheilitis: clinical and pathologic characteristics in 65 cases. Oral Dis 2004;10:212–6.

29 Menta Simonsen Nico M, Rivitti EA, Lourenco SV. Actinic cheilitis: histologic study of the entire vermilion and comparison with previous biopsy. J Cutan Pathol 2007;34:309–14.

30 Neto Pimentel DR, Michalany N, Alchorne M, et al. Actinic cheilitis: histopathology and p53. J Cutan Pathol 2006;33:539–44.

31 Clear AS, Chirambo MC, Hutt MS. Solar keratosis, pterygium, and squamous cell carcinoma of the conjunctiva in Malawi. Br J Ophthalmol 1979;63:102–9.

32 Mortemousque B, Leger F, Brindeau C, et al. [Actinic keratosis of the conjunctiva. Apropos of a clinical case]. J Fr Ophtalmol 1998;21:458–61.

33 Carapeto FJ, Garcia-Perez A. Acantholytic keratosis. Dermatologica 1974;148:233–9.

34 Graham JH. Selected precancerous skin and mucocutaneous lesions. In: Neoplasms of skin and malignant melanoma. Chicago: Year Book Medical Publishers; 1976. p. 69–121.

35 Ackerman AB, Reed RJ. Epidermolytic variant of solar keratosis. Arch Dermatol 1973;107:104–6.

36 Rosamilia LL, Helm KF. Clinical recurrence of actinic keratosis following marginal biopsy: a retrospective study. Int J Dermatol 2006;45:1114–5.

37 Lambert WC, Schwartz RA. Evidence for origin of basal cell carcinomas in solar (actinic) keratoses. J Cutan Pathol 1988;15:322.

38 Ansai S, Mihara I. Sebaceous carcinoma arising on actinic keratosis. Eur J Dermatol 2000;10:385–8.

39 Mai KT, Alhalouly T, Landry D, et al. Pagetoid variant of actinic keratosis with or without squamous cell carcinoma of sun-exposed skin: a lesion simulating extramammary Paget's disease. Histopathology 2002;41:331–6.

40 Santos-Juanes J, Galache C, Miralles M, et al. Primary cutaneous extraskeletal osteosarcoma under a previous electrodessicated actinic keratosis. J Am Acad Dermatol 2004;51:S166–8.

41 Harvey I, Frankel S, Marks R, et al. Non-melanoma skin cancer and solar keratoses. I. Methods and descriptive results of the South Wales Skin Cancer Study. Br J Cancer 1996;74:1302–7.

42 Marks R, Foley P, Goodman G, et al. Spontaneous remission of solar keratoses: the case for conservative management. Br J Dermatol 1986;115:649–55.

43 Bendl BJ, Graham JH. New concepts of the origin of squamous cell carcinomas of the skin: solar (senile), keratosis with squamous cell carcinoma. A clinicopathologic and histochemical study. In: Sixth national cancer conference proceedings. Philadelphia: JB Lippincott; 1968. p. 471–88.

44 Dinehart SM, Nelson-Adesokan P, Cockerell C, et al. Metastatic cutaneous squamous cell carcinoma derived from actinic keratosis. Cancer 1997;79:920–3.

45 de Berker D, McGregor JM, Hughes BR. Guidelines for the management of actinic keratoses. Br J Dermatol 2007;156:222–30.

46 Lober BA, Fenske NA. Optimum treatment strategies for actinic keratosis (intraepidermal squamous cell carcinoma). Am J Clin Dermatol 2004;5:395–401.

47 Lubritz RR, Smolewski SA. Cryosurgery cure rate of actinic keratoses. J Am Acad Dermatol 1982;7:631–2.

48 Jorizzo J, Weiss J, Furst K, et al. Effect of a 1-week treatment with 0.5% topical fluorouracil on occurrence of actinic keratosis after cryosurgery: a randomized, vehicle-controlled clinical trial. Arch Dermatol 2004;140:813–6.

49 Schwartz RA. Edmund Klein (1921–1999). J Am Acad Dermatol 2001;44:716–8.

50 Klein E, Stoll HL Jr, Milgrom H, et al. Tumors of the skin. XII. Topical 5-fluorouracil for epidermal neoplasms. J Surg Oncol 1971;3:331–49.

51 Klein E, Holtermann OA, Helm F, et al. Topical therapy for cutaneous tumors. Transplant Proc 1984;16:507–15.

52 Klein E. Local chemotherapy of cutaneous neoplasms. Proc Natl Cancer Conf 1970;6:501–15.

53 Klein E. Tumors of skin. IX. Local cytostatic therapy of cutaneous and mucosal premalignant and malignant lesions. N Y State J Med 1968;68:886–9.

54 Du Vivier A. Topical cytostatic drugs in the treatment of skin cancer. Clin Exp Dermatol 1982;7:89–92.

55 Jorizzo JL, Carney PS, Ko WT, et al. Fluorouracil 5% and 0.5% creams for the treatment of actinic keratosis: equivalent efficacy with a lower concentration and more convenient dosing schedule. Cutis 2004;74:18–23.

56 Bercovitch L. Topical chemotherapy of actinic keratoses of the upper extremity with tretinoin and 5-fluorouracil: a double-blind controlled study. Br J Dermatol 1987;116:549–52.

57 Peck GL. Topical tretinoin in actinic keratosis and basal cell carcinoma. J Am Acad Dermatol 1986;15:829–35.

58 Tanghetti E, Werschler P. Comparison of 5% 5-fluorouracil cream and 5% imiquimod cream in the management of actinic keratoses on the face and scalp. J Drugs Dermatol 2007;6:144–7.

59 Gupta AK, Davey V, McPhail H. Evaluation of the effectiveness of imiquimod and 5-fluorouracil for the treatment of actinic keratosis: critical review and meta-analysis of efficacy studies. J Cutan Med Surg 2005;9:209–14.

60 Lee PK, Harwell WB, Loven KH, et al. Long-term clinical outcomes following treatment of actinic keratosis with imiquimod 5% cream. Dermatol Surg 2005;31:659–64.

61 Merk HF. Topical diclofenac in the treatment of actinic keratoses. Int J Dermatol 2007;46:12–8.

62 Torres A, Storey L, Anders M, et al. Immune-mediated changes in actinic keratosis following topical treatment with imiquimod 5% cream. J Transl Med 2007;5:7.

63 Hadley G, Derry S, Moore RA. Imiquimod for actinic keratosis: systematic review and meta-analysis. J Invest Dermatol 2006;126:1251–5.

64 Chakrabarty AK, Mraz S, Geisse JK, et al. Aphthous ulcers associated with imiquimod and the treatment of actinic cheilitis. J Am Acad Dermatol 2005;52:35–7.

65 Korman N, Moy R, Ling M, et al. Dosing with 5% imiquimod cream 3 times per week for the treatment of actinic keratosis: results of two phase 3, randomized, double-blind, parallel-group, vehicle-controlled trials. Arch Dermatol 2005;141:467–73.

66 Ooi T, Barnetson RS, Zhuang L, et al. Imiquimod-induced regression of actinic keratosis is associated with infiltration by T lymphocytes and dendritic cells: a randomized controlled trial. Br J Dermatol 2006;154:72–8.

67 Rivers JJ, Wolf J. Assessing clinically meaningful end points for the management of actinic keratosis with

diclofenac 3% gel. Acta Derm Venereol 2007;87:188–9.

68 Winton GB, Salasche SJ. Dermabrasion of the scalp as a treatment for actinic damage. J Am Acad Dermatol 1986;14:661–8.

69 Fulton JE, Porumb S. Chemical peels: their place within the range of resurfacing techniques. Am J Clin Dermatol 2004;5:179–87.

70 Gold MH, Nestor MS. Current treatments of actinic keratosis. J Drugs Dermatol 2006;5:17–25.

71 Alexiades-Armenakas M. Aminolevulinic acid photodynamic therapy for actinic keratoses/actinic cheilitis/ acne: vascular lasers. Dermatol Clin 2007;25: 25–33.

72 Rivard J, Ozog D. Henry Ford Hospital dermatology experience with Levulan Kerastick and blue light photodynamic therapy. J Drugs Dermatol 2006;5: 556–61.

73 Zelickson B, Counters J, Coles C, et al. Light patch: preliminary report of a novel form of blue light delivery for the treatment of actinic keratosis. Dermatol Surg 2005;31:375–8.

74 Kligman AM, Grove GL, Hirose R, et al. Topical tretinoin for photoaged skin. J Am Acad Dermatol 1986;15:836–59.

75 Campanelli A, Naldi L. A retrospective study of the effect of long-term topical application of retinaldehyde (0.05%) on the development of actinic keratosis. Dermatology 2002;205:146–52.

76 Alberts D, Ranger-Moore J, Einspahr J, et al. Safety and efficacy of dose-intensive oral vitamin A in subjects with sun-damaged skin. Clin Cancer Res 2004;10:1875–80.

77 Edwards L, Levine N, Weidner M, et al. Effect of intralesional alpha 2-interferon on actinic keratoses. Arch Dermatol 1986;122:779–82.

78 Yarosh DB. DNA repair, immunosuppression, and skin cancer. Cutis 2004;74:10–3.

79 Abo-Darub JM, Mackie R, Pitts JD. DNA repair deficiency in lymphocytes from patients with actinic keratosis. Bull Cancer 1978;65:357–62.

80 Sbano E, Andreassi L, Fimiani M, et al. DNA-repair after UV-irradiation in skin fibroblasts from patients with actinic keratosis. Arch Dermatol Res 1978;262:55–61.

81 Rollman O, Vahlquist A. Cutaneous vitamin A levels in seborrheic keratosis, actinic keratosis, and basal cell carcinoma. Arch Dermatol Res 1981;270:193–6.

82 Esmann S, Jemec GB. Management of actinic keratosis patients: a qualitative study. J Dermatolog Treat 2007;18:53–8.

CHAPTER 3

Other premalignant cutaneous dysplasias

Robert A. Schwartz

Arsenical keratoses

Arsenic has been characterized as the number one toxic environmental contaminant [1]. It is a human carcinogen but not a potent mutagen, probably acting by modifying DNA methylation patterns. Arsenical keratoses may disclose a cryptic exposure to arsenic many years earlier [2–4]. They usually appear on the palms and soles but may occur elsewhere as cornlike, hard, yellowish papulonodules, with a predisposition along sites of trauma and friction. They may coalesce into verrucous plaques and may evolve into full-thickness dysplasia or Bowen's disease (in situ squamous cell carcinoma [SCC]).

As Bowen's disease, the eruption may be on sun-exposed or non–sun-exposed sites and may display pigmentation. Whenever one sees Bowen's disease on a non–sun-exposed site, the carcinogen is unlikely to be ultraviolet light. Accordingly, one should search for a history of previous arsenic exposure years earlier. Arsenically induced Bowen's disease may progress into metastatic invasive SCC. This point was amply illustrated by Sir Jonathan Hutchinson [5] when in 1887 he presented to the Pathologic Society of London, with Sir James Paget chairing the meeting, the proposition that arsenic can induce cancer. Hutchinson presented two patients, one an American physician who had been treated with oral potassium arsenite (Fowler's solution) for psoriasis. Yet, even with its carcinogenicity known for so long, arsenic exposure has continued medicinally, occupationally, and environmentally [6,7]. Paradoxically, this carcinogen's dramatic effect in the treatment of acute promyelocytic leukemia has returned it to mainstream medicine. Interestingly, the trivalent inorganic arsenic is the principal offender, whereas organic arsenical compounds, such as those previously used against syphilis, are not carcinogenic. Nevertheless, the use of offending forms of arsenic in Asian pills and Chinese traditional medicine for asthma continues [8]. In addition, seafood such as kelp and clams may concentrate arsenic [9,10]. Arsenic may appear in contaminated well water from insecticides or from mining by-products [11,12]. Chromium-copper-arsenate–treated plywood has a toxic legacy [13].

The key is to catch arsenicism as early as possible, before the cutaneous and systemic stigmata present serious problems. Arsenical keratoses and Bowen's disease will otherwise gradually extend, forming a large erosion or ulceration that may be difficult to treat, even without metastases [14]. The first problem is the diagnosis. Most patients referred to me with a possible diagnosis of arsenical keratoses have the relatively common autosomal dominant hyperkeratosis of the palms and soles, with small craterlike pits evident or easily produced when keratinous plugs are pulled [15] (Figs. 3.1 and 3.2). The plugs of arsenical keratoses, if removed, do not leave pits.

Other stigmata of chronic arsenicism include pigmented changes in the skin, with hyperpigmented patches often displaying small areas of depigmentation resembling raindrops (Fig. 3.3). Such pigmented patches tend to affect most commonly the nipples, axillae, groin, and other pressure points. In contrast with the hyperpigmentation of Addison's disease, the oral mucosa tends to be spared with

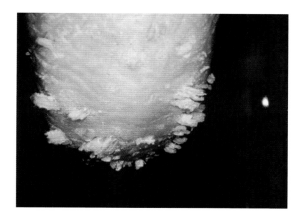

Fig. 3.1 Arsenical keratosis on the sole.

arsenicism. Other cutaneous signs of arsenicism include Mees' lines, transverse whitish narrow fingernail bands seen in both acute and chronic arsenicism. These can be used to date the episodes of exposure, with 30 to 40 days required for the lines to first appear above the lunulae of the fingernails. In addition, a diffuse alopecia of scalp, acrodermatitis, and thromboangiitis-like changes of the legs may be seen, with gangrene resulting. These destructive leg changes are called blackfoot disease.

Arsenicism is a systemic disease, with neuropathy often the hallmark [16]. One may see a symmetrical polyneuropathy resembling Guillain-Barré syndrome or paresthesias, numbness, and pain on the soles of the feet. Hematologically, anemia and leukopenia may be accompanied by thrombocytopenia, with red blood cells displaying a "cloverleaf" nucleus. The patient may exhibit a metallic breath odor and may have diarrhea and malabsorption as well as hepatic cirrhosis. Arsenic is also a myocardial toxin, producing electrocardiographic changes.

Although arsenic is known to predispose to Bowen's disease and SCC, there has been debate as to whether it may produce multiple superficial-type basal cell carcinomas (BCCs). There is no doubt that arsenicism predisposes to cancer of the respiratory, gastrointestinal, and genitourinary tracts [17,18]. Long-term exposure to inorganic arsenic, mainly from drinking water, has been documented to induce cancers in lung, urinary bladder, kidney, liver, and skin in a dose–response relationship. In addition, it is linked with liver angiosarcoma [19] and hepatoma [20]. Thus, arsenical keratoses and bowenoid arsenical keratoses should be viewed as representing arsenicism, a cutaneous marker of internal malignancy. The features of chronic arsenicism are summarized in Table 3.1. Table 3.2 lists some curiosities of arsenicism.

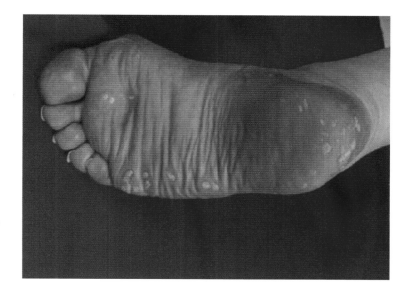

Fig. 3.2 Autosomal dominant punctate hyperkeratosis of the palms and soles, to be distinguished from arsenical keratoses. (Reprinted with permission from Rubenstein et al. [15].)

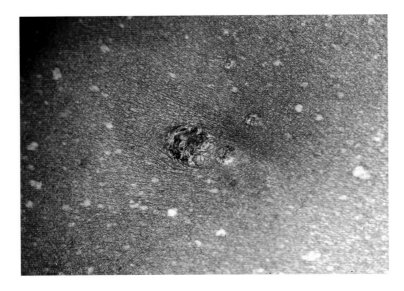

Fig. 3.3 Arsenical pigmentary changes, showing hyperpigmented patches with "raindrop" hypopigmentation. Note the plaque of Bowen's disease.

The chronology of the appearance of cutaneous and visceral findings in arsenicism is noteworthy. Arsenic does not remain in the tissues for the 10 to 20 years required for arsenical keratoses to manifest. In one series, Bowen's disease began within 10 years of exposure, invasive cutaneous SCC after 20 years, and lung cancer after 30 years [21].

Pathology

Arsenical keratoses show thick, compact parakeratotic hyperkeratosis and other epidermal changes characteristic of hypertrophic actinic keratoses [2]. The histology is most reminiscent of hypertrophic actinic keratoses. The presence of numerous vacuolated keratinocytes is suggestive of arsenical keratoses, but this is not a reliable criterion. Likewise, although basophilic degeneration of the dermis may be absent, it also may be present with arsenical keratoses, regardless of anatomic location. Actinic and arsenical keratoses may spare adnexal epithelium, so there are no pathognomonic histologic findings to separate arsenical keratoses or bowenoid arsenical keratoses from their solar equivalents. Arsenic may induce abnormal differentiation in arsenical keratosis via the effects of integrin expression in keratinocytes [22].

Proving arsenic exposure

Establishing the arsenic exposure may be difficult. Analysis of body tissues, nails, and hair may be

Table 3.1 Features of chronic arsenicism

Often cryptic exposure
Long latent period, up to 50 years
Punctate hyperkeratosis of palms and soles
Bowen's disease on sun- and non–sun-exposed skin
Hyperpigmented patches, which may be mottled
"Raindrop" hypopigmentation
Mees' lines
Diffuse alopecia
Peripheral neuropathy
Cancers of the respiratory, gastrointestinal, and genitourinary tracts; hepatic angiosarcoma
Peripheral circulatory disorders

Table 3.2 Curiosities about arsenic

Animal models for arsenic-induced carcinogenesis are lacking, yet in humans, arsenic is carcinogenic

Napoleon Bonaparte's hair was exposed to considerable arsenic during 1816 in his exile at St. Helena

Trivalent inorganic arsenic is carcinogenic; organic arsenic may not be attempted, but only relatively recent exposure will be detected. To evaluate hairs, only a few are necessary, with pubic ones being preferable. Neutron activation analysis was employed with the well-preserved remains of Napoleon Bonaparte, which revealed that he was apparently exposed to considerable amounts of arsenic during his second exile on the island of St. Helena [18,23].

Therapy

Arsenic can be chelated with dimercaprol, but by the time cutaneous and other neoplasms have developed, there are likely to be no traces of arsenic left to remove. Thus, one usually approaches arsenical keratoses and bowenoid ones by destructive means, such as excision, cryosurgery, and other modalities as delineated in the chapters on Bowen's disease and SCC, including 5-fluorouracil [24] and acitretin [25].

Cutaneous horns

A cutaneous horn is a protuberant skin growth that morphologically resembles the horn of an animal. The diagnosis of a cutaneous horn requires that the keratotic mass comprise the dominant feature, with its height being at least one half its diameter [26]. This designation does not imply any histologic pattern per se, although most cutaneous horns in elderly, light-complexioned people are actinic keratoses. Cutaneous horns are variable in size. Horns overlying seborrheic keratoses tend to be dark brown with a greasy verrucous surface. Cutaneous horns may be distributed almost anywhere on the body, including the penis [27]. From pinpoint to several centimeters, they tend to be a conical projection of cohesive keratinized material, which is of variable coloration and may be straight or curved in growth (Fig. 3.4). In young patients, most cutaneous horns are filiform warts.

In the biopsy of cutaneous horns, it is very important to include its base, to be sure that an actinic keratosis has not become an invasive SCC. In one study of eyelid cutaneous horns in 24 men and 19 women, with a mean age of 62 years (range 16 to 90), treated surgically, histopathologic examination showed 77.1% were benign, 14.6% premalignant,

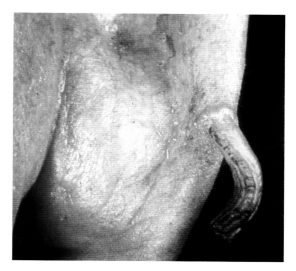

Fig. 3.4 Cutaneous horn of the ear.

and 8.3% malignant [28]. The most common benignity was seborrheic keratosis. Non-benign cutaneous horns were actinic keratosis, BCC, and SCC. Other types of cancer may also form cutaneous horns, including Kaposi's sarcoma, sebaceous carcinoma, penile SCC, penile verrucous carcinoma, and metastatic renal cell carcinoma [29,30]. A variety of benign histologic patterns may be seen, including melanoacanthoma, pilomatricoma, hemangioma, and a granular cell tumor [31–33]. The horn itself may show trichilemmomal or trichilemmal horn keratinization.

Tar keratoses

Hydrocarbon (tar) keratoses are an occupational and iatrogenic hazard [34]. The earliest probable report was that of Sir Percivall Pott [35], who in 1775 linked cancer in chimney sweeps with persistent chemical carcinogens on the rugae of the scrotum. Tars and other polycyclic aromatic hydrocarbons are used by workers in a number of occupations, including cotton workers, whose scrotums and vulvae were soaked with carcinogens when operating a machine to spin the cotton (the "mule," hence the name *mule-spinners' cancer*). Workers in other occupations associated with cutaneous SCC induced by hydrocarbons are machinists who use cutting (mineral) oil, pesticide manufacturers who use 4,4'-bipyridyl, and petrochemical workers who are exposed to polychlorinated biphenyls [36]. Iatrogenically, nitrogen mustard used for mycosis fungoides is a good example.

Tar keratoses are cutaneous dysplasias that appear as grayish oval papules on sites of exposure to carcinogenic hydrocarbons. There may be hyperpigmented patches near these tar keratoses, at the site of occupational exposure. Just as chimney sweeps developed "soot warts," workers who handle pitch today develop pitch warts [37]. They may sometimes be keratoacanthomas, although cutaneous SCCs have been noted on the exposed face and hands as well as on the scrotum. A study of occupational exposure to "tarry" by-products during manufacture of 4,4'-bipyridyl for use in paraquat production noted the progression from tar keratosis to Bowen's disease to SCC in 20 light-complexioned workers [38].

It is important to put the carcinogenicity and mutagenicity of crude coal tar into a proper perspective [39]. There are scattered reports of patients who received repetitive long-term exposure to crude coal tars and developed SCC [40]. Although studies in certain animal models suggest that the standard therapy of ultraviolet light in the "B" range and crude coal tar (the Goeckerman regimen) may be carcinogenic, the risk of developing SCC appears to be the same as in control populations [41]. Further long-term study is still needed. On the other hand, the photochemotherapy treatment of psoriasis with methoxypsoralen and ultraviolet light in the "A" range has been linked with increased risk of developing nonmelanoma skin cancer in humans as well as in animal models [42], although an 8-year follow-up of 1643 European patients failed to demonstrate increased risk [43]. Treatment of psoriasis with cyclosporine is associated with an increased risk of nonmelanoma skin cancer [44].

Thermal keratoses

As with ultraviolet-induced cutaneous dysplasias, infrared radiation—which we appreciate as the sensation of warmth—may, after a carcinogenic lag of up to 20 years or more, produce dysplastic keratoses; later, bowenoid ones; and ultimately SCCs [2]. However, the tendency to malignant degeneration of burn scars in general is not a common phenomenon [45]. It is rare but not exceptional, with 95% being SCCs in one North African series of 45 patients [46]. It also occurs among albinos [47]. Years of warming close to a fire or other heat source may be a cause [48]. A similar thermal-induced situation has been documented in rural Ireland, where 162 elderly women were identified with evidence of chronic cutaneous thermal damage (erythema ab igne, a reticulated telangiectatic pigmented eruption) and cutaneous SCCs of the lower legs [49]. These women had experienced years of exposure to an open fire, sitting close as it burned inefficient peat and, unlike men, not wearing thick trousers. Many heat-induced skin cancers in men are associated with exotic situational phenomena, such as the kangri basket cancers in Kashmir, the kang cancers in China, and the oral SCCs induced in India by the habit of reverse smoking [50]. The kangri is a pot containing burning charcoal or another fuel held to the thigh for heat. Thermal keratoses and in situ SCC have been noted in the United States after long-term use of coal and wood-burning stoves for heating and cooking [51].

It is important to recall that other cancers besides SCCs may develop in burn scars [46]. In a series of 45 burn scar patients, there were a few basal cell epitheliomas (BCCs) and one melanoma. An earlier work showed that SCCs developed on average 32.5 years after the scar [52]. Whether burn scars are best considered thermal-induced or scar-induced keratoses and carcinomas is unclear. Thermal keratoses are histologically similar to actinic keratoses, showing hyperkeratosis, parakeratosis, and keratinocyte atypia. The acrosyringium and acrotrichium are spared except in areas most severely affected. Dermal elastosis, vascular ectasia, and a mild perivascular lymphocytic infiltrate occur and have been demonstrated in albino guinea pigs as well [53]. Interestingly, skin biopsy specimens from 20 patients with erythema ab igne but without apparent thermal keratoses consistently revealed marked epidermal cellular atypia and nuclear irregularity [54]. The

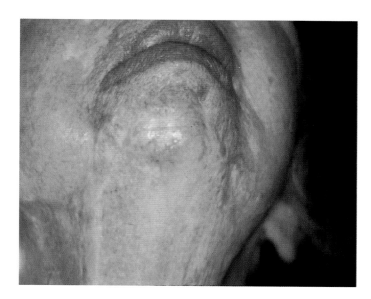

Fig. 3.5 Chronic cutaneous radiation damage on lower face and neck of woman irradiated for hirsutism and acne. Note telangiectasias, mottled pigmentary alterations, and multiple scars from excisions of basal cell carcinomas.

carcinogenicity of infrared light has been postulated and proven [55].

Chronic radiation keratoses

Chronic radiation keratoses are cutaneous dysplasias induced by that portion of the electromagnetic spectrum called x-radiation, as distinct from but parallel to those lesions induced by ultraviolet radiation (solar or actinic keratoses) or by infrared radiation (thermal keratoses). They appear up to 20 years or longer after x-ray exposure, usually as discrete keratoses or hyperkeratotic plaques on a background of chronic cutaneous radiation damage. They are distinct from early verrucous papules that may appear weeks rather than years after x-ray exposure, as well as from BCC that may also be induced from x-ray exposure [56]. In children given x-ray therapy for tinea capitis, light complexion, severe sunburning, and northern European ancestry were predictive of BCC risk [57]. In addition, chronic cutaneous damage should be viewed as a marker for the eventual development of skin cancer at or adjacent to the radiation site (Fig. 3.5). These malignancies may occur both cutaneously and viscerally, as in a BCC overlying a breast or in thyroid cancer [56].

Radiation exposure, with its long latent period of carcinogenesis, may produce a diagnostic dilemma, as the casual connection may be cryptic. For example, the occurrence of a number of cases of apparent contact dermatitis to gold rings was ultimately proven to be radiation-induced SCC; these rings contained gold that had previously been used in radiation therapy and was contaminated with breakdown products from radon "seeds" [58]. Bowenoid chronic radiation keratoses and SCCs may result from radiation exposure. Given a latency period of 20 to 50 years, one should recall how popular radiation therapy was years ago, including systems used to remove excess body hair that were often used by non-physicians in the same way that skin-tanning salons operate now. Cancers induced by properly administered radiotherapy are not rare, as exemplified by two patients treated for penile SCC who, about 20 years later, developed radiation-induced penile SCCs [59]. Even "soft" or superficial (Grenz) x-ray therapy employed in the past for benign inflammatory diseases such as psoriasis may have produced cutaneous SCCs [60,61]. However, a retrospective study of 14,140 patients who had received Grenz ray therapy with an average follow-up of 15 years demonstrated no increased incidence of melanoma and suggested that the risk of nonmelanoma malignancy is small or nonexistent [62].

Histologically, chronic radiation keratoses resemble solar keratoses, but the dermis shows the stigmata of chronic x-ray damage, including dilated capillaries, sclerosis, clumped elastic fibers, thickened vascular walls with obliteration of large vessels, and the presence of so-called radiation or giant fibroblasts [63]. SCCs developing as a result of chronic x-ray exposure are sometimes of the spindle cell type. Because other spindle cell tumors, especially the atypical fibroxanthoma, may also be induced by x-rays, difficult diagnostic problems may ensue [64]. The potential for metastases in chronic x-ray–induced SCCs is much greater than from solar-induced ones and should be viewed as comparable to those of scar SCCs.

Chronic cicatrix keratoses

Chronic cicatrix keratoses, or scar keratoses, and scar carcinomas are important because of their metastatic potential. The first description of carcinoma formation in chronic ulcers is credited to the French surgeon Jean-Nicolas Marjolin, who in 1828 described the degeneration of scars into carcinomatous ulcers, resulting in the eponym "Marjolin's ulcer" [52]. A large number of scarring and inflammatory processes have been implicated, including chronic osteomyelitis [65,66], chronic leg ulcers [67,68], discoid lupus erythematosus [68,69], acne conglobata [70,71], pilonidal sinuses [72], gunshot wounds and operative scars [73], burn scars (see above) [74], old frostbite injuries [75], smallpox vaccination scars [76], hidradenitis suppurativa including dissecting perifolliculitis of the scalp [77], hereditary ectodermal dysplasia [78], epidermolysis bullosa [79–82], porokeratosis of several types [83,84], erythema elevatum diutinum [85], granuloma inguinale [86], chromoblastomycosis [87], hypertrophic oral candidiasis [88], branchial cleft cyst [89], pemphigus vulgaris [90], cutaneous and mucosal lichen planus [91,92], lichen sclerosus et atrophicus [93], epidermal nevi [94], and tuberculosis of the skin (lupus vulgaris) [95]. When followed sequentially, evidence of a gradual progression from dysplasia and possible pseudoepitheliomatous hyperplasia to full-thickness in situ SCC

(Bowen's disease) may or may not be observed. However, when invasion through the basement membrane of the epidermis occurs, metastases may result and may rarely be evident before the primary is apparent.

The distinction between scar keratoses, scar carcinoma, and pseudoepitheliomatous hyperplasia may be difficult [96–98]. In healing debrided wounds, reactive infiltrating squamous metaplasia may mimic cutaneous SCC. Pseudoepitheliomatous hyperplasia is exhibited by a large number of inflammatory and scarring processes, including deep fungal infections, iododerma, tularemia, tungiasis, syphilis, and tuberculosis [99,100]. At times, the histology may simulate invasive SCC, although there is rarely evidence of bowenoid change. I believe that long-standing pseudoepitheliomatous hyperplasia is premalignant and warn my patients to avoid possible carcinogenic stimuli such as sun exposure.

The carcinogenic lag may be up to 20 years or more. A study of 21 burn scar SCCs showed the average time between scar and cancer to be 32.5 years [52]. Many had metastases (regional lymph node and/or visceral). Other tumors, including sarcomas, may be seen in chronic osteomyelitis and other scars, so spindle cell SCCs may need distinction from other spindle cell tumors in the setting of chronic scars [101,102].

Xeroderma pigmentosum

Xeroderma pigmentosum (XP) is a rare disorder characterized by marked hypersensitivity to ultraviolet light, resulting in multiple skin precancers and cancers at a very early age, mimicking findings seen in elderly, excessively sun-exposed, light-complexioned people [103–105]. This inherited disorder is of tremendous interest, because it represents a model for cutaneous aging and carcinogenesis. In XP, it is not unusual for a child to develop multiple freckles and actinic keratoses at age 5 years, then multiple BCCs, keratoacanthomas, and SCCs by age 12 years. Other cutaneous tumors, such as potentially lethal melanomas and sarcomas—including the atypical fibroxanthoma and angiosarcoma—may occur [106–109].

The original description of XP is credited to Kaposi, who in 1874 described and in 1882 named this

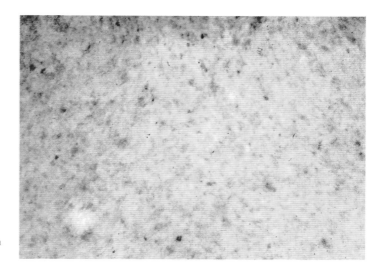

Fig. 3.6 Xeroderma pigmentosum in a 17-year-old girl with metastatic melanoma to the brain.

disorder for the patients' parchment-like skin and checkered pigmentation (Fig. 3.6) [104]. It occurs in about one in 250,000 births in most of the world, although it may be more common in Japan, Israel, and Holland. Traditionally, it is divided clinically into two forms, one limited primarily to the skin and another, rarer type (De Sanctis-Cacchione syndrome) with skeletal and genital underdevelopment, mental retardation, and severe neurologic deficits. Although the inheritance has been considered to be autosomal recessive, the modern breakdown of XP into multiple complementation groups and an XP variant can be best explained by the co-recessive inheritance model of Lambert and Lambert [110].

Clinically, XP tends to be evident in infancy by prolonged erythema after solar exposure, with the development of multiple irregular freckles and dry scaly skin followed by telangiectasia, mottled hyperpigmented and hypopigmented macules, and actinic keratoses. Ocular findings resulting from solar exposure include photophobia, keratitis, and conjunctivitis. The cutaneous tumors mentioned require prompt treatment, especially melanoma, which may be fatal in these patients. One evaluation of 132 XP patients found malignant skin neoplasms in 70% at a median age of 8 years [111]. Fifty-seven percent had BCC or SCC, and 22% had melanoma. The frequency of melanomas, like that of nonmelanoma skin cancers (BCCs and SCCs), anterior eye cancers, and tongue cancers was increased 1000-fold or more in patients with XP who

were younger than 20 years. The median age of nonmelanoma skin cancers is 8 years [103]. Internal cancers rarely seen in XP patients include brain sarcoma, acute lymphatic leukemia, myelogenous leukemia, choroidal melanoma, pancreatic adenocarcinoma, testicular sarcoma, bronchogenic carcinoma, and gastric cancer [111]. Some XP group D polymorphisms may have increased susceptibility to ovarian cancer [112]. Mild neurologic abnormalities, such as absent deep tendon reflexes and reduced hearing, are common in XP.

In 1968, Cleaver [113] noted that skin fibroblasts from these patients could not repair a certain type of ultraviolet light–induced DNA damage. Since then, this disease has been studied extensively as a prototype for genetic mutations, aging, and carcinogenesis. In most patients, the specific defect in XP occurs in the initial incision step of the nucleotide excision–repair pathway acting on pyrimidine dimers, formed after ultraviolet light–induced damage. This pathway is mediated by an endonuclease that incises the single strand of defective DNA at or near the damage site. Nevertheless, the exact defect in DNA repair is unclear. In addition, a subset of patients exhibit a defect in postreplication DNA repair; these have the XP variant.

Fibroblast fusion studies have shown that the fusing of cells from different XP patients may at times correct the DNA repair defect, indicating that separate and multiple DNA repair defects are involved. By such studies, nine complementation groups have been identified, labeled A through I. There is some correlation between the level of DNA repair and complementation groups A through E. Heterozygotes usually have normal DNA repair levels, although some may have reduced levels. Severe XP with a distinct and separate genetic disease called Cockayne syndrome is caused by mutations in the *XPB*, *XPD*, and *XPG* genes that encode specific helicase subunits and the 3′-endonuclease of nucleotide excision repair [114]. A cluster of XP-C patients within an isolated Guatemalan community was recently found to have a new mutation [115]. An American XP-C patient was identified as a compound heterozygote for two novel mutations in the *XPC* gene. The XP variant, constituting about 10% to 20% of patients with clinical XP, have normal excision repair, with the DNA repair deficit occurring after DNA replication.

The therapeutic approach in XP patients begins by making the diagnosis as early as possible, ideally in utero by amniocentesis [116]. These patients must be kept out of the sun, with the eyes and skin protected by special glasses, clothes, and sunscreens or sun blocks, if sun exposure cannot be avoided. The prophylactic use of systemic retinoids (0.5 mg of etretinate per kilogram body weight) may also be helpful. Topical application of the bacterial DNA repair enzyme T4 endonuclease V to sun-damaged skin of patients with XP has shown considerable promise, as it lowered the rate of development of actinic keratoses and BCCs during a year of treatment [117]. In America, many XP patients can modify their lifestyle to avoid sun exposure and achieve a near normal life span. However, XP presents a major health crisis in poor, isolated tropical communities, where life-threatening skin cancers result in death in the early teenage years [115].

Epidermodysplasia verruciformis

Epidermodysplasia verruciformis (EV) is a rare, usually autosomal recessive disorder first described by Lewandowsky and Lutz in 1922 [118,119]. This lifelong disease usually begins in infancy or early childhood with an eruption of widespread flat warts, some of which may evolve into cutaneous dysplasias, Bowen's disease, or invasive SCC. EV may

be a prototype for viral oncogenesis. It is associated with a high risk of skin cancer and results from a genetically determined abnormal susceptibility to a specific group of related human papillomavirus (HPV) genotypes, some with considerable oncogenic potential, such as HPV type 5 (HPV5). Its susceptibility locus was mapped to chromosomal region 17q25. EV seems to be caused by invalidating mutations in two adjacent, related, novel genes—*EVER1/TMC6* and *EVER2/TMC8*—that encode transmembrane proteins located in the endoplasmic reticulum [120–122]. EV may represent a primary defect of innate immunity, a primary deficiency of intrinsic immunity against certain papillomaviruses. However, only 75% of the patients studied harbor an *EVER* mutation, pointing to a genetic heterogeneity of the disease. EV, characterized by an abnormal susceptibility to a subset of HPV genotypes considered as harmless for the general population, leads to the lifelong persistence of benign macular and flat wartlike cutaneous papillomas and the early development of cutaneous carcinomas in some of them.

The average age of onset is 9 years, although in a few patients, delay until middle age may occur [123]. The principal EV finding resembles flat warts, seen as small scaly maculopapules that tend to involve the dorsal hands, face, neck, extremities, and trunk and spare the scalp, palms, and soles. Scaly macules or patches may also be seen, reddish brown in color, with a fine wrinkled or atrophic quality resembling macules and patches of tinea versicolor. They may coalesce into psoriasiform plaques or become quite verrucous and exophytic (Fig. 3.7). In addition, certain ones may transform into SCC, which occurs in 34% of EV patients, most frequently those in their 20s to 40s and predominately, but not exclusively, on sun-exposed cutaneous plaques. These cancers begin as thickened plaques and evolve into frank tumors. The time to evolve from wart to cancer averages 24 years, with a period as short as 2 years. These SCCs may metastasize or become lethal by locally aggressive invasion through the skull into the brain. Many of the SCCs tend to develop on sun-exposed sites, suggesting the possibility of ultraviolet light serving as a cofactor or cocarcinogen. A worsening

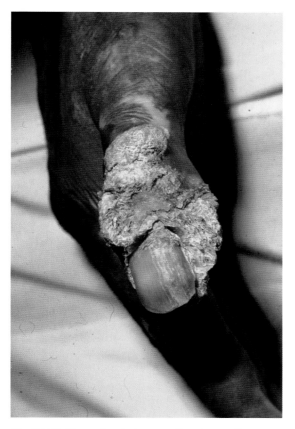

Fig. 3.7 Epidermodysplasia verruciformis on a finger.

genotype worldwide, some typical EV patients are infected with EV HPVs plus HPV3 or HPV10, both of which cause common flat warts in the general population. Patients with EV are usually infected with more than one genotype, up to 10. Not surprisingly, EV patients often have deficits in cell-mediated immunity; however, in a few it appears well preserved. Other problems reported to occur in EV include mental retardation in about 8% of patients, sweat gland and duct adenomas, and enlarged pituitary glands, evident as demonstrated by a widened sella turcica [123].

Epidermodysplasia verruciformis, a rare example of a mendelian disorder whose phenotypic expression is a narrow susceptibility to a single type of weakly pathogenic infectious agent, is associated with perplexing therapeutic options. EV patients do not usually respond to conventional wart therapy, such as liquid nitrogen cryosurgery, or to intralesional bleomycin. However, because some may respond, conservative therapy should be the first option considered. Topical imiquimod may also be a good choice [122,125].

Other therapeutic options include interferon-α with or without acitretin [126], cimetidine [127], and tacalcitol ointment [128]. Suspicious lesions should be biopsied. Bowen's disease or cutaneous SCC should be treated as in other patients.

effect of x-ray irradiation has been stressed. An SCC described developing on old surgical scar in an EV patient suggests other cofactors too [124].

At least 118 HPV genotypes have been described so far. HPV types are distributed in five phylogenetic supergroups or genera [119]. EV HPV genotypes constitute the β-papillomavirus genus and are distributed into five species, comprising the potentially oncogenic types B1 (HPV5, -8, -14, -20, and -47) and B2 (HPV9, -15, -17, -22, -23, -37, and -38). The commonest phenotype, comprising about 75% of EV patients, has multiple flat warts on the face and extremities together with tinea versicolor-like plaques on the trunk. This phenotype is associated with HPV5 infection. HPV5 appears to have significant potential for malignant transformation. Although HPV5 is the most frequently found EV HPV

Albinism

A good illustrative example of the deleterious effects of ultraviolet light is the patient with oculocutaneous albinism, characterized by photophobia, nystagmus, and poor vision (Figs. 3.8 and 3.9) [129,130]. This complex genetic disease with considerable clinical heterogeneity is divided into four different types. There are 12 different genes identified that, when mutated, result in a different type of albinism [131]. Albinos require meticulous protection from the sun. An excellent study of 1000 African albinos in Nigeria detailed the consequences of an uninformed society that ostracized albinos, forcing them to undertake menial outdoor work [132]. None of these 1000 people over the age of 20 years was free of premalignant or malignant skin lesions, which were BCCs or SCCs. Five of these

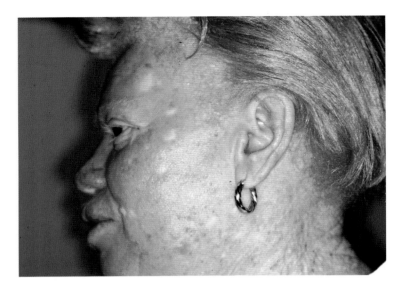

Fig. 3.8 Albino of sub-Saharan African lineage with multiple skin cancers.

albinos died of skin cancer eroding through the eyes, skull, or large blood vessels. A study of 350 African albinos from Tanzania observed chronic cutaneous damage in all albinos by the first year of life [133]; the overwhelming majority of skin cancers were SCCs, with only a few BCCs and one melanoma. Albinism among certain American Indians, including the Cuña Indians of Panama and the Hopi population in the southwestern United States, is rela-tively common [134]. Fortunately, in Cuña soci-ety, the surviving albinos are generally treated with tolerance. Up to ten different types of oculocu-taneous albinism have been described, with the type I (tyrosinase-negative) and type II (tyrosinase-positive) being the most common; the latter may have golden blond hair. Most American albinos are compound heterozygotes, each parent having a dif-ferent mutation.

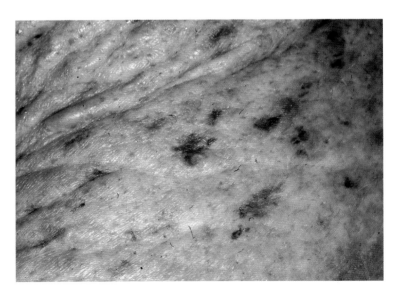

Fig. 3.9 Close-up of the skin of a woman with tyrosine-positive albinism.

Albinos tend to have the stigmata of chronic cutaneous solar damage, including atrophy, hyperpigmented patches, and telangiectasia (compare with Fig. 3.5). Although melanoma is uncommon in albinos, it occurs in both tyrosinase-positive and tyrosinase-negative forms [135]. Ocular melanomas may also develop [136]. The study of 350 albinos from Tanzania stressed that the SCCs in these patients are often clinically aggressive, with metastases and death unless treated [133].

Treatment of premalignant cutaneous dysplasias

Therapeutic options for these precancerous dysplasias are similar but more aggressive, given their enhanced malignant potential, to those for the most common type of cutaneous dysplasia, the actinic keratosis. Modalities include excision, photodynamic therapy, curettage and electrodessication, topical chemotherapy, topical immunotherapy, and cryosurgery. Of topical agents, 5-fluorouracil (5-FU) and imiquimod merit the most consideration, as discussed in the previous chapter on actinic keratosis. Locally administered 5-FU has been employed for accessible dysplasias since Klein's pioneering work in the 1960s [137–139]. Imiquimod 5% cream daily for 2 to 3 weeks or more is beneficial for arsenical keratoses [140] and chronic radiation dermatitis [141]. It is being used with enthusiasm for all types of cutaneous dysplasias. Oral retinoid therapy may be useful in patients with arsenicism, XP, and the basal cell nevus syndrome, because it seems to reduce the formation of new skin cancers and the enlargement of preexistent ones. Chemoprevention, including the topical application of the bacterial DNA repair enzyme T4 endonuclease V, has considerable promise [142].

In general, the greater the malignant potential of a precancer, the more desirable is its excision. Radiodermatitis constitutes a special clinical challenge, as there may be a relatively large, potentially premalignant area and, moreover, radiation-damaged skin tends to heal poorly. In such an instance, the use of microscopically controlled excision (Mohs surgery) to delineate the extent of involvement and remove affected tissue as conservatively as possible may be advisable.

References

1 Reichard JF, Schnekenburger M, Puga A. Long term low-dose arsenic exposure induces loss of DNA methylation. Biochem Biophys Res Commun 2007;352:188–92.
2 Schwartz RA. Premalignant keratinocytic neoplasms. J Am Acad Dermatol 1996;35:223–42.
3 Schwartz RA. Arsenic and the skin. Int J Dermatol 1997;36:241–50.
4 Rossy KM, Janusz CA, Schwartz RA. Cryptic exposure to arsenic. Indian J Dermatol Venereol Leprol 2005;71:230–5.
5 Hutchinson J. Arsenical cancer. Br Med J 1887; 2:1280–1.
6 Fukai Y, Hirata M, Ueno M, et al. Clinical pharmacokinetic study of arsenic trioxide in an acute promyelocytic leukemia (APL) patient: speciation of arsenic metabolites in serum and urine. Biol Pharm Bull 2006;29:1022–7.
7 Chou WC, Dang CV. Acute promyelocytic leukemia: recent advances in therapy and molecular basis of response to arsenic therapies. Curr Opin Hematol 2005;12:1–6.
8 Lee L, Bebb G. A case of Bowen's disease and small-cell lung carcinoma: long-term consequences of chronic arsenic exposure in Chinese traditional medicine. Environ Health Perspect 2005;113:207–10.
9 Liu CW, Liang CP, Huang FM, et al. Assessing the human health risks from exposure of inorganic arsenic through oyster (Crassostrea gigas) consumption in Taiwan. Sci Total Environ 2006;361:57–66.
10 Koch I, McPherson K, Smith P, Easton L, Doe KG, Reimer KJ. Arsenic bioaccessibility and speciation in clams and seaweed from a contaminated marine environment. Mar Pollut Bull 2007;54:586–94.
11 Ahsan H, Chen Y, Parvez F, et al. Arsenic exposure from drinking water and risk of premalignant skin lesions in Bangladesh: baseline results from the Health Effects of Arsenic Longitudinal Study. Am J Epidemiol 2006;163:1138–48.
12 Ahamed S, Kumar Sengupta M, Mukherjee A, et al. Arsenic groundwater contamination and its health effects in the state of Uttar Pradesh (UP) in upper and middle Ganga plain, India: a severe danger. Sci Total Environ 2006;370:310–22.
13 Christen K. Arsenic-treated wood may have a toxic legacy. Environ Sci Technol 2006;40:634–5.

14 Southwick GJ, Schwartz RA. Arsenically associated cutaneous squamous cell carcinoma with hypercalcemia. J Surg Oncol 1979;12:115–8.

15 Rubenstein DJ, Schwartz RA, Hansen RC, et al. Punctate hyperkeratosis of the palms and soles. An ultrastructural study. J Am Acad Dermatol 1980;3:43–9.

16 Perriol MP, Devos D, Hurtevent JF, et al. A case of neuropathy mimicking Guillain-Barre syndrome after arsenic intoxication [in French]. Rev Neurol (Paris) 2006;162:374–7.

17 Tapio S, Grosche B. Arsenic in the aetiology of cancer. Mutat Res 2006;612:215–46.

18 Yu HS, Liao WT, Chai CY. Arsenic carcinogenesis in the skin. J Biomed Sci 2006;13:657–66.

19 Ho SY, Tsai CC, Tsai YC, Guo HR. Hepatic angiosarcoma presenting as hepatic rupture in a patient with long-term ingestion of arsenic. J Formos Med Assoc 2004;103:374–9.

20 Centeno JA, Mullick FG, Martinez L, et al. Pathology related to chronic arsenic exposure. Environ Health Perspect 2002;110 Suppl 5:883–6.

21 Miki Y, Kawatsu T, Matsuda K, et al. Cutaneous and pulmonary cancers associated with Bowen's disease. J Am Acad Dermatol 1982;6:26–31.

22 Lee CH, Chen JS, Sun YL, et al. Defective beta1-integrins expression in arsenical keratosis and arsenic-treated cultured human keratinocytes. J Cutan Pathol 2006;33:129–38.

23 Lin X, Alber D, Henkelmann R. Elemental contents in Napoleon's hair cut before and after his death: did Napoleon die of arsenic poisoning? Anal Bioanal Chem 2004;379:218–20.

24 Khandpur S, Sharma VK. Successful treatment of multiple premalignant and malignant lesions in arsenical keratosis with a combination of acitretin and intralesional 5-fluorouracil. J Dermatol 2003;30:730–4.

25 Yerebakan O, Ermis O, Yilmaz E, et al. Treatment of arsenical keratosis and Bowen's disease with acitretin. Int J Dermatol 2002;41:84–7.

26 Bart RS, Andrade R, Kopf AW. Cutaneous horns. A clinical and histopathologic study. Acta Derm Venereol 1968;48:507–15.

27 Cruz Guerra NA, Saenz Medina J, Ursua Sarmiento I, et al. Malignant recurrence of a penile cutaneous horn [in Spanish]. Arch Esp Urol 2005;58:61–3.

28 Mencia-Gutierrez E, Gutierrez-Diaz E, Redondo-Marcos I, et al. Cutaneous horns of the eyelid: a clinicopathological study of 48 cases. J Cutan Pathol 2004;31:539–43.

29 Kitagawa H, Mizuno M, Nakamura Y, et al. Cutaneous horn can be a clinical manifestation of underlying sebaceous carcinoma. Br J Dermatol 2007;156:180–2.

30 Zhu JW, Luo D, Li CR, et al. A case of penile verrucous carcinoma associated with cutaneous horn. Clin Exp Dermatol 2007;32:213–4.

31 Kihiczak GG, Centurion SA, Schwartz RA, et al. Giant cutaneous melanoacanthoma. Int J Dermatol 2004;43:936–7.

32 de la Torre JP, Saiz A, Garcia-Arpa M, et al. Pilomatricomal horn: a new superficial variant of pilomatricoma. Am J Dermatopathol 2006;28:426–8.

33 Mooney MA, Meine J, Li H, et al. Exophytic pilomatricoma, clinically resembling keratoacanthoma, with peri-pilar differentiation: peripilomatricoma. J Cutan Pathol 1999;26:466.

34 Lei U, Masmas TN, Frentz G. Occupational non-melanoma skin cancer. Acta Derm Venereol 2001;81:415–7.

35 Pott P. Cancer scroti. In: Hawes L, Clarke W, Collins R, editors. Chirurgical observations relative to the cataract, the polypus of the nose, the cancer of the scrotum, the different kinds of ruptures, and the mortification of the toes and feet. London: T.J. Carnegy; 1775. p. 63–8.

36 Jarvholm B, Easton D. Models for skin tumour risks in workers exposed to mineral oils. Br J Cancer 1990;62:1039–41.

37 Waldron HA, Waterhouse JA, Tessema N. Scrotal cancer in the West Midlands 1936–76. Br J Ind Med 1984;41:437–44.

38 Bowra GT, Duffield DP, Osborn AJ, et al. Premalignant and neoplastic skin lesions associated with occupational exposure to "tarry" byproducts during manufacture of 4,4'-bipyridyl. Br J Ind Med 1982;39:76–81.

39 Pion IA, Koenig KL, Lim HW. Is dermatologic usage of coal tar carcinogenic? A review of the literature. Dermatol Surg 1995;21:227–31.

40 Take N, Kiryu H. Semi-malignant pitch-acanthoma on the hand of a coke oven worker [in Japanese]. J UOEH 1989;11:189–92.

41 Fiala Z, Borska L, Pastorkova A, et al. Genotoxic effect of Goeckerman regimen of psoriasis. Arch Dermatol Res 2006;298:243–51.

42 Raiss M, Templier I, Beani JC. Skin cancer and psoralen plus UVA: a retrospective study of 106 patients exposed to a great number of PUVA treatments [in French]. Ann Dermatol Venereol 2004;131:437–43.

43 Henseler T, Christophers E, Honigsmann H, et al. Skin tumors in the European PUVA Study. Eight-year

follow-up of 1643 patients treated with PUVA for psoriasis. J Am Acad Dermatol 1987;16:108–16.

44 Paul CF, Ho VC, McGeown C, et al. Risk of malignancies in psoriasis patients treated with cyclosporine: a 5 y cohort study. J Invest Dermatol 2003;120:211–6.

45 Mellemkjaer L, Holmich LR, Gridley G, et al. Risks for skin and other cancers up to 25 years after burn injuries. Epidemiology 2006;17:668–73.

46 Jellouli-Elloumi A, Kochbati L, Dhraief S, Ben Romdhane K, Maalej M. Cancers arising from burn scars: 62 cases [in French]. Ann Dermatol Venereol 2003;130:413–6.

47 Onuigbo WI. Epidemiology of skin cancer arisen from the burn scars in Nigerian Ibos. Burns 2006;32:602–4.

48 Rudolph CM, Soyer HP, Wolf P, Kerl H. Squamous epithelial carcinoma in erythema ab igne [in German]. Hautarzt 2000;51:260–3.

49 Cross F. On a turf (peat) fire cancer: malignant change superimposed on erythema ab igne. Proc R Soc Med 1967;60:1307–8.

50 Chowdri NA, Darzi MA. Postburn scar carcinomas in Kashmiris. Burns 1996;22:477–82.

51 Arrington JH 3rd, Lockman DS. Thermal keratoses and squamous cell carcinoma in situ associated with erythema ab igne. Arch Dermatol 1979;115:1226–8.

52 Treves N, Pack GT. The development of cancer in burn scars. An analysis and report of 34 cases. Surg Gynecol Obstet 1930;51:749–82.

53 Kligman LH. Full spectrum solar radiation as a cause of dermal photodamage: UVB to infrared. Acta Derm Venereol Suppl (Stockh) 1987;134:53–61.

54 Kligman LH. Intensification of ultraviolet-induced dermal damage by infrared radiation. Arch Dermatol Res 1982;272:229–38.

55 Schwartz RA. Infrared radiation as a carcinogenic agent. Br J Dermatol 1978;99:460–1.

56 Schwartz RA, Burgess GH, Milgrom H. Breast carcinoma and basal cell epithelioma after x-ray therapy for hirsutism. Cancer 1979;44:1601–5.

57 Shore RE, Moseson M, Xue X, et al. Skin cancer after x-ray treatment for scalp ringworm. Radiat Res 2002;157:410–8.

58 Stutzman CD, Schmidt GD. Squamous cell carcinoma of the skin associated with radioactive gold rings. J Am Acad Dermatol 1984;10:1075–7.

59 Wells AD, Pryor JP. Radiation-induced carcinoma of the penis. Br J Urol 1986;58:325–6.

60 Dabski K, Stoll HL Jr. Skin cancer caused by Grenz rays. J Surg Oncol 1986;31:87–93.

61 Frentz G. Grenz ray-induced nonmelanoma skin cancer. J Am Acad Dermatol 1989;21:475–8.

62 Lindelof B, Eklund G. Incidence of malignant skin tumors in 14,140 patients after Grenz-ray treatment for benign skin disorders. Arch Dermatol 1986;122:1391–5.

63 Brownstein MH, Rabinowitz AD. The precursors of cutaneous squamous cell carcinoma. Int J Dermatol 1979;18:1–16.

64 Kuwano H, Hashimoto H, Enjoji M. Atypical fibroxanthoma distinguishable from spindle cell carcinoma in sarcoma-like skin lesions. A clinicopathologic and immunohistochemical study of 21 cases. Cancer 1985;55:172–80.

65 Altay M, Arikan M, Yildiz Y, et al. Squamous cell carcinoma arising in chronic osteomyelitis in foot and ankle. Foot Ankle Int 2004;25:805–9.

66 Smidt LS, Smidt LF, Chedid MB, et al. Radical surgical treatment for Marjolin ulcer occurring after chronic osteomyelitis. South Med J 2005;98:1053.

67 Bachmeyer C, Cazier A, Rohaut B, Turc Y. Squamous cell carcinoma complicating chronic venous leg ulceration [in French]. Ann Dermatol Venereol 2005;132:589–90.

68 Dieng MT, Diop NN, Deme A, Sy TN, Niang SO, Ndiaye B. Squamous cell carcinoma in black patients: 80 cases [in French]. Ann Dermatol Venereol 2004;131:1055–7.

69 Gupta U, Barman KD, Saify K. Squamous cell carcinoma complicating an untreated chronic discoid lupus erythematosus (CDLE) lesion in a black female. J Dermatol 2005;32:1010–3.

70 Quintal D, Jackson R. Aggressive squamous cell carcinoma arising in familial acne conglobata. J Am Acad Dermatol 1986;14:207–14.

71 Whipp MJ, Harrington CI, Dundas S. Fatal squamous cell carcinoma associated with acne conglobata in a father and daughter. Br J Dermatol 1987;117:389–92.

72 Agir H, Sen C, Cek D. Squamous cell carcinoma arising adjacent to a recurrent pilonidal disease. Dermatol Surg 2006;32:1174–5.

73 Yuste Garcia P, Villarejo Campos P, Menendez Rubio JM, et al. Marjolin's ulcer arising from a laparostomy scar. Int Surg 2006;91:207–10.

74 Jamabo RS, Ogu RN. Marjolin's ulcer: report of 4 cases. Niger J Med 2005;14:88–91.

75 Uysal A, Kocer U, Sungur N, et al. Marjolin's ulcer on frostbite. Burns 2005;31:792–4.

76 Marmelzat WL. Malignant tumors in smallpox vaccination scars: a report of 24 cases. Arch Dermatol 1968;97:400–6.

77 Rosenzweig LB, Brett AS, Lefaivre JF, et al. Hidradenitis suppurativa complicated by squamous

cell carcinoma and paraneoplastic neuropathy. Am J Med Sci 2005;329:150–2.

78 McGregor JM, Hawk JL. Increased risk of skin cancer in patients with ectodermal dysplasia—a contraindication to psoralen and UVA (PUVA) therapy? Clin Exp Dermatol 1997;22:56.

79 Schwartz RA, Birnkrant AP, Rubenstein DJ, et al. Squamous cell carcinoma in dominant type epidermolysis bullosa dystrophica. Cancer 1981;47:615–20.

80 Fine JD, Johnson LB, Weiner M, et al. Chemoprevention of squamous cell carcinoma in recessive dystrophic epidermolysis bullosa: results of a phase 1 trial of systemic isotretinoin. J Am Acad Dermatol 2004;50:563–71.

81 Yamada T, Suzuki M, Hiraga M, et al. Squamous cell carcinoma arising on scars of epidermolysis bullosa acquisita. Br J Dermatol 2005;152:588–90.

82 Saxena A, Lee JB, Humphreys TR. Mohs micrographic surgery for squamous cell carcinoma associated with epidermolysis bullosa. Dermatol Surg 2006;32:128–34.

83 Sengupta S, Das JK, Gangopadhyay A. Multicentric squamous cell carcinoma over lesions of porokeratosis palmaris et plantaris disseminata and giant porokeratosis. Indian J Dermatol Venereol Leprol 2005;71:414–6.

84 Lin JH, Hsu MM, Sheu HM, et al. Coexistence of three variants of porokeratosis with multiple squamous cell carcinomas arising from lesions of giant hyperkeratotic porokeratosis. J Eur Acad Dermatol Venereol 2006;20:621–3.

85 Idemori M, Arao T. Erythema elevatum diutinum developing squamous cell carcinoma. J Dermatol 1979;6:75–80.

86 Hubbell CR, Rabin VR, Mora RG. Cancer of the skin in blacks. V. A review of 175 black patients with squamous cell carcinoma of the penis. J Am Acad Dermatol 1988;18:292–8.

87 Esterre P, Pecarrere JL, Raharisolo C, Huerre M. Squamous cell carcinoma arising from chromomycosis. Report of two cases [in French]. Ann Pathol 1999;19:516–20.

88 Rautemaa R, Hietanen J, Niissalo S, Pirinen S, Perheentupa J. Oral and oesophageal squamous cell carcinoma—a complication or component of autoimmune polyendocrinopathy-candidiasis-ectodermal dystrophy (APECED, APS-I). Oral Oncol 2007;43:607–13.

89 Jereczek-Fossa BA, Casadio C, Jassem J, et al. Branchiogenic carcinoma—conceptual or true clinico-pathological entity? Cancer Treat Rev 2005;31:106–14.

90 Mahomed Y, Mandel MA, Cramer SF, et al. Squamous cell carcinoma arising in pemphigus vulgaris during immunosuppressive therapy. Cancer 1980;46:1374–7.

91 Alvarez Alvarez C, Meijide Rico F, Rodriguez Gonzalez L, Anton Badiola I, Zungri Telo E, Antonio Ortiz-Rey J. Verrucous carcinoma of the penis arising from a lichen planus. A true preneoplastic lesion? [in Spanish]. Actas Urol Esp 2006;30:90–2.

92 Singh SK, Saikia UN, Ajith C, et al. Squamous cell carcinoma arising from hypertrophic lichen planus. J Eur Acad Dermatol Venereol 2006;20:745–6.

93 Barbagli G, Palminteri E, Mirri F, et al. Penile carcinoma in patients with genital lichen sclerosus: a multicenter survey. J Urol 2006;175:1359–63.

94 Affleck AG, Leach IH, Varma S. Two squamous cell carcinomas arising in a linear epidermal naevus in a 28-year-old female. Clin Exp Dermatol 2005;30:382–4.

95 Kimmritz J, Hermes B, Schewe C, Haas N. Squamous cell carcinoma in lupus vulgaris [in German]. J Dtsch Dermatol Ges 2004;2:116–9.

96 Fatima A, Matalia HP, Vemuganti GK, et al. Pseudoepitheliomatous hyperplasia mimicking ocular surface squamous neoplasia following cultivated limbal epithelium transplantation. Clin Experiment Ophthalmol 2006;34:889–91.

97 Fu X, Jiang D, Chen W, et al. Pseudoepitheliomatous hyperplasia formation after skin injury. Wound Repair Regen 2007;15:39–46.

98 Pui JC. Distinguishing pseudoepitheliomatous hyperplasia from squamous cell carcinoma in mucosal biopsy specimens from the head and neck [author reply]. Arch Pathol Lab Med 2006;130:764.

99 Kaminagakura E, Bonan PR, Lopes MA, et al. Cell proliferation and p53 expression in pseudoepitheliomatous hyperplasia of oral paracoccidioidomycosis. Mycoses 2006;49:393–6.

100 Heukelbach J, Sahebali S, Van Marck E, et al. An unusual case of ectopic tungiasis with pseudoepitheliomatous hyperplasia. Braz J Infect Dis 2004;8:465–8.

101 Nara T, Hayakawa A, Ikeuchi A, et al. Granulocyte colony-stimulating factor-producing cutaneous angiosarcoma with leukaemoid reaction arising on a burn scar. Br J Dermatol 2003;149:1273–5.

102 Ghorbani Z, Dowlati Y, Mehregan AH. Amelanotic spitzoid melanoma in the burn scar of a child. Pediatr Dermatol 1996;13:285–7.

103 Lambert WC, Kuo HR, Lambert MW. Xeroderma pigmentosum. Dermatol Clin 1995;13:169–209.

104 Leibowitz E, Janniger CK, Schwartz RA, et al. Xeroderma pigmentosum. Cutis 1997;60:75–7, 81–4.

105 Papadopoulos AJ, Schwartz RA, Sarasin A, et al. The xeroderma pigmentosum variant in a Greek patient. Int J Dermatol 2001;40:442–5.

106 Marcon I, Collini P, Casanova M, et al. Cutaneous angiosarcoma in a patient with xeroderma pigmentosum. Pediatr Hematol Oncol 2004;21:23–6.

107 Dilek FH, Akpolat N, Metin A, et al. Atypical fibroxanthoma of the skin and the lower lip in xeroderma pigmentosum. Br J Dermatol 2000;143:618–20.

108 Fazaa B, Zghal M, Bailly C, et al. Melanoma in xeroderma pigmentosum: 12 cases [in French]. Ann Dermatol Venereol 2001;128:503–6.

109 Shao L, Newell B, Quintanilla N. Atypical fibroxanthoma and squamous cell carcinoma of the conjunctiva in xeroderma pigmentosum. Pediatr Dev Pathol 2007;10:149–52.

110 Lambert WC, Lambert MW. Co-recessive inheritance: a model for DNA repair, genetic disease and carcinogenesis. Mutat Res 1985;145:227–34.

111 Kraemer KH, Lee MM, Andrews AD, et al. The role of sunlight and DNA repair in melanoma and nonmelanoma skin cancer. The xeroderma pigmentosum paradigm. Arch Dermatol 1994;130:1018–21.

112 Costa S, Pinto D, Pereira D, et al. Importance of xeroderma pigmentosum group D polymorphisms in susceptibility to ovarian cancer. Cancer Lett 2007;246:324–30.

113 Cleaver JE. Defective repair replication of DNA in xeroderma pigmentosum. 1968. DNA Repair (Amst) 2004;3:183–87.

114 Clement V, Dunand-Sauthier I, Clarkson SG. Suppression of UV-induced apoptosis by the human DNA repair protein XPG. Cell Death Differ 2006;13:478–88.

115 Cleaver JE, Feeney L, Tang JY, et al. Xeroderma pigmentosum group C in an isolated region of Guatemala. J Invest Dermatol 2007;127:493–6.

116 Regan JD, Setlow RB, Kaback MM, et al. Xeroderma pigmentosum: a rapid sensitive method for prenatal diagnosis. Science 1971;174:147–50.

117 Yarosh D, Klein J, O'Connor A, et al. Effect of topically applied T4 endonuclease V in liposomes on skin cancer in xeroderma pigmentosum: a randomised study. Xeroderma Pigmentosum Study Group. Lancet 2001;357:926–9.

118 Majewski S, Jablonska S. Why epidermodysplasia verruciformis—a rare genetic disease—has raised such great interest. Int J Dermatol 2004;43:309–11.

119 Orth G. Genetics of epidermodysplasia verruciformis: insights into host defense against papillomaviruses. Semin Immunol 2006;18:362–74.

120 Akgul B, Kose O, Safali M, et al. A distinct variant of epidermodysplasia verruciformis in a Turkish family lacking EVER1 and EVER2 mutations. J Dermatol Sci 2007;46:214–6.

121 Gober MD, Rady PL, He Q, et al. Novel homozygous frameshift mutation of EVER1 gene in an epidermodysplasia verruciformis patient. J Invest Dermatol 2007;127:817–20.

122 Berthelot C, Dickerson MC, Rady P, et al. Treatment of a patient with epidermodysplasia verruciformis carrying a novel EVER2 mutation with imiquimod. J Am Acad Dermatol 2007;56:882–6.

123 Lutzner MA. Epidermodysplasia verruciformis. An autosomal recessive disease characterized by viral warts and skin cancer. A model for viral oncogenesis. Bull Cancer 1978;65:169–82.

124 Ozyazgan I, Kontas O, Gokahmetoglu S, et al. An epidermoid carcinoma case developed on old surgical scar in an epidermodysplasia verruciformis patient. J Eur Acad Dermatol Venereol 2005;19:640–2.

125 Baskan EB, Tunali S, Adim SB, et al. A case of epidermodysplasia verruciformis associated with squamous cell carcinoma and Bowen's disease: a therapeutic challenge. J Dermatolog Treat 2006;17:179–83.

126 Anadolu R, Oskay T, Erdem C, et al. Treatment of epidermodysplasia verruciformis with a combination of acitretin and interferon alfa-2a. J Am Acad Dermatol 2001;45:296–9.

127 Micali G, Nasca MR, Dall'Oglio F, et al. Cimetidine therapy for epidermodysplasia verruciformis. J Am Acad Dermatol 2003;48:S9–10.

128 Hayashi J, Matsui C, Mitsuishi T, et al. Treatment of localized epidermodysplasia verruciformis with tacalcitol ointment. Int J Dermatol 2002;41:817–20.

129 Okulicz JF, Shah RS, Schwartz RA, et al. Oculocutaneous albinism. J Eur Acad Dermatol Venereol 2003;17:251–6.

130 Centurión SA, Schwartz RA. Oculocutaneous albinism type 2. Acta Dermatovenerol Alp Panonica Adriat 2003;12:32–6.

131 Oetting WS, Fryer JP, Shriram S, et al. Oculocutaneous albinism type 1: the last 100 years. Pigment Cell Res 2003;16:307–11.

132 Okoro AN. Albinism in Nigeria. A clinical and social study. Br J Dermatol 1975;92:485–92.

133 Luande J, Henschke CI, Mohammed N. The Tanzanian human albino skin. Natural history. Cancer
1985;55:1823–8.

134 Woolf CM. Albinism (OCA2) in Amerindians. Am J
Phys Anthropol 2005;Suppl 41:118–40.

135 Terenziani M, Spreafico F, Serra A, et al. Amelanotic
melanoma in a child with oculocutaneous albinism.
Med Pediatr Oncol 2003;41:179–80.

136 Harasymowycz P, Boucher MC, Corriveau C, et al.
Choroidal amelanotic melanoma in a patient
with oculocutaneous albinism. Can J Ophthalmol
2005;40:754–8.

137 Klein E. Tumors of skin. IX. Local cytostatic therapy of
cutaneous and mucosal premalignant and malignant
lesions. N Y State J Med 1968;68:886–9.

138 Klein E. Local chemotherapy of cutaneous neoplasms. Proc Natl Cancer Conf 1970;6:501–15.

139 Klein E, Schwartz RA, Case RW, et al. Accessible tumors. In: LoBuglio AF, editor. Clinical immunotherapy. New York: Marcel Dekker; 1980. p. 31–71.

140 Boonchai W. Treatment of precancerous and cancerous lesions of chronic arsenicism with 5% imiquimod
cream. Arch Dermatol 2006;142:531–2.

141 Sachse MM, Zimmermann J, Bahmer FA. Efficiency
of topical imiquimod 5% cream in the management
of chronic radiation dermatitis with multiple neoplasias. Eur J Dermatol 2006;16:56–8.

142 Wright TI, Spencer JM, Flowers FP. Chemoprevention
of nonmelanoma skin cancer. J Am Acad Dermatol
2006;54:933–46; quiz 947–50.

CHAPTER 4

Bowen's disease

Robert A. Schwartz

John T. Bowen [1] in 1912 described two patients with cutaneous chronic atypical epithelial proliferation, for which Darier in 1914 coined the term *la dermatose precancereuse de Bowen, dyskeratose lenticulaire et en disques* in describing further patients with this disorder [2,3]. Bowen himself also reported additional patients with this condition [2], which he described clinically as follows:

> It may apparently attack any portion of the integument and begins as a firm papule, pale red or nearly of the color of the normal skin. This papule is covered by a thickened horny layer, which may become excessive, and usually is combined with a serous exudation to form a cornified crust. These papules increase to form lenticular, or rounded, nodular lesions, which may remain discrete, or often tend to become grouped or confluent. When the crust is removed, the surface beneath is found to be red and oozing, granular, and sometimes slightly papillomatous in appearance.

Although Bowen had predicted that these lesions had "imminent" malignant potential, he also observed that they were typically solitary and of many years' duration. Bowen's disease tends to appear most commonly on light-complexioned middle-aged or elderly men, on both sun-exposed and non–sun-exposed skin. In the latter case, one should consider the possibility of arsenic induction [4]. Likewise, Bowen's disease in blacks, a relatively rare occurrence, should prompt evaluation for arsenic exposure [5].

Clinical features

As characterized by Bowen himself, the disease appears as lenticular papules or circular longstanding plaques (Figs. 4.1 and 4.2). Other morphologic patterns occur. For example, at times Bowen's disease may be so hyperkeratotic and verrucous as to suggest a wart (verruca vulgaris) or an inflamed seborrheic keratosis [6]. This morphologic pattern of a well-circumscribed, papillated, exophytic and endophytic, sometimes keratotic plaque has been called papillated Bowen's disease [7]. On the breast, it may mimic Paget's disease both clinically and histologically [8]; when pigmented, Bowen's disease may resemble a melanoma [9–11]. It may also resemble a cutaneous T cell lymphoma [12]. It is often misdiagnosed as superficial basal cell carcinoma (BCC), dermatitis, psoriasis, lichen planus, actinic keratosis, benign lichenoid keratosis, irritated seborrheic keratosis, viral wart, amelanotic melanoma, or melanoma. Rarely, it may be first evident as purpura on the scalp in the elderly, suggesting an angiosarcoma [13].

Bowen's disease on the nail beds, on the mucosa, and in intertriginous body areas may be strikingly different in appearance from that on other cutaneous surfaces. It may appear as periungual erythema with scaling and erosion, a white-colored cuticle, a verrucous nodule, a longitudinal melanonychia, or a fissuring or crusting of the lateral fold [14,15]. Eighty percent of these cases occur in men. Any chronic, persistent eczema (dermatitis) of the hand, especially around the nail beds or on a ring finger, should be evaluated for possible Bowen's disease. Clinical differential diagnoses include the common wart, fungal infections, paronychia, dermatitis, pyogenic granuloma, verrucous tuberculosis, subungual exostosis, glomus tumor, dermatitis vegetans, amelanotic melanoma, onychomatricoma, keratoacanthoma, and squamous cell carcinoma

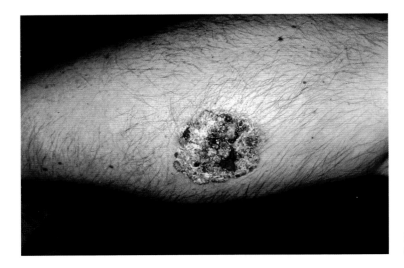

Fig. 4.1 Bowen's disease of the leg in a middle-aged woman.

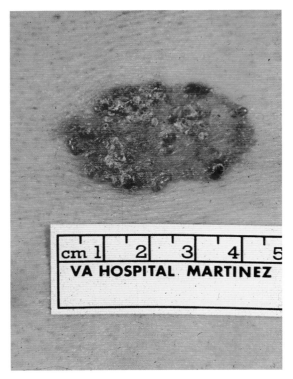

Fig. 4.2 Psoriasiform plaque of Bowen's disease beside an eroded plaque of cutaneous SCC.

(SCC) [16,17]. In one study, its dermoscopic features showed a multicomponent pattern (100%), atypical vascular structures (86.6%), absence of pigmented network (64.3%) or presence of pseudonetwork (35.7%), irregular diffuse pigmentation or blotches of pigment (64.2%), irregularly distributed dots and globules (64.2%), focal/multifocal hypopigmentation (78.5%), scaly surface (64.2%), and hemorrhages (26.6%). Thus, Bowen's disease is mainly characterized by a multicomponent global pattern associated with a prominent vascular pattern (mainly dotted vessels) and a scaly surface [18,19].

Bowen's disease in the intertriginous regions of the body may resemble an acute dermatitis, a chronic nonspecific dermatitis, or black pigmented patches [20]. Thus, such lesions in the axilla, the perianal area, the perigenital region, or the interweb spaces of the fingers or toes must be carefully evaluated [21,22] (Fig. 4.3). On the genitalia, Bowen's disease may appear as a red patch (erythroplasia) with or without a velvety quality or may be verrucous or polypoid. The clinical types of Bowen's disease are summarized in Table 4.1.

The biologic behavior of untreated Bowen's disease is noteworthy, with 3% to 5% of patients developing invasive SCC, which has considerable metastatic potential [23] (Fig. 4.3). This entity is uncommon and often misdiagnosed as seborrheic

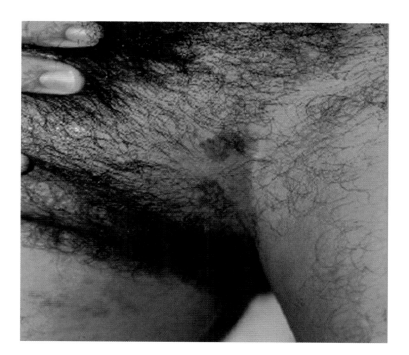

Fig. 4.3 Bowen's disease as intertriginous pigmented patches of the interweb spaces in a middle-aged missionary from Mexico, who had similar lesions in the groin and erythroplasia of Queyrat of the penis.

keratosis, BCC, metastatic carcinoma, or glomus tumor. The most frequent warning sign of an in situ SCC (Bowen's disease) undergoing spread below the basement membrane is a relatively rapidly evolving erosion or ulceration developing within it. Bowen's original description of imminent malignant potential is supported by follow-up studies showing a 13% metastatic rate for carcinoma arising within Bowen's disease, with death from generalized metastases in about 10% of patients [23]. There is no evidence in population-based cohort data of an increased risk of subsequent internal cancer associated with non-vulvar Bowen's disease [24].

Table 4.1 Clinical types of Bowen's disease

Annular Bowen's disease
Verrucous Bowen's disease
Genital erythroplasia of Queyrat
Oral erythroplakia
Pigmented Bowen's disease
Bowen's disease of nail beds
Bowenoid papulosis (?)

Bowen's disease of the hands is also frequently associated with mucosal human papillomavirus (HPV) infection [25].

Bowenoid conditions

A number of cutaneous processes may evolve into full-thickness SCC. It is implied from John T. Bowen's [1,2] original descriptions of what is now called Bowen's disease that the lesions did not arise from an obvious preexistent one. Thus, purists may wish to avoid invoking Dr. Bowen's name for full-thickness epidermal change as in "bowenoid actinic keratosis" or "bowenoid arsenical keratosis." Similarly, when in situ SCC occurs on mucosal surfaces, the invocation of "Bowen's disease" may be challenged, because Dr. Bowen described only cutaneous disease. I choose to adopt a permissive terminology, which is useful in highlighting the continuum from cutaneous dysplasia to full-thickness SCC to invasive SCC.

Bowenoid disease may develop within a number of preexistent conditions, especially in scarring and chronic inflammatory processes, perhaps as the result of reduced mutagen resistance, and may progress to invasive SCC. In any disorder associated with SCC, one presumes that at some stage it was Bowen's disease or a bowenoid keratosis. Such bowenoid alterations are associated with porokeratosis of Mibelli [26], poikiloderma congenitale [27], epidermal nevi [28], and epidermal inclusion cysts [29]; the potential for Bowen's disease in these settings and the risk of subsequent metastatic spread must be considered.

Penile intraepithelial neoplasia is a term used by some to describe erythroplasia of Queyrat, penile Bowen's disease, and bowenoid papulosis.

Erythroplasia of Queyrat

Erythroplasia of Queyrat (EQ) refers to a velvety, bright red, sharply demarcated patch or plaque on the penis as described in four patients by M. Queyrat in 1911 in French as *erythroplasie du gland* [30], which represents SCC in situ (Bowen's disease). The French word *erythroplasie* in English would be *erythroplakia*, denoting a red plaquelike growth [31]. Queyrat in 1911 chose his term to be analogous with the term *leukoplasia*, or *leukoplakia* in English [30]. Nevertheless, by common usage, we use the term *erythroplasia* rather than the correct French or its English translation, a minor linguistic anomaly [31]. A similar morphologic pattern may be seen on several mucosal surfaces, such as the oral mucosa, the vulva, the urethra, the tongue, and the conjunctivae [32] (Table 4.2). Erythroplasia of the oral cavity is discussed separately in Chapter 18.

Erythroplasia of Queyrat occurs almost exclusively in uncircumcised men or those circumcised later in life (Fig. 4.4); it has been noted in a man who was only partially circumcised [33]. It is most

Table 4.2 Sites of erythroplasia

Penis (erythroplasia of Queyrat)
Conjunctivae
Oral cavity
Vulva
Urethra
Tongue

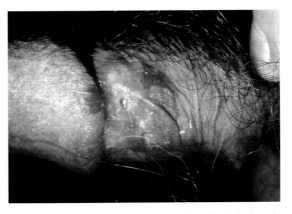

Fig. 4.4 Erythroplasia of Queyrat on the distal shaft and glans of an uncircumcised man. (Reprinted with permission from Schultze et al. [36].)

common in the second through sixth decade of life, although its occurrence in patients in their 20s is not rare [34]. EQ involves the distal penis, including the glans, urethral meatus, frenulum, corona, sulcus, and prepuce. About one half of the 100 patients in one large series had involvement in several of these sites [34]. Most patients complain of crusting, redness, and scaling; some experience bleeding or difficulty retracting the foreskin. Many EQ patients note pruritus or discomfort at the involved site. Leukoplakia may be seen in association with EQ [31], but is itself much less likely to be malignant.

Histologically, EQ is typical Bowen's disease [31,32,34] (Fig. 4.5). Approximately 5% of cutaneous SCCs in situ have a nested pattern, referred to as pagetoid SCC in situ or pagetoid Bowen's disease. It may simulate extramammary Paget's disease when the external genitalia are involved [35]. The factors producing EQ are probably local environmental carcinogens and cofactor(s) in uncircumcised men, such as smegma, poor hygiene, genital herpes simplex, genital papillomavirus, heat, friction, and trauma [34,36]. Mucosal oncogenic HPV is detected by in situ hybridization in almost 30% of extragenital Bowen's disease specimens [37,38]. Bowen's disease of the scrotum has been linked to HPV type 82 [39]. There has been no association observed between arsenic intake or internal cancer and EQ [34].

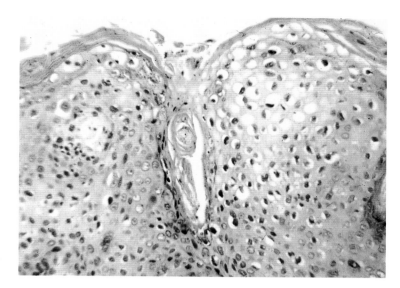

Fig. 4.5 Histologic view of Bowen's disease showing full-thickness epidermal dysplasia (Bowen's disease) with some loss of polarity.

Clinically, a number of benign processes may resemble EQ (Table 4.3), including psoriasis, lichen planus, lichen sclerosus et atrophicus, drug eruptions, bacterial and traumatic balanitides, keratoderma blennorrhagicum, granuloma inguinale, lymphogranuloma venereum, candidiasis, pemphigus, dermatitis, distinctive exudative discoid and lichenoid chronic dermatosis (oid-oid disease), familial pemphigus, Kaposi's sarcoma, leukoplakia, SCC, and Zoon's plasma cell balanitis [36,40,41]. These disorders can be distinguished by the patient's history, response to therapy, bacteriologic studies, and/or a biopsy specimen. I have found that the most frequent disorder in the differential diagnosis of EQ is Zoon's balanitis, a benign genital eruption of elderly patients [42].

Table 4.3 Principle considerations in the differential diagnosis of erythroplasia of Queyrat

Psoriasis
Lichen planus
Candidiasis
Zoon's balanitis
Contact dermatitis
Drug eruptions
Keratoderma blennorrhagica (Reiter's syndrome)

Erythroplasia of Queyrat should be regarded as having metastatic potential [34,43]. Thus, any question of a diagnosis of EQ merits a prompt biopsy and therapeutic measures if EQ is proven. The therapeutic options for EQ are the same as those for Bowen's disease of the skin, including topical fluorouracil, imiquimod [44,45], radiotherapy [46,47], liquid nitrogen cryosurgery [48], photodynamic therapy [49–51], and—recognizing the concern for conserving tissue in this region—Mohs microscopically controlled excision [52].

Leukoplakia

Leukoplakia refers to the appearance of a white plaque on mucosal surfaces. The white color results from the hydration of the keratin of the normally nonkeratinized mucosa rather than the increased thickness of the stratum corneum per se [53]. Leukoplakia is most commonly seen on the oral, anal, and genital mucosa, where it invariably raises the question of SCC. Fortunately, leukoplakia is now known not to be an ominous sign. For example, in one series of 782 patients with oral or lip leukoplakia evaluated at regular intervals, oral cancer developed in only 2.4% in 10 years and 4% in 20 years [54]. The conventional wisdom for years has been to emphasize the significance of leukoplakia as a marker for oral cancer. When both leukoplakia and erythroplasia occur together in oral cancers, the leukoplakia is what often draws comment [55].

Oral leukoplakia may appear homogenous, verrucous, or speckled; the latter pattern of white flecks on an erythematous or eroded base is said to have the highest malignant potential [56] and underscores that erythroplasia, and not leukoplakia per se, is the marker of malignancy. In my experience, most oral leukoplakias represent candidiasis or mucosal hyperkeratosis due to mechanical factors such as poorly fitting dentures or pipe smoking. The leukoplakia of tobacco users often has a pumice-like morphology [57]. Benign or atrophic inflammatory causes of leukoplakia include lichen planus, lupus erythematosus, psoriasis, erythema multiforme, leukoedema, syphilis, and lichen sclerosis et atrophicus (LS&A). Other causes of leukoplakia include autosomal dominant congenital diseases such as oral epidermal nevi, either by itself or as part of the syndrome called pachyonychia congenita. X-ray therapy may also induce a benign leukoplakia [58]. Proliferative verrucous leukoplakia is a multifocal oral premalignant form, proliferative in nature, with a tendency to recur despite adequate therapy and has a high rate of malignant transformation. The field cancerization phenomenon may explain its behavior [59]. Because oral SCC is a highly malignant process, a biopsy is mandatory if there is any question.

It is important to recall that even apparently benign inflammatory processes, such as lichen planus and LS&A, may undergo malignant degeneration [60,61]. LS&A is said to undergo malignant degeneration from a penile leukoplakia, with an incidence varying from 2% up to 18% [61,62]; the former is probably the more accurate. However, evidence linking LS&A to SCC is debatable [61]. One large series of 107 patients observed that when the two disorders are linked, the cancer tends to arise on areas of minimal LS&A or on isolated areas of normal vulva. Leukoplakia may also be seen in dyskeratosis congenita, which is often associated with Fanconi syndrome. In both of these conditions, leukoplakia may become SCC [63].

Thus, an index of suspicion in all leukoplakias needs to be maintained, even though these patients are at much less risk than those with erythroplasia. The diagnosis of cutaneous precancer or cancer itself is always a histologic one. An interesting lectin-staining study of oral leukoplakias showed dysplastic and in situ SCC had a loss of lectin binding in intercellular spaces and cellular membranes [64].

Vulvar dysplasia and Bowen's disease

Vulvar neoplasms have undergone a number of terminology changes in the gynecologic literature [62,65–67]. The basic alteration has been the elimination of the terms *leukoplakia* and *kraurosis* in favor of *hyperplastic dystrophy* with or without dysplasia and *lichen sclerosis*. Whether these two types of so-called vaginal dystrophies are premalignant is unknown [61,65,66]. Certainly, any persistent vulvar lesion deserves a biopsy if the diagnosis is unclear. A large number of benign inflammatory processes may resemble these vaginal dystrophies. A 1% solution of toluidine blue dye may be painted on to identify areas of abnormal nuclear maturation for biopsy [66]; unfortunately, this test is relatively inaccurate.

In situ SCC of the vulva tends to become evident as a patch or plaque of red and white coloration (erythroleukoplakia), although it may appear as a hypertrophic plaque and may sometimes be pigmented. As discussed above, the older literature emphasized leukoplakia [68], which indeed may appear concurrently with erythroplasia, the more significant finding. Vaginal Bowen's disease tends to affect women aged 20 to 40 years. However, because the average age for invasive vaginal SCC is 60 to 70 years, perhaps in situ SCC in these younger women may not progress [65,67]. Nevertheless, it should be treated by elimination. Importantly, vulvar Bowen's disease may be a marker for internal cancer. In one series of 24 patients with vulvar Bowen's disease, 37.5% had other cancers, especially SCC of the cervix and upper vagina (25%) [69].

Bowenoid papulosis

Because genital and especially penile SCC is a major killer in much of the world, dysplasia in the genital region must be viewed with careful scrutiny. It is a sound principle that SCC of any mucosal surface is more likely to metastasize than SCC on the skin itself. Nevertheless, there is a specific disorder called bowenoid papulosis that appears clinically benign, though histologically malignant [5,29,70]. It may be linked to a high risk of cervical neoplasia in female patients and in women who are the sexual partners of affected males [71]. Bowenoid papulosis may also be classified as grade 3 vulvar intraepithelial neoplasia.

Bowenoid papulosis is an eruption of one or more reddish brown and sometimes verrucous papules usually on the male or female genitalia of predominately young adults. Isolated extragenital bowenoid papulosis is rare [72]. Bowenoid papulosis may also occur in the oral cavity [73] and in an epidermal inclusion cyst [29]. It tends to clinically resemble verrucae vulgaris, melanocytic nevi, condyloma acuminata, lichen planus, or psoriasis [29], sometimes evolving into pigmented plaques. It has been described in a child only 3 years of age [74]. It appears that bowenoid papulosis responds to conservative therapy but may be a marker for malignancy. Spontaneous regression of bowenoid papulosis as well as progression to Bowen's disease has been documented; thus, the biological behavior of bowenoid papulosis remains poorly understood [29,75]. HPV types 16 and 31 have been found in association with bowenoid papulosis [76,77]. The salient features of bowenoid papulosis are summarized in Table 4.4.

In bowenoid papulosis, there may be scattered dysplastic keratinocytes, but there remains a background of ordered keratinocyte maturation. This distinction is not helpful on mucosal surfaces, which tend to lack hair and eccrine glands. Significant differences were found morphometrically between Bowen's disease and bowenoid papulosis. Bowen's

Table 4.4 Essentials of bowenoid papulosis

Reddish brown or violaceous papules
Often warty and multiple
Usually on penile shaft; seen on vulva also
Histologically resembles Bowen's disease
Associated with HPV
Biologic behavior unclear

---

disease has nuclei that are larger and more oval and irregular than those of bowenoid papulosis [78].

Histology

Bowen's disease is an intraepithelial SCC (Fig. 4.5). It represents full-thickness–change SCC in situ. The keratinocytes show loss of polarity, atypia, and mitoses. There may be a large number of atypical cells with pale-staining cytoplasm, at times appearing arranged in nests. Often, there is prominent acanthosis with elongation and thickening of the rete ridges. One commonly sees individual cell keratinization; such cells are large and rounded, with eosinophilic cytoplasm and a pyknotic nucleus. Actual horn pearls may be evident. Cells with large hyperchromatic nuclei and multinucleated keratinocytes may be seen. Bowen's disease may have marked hyperkeratosis and papillomatosis, to the extent that the clinical appearance of a cutaneous horn may be produced, or may display hyperkeratosis with epidermal thinning. Papillated Bowen's disease shows keratinocytes with prominent perinuclear halos suggestive of koilocytic change associated with HPV infection [7]. Bowenoid actinic keratosis may in addition spare appendageal structures and be more clearly demarcated than de novo Bowen's disease.

When Bowen's disease evolves into invasive SCC, islands of neoplastic keratinocytes tend to extend into the dermis. At times, these invasive components may resemble a BCC or show pilar, pilosebaceous, or adenoid differentiation [23]; thus, the impression of a BCC [3], or of an adnexal carcinoma with pilar differentiation may be suggested [79]. It is important to have a complete specimen so that the overlying Bowen's disease can be evaluated. At times, it may be difficult to distinguish a primary cutaneous appendageal carcinoma or a metastatic adenoid carcinoma from Bowen's disease showing multi-pluripotential differentiation. A reported case of sebaceous carcinoma arising from Bowen's disease of the vulva [80] may in fact be an example of Bowen's disease with pilosebaceous differentiation [23].

Clearly, when two distinct histologic patterns appear concurrently, the biology may be difficult to interpret. Whether the coexistence of Merkel cell carcinoma and intraepidermal SCC is significant or simply a chance collision of two tumors is unknown [81,82]. Nevertheless, the possibility of a Merkel cell carcinoma deriving from Bowen's disease, with its multipotential for differentiation, is still difficult to exclude given our incomplete knowledge regarding Merkel cell carcinoma, the subject of Chapter 13.

Distinguishing Bowen's disease from bowenoid papulosis is usually not difficult if one correlates the clinical and histologic patterns. Microscopically, bowenoid papulosis lacks the full-thickness dysplasia and disordered maturation characteristic of Bowen's disease; rather, it has dysplastic keratinocytes "shot-gunned" throughout the epidermis, often with keratinocytes in metaphase [70]. In bowenoid papulosis on the skin, the acrotrichia are frequently spared, whereas in Bowen's disease they are regularly involved, an important diagnostic criterion [70]. In addition, when biopsying genital papules, one need inquire whether podophyllin has been employed topically, because it causes metaphase arrest with bizarre keratinocyte forms and sometimes a pattern of pseudo-epitheliomatosis hyperplasia [83]. It is doubtful whether what appears to be Bowen's disease developing with a seborrheic keratosis is meaningful [84].

Within cutaneous cysts, Bowen's disease may be mimicked when proliferating trichilemmal cysts display pseudo-epitheliomatosis hyperplasia with cellular atypia [85]. In addition, occult Bowen's disease within epidermal inclusion cysts [86] and bowenoid papulosis within a penile epidermal inclusion cyst have been documented [29].

At times, the distinction of Bowen's disease from Paget's disease may be difficult. Both are intraepithelial carcinomas. When Bowen's disease exhibits plentiful clear cells, it may be confused with Paget's disease. Both may show atypical cells with abundant pale-staining cytoplasm arranged singly or in apparent nests. "Pagetoid Bowen's disease" is a distinctive histologic subtype of Bowen's disease.

However, when doubt exists, special stains can be easily and effectively employed. Although both Paget's disease cells and those of pagetoid Bowen's disease may contain periodic acid-Schiff (PAS)-positive neutral mucopolysaccharides, in the latter disorder, they are eliminated by pretreatment with

Table 4.5 Histologic differential diagnosis of Bowen's disease

Bowenoid actinic keratosis
Paget's disease vs. pagetoid Bowen's disease
Pagetoid in situ melanoma vs. pagetoid Bowen's disease
Primary adnexal carcinoma
Sebaceous carcinoma arising in Bowen's disease
Metastatic carcinoma with adenoid features

diastase. The cytoplasm of Paget's disease contains acid mucopolysaccharides, so it is positive with colloidal iron and mucicarmine stains. In addition, antibodies against keratin are positive in Bowen's disease yet negative in Paget's disease; staining for carcinoembryonic antigen is positive in Paget's disease and negative in Bowen's disease [87].

Pagetoid melanoma in situ must also be distinguished. The presence of melanin is not necessarily helpful, as the pagetoid cells of Paget's disease and of pagetoid Bowen's disease may at times contain melanin in their cytoplasm. However, the characteristic nesting at or just above the basal cell layer in melanoma usually provides distinction. In addition, the pagetoid cells of melanoma are PAS negative and DOPA (3,4-dihydroxy-phenylalanine) positive. Melanoma cells are usually S-100 protein positive, unlike Paget's disease or Bowen's disease.

On occasion, tissue peripheral to the clear histologic pattern of Bowen's disease may exhibit intraepidermal nests of malignant-appearing keratinocytes surrounded by normal epidermis, at times suggesting superficial spreading melanoma [87]. However, careful evaluation of the entire specimen distinguishes it from intraepithelial epitheliomas of other types. Table 4.5 lists important considerations in the differential diagnosis.

Immunohistochemistry

In an effort to distinguish the essential characteristics of benign versus malignant lesions and to more effectively predict biological behavior, a number of special stains and techniques have been employed. These technologies are yielding prolific data, both from the reactions of the keratinocytes themselves and from the inflammatory cells that altered keratinocytes presumably stimulate

[64,88–91]. Whether any clinically useful diagnostic stains or observations will ultimately derive from these studies remains to be seen. Probably the most useful staining techniques so far are for the lectins, especially those using peanut lectin [64,89]. The use of flow cytometry to detect aneuploidy as a predictive index of malignant change in Bowen's disease may also prove of value [88].

Etiologic considerations

Whether chemical carcinogens besides arsenic can induce Bowen's disease is unknown. A number of former poison-gas workers in Japan developed Bowen's disease, suggesting that mustard gas may predispose [92]. Because some HPVs may induce Bowen's disease [93,94], the possibility of the patient having the rare inherited disorder called epidermodysplasia verruciformis must be considered [95].

Bowen's disease and internal malignancy

Whether Bowen's disease is a marker for internal malignancy remains an unanswered controversy. The relationship is most convincing for female genital Bowen's disease and when Bowen's disease produced as a result of arsenic-induced carcinogenesis is associated with visceral malignancies [96–99]. Graham's [98] report of at least 38% of women with anogenital Bowen's disease having genitourinary tract cancer makes this site for Bowen's disease one of special concern. An earlier study of 24 women with vulvar Bowen's disease showed 37.5% with visceral cancer, especially SCC of the cervix and upper vagina [69].

Callen and Headington [100] studied 72 patients with Bowen's disease and found the incidence of internal cancer to be 29%. They detected no significant difference in the incidence of internal cancer when the Bowen's disease was maximally or minimally on sun-exposed sites. Most studies have found an incidence of 15% to 30% [69,98,100,101]. Yet other works employing matched populations from registry data have shown no increased incidence of internal cancer with Bowen's disease [98,102]; however, I concur with Callen and Head-

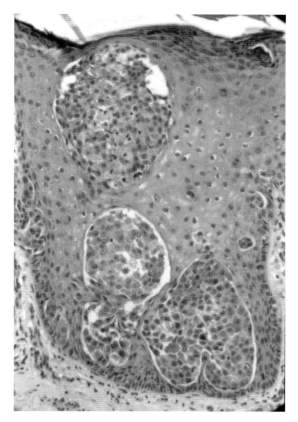

Fig. 4.6 Histologic view of a Borst-Jadassohn tumor showing malignant-appearing cells within an epidermis with its architecture preserved.

ington [100] that such registry studies have inherent flaws.

Internal malignancy, Bowen's disease, SCC, and BCC are all linked through the mutually predisposing mechanism of immunosuppression [103,104]. Thus, it is not surprising that Bowen's disease has been noted in association with lymphoma and myeloma [104,105], though it is not considered a marker for either. Such immunosuppression may occur in patients after renal transplantation or with lymphoma itself [105].

Intraepidermal carcinoma

Intraepidermal collections of malignant-appearing cells within an epidermis where the normal architecture is preserved is a rare phenomenon (Fig. 4.6). In 1904, Borst [106] described this pattern at the border of an ulcerated "ordinary carcinoma of the lip" [107]. In 1922, Jadassohn, in discussing the superficial type of BCC, commented that he had observed intraepidermal BCCs [107]. Thus, the process noted above has been labeled intraepidermal carcinoma of Borst-Jadassohn, or the Borst-Jadassohn tumor, a misnomer [108].

The intraepidermal carcinoma of Borst-Jadassohn is probably best viewed as a heterogeneous collection of both benign and malignant entities, including irritated seborrheic keratoses with squamous eddies simulating SCC, eccrine poromas, hidradenoma simplex, hidradenoma simplex with porocarcinoma, Bowen's disease, and rarely melanoma [109–113]. Clearly, malignant-appearing intraepidermal cell nests may signify a focal dysplastic process (actinic keratoses, thermal keratoses, scar keratoses, chronic radiation keratoses), a malignant metastatic process (melanoma, SCC), or Paget's disease. Rarely, such dysplastic changes may be seen within seborrheic keratoses or an epidermal nevus [114]. However, there is still debate as to whether the Borst-Jadassohn tumor constitutes a distinct entity, because at least some Borst-Jadassohn tumors have a characteristic clinical and histologic pattern [115–117]. Such tumors clinically resemble seborrheic keratoses but are flattened and less polypoid, tending to appear anywhere on the body as a sharply demarcated plaque.

Treatment of premalignant cutaneous dysplasias

Therapeutic options for Bowen's disease include excision, photodynamic therapy, curettage and electrodesiccation, topical 5-fluorouracil (5-FU), topical imiquimod, topical immunotherapy, cryosurgery, and Grenz-ray therapy [45,47,118–123]. If histologic evidence of deep follicular involvement by the in situ carcinoma is present, local destruction may be necessary and modalities such as topical chemotherapy may be ineffective. Locally administered 5-FU has been employed for accessible dysplasias and Bowen's disease since Klein's pioneering work in the 1960s [124]. Topical 5% 5-FU cream may be of value in treating EQ, vulvar and intraoral leukoplakia, bowenoid papulosis, and Bowen's

disease [125,126]. However, at present, topical 5% imiquimod cream is becoming fashionable [44]. There are some special options for vulvar and other dysplasias, including imiquimod [127] and focused ultrasound therapy [128]. The physician must evaluate each in situ SCC individually, basing the choice of modality on location, size, extent, clinical and histologic diagnosis, metastatic potential, and physician and patient experience with the therapeutic technique. These nonsurgical options are covered in detail in Chapter 2, the surgical ones in the chapters devoted to them.

Prevention

Prevention may be the best treatment. HPV quadrivalent recombinant vaccine, a mixture of viruslike particles derived from the L1 capsid proteins of HPV types 6, 11, 16, and 18, is indicated for use in the prevention of cervical cancer, vulvar and vaginal precancer and cancers, precancerous lesions, and genital warts associated with HPV types 6, 11, 16, or 18 infection in adolescents and young women [129]. Results of such efforts are eagerly anticipated.

References

1 Bowen JT. Precancerous dermatoses: a study of two cases of chronic atypical epithelial proliferation. J Cutan Pathol 1912;30:241–55.

2 Bowen JT. Precancerous dermatoses: a sixth case of a type recently described. J Cutan Pathol 1915;33:787–802.

3 Montgomery H. Precancerous dermatosis and epithelioma in situ. Arch Dermatol Syphilol 1939;39:387–408.

4 Watson K, Creamer D. Arsenic-induced keratoses and Bowen's disease. Clin Exp Dermatol 2004;29:46–8.

5 Schwartz RA, Janniger CK. Bowenoid papulosis. J Am Acad Dermatol 1991;24:261–4.

6 Mitsuishi T, Kawashima M, Sata T. Human papillomavirus associated Bowen's disease of the foot: unique clinical features mimicking a common wart. Eur J Dermatol 2001;11:463–5.

7 Sun JD, Barr RJ. Papillated Bowen disease, a distinct variant. Am J Dermatopathol 2006;28:395–8.

8 Blobstein SH, Wolfin NS, Urmacher C, et al. Pagetoid Bowen's disease on the breast. Int J Dermatol 1986;25:381–2.

9 Krishnan R, Lewis A, Orengo IF, et al. Pigmented Bowen's disease (squamous cell carcinoma in situ): a mimic of malignant melanoma. Dermatol Surg 2001;27:673–4.

10 Fisher GB Jr, Greer KE, Walker AN. Bowen's disease mimicking melanoma. Arch Dermatol 1982;118:444–5.

11 Firooz A, Farsi N, Rashighi-Firoozabadi M, et al. Pigmented Bowen's disease of the finger mimicking malignant melanoma. Arch Iran Med 2007;10:225–7.

12 Yoo SS, Viglione M, Moresi M, et al. Unilesional mycosis fungoides mimicking Bowen's disease. J Dermatol 2003;30:417–9.

13 Yoon TY, Kim HJ, Kim JW, et al. Bowen's disease concealed by purpura. J Dermatol 2007;34:65–7.

14 Koch A, Schonlebe J, Haroske G, et al. Polydactylous Bowen's disease. J Eur Acad Dermatol Venereol 2003;17:213–5.

15 Lambiase MC, Gardner TL, Altman CE, et al. Bowen disease of the nail bed presenting as longitudinal melanonychia: detection of human papillomavirus type 56 DNA. Cutis 2003;72:305–9; quiz 296.

16 Usmani N, Stables GI, Telfer NR, et al. Subungual Bowen's disease treated by topical aminolevulinic acid-photodynamic therapy. J Am Acad Dermatol 2005;53:S273–6.

17 Baran R, Perrin C. Bowen's disease clinically simulating an onychomatricoma. J Am Acad Dermatol 2002;47:947–9.

18 Bugatti L, Filosa G, De Angelis R. Dermoscopic observation of Bowen's disease. J Eur Acad Dermatol Venereol 2004;18:572–4.

19 Zalaudek I, Di Stefani A, Argenziano G. The specific dermoscopic criteria of Bowen's disease. J Eur Acad Dermatol Venereol 2006;20:361–2.

20 Marchesa P, Fazio VW, Oliart S, et al. Perianal Bowen's disease: a clinicopathologic study of 47 patients. Dis Colon Rectum 1997;40:1286–93.

21 Burns DA. Bilateral pigmented Bowen's disease of the web-spaces of the feet. Clin Exp Dermatol 1981;6:435–7.

22 Masuda T, Hara H, Shimojima H, et al. Spontaneous complete regression of multiple Bowen's disease in the web-spaces of the feet. Int J Dermatol 2006;45:783–5.

23 Kao GF. Carcinoma arising in Bowen's disease. Arch Dermatol 1986;122:1124–6.

24 Braverman IM. Bowen's disease and internal cancer. JAMA 1991;266:842–3.

25 Mitsuishi T, Sata T, Matsukura T, et al. The presence of mucosal human papillomavirus in Bowen's disease of the hands. Cancer 1997;79:1911–7.

26 James WD, Rodman OG. Squamous cell carcinoma arising in porokeratosis of Mibelli. Internat J Dermatol 1986;25:389–91.

27 Haneke E, Gutschmidt E. Premature multiple Bowen's disease in poikiloderma congenitale with warty hyperkeratoses. Dermatologica 1979;158:384–8.

28 Swint RB, Klaus SN. Malignant degeneration of an epithelial nevus. Arch Dermatol 1970;101:56–8.

29 Masessa JM, Schwartz RA, Lambert WC. Bowenoid papulosis in a penile epidermal inclusion cyst. Br J Dermatol 1987;116:237–9.

30 Queyrat M. Erythroplasie du gland. Soc Dermatol Syphilol 1911;22:378–82.

31 Blau S, Hyman AB. Erythroplasia of Queyrat. J Am Acad Dermatol 1955;35:341–73.

32 Dixon RS, Mikhail GR. Erythroplasia (Queyrat) of conjunctiva. J Am Acad Dermatol 1981;4:160–5.

33 Milstein HG. Erythroplasis of Queyrat in a partially circumcised man. J Am Acad Dermatol 1982;6:398.

34 Graham JH, Helwig EB. Erythroplasia of Queyrat. A clinicopathologic and histochemical study. Cancer 1973;32:1396–414.

35 Raju RR, Goldblum JR, Hart WR. Pagetoid squamous cell carcinoma in situ (pagetoid Bowen's disease) of the external genitalia. Int J Gynecol Pathol 2003;22:127–35.

36 Schulze K, Schwartz RA, Lambert WC. Erythroplasia of Queyrat. Am Family Phys 1984;29:185–6.

37 Zheng S, Adachi A, Shimizu M, et al. Human papillomaviruses of the mucosal type are present in some cases of extragenital Bowen's disease. Br J Dermatol 2005;152:1243–7.

38 Derancourt C, Mougin C, Chopard Lallier M, Coumes-Marquet S, Drobacheff C, Laurent R. Oncogenic human papillomaviruses in extra-genital Bowen disease revealed by in situ hybridization [in French]. Ann Dermatol Venereol 2001;128:715–8.

39 Ueda M, Ashida M, Kunisada M, et al. Bowen's carcinoma of the scrotal skin associated with human papillomavirus type 82. J Eur Acad Dermatol Venereol 2005;19:232–5.

40 Alessi E, Coggi A, Gianotti R. Review of 120 biopsies performed on the balanopreputial sac. From Zoon's balanitis to the concept of a wider spectrum of inflammatory non-cicatricial balanoposthitis. Dermatology 2004;208:120–4.

41 Porter WM, Francis N, Hawkins D, et al. Penile intraepithelial neoplasia: clinical spectrum and treatment of 35 cases. Br J Dermatol 2002;147:1159–65.

42 Toonstra J, van Wichen DF. Immunohistochemical characterization of plasma cells in Zoon's balanoposthitis and (pre)malignant skin lesions. Dermatologica 1986;172:77–81.

43 Avrach WW, Christensen HE. Metastasizing erythroplasia of Queyrat. Acta Derm Venereol 1976;56:409–12.

44 Micali G, Nasca MR, De Pasquale R. Erythroplasia of Queyrat treated with imiquimod 5% cream. J Am Acad Dermatol 2006;55:901–3.

45 Arlette JP. Treatment of Bowen's disease and erythroplasia of Queyrat. Br J Dermatol 2003;149 Suppl 66:43–9.

46 Davis-Daneshfar A, Trueb RM. Bowen's disease of the glans penis (erythroplasia of Queyrat) in plasma cell balanitis. Cutis 2000;65:395–8.

47 Blank AA, Schnyder UW. Soft-X-ray therapy in Bowen's disease and erythroplasia of Queyrat. Dermatologica 1985;171:89–94.

48 Sonnex TS, Ralfs IG, Plaza de Lanza M, et al. Treatment of erythroplasia of Queyrat with liquid nitrogen cryosurgery. Br J Dermatol 1982;106:581–4.

49 Del Losada JP, Ferre A, San Roman B, et al. Erythroplasia of Queyrat with urethral involvement: treatment with carbon dioxide laser vaporization. Dermatol Surg 2005;31:1454–7.

50 Conejo-Mir JS, Munoz MA, Linares M, et al. Carbon dioxide laser treatment of erythroplasia of Queyrat: a revisited treatment to this condition. J Eur Acad Dermatol Venereol 2005;19:643–4.

51 Lee MR, Ryman W. Erythroplasia of Queyrat treated with topical methyl aminolevulinate photodynamic therapy. Australas J Dermatol 2005;46:196–8.

52 Bernstein G, Forgaard DM, Miller JE. Carcinoma in situ of the glans penis and distal urethra. J Dermatol Surg Oncol 1986;12:450–5.

53 Payne TF. Why are white lesions white? Observations on keratin. Oral Surg Oral Med Oral Pathol 1975;40:652–8.

54 Einhorn J, Wersall J. Incidence of oral carcinoma in patients with leukoplakia of the oral mucosa. Cancer 1967;20:2189–93.

55 Shibuya H, Amagasa T, Seto K, et al. Leukoplakia-associated multiple carcinomas in patients with tongue carcinoma. Cancer 1986;57:843–6.

56 Dorey JL, Blasberg B, Conklin RJ, et al. Oral leukoplakia. Current concepts in diagnosis, management, and malignant potential. Int J Dermatol 1984;23:638–42.

57 Pindborg JJ, Reibel J, Roed-Peterson B, et al. Tobacco-induced changes in oral leukoplakic epithelium. Cancer 1980;45:2330–6.

58 Kopf AW, Allyn B, Andrade R, et al. Leukoplakia of the conjunctiva. A complication of x-ray therapy for carcinoma of the eyelid. Arch Dermatol 1966;94:552–7.

59 Feller L, Wood NH, Raubenheimer EJ. Proliferative verrucous leukoplakia and field cancerization: report of a case. J Int Acad Periodontol 2006;8:67–70.

60 Krutchkoff DJ, Cutler L, Laskowski S. Oral lichen planus: the evidence regarding potential malignant transformation. J Oral Pathol 1978;7:1–7.

61 Hart WR, Norris HJ, Helwig EB. Relation of lichen sclerosus et atrophicus of the vulva in development of carcinoma. Obstet Gynecol 1975;45:369–77.

62 Sanchez NP, Mihm MC Jr. Reactive and neoplastic epithelial alterations of the vulva. A classification of the vulvar dystrophies from the dermatopathologist's viewpoint. J Am Acad Dermatol 1982;6:378–88.

63 Kennedy AW, Hart WR. Multiple squamous-cell carcinomas in Fanconi's anemia. Cancer 1982;50:811–4.

64 Hyun K-H, Nakai M, Kawamura K, et al. Histochemical studies of lectin binding in keratinized lesions, including malignancy. Virchows Archiv (Pathol Anat) 1984;402:337–51.

65 Noumoff JS, Farber M. Tumors of the vulva. Internat J Dermatol 1986;25:552–63.

66 Woodruff JD. Carcinoma in situ of the vulva. Clin Obstet Gynecol 1985;28:230–9.

67 Renaud-Vilmer C, Dehen L. Single erythroplastic vulvar lesion in a 70-year-old woman: Bowen disease [in French]. Ann Dermatol Venereol 2001;128:1361–2.

68 McAdams AJ, Kistner RW. The relationship of chronic vulvar disease, leukoplakia, a carcinoma in situ to carcinoma of the vulva. Cancer 1958;11:740–57.

69 Abell MR, Gosling JR. Intraepithelial and infiltrative carcinoma of vulva: Bowen's type. Cancer 1961;14:318–29.

70 Patterson JW, Kao GF, Graham JH, Helwig EB. Bowenoid papulosis: a clinicopathologic study with ultrastructural observations. Cancer 1986;57:823–36.

71 Obalek S, Jablonska S, Beaudenon S. Bowenoid papulosis of the male and female genitalia: risk of cervical neoplasia. J Am Acad Dermatol 1986;14:433–44.

72 Papadopoulos AJ, Schwartz RA, Lefkowitz A, et al. Extragenital bowenoid papulosis associated with atypical human papillomavirus genotypes. J Cutan Med Surg 2002;6:117–21.

73 Rinaggio J, Glick M, Lambert WC. Oral bowenoid papulosis in an HIV-positive male. Oral Surg Oral Med Oral Pathol Oral Radiol Endod 2006;101:328–32.

74 Halasz C, Silvers D, Crum CP. Bowenoid papulosis in three-year-old girl. J Am Acad Dermatol 1986;14:326–30.

75 DeVillez RL, Stevens CS. Bowenoid papules of the genitalia: a case progressing to Bowen's disease. J Am Acad Dermatol 1980;3:149–52.

76 Lookingbill DP, Kreider JW, Howett MK, Olmstead PM, Conner GH. Human papillomavirus type 16 in bowenoid papulosis, intraoral papillomas, and squamous cell carcinoma of the tongue. Arch Dermatol 1987;123:363–8.

77 Hama N, Ohtsuka T, Yamazaki S. Detection of mucosal human papilloma virus DNA in bowenoid papulosis, Bowen's disease and squamous cell carcinoma of the skin. J Dermatol 2006;33:331–7.

78 Yu DS, Kim G, Song HJ, et al. Morphometric assessment of nuclei in Bowen's disease and bowenoid papulosis. Skin Res Technol 2004;10:67–70.

79 Slater DN, Parsons MA, Mudhar H. In-situ squamous cell carcinoma (Bowen's disease) with divergent adnexal differentiation. Histopathology 2003;43:100.

80 Jacobs DM, Sandles LG, Leboit PE. Sebaceous carcinoma arising from Bowen's disease of the vulva. Arch Dermatol 1986;122:1191–3.

81 Ohnishi Y, Murakami S, Ohtsuka H, et al. Merkel cell carcinoma and multiple Bowen's disease: incidental association or possible relationship to inorganic arsenic exposure? J Dermatol 1997;24:310–6.

82 Tsuruta D, Hamada T, Mochida K, et al. Merkel cell carcinoma, Bowen's disease and chronic occupational arsenic poisoning. Br J Dermatol 1998;139:291–4.

83 Miller RA. Podophyllin. Internat J Dermatol 1985;24:491–8.

84 Clemmensen OJ, Sjolin K-E. Malignancy in seborrheic keratoses. Acta Derm Venereol 1986;66:158–61.

85 Brownstein MH, Rabinowitz AD. Precursors of cutaneous squamous cell carcinoma. Int J Dermatol 1979;18:1–16.

86 Shelley WB, Wood MG. Occult Bowen's disease in keratinous cysts. Br J Dermatol 1981;105:105–8.

87 Rosen L, Amazon K, Frank B. Bowen's disease, Paget's disease, and malignant melanoma in situ. South Med J 1986;79:410–3.

88 Newton JA, Camplejohn RS, McGribbon DH. Aneuploidy in Bowen's disease. Br J Dermatol 1986;114:691–4.

89 Ariano MC, Wiley EL, Ariano LH. Peanut lectin receptor, and carcinoembryonic antigen distribution in keratoacanthomas, squamous dysplasias, and carcinomas of skin. J Dermatol Surg Oncol 1985;11:1076–83.

90 Zambruno G, Reano A, Meissner K, et al. GP37 expression in normal and diseased human epidermis: a marker for keratinocyte distribution. Acta Derm Venereol 1986;66:185–92.

91 Morita H, Haneda T, Sagami S. OKT 6-positive cells and lymphocyte subsets within tumors before and after therapy with local injection of interferon-alpha. Acta Dermatol (Kyoto) 1986;81:241–6.

92 Inada S, Hiragun K, Seo K, Yamura T. Multiple Bowen's disease in former workers of a poison gas factory in Japan, with special reference to mustard gas exposure. J Dermatol 1978;5:49–60.

93 Kawashima M, Jablonska S, Favre M, Obalek S, Croissant O, Orth G. Characterization of a new type of human papillomavirus found in a lesion of Bowen's disease of the skin. J Virol 1986;57:688–92.

94 Maeda K, Jimbow K, Fukushima M. Epidermodysplasia verruciformis associated with Bowen's carcinoma, B lymphocytopenia and decreased functions. Dermatologica 1985;171:478–85.

95 Baskan EB, Tunali S, Adim SB, et al. A case of epidermodysplasia verruciformis associated with squamous cell carcinoma and Bowen's disease: a therapeutic challenge. J Dermatolog Treat 2006;17:179–83.

96 Anderson SLC, Nielsen A, Reymann F. Relationship between Bowen disease and internal malignant tumors. Arch Dermatol 1973;108:367–70.

97 Peterka ES, Lynch FW, Goltz RW. An association between Bowen's disease and internal cancer. Arch Dermatol 1961;84:623–9.

98 Graham JH. Selected precancerous skin and mucocutaneous lesions. In: Neoplasms of the skin and malignant melanoma. Chicago: Year Book Medical Publishers; 1976. p. 69–121.

99 Miki Y, Kawatsu T, Matsuda K, Machino H, Kubo K. Cutaneous and pulmonary cancers associated with Bowen's disease. J Am Acad Dermatol 1982;6:26–31.

100 Callen JP, Headington JT. Bowen's disease and non-Bowen's squamous intraepidermal neoplasia of the skin. Arch Dermatol 1980;116:422–6.

101 Epstein E. Association of Bowen's disease with visceral cancer. Arch Dermatol 1960;82:349–51.

102 Hugo NE, Conway H. Bowen's disease: its malignant potential and relationship to systemic cancer. Plastic Reconstruct Surg 1967;39:190–4.

103 Moller R, Nielsen A, Reymann F. Multiple basal cell carcinoma and internal malignant tumors. Arch Dermatol 1975;111:584–5.

104 Schwartz RA, Stoll HL Jr. Epithelial precancerous lesions. In: Fitzpatrick TB, Freedberg IM, Eisen AZ, Austin KF, Wolffe K, editors. Dermatology in general medicine. 3rd ed. New York: McGraw-Hill; 1987. p. 733–48.

105 Kanoh T, Morita T, Horii S, et al. Bowen's disease associated with multiple myeloma. Tohoku J Exper Med 1986;148:403–9.

106 Borst M. Ueber die Moglichkeit einer ausgedehnten intraepidermalen. Verbreitung des Hautkrebses Verh Deutsch Ges Pathol 1904;7:118–23.

107 Mehregan AH, Pinkus H. Intraepidermal epithelioma: a critical study. Cancer 1964;17:609–36.

108 Holubar K, Wolff K. Borst (Jadassohn): a misnomer [author reply]. Dermatology 2004;209:348.

109 Amichai B, Grunwald MH, Halevy S. A seborrheic keratosislike lesion. Intraepidermal epithelioma of Borst-Jadassohn. Arch Dermatol 1995;131:1331, 4.

110 Helm KF, Helm TN, Helm F. Borst-Jadassohn phenomenon associated with an undifferentiated spindle cell neoplasm. Int J Dermatol 1994;33:563–5.

111 Watanabe T, Murakami T, Okochi H, et al. Eccrine poroma associated with Bowen's disease. Int J Dermatol 2004;43:472–3.

112 Stante M, de Giorgi V, Massi D, et al. Pigmented Bowen's disease mimicking cutaneous melanoma: clinical and dermoscopic aspects. Dermatol Surg 2004;30:541–4.

113 Vun Y, De'Ambrosis B, Spelman L, et al. Seborrhoeic keratosis and malignancy: collision tumour or malignant transformation? Australas J Dermatol 2006;47:106–8.

114 Kwittken J. Squamous cell carcinoma arising in seborrheic keratosis. Mt. Sinai J M 1981;48:61–2.

115 Steffen C, Ackerman AB. Intraepidermal epithelioma of Borst-Jadassohn. Am J Dermatopathol 1985;7:5–24.

116 Cook MG, Ridgway HA. The intra-epidermal epithelioma of Jadassohn: a distinct entity. Br J Dermatol 1979;101:659–67.

117 Sampson DD, Kelly AP. Intraepidermal epithelioma of Jadassohn. Cutis 1986;37:339–41.

118 Braathen LR, Szeimies RM, Basset-Seguin N, et al. Guidelines on the use of photodynamic therapy for nonmelanoma skin cancer: an international consensus. International Society for Photodynamic Therapy in Dermatology, 2005. J Am Acad Dermatol 2007;56:125–43.

119 Cox NH, Eedy DJ, Morton CA. Guidelines for management of Bowen's disease: 2006 update. Br J Dermatol 2007;156:11–21.

120 Ko H-C, Oh C-K, Kim S-J, et al. The effects of 5% imiquimod cream on Bowen's disease. Korean J Dermatol 2006;44:1410–6.

121 van Egmond S, Hoedemaker C, Sinclair R. Successful treatment of perianal Bowen's disease with imiquimod. Int J Dermatol 2007;46:318–9.

122 Moreno G, Chia AL, Lim A, et al. Therapeutic options for Bowen's disease. Australas J Dermatol 2007;48:1–8; quiz 9–10.

123 Morton CA. Methyl aminolevulinate: actinic keratoses and Bowen's disease. Dermatol Clin 2007;25:81–7.

124 Klein E, Stoll HL Jr, Milgrom H, et al. Tumors of the skin. XII. Topical 5-fluorouracil for epidermal neoplasms. J Surg Oncol 1971;3:331–49.

125 Bargman H, Hochman J. Topical treatment of Bowen's disease with 5-fluorouracil. J Cutan Med Surg 2003;7:101–5.

126 Graham BD, Jetmore AB, Foote JE, et al. Topical 5-fluorouracil in the management of extensive anal Bowen's disease: a preferred approach. Dis Colon Rectum 2005;48:444–50.

127 Baulon E, Vautravers A, Rodriguez B, Nisand I, Baldauf JJ. Imiquimod and immune response modifiers in gynaecology [in French]. Gynecol Obstet Fertil 2007;35:149–57.

128 Li C, Bian D, Chen W, et al. Focused ultrasound therapy of vulvar dystrophies: a feasibility study. Obstet Gynecol 2004;104:915–21.

129 Siddiqui MA, Perry CM. Human papillomavirus quadrivalent (types 6, 11, 16, 18) recombinant vaccine (Gardasil). Drugs 2006;66:1263–71; discussion 1272–3.

CHAPTER 5
Squamous cell carcinoma

Robert A. Schwartz

Cutaneous squamous cell carcinoma (SCC) is the most common skin cancer in much of the world [1–3]. Although it may occur in any anatomic location on the body, it tends to develop from a predisposing cutaneous dysplasia rather than de novo. The overwhelming majority of cutaneous SCCs evolve within solar (actinic) keratoses and rarely are aggressive. However, de novo SCCs and those that develop from scar keratoses, chronic radiation keratoses, chemical keratoses, or thermal keratoses or on mucosal surfaces have greater malignant potential [4,5]. These invasive SCCs may be biologically aggressive and are prone to recur [6]. In addition, SCC of the scalp in organ transplant recipients should be considered a high-risk tumor [7]. Cutaneous SCC is an important malignant complication of renal transplantation [8].

The SCC is a malignant proliferation of epidermal keratinocytes, the most abundant epidermal cell type. The natural history of SCC may be modified substantially by the patient's immunologic status [9–11]. For example, patients with cutaneous T cell lymphomas on chemotherapy are at increased risk of developing aggressive cutaneous SCCs.

Incidence and etiology

In the United States alone, more than 1 million cases of nonmelanoma skin cancer are anticipated to develop in 2007, with about one fifth of these skin cancers being SCCs [12–14]. The age-adjusted SCC incidence per 100,000 for non-Hispanic whites was 364 in men and 153.5 in women in Arizona in 1996, as compared with a rate in New Hampshire of 97 and 32 and in North Queensland of 1332 and 755, all from that same year [15]. In all of America for 1994, the incidence was 81 and 26 in 100,000. The risk of SCC is principally related to two factors: the amount of sun exposure and the degree of pigmentation. Those at greatest risk are light-complexioned individuals with excessive sun exposure, because SCC is most often sun induced, evolving from actinic keratoses (AKs) in these individuals. In Holland, the annual incidence in the past few decades has been 1.2% in men and 3.4% in women for cutaneous SCC [16]. The mortality rate has increased less rapidly. Of 208 patients with SCC, an AK was contiguous with an SCC in 72%, evidence that the SCC arose in the AK [17]. In Spain, the mean age for SCC was 77.3 years, with photoexposed skin areas accounting for 93.8% of them [18].

The annual age-adjusted incidence for cutaneous SCCs in white men in metropolitan New Orleans was 154 per 100,000 in 1977 to 1978, as opposed to 30 per 100,000 in Detroit [13]. Detroit is situated at a latitude of 42° north, versus 30° for New Orleans, in conformity with the principal that the estimated annual count of ultraviolet (UV) light in its principal carcinogenic range (UV-B) reaching the earth's surface tends to increase with decreasing latitude, producing a higher incidence of sun-induced skin cancers. However, other factors, such as altitude and low annual precipitation, may affect UV-B levels, so Albuquerque, New Mexico, has a higher UV-B index than New Orleans despite being more northerly in latitude. In fact, the incidence of SCC in Albuquerque among so-called Anglos was 180 per 100,000. By way of comparison, the annual age-adjusted rate for nonmelanoma skin cancer among whites was 233 per 100,000 (four fifths of which were basal cell carcinomas [BCCs] and one fifth, SCCs), whereas the corresponding rate for black

Americans was only three per 100,000. An evaluation of the Tumor Registry of Charity Hospital in New Orleans showed 163 black patients with a total of 176 SCCs of the skin between 1948 and 1979 [19]. SCCs were noted to be about 20% more common in this group than BCCs. Strikingly, a mortality of 18% was observed, which was attributed to the fact that these SCCs occurred in chronic scarring processes rather than in AKs. Some advocate that the AK does not transform, convert, or progress into cutaneous SCC but is its earliest clinically recognizable manifestation [20]. I consider the AK to be an SCC grade $\frac{1}{4}$ to 1.

Actinic keratoses can and do occur in blacks, who are sometimes predisposed by hereditary factors, such as a light complexion, or albinism. People of intermediate pigmentation, such as Polynesians and Asians, have an SCC incidence rate between that of light-complexioned whites and that of dark-complexioned blacks [21]. However, one group at very high risk of skin cancer, whether residing in their country or elsewhere, are the Celts, who genetically tend to burn and not tan [22]. Such skin cancer–prone individuals tend to be fair complexioned, have light-colored hair and blue eyes, and tan poorly. Prolonged erythema after UV light exposure may help to identify such individuals.

Cutaneous SCCs are about one third more common in white women than they are in men. For example, among white women in Detroit, the annual age-adjusted incidence per 100,000 for 1977 to 1978 was 11, versus 49 for white women in New Orleans and 63 for those in Albuquerque [13], about one third the incidence for white men in those cities. Overall, men have greater solar exposure than do women owing to differences in clothing usage patterns and leisure activities. Among light-complexioned people, the areas of predilection for SCC vary with sex and correspond to exposed areas. In blacks, SCCs tend to display no preference for sun-exposed areas [19], probably reflecting the lack of importance of solar induction for them.

Chronic immunosuppression predisposes to the development of nonmelanoma skin cancers, both BCCs and SCCs [9,23–26]. Immunosuppression by UV radiation is important; new and existing agents are being developed to protect the skin's immune response [27]. In a recent study [28], 523 white patients were evaluated after renal transplantation, which was found to increase the risk for developing nonmelanoma skin cancer. SCCs predominated over BCCs by a ratio of 2.3 to 1, versus the expected ratio for the general white population of 0.2 to 1. In addition, both types of skin cancers developed at an earlier age in transplant recipients than it did in the general population. SCCs tended to be more aggressive clinically, with a greater chance of exhibiting metastatic behavior. This study confirmed earlier ones. Immunosuppression, UV light, and other carcinogenic stimuli, such as human papillomavirus (HPV) infections, may act synergistically to increase the potential for skin cancers in these patients. HPV-linked digital SCC may be associated with genital–digital spread as a mechanism of tumor genesis [29]. Anorectal SCCs in homosexual men may be associated with HPV infection and immunosuppression [30]. The use of cyclosporine as a chronic immunosuppressive therapy may further favor the tendency to develop nonmelanoma skin cancers [26]. Previous exposure to cutaneous carcinogens and continued exposure after immunosuppressive therapy may be an important predisposing factor, especially in patients who have received long-term photochemotherapy for psoriasis [25]. In immunosuppressed patients, multiple SCCs may appear at once and exhibit an eruptive quality [23,31].

The incidence of SCC increases with age [13,21]. For example, it seems to rise rapidly after the age of 40 in white persons in the United States and New Zealand [13,21]. The prevalence of cutaneous SCC in whites 75 years of age or older in New Zealand was 1228 per 100,000 [21]. BCCs and SCCs seem to be increasing in recent years, the former more than the latter. Cutaneous SCCs on the upper extremities, in particular, seem to be increasing in incidence, although eyelid SCCs and BCCs have been decreasing [13].

In evaluating a cutaneous SCC, one should consider the possible carcinogenic agents involved. Exposure to ionizing radiation or arsenic years earlier may explain a new skin cancer [32,33]. Sometimes the clinical stigmata of arsenic exposure may be present. A lack of histologic evidence of solar elastosis should alert the clinician that the SCC is not

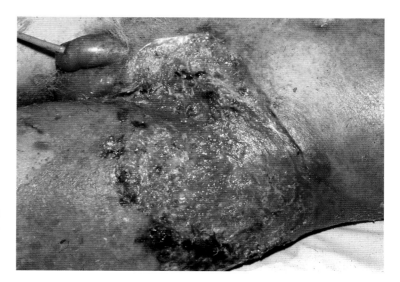

Fig. 5.1 Massive cutaneous squamous cell carcinoma in a psoriatic man with a history of medicinal arsenic intake. (Reprinted with permission from Southwick and Schwartz [33].)

actinically induced (Figs. 5.1, 5.2, and 5.3). Other carcinogenic stimuli include low-energy Grenz irradiation given for psoriasis [34], therapeutically used x-rays [35], and possibly viral oncogenesis, either by itself or combined with inherited or acquired immunosuppression [36]. A combination of potentially carcinogenic stimuli, such as x-rays, chronic scar formation, chemical carcinogens, and UV light, may be at work in the same patient [37]. For example, a person with a congenital hemangioma of the lip that has been treated with x-rays may be exposed to nicotine and sunlight; these factors may

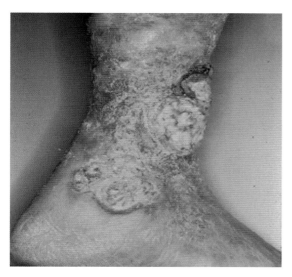

Fig. 5.2 Squamous cell carcinoma developing within a chronic inherited scar process (epidermolysis bullosa dystrophica).

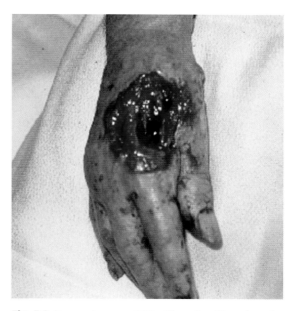

Fig. 5.3 Huge cutaneous SCC with regional lymph node metastases in a dentist who for years exposed his hand to x-rays.

superimpose, with lip SCC ultimately developing. In organ transplant recipients, the level of sun exposure is considered the most important factor in explaining differences in the anatomic site distribution and highlights the importance of sun avoidance in this group [38].

Squamous cell carcinomas may arise in a number of chronic inflammatory or scarring dermatoses, including chronic ulcers, burn scars, chronic osteomyelitis, colocutaneous fistula, hidradenitis suppurativa, epidermolysis bullosa dystrophica, granuloma inguinale, lymphogranuloma venereum, lupus vulgaris (cutaneous tuberculosis) [19, 39–41], lupus erythematosus [42], porokeratoses of various types, lichen sclerosis et atrophicus, and lichen planus [19,43,44]. There is a special name—Marjolin's ulcer—for a rare and often aggressive cutaneous malignancy that arises in a previously traumatized or chronically inflamed skin, particularly after burns [45]. In oil-rich countries, an increasing incidence of petrochemical burns may increase the incidence of Marjolin's ulcer. Other genodermatoses may also predispose to SCC [46]. There are four to six types of porokeratoses, with some intermixing [43]. The rare classic form described by Mibelli presents as a few prominent annular plaques with atrophic centers and an expanding keratinous border [47]. The most common form, disseminated superficial actinic porokeratoses, consists of multiple small superficial papules limited to exposed areas of sun-damaged skin [48]. Within both these types of porokeratoses, SCC may develop. Patients with porokeratoses should probably be instructed to avoid excessive solar exposure, use sunscreens, and be monitored periodically by a dermatologist [48]. I have adopted this approach for my patients with cutaneous lupus erythematosus, lichen sclerosis et atrophicus, and lichen planus. In another type of genodermatosis—congenital ichthyosis—bilateral fungating SCCs were reported [49]. SCC may also arise within an epidermal inclusion cyst [50].

Molecular analyses of solar keratosis, a prototype of early SCC, show that loss of *p16 (INK4a)/p14 (ARF)* and dysfunction of *p53* play a critical role [51]. The SCC precursor cells have minimal but critical genetic alterations, such as cyclin D1 amplification and *p53* mutation, and can be identified using fluorescent in situ hybridization and immunostaining with p53 antibodies. These precursor cells may be defective in repair response to DNA damage and would have proliferative or survival advantages over their normal neighboring counterparts in the presence of growth factor stimulation or genotoxic events, such as UV irradiation. SCCs arising in sun-exposed areas showed less frequent *p53* gene mutations compared with SCCs arising in non–sun-exposed areas [52]. The frequency of loss of heterozygosity on *D5S178* in non–sun-exposed SCC was significantly higher than in sun-exposed SCC. Furthermore, the incidence of fractional allelic loss was markedly elevated in non–sun-exposed SCC than in sun-exposed SCC. These findings suggest that sun-exposed SCC in Japan may be relatively less involved with *p53* mutation and that non–sun-exposed SCC requires more genetic alterations than does sun-exposed SCC.

Matrix metalloproteinase enzymes are involved in degradation of the extracellular matrix, through which tumor cells must penetrate the basement membrane and traverse the extracellular matrix to invade surrounding structures and metastasize to distant sites [53]. Gelatinases, particularly gelatinase A (matrix metalloproteinase-2), demonstrate degradative activity against components of the basement membrane and may be involved in the progression of in situ SCC. The intensity of matrix metalloproteinase-2 staining has been found to correlate with cellular atypia, inflammation, neovascularization, and the invasive tumor front, as well as tumor aggressiveness, and may play a role in the pathogenesis, invasion, and metastasis of cutaneous SCC.

Clinical features

Cutaneous SCC may develop from preexistent cutaneous dysplasias or in situ SCCs, or it may develop de novo. The de novo form, developing in apparently previously unaltered skin, is aggressive [28,54]. SCCs developing in preexistent lesions that are not AKs should be similarly regarded (Figs. 5.1 through 5.3). Most SCCs develop within bowenoid AKs on sun-exposed skin, appearing about 25%

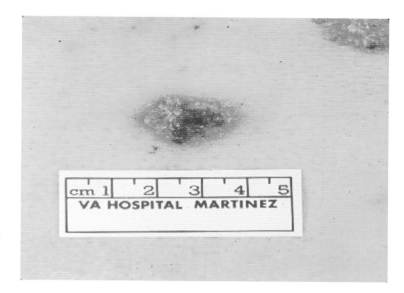

Fig. 5.4 Squamous cell carcinoma on the upper back of an elderly light-complexioned man. Note the erosion of the nodule.

more often than BCCs in the head and neck area. However, over the pinna, the SCC/BCC ratio is 1.3 to 1 [54,55].

When a hyperkeratotic nodule or plaque of Bowen's disease ulcerates, it is an important diagnostic clue to the transition into invasive SCC (Fig. 5.4). The earliest evidence of invasive SCC extending beyond the epidermal basal membrane may actually be the formation of a distinct firm, often erythematous nodule, which may be quite small. The surface may be smooth but often becomes rather verrucous and at times may be so protuberant as to resemble a horn of an animal (and thus be called a cutaneous horn; Fig. 5.5). The cutaneous SCC lacks the cutaneous telangiecta and the translucency seen in the BCC, allowing distinction.

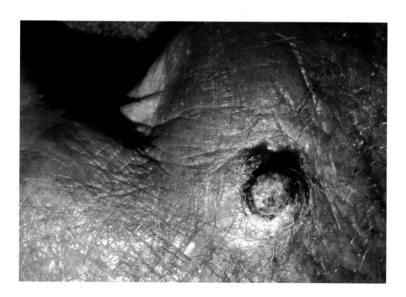

Fig. 5.5 Squamous cell carcinoma on the back of a hand demonstrating a slow-growing hyperkeratotic nodule resembling a keratoacanthoma.

Occasionally, it may appear as a large dermatitis-like plaque with a raised border, resembling persistent tinea corporis [56].

Clinical behavior

The natural history of an invasive SCC is variable, with its mode of induction perhaps the most important biologic clue. Although the invasive SCC developing within an AK of a nonimmunologically compromised light-complexioned man is usually not aggressive, some SCCs exhibit progressive growth in all directions, including downward into soft tissue and bone. SCCs arising on mucosal membranes are especially likely to be locally invasive and to metastasize [57]. Every SCC should be viewed as potentially aggressive and treated accordingly. Cutaneous SCC behavior may correlate best with the level of dermal invasion and the vertical tumor thickness [4]. Deeper lesions tend to recur and then metastasize to regional lymph nodes, even if they have been associated with actinic skin changes [58]. Cutaneous SCC may become clinically aggressive during treatment with prolonged administration of rituximab [59].

One series of 7000 patients with cutaneous SCC noted that 2% manifested metastatic disease at time of diagnosis [60]. This California Tumor Registry survey noted that regional lymph nodes were the most likely site of spread, but distant viscera were involved in 5% to 10% of patients with metastatic cutaneous SCC. Another study of 3700 SCCs in a dermatopathology practice showed that 0.1% metastasized [61]. In this study, the vast majority of sun-induced cutaneous SCCs were found to be only locally aggressive; metastases appeared related to antecedent lesions, such as burns, chronic scars, chronic ulcers, arsenical keratoses, or x-ray injury. A survey of 31 cases of SCC arising within scars found an average time of 23 years from injury to diagnosis. The 3-year survival rate was 94% for patients with histologically well-differentiated scar SCCs versus 38% for those with poorly differentiated scar SCCs, which were more likely to metastasize [62].

Tumor spread may occur in many ways. Invasion of trigeminal and facial perineural spaces is a recognized complication of cutaneous SCC. Centripetal spread along the trigeminal nerve axis and into the cavernous sinus and the gasserian ganglion is rare [63]. Fine-needle aspiration biopsy is an excellent noninvasive diagnostic tool for evaluating possible SCC metastases within a salivary gland [64]. Renal transplant recipients need extra vigilance, as unusual complications, such as ileal obstruction as a consequence of cutaneous SCC metastases to the small intestine, may occur [8].

Based on the malignant potential of SCC variants, one can separate SCC into categories of low ($\leq$2% metastatic rate), intermediate (3% to 10%), high (>10%), and indeterminate behavior [65,66]. Low-risk SCCs include SCC arising in AK, HPV-associated SCC, trichilemmal carcinoma, and spindle cell SCC unassociated with radiation. Intermediate-risk SCCs include adenoid (acantholytic) SCC, intraepidermal epithelioma with invasion, and lymphoepithelioma-like carcinoma of the skin. High-risk subtypes include de novo SCC, SCC arising in association with predisposing factors (radiation, burn scars, and immunosuppression), invasive Bowen's disease, adenosquamous carcinoma, and malignant proliferating pilar tumors. The indeterminate category includes signet-ring cell SCC, follicular SCC, papillary SCC, SCC arising in adnexal cysts, squamoid eccrine ductal carcinoma, and clear-cell SCC.

Recurrent disease and metastasis are more likely with deeply invasive SCCs, even those associated with actinic skin changes [58]. Years ago, Mohs and Lathrop [67] meticulously traced the local tendencies of both SCCs and BCCs. They observed lateral spread along periosteum and perichondrium, followed by invasion into bone or cartilage, as well as deep spread along embryonic fusion lines on the face. Metastatic disease from facial SCCs, as well as BCCs, may appear long after these apparently have been successfully treated and may become evident as a trigeminal or facial neuropathy arising from perineural metastases. A high level of suspicion for perineural invasion should be maintained, even if there is no sequential evidence on magnetic resonance imaging [68]. Perineural invasion of the facial nerve by a cutaneous SCC may result in a slowly progressive facial paralysis [69]. This diagnosis may be suspected when signs and symptoms are initially confined to superficial nerve branches and later extend to more central ones.

Humoral hypercalcemia of malignancy, hypercalcemia secondary to the production of humoral factors by malignant cells in patients without bone metastases, has been documented to occur in association with advanced primary cutaneous SCC [33,70]. This rare but important paraneoplastic complication needs to be promptly recognized and treated. Parathyroid hormone–related protein levels provide high diagnostic sensitivity, seem to reflect tumor bulk, and may also be useful in monitoring response to treatment or tumor progression in these patients.

Unusual possible squamous cell carcinoma variants

Lymphoepithelioma-like carcinoma of the skin is a rare cutaneous neoplasm with histologic features resembling lymphoepitheliomatous tumors of the nasopharynx [71–73]. It may appear as a non-specific slow-growing nodule on the forehead or back that may metastasize to lymph nodes. Differential diagnoses include SCC, adnexal carcinoma, Merkel cell carcinoma, lymphomas, and cutaneous metastatic disease. An association of lymphoepitheliomas with Epstein-Barr virus (EBV) has been observed. Histologically, the entire dermis is occupied by lobules composed of atypical epithelial cells with a moderate amount of eosinophilic cytoplasm and vesicular nuclei with prominent nucleoli. A heavy lymphoplasmacytic infiltrate is usually evident. No dysplasia is noted in the epidermis. Immunohistochemical examination shows the epithelial tumor cells positive for cytokeratin and epithelial membrane antigen. In situ hybridization investigations for the presence of EBV-encoded RNA have yielded negative results. No EBV genomic sequences were detected by in situ hybridization in one study, a result that may help in its distinction from metastatic lymphoepitheliomatous nasopharyngeal carcinoma.

Cutaneous carcinosarcoma tends to be seen on the head and neck region of older individuals [74,75]. It tends to occur on sun-damaged skin as a keratotic papule of short duration. Microscopi-cally, the more common carcinoma part is an SCC followed by BCC, whereas the most frequent sarcoma section is an osteosarcoma or a malignant mesenchymal tumor that is most consistent with malignant fibrous histiocytoma [76]. The epithelial component exhibits a positive immunohistochemical reaction to cytokeratin and a negative one to vimentin, whereas the mesenchymal area shows a positive immunohistochemical reaction to vimentin and a negative one to cytokeratin.

Verrucous carcinoma

Verrucous carcinoma (VC) of the skin is an unusual variety of low-grade SCC that clinically appears as a slowly enlarging warty mass that is both exophytic and endophytic, extending deeply locally [77–81] (Figs. 5.6 and 5.7). Histologically, it is well-differentiated SCC that displays local invasion and little if any dysplasia [82]. VC has certain characteristic sites of predilection, such as the dorsum of the foot, where it was named epithelioma cuniculatum because of its resemblance histologically to multiple crypts of a rabbit burrow. The condylomata acuminatum–like carcinoma of the penis described by Buschke and Löwenstein in 1925 [83] was a VC (Fig. 5.8). It also occurs perianally and on the vagina and may rarely be seen anywhere on the body, including the face, scalp, buttocks, palms, or fingers [84–91]. Other names for VC employed include papillomatosis cutis carcinoides, papillomatosis cutis, and Ackerman tumor (VC of the oral cavity).

This tumor occurs predominately in middle-aged men, although it may be seen in both sexes and in a wide age range (23 to 85 years). Etiologically, it is most likely related to an HPV infection and may also be associated with chemical carcinogens or cocarcinogens [82,85,92]. VC may develop at the site of longstanding cutaneous scars. It may occur at the site of a leg amputation stump scar [93] (Fig. 5.6). Clinically, this tumor may become quite bulky, as it enlarges with extensive compression of underlying tissues. It may be evident as giant plantar horns [94]. It may become a large foul-smelling tumor with the consistency of an overripe orange. Eventually, it will penetrate underlying bone. It may rarely appear as a large pedunculated tumor [95]. Metastases of this well-differentiated cancer are rare, although

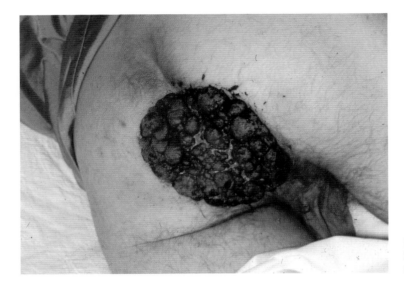

Fig. 5.6 Perianal verrucous carcinoma in an elderly man. (Reprinted from Schwartz et al. [79].)

in longstanding or irradiated tumors, spread to the regional lymph nodes has occurred [96,97].

Scrotal squamous cell carcinoma

Cutaneous SCC may appear verrucous at times, especially on the scrotum. In fact, scrotal SCC was the first occupationally related cancer described, when in 1775 Sir Percivall Pott [98] noted:

[T]here is a disease as peculiar to a certain set of people which has not, at least to my knowledge, been publicly noticed; I mean the chimney-sweepers' cancer.

It is a disease which always makes its first attack on, and its first appearance in the inferior part of the scrotum; where it produces a superficial, painful, ragged, ill-looking sore, with hard and rising edges. The trade call it the soot-wart... [I]n no great length of time, it pervades the skin, dartos, and the membranes of the scrotum, and seizes the testicle, which it inlarges, hardens and renders truly and thoroughly distempered... [T]he fate of these people seems singularly hard; in their infancy, they are frequently treated

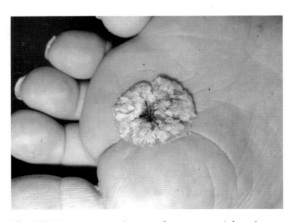

Fig. 5.7 Verrucous carcinoma of many years' duration on the sole of a foot.

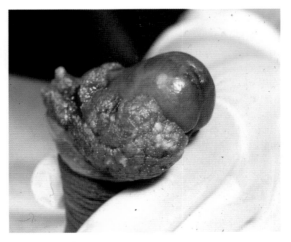

Fig. 5.8 Penile SCC.

Table 5.1 Scrotal squamous cell carcinoma

Described in 1775 as soot-wart by Sir Percivall Pott
Carcinogen said to be tar (arsenic possible)
Occurs in mule spinners (cotton workers)
Starts as wartlike lesion; may metastasize and kill

with great brutality; and almost starved with cold and hunger; they are thrust up narrow, and sometimes hot chimnies, where they are bruised, burned, and almost suffocated; and when they get to puberty, become peculiarly liable to a most noisome, painful, and fatal disease.

Fortunately, children today are not forced to work in chimneys. Nevertheless, scrotal and vulvar SCC persists as an occupational hazard in paraffin and tar workers, shale oil workers, and cotton textile workers, in whom it is called mule-spinners' disease [99–101]. This colorful name derives from the oiled turning axle of the cotton-spinning machine (the "mule"), which the employee straddles. The mineral oil, which lubricates the axle, soaks the workers pants and genitalia, adhering to the scrotal or vulvar rugae. Clinically, a wartlike lesion develops and may be removed and disregarded; 1 or 2 years later, lymph node metastases may appear. As with chimney-sweeps' cancer, the exact carcinogen(s) is (are) not known.

Probably the best description of mule-spinners' cancer is the original one in 1922, in which 141 cases of scrotal cancer in the Manchester (England) Royal Infirmary were described, 69 of which were in mule spinners [99]. This and other descriptions emphasized the potential for regional lymph node metastases [99,100]. Psoriatic patients may develop scrotal SCC as a result of coal tar therapy on the scrotum [101]. Clearly, a verrucous nodule of the scrotum or vulva is not always benign; biopsy may be indicated, especially if there is a history of possible exposure to carcinogens. Some highlights of scrotal SCC are summarized in Table 5.1.

Vulvar squamous cell carcinoma

As mentioned above, mule-spinners' cancer occurs on the scrotum and its counterpart, the vulva. More commonly, however, vulvar SCC occurs in women in their 60s and 70s, with an average age of 62 years. Because in situ changes have been observed in women in their 20s and 30s, this implies a latent period of 30 to 35 years between in situ and invasive changes or that these in situ changes are unrelated in vulvar SCC [102,103]. Vulvar SCC is a serious malignancy, with 5-year disease-specific survival rates after appropriate surgical therapy of 100%, 100%, 86%, and 29% for stages I through IV, respectively [104]. Besides systemic metastases, cutaneous ones may occur as well [105].

Vulvar SCC tends to appear as a nodule or erosion on the background of erythroplasia. Leukoplakia may be present but is less significant as a sign of malignancy. The patient often complains of vulvar pruritus; local bleeding and discomfort are common. Vulvar SCC may also be seen in Fanconi syndrome [106]. VC may also occur on the vulva [82] (*vide supra*, VC). A series of 48 excised thin invasive vulvar SCCs 5 mm or less in tumor thickness in 44 patients were studied to determine the interrelationships of tumor type and adjacent vulvar intraepithelial neoplasia and lichen sclerosus [107]. Vulvar intraepithelial neoplasia is the most likely precursor of conventional keratinizing SCC, the most common type of vulvar invasive carcinoma.

Lip squamous cell carcinoma

The lower lip is the principal mucosal site of solar exposure [108]. As such, it is the most dangerous spot for a sun-induced SCC. Upper lip SCC is a different disease than lower lip SCC, with a different epidemiology [109]. In this section, lip cancer refers to that of the lower lip. Light-complexioned men have the most risk, which rises with increasing age. Women tend to be less affected by lip SCC because they have less solar exposure and tend to use lipstick, which serves as a sun block. Smoking has been implicated as a risk factor in lip SCC, and recurrent lip herpetic infections may also have a role [109]. In fisherman, in the days when tar was used to prevent ropes from rotting, lip SCC may have been associated with tar as well as solar exposure [110].

Actinically induced lip SCC begins as a roughened papule (actinic cheilitis, i.e., AK of the lip) (Fig. 5.9), which is discussed in Chapter 2. Lip SCC may

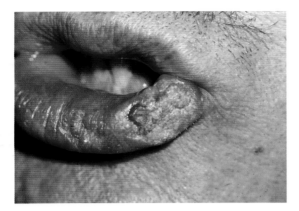

Fig. 5.9 Lip SCC in an elderly light-complexioned man.

also evolve within chronic scarring or inflammatory processes such as discoid lupus erythematosus [111]. Beginning as roughened papules or plaques, they may progress to large fungating tumors, or their evolution into invasive SCC may be subtle. Clinical clues include a generalized variegated, red and white, blotchy vermilion lip; a dry atrophic-appearing vermilion lip with focal areas of leukoplasia; persistent chapping with localized flaking and crusting; and an indistinct or wandering vermilion lip border [112].

A skin biopsy specimen is mandatory to evaluate lip SCC. Prognostic factors in lip SCC include a number of histologic parameters [57]. Thicker tumors are more likely to be metastatic. Metastases occurred in 74% of lip SCCs measuring 6 mm or more in thickness, in 60% with perineural invasion, and in 92% with a Broders grade 4 (extremely poorly differentiated) pattern. The histologic patterns were best evaluated in the deeper portions of the biopsy specimen. The inflammatory infiltrate was not found to be of prognostic importance [57,113]. These microscopic parameters may be useful in deciding to do a prophylactic regional lymph node dissection.

Identifying lip SCCs in their early stages is paramount, because they can be cured easily [108,114]. However, once metastatic disease has occurred, the prognosis is not good. Metastases tend to appear first in the regional lymph nodes, usually in ipsilateral submandibular or submental nodes [57]. Metastatic disease in younger patients appears to portend a worse prognosis than in older ones. A study of lip SCC patients from Texas under the age of 40 years showed a 5-year mortality rate from metastatic disease of 21% [115]. Although this younger group constituted only 7% of a series of 1308 lip SCC patients, it showed a higher incidence of neck node metastases and late recurrences and a higher mortality rate than those seen in elderly patients with lip cancer. In a more recent study of 223 patients, local recurrence occurred in 10.8% whereas regional metastases developed in 4.5%, with a mortality rate from lip SCC of only 2.2% [108]. Neck lymph node metastases were detected at presentation in 26.5% of patients, mandating neck dissection.

The differential diagnosis of lip SCC includes factitious lip crusting [116], malignant salivary gland tumors [117], plasma cell orificial mucositis [118,119], and congenital arterial malformations of the lip [120].

Penile squamous cell carcinoma

Penile SCC has high malignant potential and at times requires distinction from verrucous penile carcinoma [121]. Penile SCC is a major problem in much of the world, responsible for up to 20% of cancers in men [122]. Yet it accounts for only about 1% of all cancers in American and European men. Penile SCC usually appears on the glans. Men circumcised early in life rarely get penile SCC [123]. Interestingly, a series of 15 patients with post-circumcision penile SCC was documented in a certain part of Saudi Arabia where aggressive circumcision performed by laymen was practiced [124]. In each case, the SCC had arisen in the circumcision scar; hence, these penile cancers were really a form of scar carcinoma. Two patients with penile SCC cured with interstitial radiation subsequently developed radiation-induced penile SCCs about 20 years later [125]. In general, lack of circumcision, poor genital hygiene, phimosis, and chronic inflammatory processes may predispose to penile SCC.

Penile SCC tends to first appear as an indurated plaque but later may become fungating (Fig. 5.8). Often there is evidence of a preexistent chronic inflammatory process, such as lichen sclerosis et atrophicus or an in situ plaque of erythroplasia of Queyrat or leukoplakia [44]. Although one study

Table 5.2 Penile squamous cell carcinoma

Up to 20% of male cancer worldwide, but only 1% in US
Clinically, usually an eroded plaque
Lichen sclerosus et atrophicus may predispose

showed adjacent leukoplakia in 17% of penile SCC [126], it is more likely simply coexistent with SCC rather than a precursor. VC may appear on the penis as a slowly growing locally destructive mass. It is also called the giant condylomata of Buschke and Löwenstein [82,85,88,127] (*vide supra*, VC). Major features of penile SCC are listed in Table 5.2. Humoral hypercalcemia of malignancy may also occur in association with advanced primary penile SCC [128].

Histology of cutaneous squamous cell carcinoma

An invasive cutaneous SCC is by definition a proliferation of malignant keratinocytes beyond the basement membrane of the epidermis. In 1932, Broders introduced the concept of grading carcinoma to correlate with tumor biologic behavior [129]. He noted that BCCs, with low metastatic potential, have only slight dedifferentiation. Morphologically, these would have to differentiate only to a small extent to be normal basal cells again. However, SCCs undergo a much wider range of differentiation, which we grade from 1 to 4. In grade 1, the proportion of differentiated cells ranges from almost 100% down to 75%; in grade 2 carcinoma, differentiated cells range from 75% to 50%; in grade 3, 50% to 25%; and in grade 4, 25% to 0%.

Grade 1 SCC often exhibits horn pearls within the mass of invading malignant squamous cells and intercellular bridges between keratinocytes—two indications of differentiation often hard to find in grade 4 SCCs. Grade 4 lesions may be so dedifferentiated as to appear as spindle cells and thus may be difficult to distinguish from melanoma or fibrosarcoma. Electron microscopy or special histochemical stains help distinguish these entities. Keratin antibodies and other keratinocyte antigen markers may be useful to show that the spindle SCC is not a fibrosarcoma or a melanoma. Within the differen-

tial diagnoses of desmoplastic melanoma, atypical fibroxanthoma, dermatofibrosarcoma protuberans, and leiomyosarcoma, p63 appears relatively specific to spindle SCC [76,130]. In addition, the cytokeratins MNF116 and CK34βE12 may be more useful than standard cytokeratins in labeling spindle cell SCC. Spindle cell morphology was found to be more common in transplant SCCs [131]. Fortunately, grade 4 SCCs are rare in the skin.

Posttransplantation SCCs commonly show verrucous and epidermal cystlike features mimicking benign conditions. The younger age of these patients, the frequent absence of solar elastosis, and the infrequent occurrence of well-differentiated verrucacystic SCC in the nontransplant population suggest a different pathogenesis and the need to evaluate small biopsy specimens from transplant recipients with particular care [132].

The microscopic thickness of the cutaneous SCC and its level of invasion are important prognostic factors [4,57]. Sometimes cutaneous SCC displays an adenoid pattern, with a definite wall of cohesive wells about areas of acantholysis and dyskeratosis [133,134]. The prognostic significance of the adenoid SCC is unknown, although some of these uncommon tumors will metastasize [133]. Rarely, acantholysis may be so extreme that, histologically, the SCC mimics a vascular tumor [135]. These pseudovascular SCCs show a higher degree of recurrence and metastasis than other variants of SCC. Adenosquamous SCC is a distinct and aggressive SCC variant with two components: conventional SCC merging with adenocarcinoma [136]. One should reserve this term carefully to avoid confusing it with SCCs having a better prognosis, such as mucoepidermoid carcinomas and acantholytic SCCs. In such circumstances, a metastatic origin must always be excluded. Spindle cell SCC associated with radiation seems to behave rather aggressively and tends to be seen in x-ray induced SCCs [137]. Clear cell SCCs and their in situ counterparts appear mainly on sun-exposed skin, most commonly on the face, followed by the upper extremity in men and the lower extremity in women [138]. There was no gender difference identified in overall frequency or age of onset. They may mimic sebaceous carcinomas [139]. It is believed that the clear cells result from hydropic degeneration.

Histologic features of HPV infection are overrepresented in transplant SCCs [131]. Features that were significantly more common in a large series of organ transplant recipients were acantholytic changes, early dermal invasion, an infiltrative growth pattern with or without desmoplasia, and Bowen's disease with carcinoma [140]. Sometimes one sees keratoacanthoma-like SCC [141].

Squamous cell carcinoma arising from the wall of hair follicles shows SCC developing in the upper part of hair follicles with or without focal involvement of the overlying epidermis at the border with the involved follicle [142]. Immunohistochemically, tumors were positive for cytokeratin and negative for a battery of immunomarkers, including antibodies against the most common carcinogenic HPVs of the skin. Most tumors were removed by simple excision.

An unusual type of well-differentiated SCC is the VC. Histologically, the tumor shows well-differentiated blunt projections extending into the dermis. Centripetal keratinization is seen at times, but not horn pearls. Individual tumor keratinocytes may be very large and have big nuclei with prominent nucleoli. Intracytoplasmic glycogen is scant in comparison with that seen in keratoacanthomas and pseudoepitheliomatous hyperplasia [82,85]. The stratum granulosum may show the characteristic changes of viral warts.

Other parameters have been studied in an effort to better understand the biology of SCC and differentiate it from other tumors. Elevated levels of prostaglandins were found in SCCs [143]. The reactive infiltrates around cutaneous SCCs display a different pattern than that around the BCC [144]. Involutin, a protein precursor of the cross-linked envelope of stratified squamous cells, may serve as a marker for preterminal squamous differentiation and be used to distinguish SCCs from keratoacanthomas [145]. Lectin staining may also hold promise [146].

The differential diagnosis of cutaneous SCC includes a number of tumors and granulomatous reactions. Among tumors, one must consider benign appendageal tumors and their malignant counterparts, atypical fibroxanthoma, epithelioid sarcoma, Merkel cell carcinoma, metastatic carcinomas, fibrosarcomas, and melanomas. Metastases from SCC, eccrine carcinoma, transitional cell carcinoma, and melanoma may simulate primary cutaneous SCC [147,148]. Granulomatous processes with overlying pseudocarcinomatous hyperplasia simulating SCC include tuberculosis, syphilis, coccidioidomycosis and other deep fungal infections, halogenoderma, leishmaniasis, and granuloma inguinale [149]. Tumors with substantial SCC-like reactions overlying them include dermatofibromas, granular cell myoblastomas, and necrotizing sialometaplasia. Necrotizing sialometaplasia is important as it is easily misdiagnosed as SCC, both clinically and histologically. Clinically it may appear as an oral ulcer; histologically it shows extensive squamous metaplasia of the salivary glands [150,151].

Lymphatic mapping and sentinel lymph node biopsy have been suggested for appropriate cutaneous SCCs in the head and neck region [152,153]. New studies are needed to focus on refinements of technique and validation of accuracy as well as biologic correlates for the prediction of metastases.

Treatment

There are a number of treatment modalities available for cutaneous SCCs. The goal is to eradicate the cancer with minimal disability and dysfunction for the patient. Each of the standard methods is effective because the SCC characteristically grows in a continuous cellular structure, enlarging by peripheral extension of narrow cellular strands rather than by uniform advancement of an entire tumor border. The four principal therapeutic options are excisional surgery, cryosurgery, curettage and electrodesiccation, and radiotherapy. Each of these techniques cures the SCC if it encompasses the entire tumor. Local destruction may be supplemented by topical 5-fluorouracil or topical imiquimod. I favor imiquimod 5% cream once daily for up to 10 to 14 weeks as a desirable option, after use of curettage and electrodessication or curettage alone. For candidates unsuitable for destructive techniques, this 5% cream may used by itself, applied once daily for 12 to 16 weeks [154,155].

The physician must evaluate each SCC individually, basing the choice of modality on location, size, extent, clinical and histologic features, metastatic potential, and physician and patient experience with the therapeutic technique. Mohs micrographic surgery has become an important method of surgical excision for selected SCCs. Sentinel lymph node biopsy for high-risk cutaneous SCC is an option whose value requires further evaluation [156]. Surgery with adjuvant radiotherapy may be beneficial for metastatic SCCs [157]. Patients with a poor prognosis should be considered for adjuvant therapy trials [158]. Patients with invasive SCCs metastatic to regional nodes are at high risk for recurrence and death. Regional metastases are often treated with comprehensive nodal dissection, sometimes followed by radiation and/or chemotherapy [159]. Systemic chemotherapy may also be useful for cutaneous and penile SCC [160]. At times, prophylactic radiotherapy of regional lymph nodes may be employed in menacing scar SCCs of high histologic grade. The role of adjuvant radiotherapy in the treatment of cutaneous SCC with perineural invasion requires additional analysis [161].

Verrucous carcinomas are approached in a manner similar to that for other SCCs [77]. Destructive methods tend to be preferred. Mohs surgery is a good modality [162]. Photodynamic therapy may be employed for extensive VCs [163]. There are no standard therapeutic guidelines as to the best treatment strategy according to different stages, including efficacy of conservative nonsurgical modalities and indications for lymph node dissection. However, for VC, radiotherapy is controversial and probably contraindicated because of the risk of its transformation into an aggressive SCC [77,164,165]. Extensive cutaneous VC may be treated successfully with systemic acitretin [166]. Topical imiquimod is also an option [167]. Intra-arterial infusion chemotherapy is a simple and effective method successfully employed with methotrexate for thumb subungual VC [168].

Prevention

Regular users of nonsteroidal anti-inflammatory agents appear to have lower risks of SCC and lower counts of AKs than do nonusers [169]. Although optimal dosing and indications for initiation of systemic retinoid therapy are not conclusive, retinoids may be effective in patients with multiple previous nonmelanoma skin cancers in the transplant population [170]. Retinoids should be initiated at a low dosage and increased as tolerated to a minimally effective dosage. However, more data are needed for both nonsteroidal anti-inflammatory agents and retinoids.

References

1 Zamanian A, Farshchian M, Meheralian A. A 10-year study of squamous cell carcinoma in Hamedan in the west of Iran (1993–2002). Int J Dermatol 2006;45:37–9.

2 Katalinic A, Kunze U, Schafer T. Epidemiology of cutaneous melanoma and non-melanoma skin cancer in Schleswig-Holstein, Germany: incidence, clinical subtypes, tumour stages and localization (epidemiology of skin cancer). Br J Dermatol 2003;149:1200–6.

3 Schwartz RA, Stoll HL Jr. Squamous cell carcinoma. In: Freedburg IM, Eisen AZ, Wolff K, Austen KF, Goldsmith LA, Katz SI, Fitzpatrick TB, editors. Fitzpatrick's dermatology in general medicine. 5th ed. New York: McGraw-Hill; 1999. p. 840–56.

4 Friedman HI, Cooper PH, Wanebo HJ. Prognostic and therapeutic use of microstaging of cutaneous squamous cell carcinoma of the trunk and extremities. Cancer 1985;56:1099–105.

5 Rudolph CM, Soyer HP, Wolf P, Kerl H. Squamous epithelial carcinoma in erythema ab igne [in German]. Hautarzt 2000;51:260–3.

6 Mullen JT, Feng L, Xing Y, et al. Invasive squamous cell carcinoma of the skin: defining a high-risk group. Ann Surg Oncol 2006;13:902–9.

7 Cooper JZ, Brown MD. Special concern about squamous cell carcinoma of the scalp in organ transplant recipients. Arch Dermatol 2006;142:755–8.

8 Abraham KA, Keeling A, McGreal G, et al. Cutaneous squamous carcinoma leading to acute abdomen after renal transplantation. J Nephrol 2002;15:589–92.

9 Abel EA, Sendagorta E, Hoppe RT. Cutaneous malignancies and metastatic squamous cell carcinoma following topical therapies for mycosis fungoides. J Am Acad Dermatol 1986;14:1029–38.

10 Pamuk GE, Turgut B, Vural O, et al. Metastatic squamous cell carcinoma of the skin in chronic myeloid leukaemia: complication of hydroxyurea therapy. Clin Lab Haematol 2003;25:329–31.

11 Agnew KL, Ruchlemer R, Catovsky D, et al. Cutaneous findings in chronic lymphocytic leukaemia. Br J Dermatol 2004;150:1129–35.

12 Jemal A, Siegel R, Ward E, et al. Cancer statistics, 2007. CA Cancer J Clin 2007;57:43–66.

13 Scotto J, Fears TR, Fraumeni J Jr. Incidence of nonmelanoma skin cancer in the United States. National Institutes of Health Publication No 83-2433; 1983.

14 Jemal A, Siegel R, Ward E, et al. Cancer statistics, 2006. CA Cancer J Clin 2006;56:106–30.

15 Harris RB, Griffith K, Moon TE. Trends in the incidence of nonmelanoma skin cancers in southeastern Arizona, 1985–1996. J Am Acad Dermatol 2001;45:528–36.

16 de Vries E, Coebergh JW, van der Rhee H. Trends, causes, approach and consequences related to the skin-cancer epidemic in the Netherlands and Europe [in Dutch]. Ned Tijdschr Geneeskd 2006;150:1108–15.

17 Czarnecki D, Meehan CJ, Bruce F, et al. The majority of cutaneous squamous cell carcinomas arise in actinic keratoses. J Cutan Med Surg 2002;6:207–9.

18 Revenga Arranz F, Paricio Rubio JF, Mar Vazquez Salvado M, et al. Descriptive epidemiology of basal cell carcinoma and cutaneous squamous cell carcinoma in Soria (north-eastern Spain) 1998–2000: a hospital-based survey. J Eur Acad Dermatol Venereol 2004;18:137–41.

19 Mora RG, Perniciaro C. Cancer of the skin in blacks. I. A review of 163 black patients with cutaneous squamous cell carcinoma. J Am Acad Dermatol 1981;5:535–43.

20 Lober BA, Lober CW. Actinic keratosis is squamous cell carcinoma. South Med J 2000;93:650–5.

21 Freeman NR, Fairbrother GE, Rose RJ. Survey of skin cancer incidence in the Hamilton area. New Zealand Med J 1982;95:529–33.

22 Tannenbaum L, Parrish JA, Haynes HA. Prolonged ultraviolet light-induced erythema and the cutaneous carcinoma syndrome. J Invest Dermatol 1976;67:513–7.

23 Kahn JR, Chalet MD, Lowe NJ. Eruptive squamous cell carcinoma following psoralen-UVA phototoxicity. Clin Exper Dermatol 1986;11:398–402.

24 Gupta AK, Cardella CJ, Haberman HF. Cutaneous malignant neoplasms in patients with renal transplants. Arch Dermatol 1986;122:1288–93.

25 Tanew A, Honigsmann H, Ortel B, et al. Non-melanoma skin tumors in long-term photochemotherapy treatment of psoriasis. An 8-year follow-up study. J Am Acad Dermatol 1986;15:960–5.

26 Bencini PL, Montagnino G, Sala F, De Vecchi A, Crosti C, Tarantino A. Cutaneous lesions in 67 cyclosporin-treated renal transplant recipients. Dermatologica 1986;172:24–30.

27 Aboutalebi S, Strickland FM. Immune protection, natural products, and skin cancer: is there anything new under the sun? J Drugs Dermatol 2006;5:512–7.

28 Schwartz RA, Klein E. Ultraviolet light-induced carcinogenesis. In: Holland JF, Frei E 3rd, editors. Cancer medicine. 2nd ed. Philadelphia: Lea & Febiger; 1982. p. 109–19.

29 Alam M, Caldwell JB, Eliezri YD. Human papillomavirus–associated digital squamous cell carcinoma: literature review and report of 21 new cases. J Am Acad Dermatol 2003;48:385–93.

30 Gal AA, Meyer PR, Taylor CR. Papillomavirus antigens in anorectal condylomata and carcinoma in homosexual men. JAMA 1987;257:337–40.

31 Neves-Motta R, Ferry FR, Basilio-de-Oliveira CA, et al. Highly aggressive squamous cell carcinoma in an HIV-infected patient. Rev Soc Bras Med Trop 2004;37:496–8.

32 Rossy KM, Janusz CA, Schwartz RA. Cryptic exposure to arsenic. Indian J Dermatol Venereol Leprol 2005;71:230–5.

33 Southwick GJ, Schwartz RA. Arsenically associated cutaneous squamous cell carcinoma with hypercalcemia. J Surg Oncol 1979;12:115–8.

34 Dabski K, Stoll HL Jr. Skin cancer caused by Grenz rays. J Surg Oncol 1986;31:87–93.

35 van Vloten WA, Hermans J, van Daal WA. Radiation-induced skin cancer and radiodermatitis of the head and neck. Cancer 1987;59:411–4.

36 Misra RS, Mukherjee A, Nath I. Extensive verrucosis, squamous cell carcinoma, and immunologic abnormalities in Klinefelter's syndrome. Internat J Dermatol 1986;25:529–30.

37 Mikhail GR. Squamous cell carcinoma in hemangioma of lip. J Dermatol Surg Oncol 1986;12:524–5.

38 Lindelof B, Dal H, Wolk K, et al. Cutaneous squamous cell carcinoma in organ transplant recipients: a study of the Swedish cohort with regard to tumor site. Arch Dermatol 2005;141:447–51.

39 Masmoudi A, Ayadi L, Turki H, et al. Squamous cell carcinoma on tuberculous lupus [in French]. Ann Dermatol Venereol 2005;132:591–2.

40 Lee YT, Hsu SD, Kuo CL, et al. Squamous cell carcinoma arising from longstanding colocutaneous fistula: a case report. World J Gastroenterol 2005;11:5251–3.

41 Schwartz RA, Birnkrant AP, Rubenstein DJ, et al. Squamous cell carcinoma in dominant type epidermolysis bullosa dystrophica. Cancer 1981;47:615–20.

42 Goh CL, Ang LC, Ho J. Squamous cell carcinoma complicating discoid lupus erythematosus. Int J Dermatol 1986;26:110–1.

43 Chernosky ME. Porokeratosis. Arch Dermatol 1986;122:869–70.

44 Innocenzi D, Nasca MR, Skroza N, et al. Penile lichen sclerosus: correlation between histopathologic features and risk of cancer. Acta Dermatovenerol Croat 2006;14:225–9.

45 Jamabo RS, Ogu RN. Marjolin's ulcer: report of 4 cases. Niger J Med 2005;14:88–91.

46 Micali G, Nasca MR, Innocenzi D, et al. Association of palmoplantar keratoderma, cutaneous squamous cell carcinoma, dental anomalies, and hypogenitalism in four siblings with 46,XX karyotype: a new syndrome. J Am Acad Dermatol 2005;53:S234–9.

47 Lozinski AZ, Fisher BK, Walker JB, et al. Metastatic squamous cell carcinoma in linear porokeratosis of Mibelli. J Am Acad Dermatol 1987;16:448–51.

48 Chernosky ME, Rapini RP. Squamous cell carcinoma in lesions of disseminated superficial actinic porokeratoses: a report of two cases. Arch Dermatol 1986;122:853–5.

49 Madariaga J, Fromowitz F, Phillips M, et al. Squamous cell carcinoma in congenital ichthyosis with deafness and keratitis. Cancer 1986;57:2026–9.

50 Wong TH, Khoo AK, Tan PH, et al. Squamous cell carcinoma arising in a cutaneous epidermal cyst—a case report. Ann Acad Med Singapore 2000;29:757–9.

51 Takata M, Saida T. Early cancers of the skin: clinical, histopathological, and molecular characteristics. Int J Clin Oncol 2005;10:391–7.

52 Hayashi M, Tamura G, Kato N, et al. Genetic analysis of cutaneous squamous cell carcinomas arising from different areas. Pathol Int 2003;53:602–7.

53 Fundyler O, Khanna M, Smoller BR. Metalloproteinase-2 expression correlates with aggressiveness of cutaneous squamous cell carcinomas. Mod Pathol 2004;17:496–502.

54 Stoll HL Jr, Schwartz RA. Basal cell epithelioma and squamous cell carcinoma. In: McKenna RJ and Murphy GP, editors. Fundamentals of surgical oncology. New York: Macmillan; 1986. p. 406–19.

55 Ahmad I, Das Gupta AR. Epidemiology of basal cell carcinoma and squamous cell carcinoma of the pinna. J Laryngol Otol 2001;115:85–6.

56 Barnett CR, Barnett JG, Schwartz RA. Dermatitis-like squamous cell carcinoma. Dermatol Surg 2004;30:334–5.

57 Frierson HF, Cooper PH. Prognostic factors in squamous cell carcinoma of the lower lip. Hum Pathol 1986;17:346–54.

58 Immerman SC, Scanlon EF, Christ M, Knox KL. Recurrent squamous cell carcinoma of the skin. Cancer 1983;51:1537–40.

59 Fogarty GB, Bayne M, Bedford P, et al. Three cases of activation of cutaneous squamous-cell carcinoma during treatment with prolonged administration of rituximab. Clin Oncol (R Coll Radiol) 2006;18:155–6.

60 Epstein E, Epstein NN, Bragg K, et al. Metastases from squamous cell carcinomas of the skin. Arch Dermatol 1968;97:245–51.

61 Lund H. How often does squamous cell carcinoma of the skin metastasize? Arch Dermatol 1965;92:635–7.

62 Stromberg BV, Keiter JE, Wray RC, Weeks PM. Scar carcinoma: prognosis and treatment. South Med J 1977;70:821–2.

63 Zhu JJ, Padillo O, Duff J, et al. Cavernous sinus and leptomeningeal metastases arising from a squamous cell carcinoma of the face: case report. Neurosurgery 2004;54:492–8; discussion 498–9.

64 Zhang C, Cohen JM, Cangiarella JF, et al. Fine-needle aspiration of secondary neoplasms involving the salivary glands. A report of 36 cases. Am J Clin Pathol 2000;113:21–8.

65 Cassarino DS, Derienzo DP, Barr RJ. Cutaneous squamous cell carcinoma: a comprehensive clinicopathologic classification. Part one. J Cutan Pathol 2006;33:191–206.

66 Cassarino DS, Derienzo DP, Barr RJ. Cutaneous squamous cell carcinoma: a comprehensive clinicopathologic classification. Part two. J Cutan Pathol 2006;33:261–79.

67 Mohs FE, Lathrop TG. Modes of spread of cancer of skin. Arch Dermatol Syphilol 1952;66:427–39.

68 Esmaeli B, Ginsberg L, Goepfert H, Deavers M. Squamous cell carcinoma with perineural invasion presenting as a Tolosa-Hunt-like syndrome: a potential pitfall in diagnosis. Ophthal Plast Reconstr Surg 2000;16:450–2.

69 Lesnik DJ, Boey HP. Perineural invasion of the facial nerve by a cutaneous squamous cell cancer: a case report. Ear Nose Throat J 2004;83:824, 826–7.

70 Kaur MR, Marsden JR, Nelson HM. Humoral hypercalcaemia of malignancy associated with primary

cutaneous squamous cell carcinoma. Clin Exp Dermatol 2007;32:237–8.

71 Fenniche S, Zidi Y, Tekaya NB, et al. Lymphoepithelioma-like carcinoma of the skin in a Tunisian patient. Am J Dermatopathol 2006;28:40–4.

72 Hall G, Duncan A, Azurdia R, et al. Lymphoepithelioma-like carcinoma of the skin: a case with lymph node metastases at presentation. Am J Dermatopathol 2006;28:211–5.

73 Clarke LE, Ioffreda MD. Lymphoepithelioma-like carcinoma of the skin with spindle cell differentiation. J Cutan Pathol 2005;32:419–23.

74 Ram R, Saadat P, Peng D, et al. Case report and literature review: primary cutaneous carcinosarcoma. Ann Clin Lab Sci 2005;35:189–94.

75 Tran TA, Muller S, Chaudahri PJ, et al. Cutaneous carcinosarcoma: adnexal vs. epidermal types define high- and low-risk tumors. Results of a meta-analysis. J Cutan Pathol 2005;32:2–11.

76 Vincek V, Mirzabeigi M, Jewett BS, et al. Primary carcinosarcoma of the helix of the ear. Ear Nose Throat J 2005;84:712–5.

77 Schwartz RA. Verrucous carcinoma of the skin and mucosa. J Am Acad Dermatol 1995;32:1–21; quiz 22–4.

78 Schwartz RA. Buschke-Loewenstein tumor: verrucous carcinoma of the penis. J Am Acad Dermatol 1990;23:723–7.

79 Schwartz RA, Nychay SG, Lyons M, et al. Buschke-Löwenstein tumor: verrucous carcinoma of the anogenitalia. Cutis 1991;47:263–6.

80 Rogozinski TT, Schwartz RA, Towpik E. Verrucous carcinoma in Unna-Thost hyperkeratosis of the palms and soles. J Am Acad Dermatol 1994;31:1061–2.

81 Barreto JE, Velazquez EF, Ayala E, et al. Carcinoma cuniculatum: a distinctive variant of penile squamous cell carcinoma: report of 7 cases. Am J Surg Pathol 2007;31:71–5.

82 Schwartz RA. Verrucous carcinoma of the skin. In: Demis DJ, editor. Clinical dermatology. 18th ed. Philadelphia: JB Lippincott; 1991. p. 1–8 (unit 20–21).

83 Löwenstein L. Carcinoma-like condylomata acuminata of the penis. Med Clin North Am 1939;23:789–95.

84 Pattee SF, Bordeaux J, Mahalingam M, et al. Verrucous carcinoma of the scalp. J Am Acad Dermatol 2007;56:506–7.

85 Kao GF, Graham JH, Helwig EB. Carcinoma cuniculatum (verrucous carcinoma of the skin): a clinicopathologic study of 46 cases with ultrastructural observations. Cancer 1982;49:2395–403.

86 Bendelac A, Grossin M, Siagal M, et al. L'epithelioma cuniculatum. Ann Pathol 1984;4:223–9.

87 Okagaki T, Clark BA, Zachow KR. Presence of human papillomavirus in verrucous carcinoma (Ackerman) of the vagina. Arch Pathol Lab Med 1984;108:567–70.

88 Balazs M. Buschke-Loewenstein tumour. A histologic and ultrastructural study of six cases. Virchows Arch A 1986;410:83–92.

89 Kumar AS, George E, Pandhi PK. Epithelioma cuniculatum palmare (verrucous carcinoma) with palmoplantar keratoderma. Indian J Dermatol Venereol Leprol 1984;50:269–70.

90 Nguyen KQ, McMarlin SL. Verrucous carcinoma of the face. Arch Dermatol 1984;120:383–5.

91 Coldiron BM, Brown FC, Freeman RG. Epithelioma cuniculatum (carcinoma cuniculatum) of the thumb: a case report literature review. J Dermatol Surg Oncol 1986;12:1150–4.

92 Okagaki T, Clark BA, Zachow KR, et al. Presence of human papillomavirus in verrucous carcinoma (Ackerman) of the vagina. Arch Pathol Lab Med 1984;108:567–70.

93 Schwartz RA, Bagley MP, Janniger CK, et al. Verrucous carcinoma of a leg amputation stump. Dermatologica 1991;182:193–5.

94 Alshahwan MA, Alghamdi KM, Alsaif FM. Verrucous carcinoma presenting as giant plantar horns. Dermatol Surg 2007;33:510–2.

95 Shimizu A, Tamura A, Tanaka S, et al. Pedunculated verrucous carcinoma of the thigh. Eur J Dermatol 2005;15:393–5.

96 Perez C, Kraus FT, Evans JC. Anaplastic transformation in verrucous carcinoma of the oral cavity after radiation therapy. Radiology 1966;86:108–15.

97 Demian SDE, Buskin FL, Echlevarria RA. Perineural invasion and anaplastic transformation of verrucous carcinoma. Cancer 1973;32:395–401.

98 Pott P. Cancer scroti. In: Hawes L, Clarke W, Collins R, editors. Chirurgical observations relative to the cataract, the polypus of the nose, the cancer of the scrotum, the different kinds of ruptures, and the mortification of the toes and feet. London: T.J. Carnegy; 1775. p. 63–8.

99 Southam AH, Wilson SR. Cancer of the scrotum. Brit Med J 1922;2:971–3.

100 Castiglione FM Jr, Selikowitz SM, Dimond RL. Mule spinner's disease. Arch Dermatol 1985;121:370–2.

101 Moy LS, Chalet M, Lowe NJ. Scrotal squamous cell carcinoma in a psoriatic patient treated with coal tar. J Am Acad Dermatol 1986;14:518–9.

102 Noumoff JS, Farber M. Tumors of vulva. Int J Dermatol 1986;25:552–63.

103 Woodruff JD. Carcinoma in situ of the vulva. Clin Obstet Gynecol 1985;28:230–9.

104 Chan JK, Sugiyama V, Pham H, et al. Margin distance and other clinico-pathologic prognostic factors in vulvar carcinoma: a multivariate analysis. Gynecol Oncol 2007;104:636–41.

105 Ghaemmaghami F, Modares M, Behtash N, et al. Multiple, disseminated cutaneous metastases of vulvar squamous cell carcinoma. Int J Gynecol Cancer 2004;14:384–7.

106 Kennedy AW, Hart WR. Multiple squamous-cell carcinomas in Fanconi's anemia. Cancer 1982;50: 811–4.

107 Chiesa-Vottero A, Dvoretsky PM, Hart WR. Histopathologic study of thin vulvar squamous cell carcinomas and associated cutaneous lesions: a correlative study of 48 tumors in 44 patients with analysis of adjacent vulvar intraepithelial neoplasia types and lichen sclerosus. Am J Surg Pathol 2006;30:310–8.

108 Vukadinovic M, Jezdic Z, Petrovic M, et al. Surgical management of squamous cell carcinoma of the lip: analysis of a 10-year experience in 223 patients. J Oral Maxillofac Surg 2007;65:675–9.

109 Lindqvist C, Teppo L. Is upper lip cancer "true" lip cancer? J Cancer Res Clin Oncol 1980;97:187–91.

110 Shambaugh P. Tar cancer of the lip in fisherman. JAMA 1935;104:2326–9.

111 Dieng MT, Ndiaye B. Squamous cell carcinoma arising on cutaneous discoid lupus erythematosus. Report of 3 cases [in French]. Dakar Med 2001;46:73–5.

112 LaRiviere W, Pickett AB. Clinical criteria in diagnosis of early squamous cell carcinoma of the lower lip. J Am Dental Assoc 1979;99:972–7.

113 Boncinelli U, Fornieri C, Muscatello U. Relationship between leukocytes and tumor cells in pre-cancerous and cancerous lesions of the lip: a possible expression of immune reaction. J Invest Dermatol 1978;71:407–11.

114 Vahtsevanos K, Ntomouchtsis A, Andreadis C, et al. Distant bone metastases from carcinoma of the lip: a report of four cases. Int J Oral Maxillofac Surg 2007;36:180–5.

115 Boddie AW Jr, Fischer EP, Byers RM. Squamous cell carcinoma of the lower lip in patients under 40 years of age. South Med J 1977;70:711–2.

116 Crotty CP, Dicken CH. Factitious lip crusting. Arch Dermatol 1981;117:338–40.

117 Byers RM, Boddie A, Luna MA. Malignant salivary gland neoplasms of the lip. Am J Surg 1977;134:528–30.

118 White JW Jr, Olsen KD, Banks PM. Plasma cell orificial mucositis. Arch Dermatol 1986;122: 1321–4.

119 Bharti R, Smith DR. Mucous membrane plasmacytosis: a case report and review of the literature. Dermatol Online J 2003;9:15.

120 Miko T, Adler P, Endes P. Simulated cancer of the lower lip attributed to a "caliber persistent" artery. J Oral Pathol 1980;9:137–44.

121 Micali G, Nasca MR, Innocenzi D, et al. Invasive penile carcinoma: a review. Dermatol Surg 2004;30:311–20.

122 Persky L, deKernion J. Carcinoma of the penis. CA Cancer J Clin 1976;26:130–42.

123 Onuigbo WI. Carcinoma of skin of penis. Br J Urol 1985;57:465–6.

124 Bissada NK, Morcos RR, El-Senoussi M. Post-circumcision carcinoma of the penis. I. Clinical aspects. J Urol 1986;135:284–5.

125 Wells AD, Pryor JP. Radiation-induced carcinoma of the penis. Br J Urol 1986;58:325–6.

126 Hanash KA, Furlow WL, Utz DC, Harrison EG Jr. Carcinoma of the penis: a clinicopathological study. J Urol 1970;104:291–7.

127 Steffen C. The men behind the eponym—Abraham Buschke and Ludwig Loewenstein: giant condyloma (Buschke-Loewenstein). Am J Dermatopathol 2006;28:526–36.

128 Ayyathurai R, Webb DB, Rowland S, et al. Humoral hypercalcemia of penile carcinoma. Urology 2007;69:184.

129 Broders AC. Practical points on the microscopic grading of carcinoma. New York J Med 1932;32:667–71.

130 Dotto JE, Glusac EJ. p63 is a useful marker for cutaneous spindle cell squamous cell carcinoma. J Cutan Pathol 2006;33:413–7.

131 Harwood CA, Proby CM, McGregor JM, et al. Clinico-pathologic features of skin cancer in organ transplant recipients: a retrospective case-control series. J Am Acad Dermatol 2006;54:290–300.

132 Stelow EB, Skeate R, Wahi MM, et al. Invasive cutaneous verruco-cystic squamous cell carcinoma. A pattern commonly present in transplant recipients. Am J Clin Pathol 2003;119:807–10.

133 Watanabe K, Mukawa A, Saito K, Nakanishi I, Tsuda H. Adenoid squamous cell carcinoma of the skin overlying the right breast. Acta Pathol Jpn 1986;36:1921–9.

134 Johnson WC, Helwig EB. Adenoid squamous cell carcinoma (adenocarcinoma). A clinicopathologic study of 155 patients. Cancer 1966;19:1639–50.

135 Nagore E, Sanchez-Motilla JM, Perez-Valles A, et al. Pseudovascular squamous cell carcinoma of the skin. Clin Exp Dermatol 2000;25:206–8.

136 Azorin D, Lopez-Rios F, Ballestin C, et al. Primary cutaneous adenosquamous carcinoma: a case report and review of the literature. J Cutan Pathol 2001;28:542–5.

137 McGilbbon D. Malignant epidermal tumours. J Cutan Pathol 1985;12:224–38.

138 Al-Arashi MY, Byers HR. Cutaneous clear cell squamous cell carcinoma in situ: clinical, histological and immunohistochemical characterization. J Cutan Pathol 2007;34:226–33.

139 Kuo T. Clear cell carcinoma of the skin. A variant of the squamous cell carcinoma that simulates sebaceous carcinoma. Am J Surg Pathol 1980;4:573–83.

140 Smith KJ, Hamza S, Skelton H. Histologic features in primary cutaneous squamous cell carcinomas in immunocompromised patients focusing on organ transplant patients. Dermatol Surg 2004;30:634–41.

141 Schwartz RA, Tarlow MM, Lambert WC. Keratoacanthoma-like squamous cell carcinoma within the fibroepithelial polyp. Dermatol Surg 2004;30:349–50.

142 Diaz-Cascajo C, Borghi S, Weyers W, et al. Follicular squamous cell carcinoma of the skin: a poorly recognized neoplasm arising from the wall of hair follicles. J Cutan Pathol 2004;31:19–25.

143 Vanderveen EE, Grekin RC, Swanson NA, et al. Arachidonic acid metabolites in cutaneous carcinomas. Evidence suggesting that elevated levels of prostaglandins in basal cell carcinomas are associated with an aggressive growth pattern. Arch Dermatol 1986;122:407–12.

144 Claudatus JC Jr, d'Ovidio R, Lospalluti M, Meneghini CL. Skin tumors and reactive cellular infiltrate: further studies. Acta Derm Venereol 1986;66:29–34.

145 Smoller BR, Kwan TH, Said JW, Banks-Schlegel S. Keratoacanthoma and squamous cell carcinoma of the skin: immunohistochemical localization of involucrin and keratin proteins. J Am Acad Dermatol 1986;14:226–34.

146 Ariano MC, Wiley EL, Ariano L, Coon JS 4th, Tetzlaff L. H, peanut lectin receptor, and carcinoembryonic antigen distribution in keratoacanthomas, squamous dysplasias, and carcinomas of skin. J Dermatol Surg Oncol 1985;11:1076–83.

147 Schwartz RA, Fleishman JS. Transitional cell carcinoma of the urinary tract presenting with cutaneous metastases. Arch Dermatol 1981;117:513–5.

148 Weidner N, Foucar E. Epidermotropic metastatic squamous cell carcinoma. Report of two cases showing histologic continuity between epidermis and metastasis. Arch Dermatol 1985;121:1041–3.

149 Friedman R, Hanson S, Goldberg LH. Squamous cell carcinoma arising in a Leishmania scar. Dermatol Surg 2003;29:1148–9.

150 Mesa ML, Gertler RS, Schneider LC. Necrotizing sialometaplasia: frequency of histologic misdiagnosis. Oral Surg Oral Med Oral Pathol 1984;57:71–3.

151 Kinney RB, Burton CS, Vollmer RT. Necrotizing sialometaplasia: a sheep in wolf's clothing. Arch Dermatol 1986;122:208–10.

152 Civantos FJ, Moffat FL, Goodwin WJ. Lymphatic mapping and sentinel lymphadenectomy for 106 head and neck lesions: contrasts between oral cavity and cutaneous malignancy. Laryngoscope 2006;112:1–15.

153 Cecchi R, Buralli L, de Gaudio C. Lymphatic mapping and sentinel lymphonodectomy in recurrent cutaneous squamous cell carcinomas. Eur J Dermatol 2005;15:478–9.

154 Peris K, Micantonio T, Fargnoli MC, et al. Imiquimod 5% cream in the treatment of Bowen's disease and invasive squamous cell carcinoma. J Am Acad Dermatol 2006;55:324–7.

155 Martin-Garcia RF. Imiquimod: an effective alternative for the treatment of invasive cutaneous squamous cell carcinoma. Dermatol Surg 2005;31:371–4.

156 Renzi C, Caggiati A, Mannooranparampil TJ, et al. Sentinel lymph node biopsy for high risk cutaneous squamous cell carcinoma: case series and review of the literature. Eur J Surg Oncol 2007;33:364–9.

157 Veness MJ, Porceddu S, Palme CE, Morgan GJ. Cutaneous head and neck squamous cell carcinoma metastatic to parotid and cervical lymph nodes. Head Neck 2007;29:621–31.

158 Mullen JT, Feng L, Xing Y, et al. Invasive squamous cell carcinoma of the skin: defining a high-risk group. Ann Surg Oncol 2006;13:902–9.

159 Vauterin TJ, Veness MJ, Morgan GJ, et al. Patterns of lymph node spread of cutaneous squamous cell carcinoma of the head and neck. Head Neck 2006;28:785–91.

160 Bermejo C, Busby JE, Spiess PE, et al. Neoadjuvant chemotherapy followed by aggressive surgical consolidation for metastatic penile squamous cell carcinoma. J Urol 2007;177:1335–8.

161 Han A, Ratner D. What is the role of adjuvant radiotherapy in the treatment of cutaneous squamous cell carcinoma with perineural invasion? Cancer 2007;109:1053–9.

162 Alkalay R, Alcalay J, Shiri J. Plantar verrucous carcinoma treated with Mohs micrographic surgery: a case report and literature review. J Drugs Dermatol 2006;5:68–73.

163 Chen HM, Chen CT, Yang H, et al. Successful treatment of an extensive verrucous carcinoma with topical 5-aminolevulinic acid-mediated photodynamic therapy. J Oral Pathol Med 2005;34:253–6.

164 Micali G, Nasca MR, Innocenzi D, et al. Penile cancer. J Am Acad Dermatol 2006;54:369–91; quiz 391–4.

165 Rush B. Radiotherapy for verrucous carcinoma of the oral cavity [author reply]. J Surg Oncol 2006;94:639.

166 Kuan YZ, Hsu HC, Kuo TT, et al. Multiple verrucous carcinomas treated with acitretin. J Am Acad Dermatol 2007;56:S29–32.

167 Schalock PC, Kornik RI, Baughman RD, et al. Treatment of verrucous carcinoma with topical imiquimod. J Am Acad Dermatol 2006;54:S233–5.

168 Sheen MC, Sheen YS, Sheu HM, et al. Subungual verrucous carcinoma of the thumb treated by intraarterial infusion with methotrexate. Dermatol Surg 2005;31:787–9.

169 Butler GJ, Neale R, Green AC, et al. Nonsteroidal anti-inflammatory drugs and the risk of actinic keratoses and squamous cell cancers of the skin. J Am Acad Dermatol 2005;53:966–72.

170 Kovach BT, Sams HH, Stasko T. Systemic strategies for chemoprevention of skin cancers in transplant recipients. Clin Transplant 2005;19:726–34.

CHAPTER 6
Keratoacanthoma

Robert A. Schwartz

The keratoacanthoma (KA) is a common and distinctive neoplasm, usually demonstrating rapid growth and a histologic pattern often resembling that of a common squamous cell carcinoma (SCC). KA most often appears on sun-exposed regions of light-complexioned persons of middle age or older. Its enlargement may suggest a highly malignant SCC variant, the de novo SCC [1–5]. The KA may be considered an abortive malignancy that only rarely progresses into an invasive SCC. Often labeled a pseudo-malignancy, the KA may be better classified as a pseudo-benignity meriting Kwittken's alternative term, *keratocarcinoma* [6,7]. It may be best viewed as an aborted malignancy that only rarely progresses into an invasive SCC. However, its unique status sometimes results in therapeutic conundrums. In fact, the clinical and histologic features it shares with the aggressive de novo type of SCC remain a concern today, as the only true test of distinction is spontaneous resolution, which sometimes requires anxiety-provoking months of waiting and a cosmetically unacceptable atrophic scar.

History

Although this neoplasm was originally described by Sir Jonathan Hutchinson in the late 1880s [8,9], Freudenthal of Wroclaw working in England coined the name *keratoacanthoma* in the late 1940s, denoting the tumor's impressive histologic changes of "acanthosis" [5,10,11]. The multiple familial type of keratoacanthomas noted by British dermatologist John Ferguson Smith (1888 to 1978) in 1934 [12], the generalized eruptive type of KAs described in 1950 by Marian Grzybowski (1895 to 1949) of Warsaw [13], and an expanding massive tumor form—keratoacanthoma centrifugum—delineated in 1962 by the Polish dermatology professors Franciszek Miedzinski and Jerzy Kozakiewicz [14] are the major subtypes [15,16]. In 1959, Maria Dąbska and Anna Madejczykowa [17] performed detailed histopathologic studies on 60 KAs, demonstrating the need for representative skin biopsies for diagnosis, with the specimen taken by incisional biopsy to include peripheral and central tumor [18].

Incidence

Keratoacanthoma occurs on sun-exposed skin, with a peak incidence in people ages 50 to 70 years [3,5,19,20]. Solitary KAs affect men equally or up to three times more frequently than they do women. However, because the KA is often presumptively treated as an SCC, its true incidence may be difficult to calculate. The Australian experience shows a relatively common tumor with an annual incidence of about 150 per 100,000, yet one not evident in Aborigines [21]. Seasonal presentation of KA in Rhode Island has been demonstrated, with a peak incidence in the summer and early autumn months [22]. KA is more frequent in pale-complexioned persons and less so with increasing pigmentation. Other signs of actinic damage are often present, including solar elastosis, actinic keratoses, solar lentigines, and other cutaneous neoplasms. The majority of KAs are seen on the face, forearms, and hands. KAs of the hand occur more frequently in men, whereas those of the calf and anterior tibial area are relatively common in women and infrequent in men. However, a KA may develop anywhere, including the male nipple [23]. A study from Hawaii found that KA had an incidence among whites of

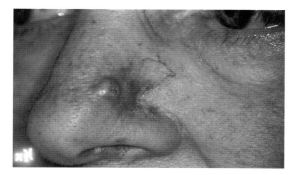

Fig. 6.1 Dome-shaped early KA of the nose anterior to chronic radiation dermatosis associated with radiotherapy of a previous KA.

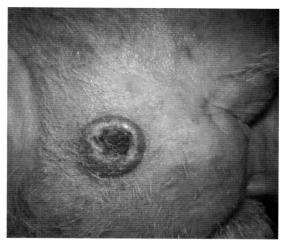

Fig. 6.2 Mature KA on a cheek, with a prominent central keratotic core.

104 per 100,000 residents, virtually the same as that of SCC in that population [20]. The incidence of KA seems to increase with advancing age [16,24,25].

The incidence of eruptive KAs of Ferguson Smith and generalized eruptive KAs of Grzybowski is rather low [4,26,27]. The familial type of multiple eruptive KAs of Ferguson Smith may have its onset in adolescence or earlier. Multiple eruptive KAs of Ferguson Smith have a three-to-one male predominance, with the incidence of generalized eruptive KAs of Grzybowski similar in men and women.

Clinical manifestations

Types of keratoacanthoma

The KA is usually solitary (Figs. 6.1 and 6.2). In one private practice, 84 of 90 patients had a solitary KA [28]. However, multiple ones may be present (Table 6.1). In fact, two solitary KAs in that study were seen in each of four patients; two patients had more than two KAs and could be classified as having the Ferguson Smith type of multiple KAs. The KA has many morphologic forms. In some, no central core is evident clinically. Rarely, the hyperkeratosis is so massive that the KA resembles a cutaneous horn. There are, in addition, several special morphologic or syndromic types:

1 Agglomerated KAs: This type, originally described by Stevanovic [29], is composed of several nodules that coalesce to form a large keratotic plaque [30]. It may persist for almost 6 months and then spontaneously involute. Some show ulceration before

healing. Stevanovic [29] coined the name *keratoacanthoma dyskeratoticum et segregans* based on the histologic findings.

2 KA centrifugum: This exhibits peripheral growth up to 20 cm in diameter with concurrent central healing. A small KA of 1 cm or less may expand to more than 5 cm in diameter. New KAs may form peripherally [31–37]. There may be no spontaneous resolution, or the KA may heal in 6 to 12 months rather than the 2 to 6 months for the common KA. It affects men and women of middle age or older and involves the face, trunk, or extremities. Only about 30 cases have been reported [32]. This variant has been reported as aggregated KA, coral-reef KA, nodulo-vegetating KA, multinodular KA, KA centrifugum marginatum, and in honor of its original describers, KA centrifugum of Miedzinski and Kozakiewicz [14,15].

3 Giant KA: The tumor may grow to more than 9 cm in diameter [38–41]. Although the KA usually does not invade below the level of the eccrine sweat glands, in some giant KAs there may be destruction of underlying tissue and cartilage. KA centrifugum is in a sense a giant KA, but its growth characteristics and morphologic features distinguish it.

4 Subungual KA: This KA may be persistent, painful, and locally destructive to underlying bone [42–45]. It originates in the nail bed, growing at

Table 6.1 The keratoacanthoma

Type	Inheritance	Onset of KA	Size	Number	Mucosal KA
Ferguson Smith	Autosomal dominant	Adolescent, adult	Up to 2 cm	Few to hundreds	Genitalia rarely
Eruptive (Grzybowski)	Probably acquired	Adult	3–6 mm	Thousands	Oral, genital
Multiple persistent	Probably acquired	Adult	2 cm or more		Conjunctivae rarely
Muir-Torre syndrome	Autosomal dominant	Adult	2–3 mm often		Not observed
Nevus sebaceus	Congenital nonhereditary	Adolescent, adult	3 mm to 1 cm		None
Xeroderma pigmentosum	Autosomal recessive	Child, adolescent	Up to 2 cm		Lips
KA centrifugum	Acquired	Adults	Up to 20 cm		None

times to erode or destroy the distal phalanx [46]. It most commonly occurs in middle-aged whites as a painful, rapidly growing tumor of the terminal phalanx [47]. Radiography consistently shows a well-defined cup-shaped erosion of the underlying bone. There is one report of spontaneous regression of subungual KA with reossification of underlying distal lytic phalanx [43].

5 Intraoral and other mucous membrane KAs [48–54]: KA may occur on the hard palate, lips, other oral sites, conjunctiva [55], nasal mucosa, anus [56], and genitalia, including the vulva [50]. Because there are no hair follicles in oral mucosa, the KA may develop from ectopic sebaceous glands. A rare type of KA, generalized eruptive KAs of Grzybowski, has a tendency to involve the mucosal surfaces (see below). Solitary KAs with localization on the lips and nose are most often derived from skin rather than mucosa.

6 Multiple KAs of Ferguson Smith type: This disorder, also called familial primary self-healing squamous epithelioma of the skin, is characterized by several KAs that suddenly appear, slowly involute, and periodically reappear for many years [36,57,58]. Each lesion starts as a red macule, becomes papular, and then grows rapidly into an ordinary solitary KA. The number of KAs varies from only a few to hundreds; they may heal with deep unsightly scars, especially on the face. They usually

begin in childhood, adolescence, or early adulthood. They may even begin in infancy. The mean age of onset in women is 25.5 years (standard deviation, 11.1 years); in men, the mean age of onset is 26.9 years (standard deviation, 12.4 years). They persist throughout life, mainly on sun-exposed areas, but the scalp and external genitalia may also be involved. They affect both sexes with equal severity, but their distribution differs in men and women because of differences in sun-exposure patterns [58]. KAs also tend to develop at sites of trauma, such as the edge of a donor site of a graft or in a fingertip puncture site [59]. Multiple KAs remained unilateral in three patients, who had involvement of the face and upper extremities [60]. This disorder appears to be inherited in an autosomal dominant manner [58]. The *MSSE* (multiple self-healing squamous epitheliomas) gene predisposes to the development of multiple invasive but self-healing skin tumors. *MSSE* (previously named *ESS1*) was mapped to chromosome 9q by linkage analysis; haplotype analysis in families then suggested a common founder mutation and indicated that the gene lies in the interval D9S1-D9S29 (9q22–q31) [61]. Molecular analysis of *MSSE* tumors shows loss of heterozygosity of the *MSSE* region, with loss of the normal allele, providing the first evidence that *MSSE* is a tumor-suppressor gene [27]. This disorder is the likely result of a single mutation occurring before

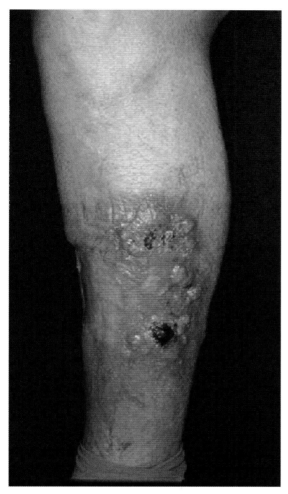

Fig. 6.3 Keratoacanthomas, in various stages of development, on the leg of a patient with multiple persistent KAs adjacent to a large skin graft site. *Left,* this solitary dome-shaped nodule is an early proliferative lesion. *Right,* mature and resolving KAs.

1790. The same mutation is probably responsible for some cases in Canada and the United States.

7 Multiple familial KAs of Witten and Zak [62,63]: This rare entity first described by Witten and Zak [64] in 1952 combines the findings of multiple small eruptive KAs of Grzybowski and large nodular KAs of Ferguson Smith.

8 Multiple persistent KAs: These KAs are slow healing and nonfamilial (Fig. 6.3). The conjunctivae,

palms, soles, and penis have been involved [65–68]. In one possible case, the KAs kept developing for 35 years and became a painful mass that extended around the underlying tendon [69]. Another developed periorally [67].

9 Generalized eruptive KAs of Grzybowski: Literally thousands of tiny disseminated 2- to 3-mm KAs are present [70–74]. Grzybowksi [13] noted the lesions to be "varying in size from a nearly invisible point to the size of a bean." These patients tended to be middle aged or older. Of these, 13 were woman and nine were men. No familial pattern has been shown. Most patients were white [75]. Individual lesions resolve spontaneously with scarring in about 6 months. Pruritus is common, as is ectropion caused by KAs of the eyelids. Corrective blepharoplasty may be required to prevent serious keratopathy. The face may become so involved as to produce a masked facies. Individual nodules may coalesce to become tumors cherry-sized or larger. Koebnerization may be evident. An unexplained hepatomegaly may be noted. KAs may appear as multiple papulonodules on the palms and soles, oral mucosa and palate, larynx, and glans penis. Cancers of the larynx and the female genital tract have been reported in association with generalized eruptive KAs [1,76–78].

10 KA in Muir-Torre syndrome (MTS): An eruption of KAs may appear in association with sebaceous neoplasms and one or more low-grade visceral cancers usually of gastrointestinal or urogenital origin [77,79–83]. The association of KAs and sebaceous neoplasms may be explained by their common derivation from pilosebaceous glands. Almost half the patients with this syndrome have at least one KA. The KAs tend to be 0.5 to 1.0 cm in diameter, three to 10 in number, and scattered on the head and trunk. Although patients with a solitary KA do not have an increased risk of concurrent or subsequent internal cancer [28], I believe that every patient with multiple KAs should be evaluated for the presence of sebaceous neoplasms, the absence of which still requires consideration of this syndrome. It is inherited as an autosomal dominant trait. KAs in possible MTS patients may be analyzed for microsatellite instability and by immunohistochemistry. KAs may show

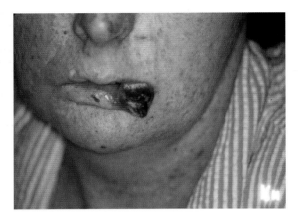

Fig. 6.4 Resolving KA of the lower lip showing abundant keratotic debris in a patient with xeroderma pigmentosum.

microsatellite instability with concomitant MSH2 or MLH1 immunostaining. However, the diagnosis of MTS, which is mainly clinical, should take into account ample phenotypic variability, which includes both cases with typical cancer aggregation in families and those characterized by the association of visceral malignancies with multiple KAs (without sebaceous neoplasms), without an apparent family history of cancer [84]. Thus, clinical, biomolecular, and immunohistochemical characterization of sebaceous neoplasms and KAs may be used to screen for the identification of families at risk of MTS [85].

11 KA in xeroderma pigmentosum [2,54,86]: This defect of DNA repair is associated with development at an early age of basal cell carcinomas (BCCs), SCCs, melanomas, and KAs on sun-exposed sites (Fig. 6.4). A KA in a child should suggest consideration of this syndrome.

12 KA in florid cutaneous papillomatosis and an underlying cancer [87]: Multiple papillomas and a KA were noted in the original report [88]. This disorder may be caused by a malignancy-secreted growth factor.

13 KA in nevus sebaceus of Jadassohn: This type of epidermal nevus tends to occur on the scalp in infants, proliferating at puberty with a wide variety of neoplasms developing within it [89–92]. Most are a basal cell epithelioma or a benign appendageal tumor, such as a trichoblastoma or a syringocystadenoma papilliferum, but occasionally a KA or an SCC. One series of 150 cases had 52 tumors, four of which in adults were KA [93]. The KA may also occur in childhood within a nevus sebaceus [90].

14 Pseudo-recidive KA: Pseudo-recidives are pseudoepitheliomatous reactions that occasionally develop after radiotherapy for skin and other cancers [94–96]. These are rapidly developing early sequelae of radiation therapy that may be confused with a recurrence of the original skin cancer, hence the name *pseudo-recidive*. They occur when the initial radiation reaction is subsiding and evolve rapidly—sometimes in a few days, at other times in a few weeks. They tend to appear granulomatous or wartlike. Their histologic pattern varies from acanthomatous (wartlike) to more typically KA-like. Pseudo-recidives may lack the typical central keratotic plug of the KA, and their exact categorization remains unclear. Nodules with both clinical and histologic features considered "classical" for KAs have been described by Baer and Kopf [24] that developed in cutaneous radiotherapy sites several years after treatment of a BCC. Multiple KAs appearing after a thermal burn from a gasoline explosion are better classified as reactive KAs [97].

15 Reactive KAs: KAs may appear at the site of scar formation [28,73,74,98,99], including healing herpes zoster sites [73,74], a surgical scar [100], and even a scar after skin cancer excision [101,102]. KA may also form in association with vitiligo during a prolonged course of ultraviolet (UV)-B–narrow band therapy [103] or after a body peel or other trauma [94,98,104] (Fig. 6.1). It may also be seen in hypertrophic lichen planus [39], cutaneous lupus erythematosus [105,106], and other benign inflammatory disorders [28], including psoriasis [65], folliculitis barbae [107], pemphigus foliaceus [108], and epidermolysis bullosa dystrophica [109]. Some of these KAs may have been associated with the underlying therapy used, such as tar. Just as crops of seborrheic keratoses may occur after an outbreak of dermatitis, so rarely may KA develop. With multiple KAs of the Ferguson Smith type, KAs tend to develop at sites of trauma (see above) (Table 6.2). Thermal burns may be the preceding trauma in the development of KAs [97], so may the cold trauma

Table 6.2 Keratoacanthomas may develop in selected benign conditions

Stasis dermatitis
Vaccination site
Lichen planus
Psoriasis
Venipuncture site
Nevus sebaceus
Epidermolysis bullosa dystrophica
Atopic dermatitis
Acne conglobata
Discoid lupus erythematosus
Radiation dermatitis
Folliculitis
Lichen simplex chronicus
Thermal burns
Nitrogen mustard patch testing site
Linear epidermal nevus
Pemphigus foliaceus
Lepromatous leprosy

Table 6.3 The keratoacanthoma: clinical stages

Proliferative stage: a rapidly enlarging papulonodule
Mature stage: a bud- or hemisphere-shaped tumor with central keratinous core
Involuting stage: a keratotic tumor, often black in coloration

of cryotherapy [110]. Radiation may be an etiologic factor in the development of multiple KAs [111].

16 Chemical induced (mainly tar) KA: In humans as well as in animals, contact with tar or pitch enhances the chance of KA development [112–114]. There is a significantly increased incidence of KAs in tar and pitch workers [113]. The frequent occurrence of KAs was found to be almost 20% among German tar refinery workers, with an earlier age relative to the general population. Occupational exposure may also occur in machinists because of chronic contact with machine oil [19]. A typical KA has been described after topical podophyllin therapy [95,115].

17 KAs in an immunosuppressed patient: The immunocompromised patient may be at increased risk of KAs as well as skin cancers [2,114,116]. At least some skin neoplasms and possibly KA may show increased aggressive potential in immunosuppressed patients.

Morphologic stages

There are three clinical stages in the natural history of the KA (Table 6.3): proliferative (Fig. 6.1), mature (Figs. 6.2 and 6.3), and resolving (Fig. 6.4).

The proliferative stage produces a firm hemispheric, smooth, enlarging papule that grows rapidly for 2 to 4 weeks, often achieving a size of 2 cm or greater. The border is skin colored or slightly erythematous. Fine telangiectasias may be evident. The mature form is a bud-, dome-, or berry-shaped, skin-colored or erythematous nodule with a central, often umbilicated, keratinous core (Fig. 6.2). It is firm, but without induration at its base or fixation to underlying structures. If the keratotic core is partially removed, the KA may appear crateriform. Involution tends to take place after a few months with tumor resorption and expulsion of the central keratotic plug, leaving a typical slightly depressed puckered, often hypopigmented scar. Some KAs persist for a year or more. In its resolving phase, it appears as a keratotic necrotic nodule (Fig. 6.4). The keratotic debris gradually becomes detached, healing with scar formation. The entire process from origin to spontaneous resolution usually takes about 4 to 6 months.

The morphologic features of the mature KA are distinctive. Ghadially's studies [117] classified it into three morphologic types: type 1, or bud-shaped; type 2, or dome-shaped; and type 3, or berry-shaped. He considered the latter two patterns to represent lower follicular origin and the former, upper follicular derivation. Histologically typical KAs are encountered in practice that are bud- or berry-shaped and resemble a hypertrophic actinic keratosis, a digitate verruca vulgaris, or at times a seborrheic keratosis.

Histogenesis

The probable derivation of KAs from hair follicles has been well documented in humans [19,114] and in animals [117–119]. In fact, the pioneer study in chemical carcinogenesis by Yamagiwa and

Ichikawa [120] in 1918 produced a number of growths that these investigators labeled folliculoepitheliomas. Many were undoubtedly KAs [2]. They observed the histologic evolution of these tumors as follows: "The epithelium, and especially that at the periphery of the hair follicles, gradually undergoes hyperplasia; (1) each layer increases considerably in thickness; (2) many symmetrical mitoses are found in its basal layer; (3) the hair follicles become cystic; (4) the basal layer grows irregular in outline, owing to the projection of processes which ramify in the surrounding subcutaneous tissues." [120].

The role of hair follicles and epidermis in the origin and evolution of cutaneous tumors in humans and animals has been elucidated and summarized by Ghadially [19]. He noted that the usual description of most benign cutaneous growths produced during experimental carcinogenesis has been a *papilloma*, an inadequate term for a variety of tumors. He illustrated diagrammatically and histologically how some of these benign neoplasms were of sebaceous gland origin and others of epidermal or hair follicle lineage. The latter began as striking cellular growth and keratinization in the upper part of the hair follicle and evolved into a KA. He also described a type of KA derived from the hair follicle below the attachment of the arrector pili muscle. Although this lower hair follicle histogenesis is not universally accepted, it serves as a model for the histogenesis of the three distinct morphologic types of KA. These deeper types displayed a consistent and rapid resolution and were derived from the cyclically evanescent hair germ rather than the permanent upper portion of the hair follicle.

Etiology

The etiology of the KA is uncertain. There may be an interaction between genetic predisposition and other cofactors, such as UV light, chemical agents, immune status, and viral infections, together with trauma or immunosuppression in the pathogenesis of KA. Clearly, trauma plays a role. KAs tend to occur or recur at or near skin graft sites [68] and surgical scars [100,101]. Ghadially's classic experiments demonstrated that trauma to the chemically pretreated experimental animal produced KAs [113,117]. Their usual occurrence on sun-exposed areas in elderly persons suggests that UV light may be of etiologic significance in the common solitary KA [5,20]. In England and Australia, the incidence of both KA and SCC shows parallel increases with increased solar exposure [3]. Also suggestive of this etiology is the presence of KAs in patients with xeroderma pigmentosum (Fig. 6.4). The defective DNA repair in xeroderma pigmentosum after UV light injury has been well characterized [121]. The role of higher electromagnetic frequencies in tumorigenesis is suggested by the possible induction of KAs with cutaneous x-ray therapy.

Chemical tumorigenesis has been documented in KAs in several animal models (rabbit, rat, hamster, mouse, hedgehog, duck, chicken) by painting their skin with tar derivatives [113,119]. p53 protein overexpression is an age-related process significantly associated with sun exposure in KA and SCC [122]. In animal studies, two main types of tumors have been noted: papillomas derived from surface epithelium and KAs of hair follicle origin. The latter were both clinically and histologically indistinguishable from the KAs of humans [117]. A somewhat greater tendency for continued local growth was observed in mice and hamsters than in rabbits [113]. The frequent occurrence of KAs among German tar refinery workers with an earlier age relative to the general population and machinists working with machine oil has been noted [19,112,123]. Yet crude coal tar, which enhances UV light carcinogenesis in animals, has been used in conjunction with UV light to treat psoriatic patients for many years, with no increase in KAs observed. The unusual development of multiple KAs in six psoriatic patients has been described [123], as has multiple KAs possibly induced by oral psoralens and UV light and the early and explosive development of nodular BCC and multiple KAs in psoriasis patients treated with cyclosporine [124]. The risk of developing a KA is increased in psoriatics using high-dose psoralen plus UV-A light therapy [125]. A higher prevalence in smokers was observed in KA patients (69.2%) than in controls (21.6%), and the odds ratio adjusted for sex and age was 9.1 (95% CI, 4.9 to 17.1; $P < 0.01$) [126]. These findings suggest that cigarette smoking is associated with the development of KA.

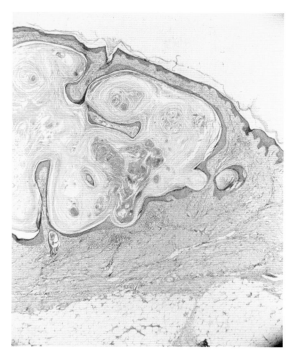

Fig. 6.5 Proliferating phase (early development) of a KA showing a keratin-filled invagination of the epidermis and a few epidermal strands extending into the dermis (hematoxylin–eosin, × 30). (Reprinted with permission from Schwartz RA [1].)

A viral etiology for KA has long been postulated. Shope virus–induced tumors of rabbits are similar to KA [19]. DNA related to human papillomavirus (HPV)-25 has been found in some solitary KAs [127,128] but not in multiple KAs of Grzybowski [26]. The low-risk HPV-6 was found in a giant KA [129]. The role, if any, of HPV in the development of KA remains unclear.

Histopathologic findings

An adequate representative biopsy specimen is important, down to subcutaneous fat, achieved either by total or by a fusiform partial excision through the entire KA to include its center and both sides [2,17,18]. Shave and incisional punch biopsy specimens are tempting but often inadequate. Awaiting spontaneous resolution is not usually a good idea, as it may require anxiety-provoking months of waiting and often a cosmetically unsightly atrophic scar.

The morphologic features and growth pattern of a KA are distinctive enough to be diagnostic in most cases (Fig. 6.5). The diagnosis of a KA is based more on architecture than on cytologic features. Although the cellular characteristics of KA and SCC are similar, the tumor architecture usually provides the distinction. There is no sufficiently sensitive and specific criterion to distinguish KA from SCC. The five most relevant criteria are epithelial lipping and sharp demarcation between tumor and stroma—favoring KA—and ulceration, numerous mitoses, and marked pleomorphism/anaplasia—favoring SCC [130]. Yet the combination of these five did not prove of value in difficult cases. Other well-described criteria, such as intraepithelial elastic fibers, extension beyond sweat glands, keratin-filled crater, intraepithelial abscess formation, lateral growth predominance, and dyskeratosis, are often not helpful. Accordingly, one good idea is a histologic diagnosis: "probable KA; SCC cannot be ruled out" or "SCC, KA type." Alternatively, one may adopt Kwittken's [6,7] term *keratocarcinoma*. KA-like tumors should be treated as a regular SCC. An acrochordon was described that contained an SCC with features resembling a KA [131].

The histologic appearance of KA can be divided into three stages: proliferative, fully developed, and involuting.

Proliferative stage

In the early, rapidly growing phase, there is a horn-filled invagination of the epidermis arising from contiguous hair follicles, from which epidermal strands may extend into the dermis (Fig. 6.4). This incipient KA shows mild hyperkeratosis, acanthosis, and premature keratinization characterized by enlarged cells of the lower portion of the malpighian layer, often with a thick granular layer and prominent keratohyalin granules [6]. There may or may not be a central depression. The hyperkeratosis forms a crenulated border with the acanthotic epidermis. The epidermal strands may be carcinoma-like, containing atypical-appearing squamous cells with multiple mitotic figures as the KA enlarges and extends downward toward the level of the eccrine sweat glands. Some of these mitotic figures may appear atypical. Abnormal mitoses in general and tripolar ones in particular strongly indicate a carcinoma. Some tumor regions may show pronounced keratinization with abundant and pale staining cytoplasm producing an eosinophilic "glassy" appearance. Eosinophils and neutrophils may be present, probably causing some of the keratinocytes to become necrotic and others to disassociate as evidenced by acantholysis. One variant, KA dyskeratoticum et segregans, was named for its marked dyskeratosis and acantholysis [29]. Collagen and elastin fiber fragments may be trapped within the expanding tumor. A sparse dermal inflammatory infiltrate may be evident at the tumor interface with the dermis [132]. Perineural invasion may occasionally be seen at this stage and should not be interpreted as a sign of malignancy. Likewise, intravascular extension and deep invasion below the eccrine glands may be present. Both are considered benign phenomena [133], although the latter may be an ominous sign. Nests of squamous cells may be located in medium-sized veins.

Fully developed stage

The fully developed dome-shaped crateriform nodule has a central depression composed of a keratotic central core. The epidermis extends around the crater sides, forming a lip. Irregular epidermal proliferations protrude both into the crater and below its base. In the mature KA, the individual squamous cells may appear somewhat atypical, but atypia is more pronounced in the rapidly growing stage. However, carcinoma-like foci appear either focally or diffusely in almost three fourths of established KAs and are more common in them than in early or regressing ones [132]. Keratinization of these squamous cells is marked, producing an eosinophilic and glassy appearance. Many keratinocytes have undergone necrosis. Microabscesses, composed of neutrophils and often eosinophils, may be evident. Horn pearls, also characteristic of cutaneous SCC, are present. These are concentric layers of squamous cells with central keratinization that increase centripetally. Lateral tumor strands projecting between collagen bundles may also be seen. There is a focally dense mixed dermal collection of lymphocytes, histiocytes, eosinophils, neutrophils, and plasma cells. This infiltrate is prominent at its advancing margins in carcinoma-like foci but does not penetrate the tumor [132]. Atypical eccrine sweat duct hyperplasia may be present.

Involuting stage

During involution, the KA becomes flattened and less crateriform, as most cells at the crater base have become keratinized. There may be shrunken cells staining intensely with eosin adjacent to tumor cells nearby and within the stroma. A mixed dermal infiltrate may contain multinucleated histiocytes, probably best considered a foreign body granuloma to keratin. Beneath the KA, granulation tissue may be evident, with fibrosis at its base. Fibroblasts at the KA base proliferate, with resultant fibrosis pushing the neoplastic remnants through the crater to the surface. A lichenoid reaction may be seen at the epidermal–dermal interface lining the regressing crater, which slowly becomes flat and heals with the formation of an irregularly shaped atrophic scar.

Ultrastructural pathology

Electron microscopic analysis of the KA has been performed on both human KAs and experimental animal ones [134,135]. There appears to be an increased number of desmosomes in a KA than in normal skin. They may be seen within abnormally keratinized cells. Intranuclear inclusions may sometimes be evident; these viruslike particles may actually be perichromatin granules and nuclear bodies [136]. The main morphologic features distinguishing the KA from the SCC are the desmosomes and the intercellular space [135]. Both the number and surface density of desmosomes are lower than in normal skin; in well-differentiated SCC, these are significantly lower than in a KA. The intercellular space, a reflection of keratinocyte cohesiveness, is significantly larger in an SCC than in a KA. KAs show a significantly larger volume-weighted mean nuclear volume than do SCCs and thus, the estimation of the volume-weighted mean nuclear volume has been suggested as a helpful tool for the differential diagnosis of KA and SCC [137].

Cellular and basement membrane features

There are two important pathologic features commonly used to separate benignity from malignancy that require consideration for KAs. These are individual cell cytology and invasiveness below the basement membrane. Premalignant tumors can be distinguished from malignant ones by whether or not the neoplasm has invaded below the basement membrane. However, a number of exceptions have reduced the value of this generalization. Immunologic, histochemical, and electron microscopic studies of KA have shown conflicting results [138,139]. Another point is that the degree of cellular atypia may be useful in separating benign from malignant neoplasms. Studies demonstrated aneuploidy in some KAs, although to a lesser extent than in well-differentiated SCC [140,141]. The majority of both were diploid.

Differential diagnosis

The most frequent consideration in the clinical and histologic differential diagnosis of the KA is SCC. Clinically, the rapid tumor growth may suggest a de novo cutaneous SCC, a relatively rare aggressive tumor that produces regional or distant metastases in at least 8% of patients [142]. A series of four such patients illustrated this point [143]. Each de novo SCC was initially diagnosed as KA, but each had an early recurrence after conservative therapy. In three of the four patients, rapidly spreading metastatic cutaneous SCC occurred, resulting in the death of two. Other examples exist [144].

Fortunately, the morphologic features and growth pattern of a KA are sufficiently distinctive to be diagnostic in most cases [17,18,145]. In distinction from SCC, KAs tend to be both exophytic and endophytic, with a central keratin-filled crater, whereas the cutaneous SCC is mainly endophytic, with ulceration often present. The crater is surrounded by overhanging epithelial "lips," which are absent in the SCC. Intraepidermal abscesses are common in KA and rarely seen in SCC. In KA, acantholytic cells and polymorphonuclear leukocytes are present in these abscesses; when abscesses occur in cutaneous SCCs, there are few, if any,

inflammatory cells. KAs have abundant pale-staining keratinocyte cytoplasm; less is seen in the SCC. Resolving KAs often show fibrosis at their base; in SCCs, fibrosis, when present, is of the desmoplastic type [146]. Sometimes a well-differentiated SCC and pseudoepitheliomatosis hyperplasia overlying certain granulomatoses may be difficult to distinguish from a KA without a clinical history.

There are a number of features that help distinguish KA from SCC, but none is absolute. For example, atypical eccrine duct hyperplasia is more common, as are actinically damaged elastic fibers and an increased content of intracytoplasmic glycogen within the epidermis of a KA [147]. Likewise, expression of keratin and involucrin in KA may be an immunohistochemical aid to diagnosis [138,148]. Other potential aids in distinction include morphometry on ultrastructural sections, DNA cytometry and content [135,140], staining for peanut agglutinin lectin [149], nucleolar organizer regions [150], and expression of proliferating cell nuclear antigen [139,151], filaggrin [152], blood group antigens [151], growth factors [153–155], and oncogenes [156–158].

There are a variety of special stains or tests, including expression of lectins, proliferating cell nuclear antigen (PCNA), vascular cell adhesion molecule (VCAM; CD-106), and intercellular adhesion molecule (ICAM; CD-54); cytokeratin 10 expression and proliferation rate as measured by Ki-67 expression; angiotensin type-1 receptor expression; oncostatin M expression; syndecan-1 expression; MIB-1 immunohistometry; immunohistochemical staining for desmogleins 1 and 2, stromelysin 3, and apoptotic and cell adhesion markers; and ultrastructural features that are said to be useful in distinguishing KA from SCC [159–163]. Sadly, none of these methods, including identification of BCCs and KAs by fluorescent lectin staining of a tumor-specific disaccharide [164], has proven of practical value. In 1981, working with Professor Peter M. Elias in his laboratory, I identified the value of peanut lectin in KA, an observation published by Kannon and Park [149] in 1990. Combining DNA image cytometry and p53 expression may enhance the distinction of KA from SCC [165]. Likewise, testing KAs for microsatellite instability and/or using MSH2 or MLH1 immunostaining may identify

KAs linked to Muir-Torre syndrome [84]. The latest technology applied to KA with speculations as to biologic significance is, as LeBoit [166] has correctly observed, a "one stain, one paper" approach. Thus, because no definitive and universally accepted criteria exist to distinguish KA from SCC, a KA should be regarded and treated clinically as an SCC.

A KA may be associated anatomically with other sun-induced neoplasms, including melanoma and BCC, with or without a transition between the two. The KA could have arisen from a preexistent BCC or superficial spreading malignant melanoma, or vice versa; however, this author views the situation as more likely a matter of histologic collision between two sun-induced tumors. When elements of sebaceous adenoma and KA occur in the same lesion, presumably caused by joint pilosebaceous proliferation within a hair follicle, it may be classified as a "seboacanthoma," reflecting the strong possibility of the Muir-Torre syndrome [167]. They show converging follicular and sebaceous proliferation, often with an epidermal buttress or collarette.

The clinical differential diagnosis besides SCC includes verrucous carcinoma, giant condyloma acuminatum of Buschke and Löwenstein, hypertrophic actinic keratosis, other causes of cutaneous horns, inverted follicular keratosis, warty dyskeratoma, giant molluscum contagiosum, fibrous histiocytoma [168], exophytic pilomatricoma [169], verruca vulgaris, metastatic cancer [170], giant molluscum contagiosum, deep fungal infections such as chromoblastomycosis or North American blastomycosis, other pseudoepitheliomatous hyperplasias, syphilis, histoid lepromas [171], and seborrheic keratosis. KA-like cutaneous metastases may also occur. Cutaneous lupus erythematosus may also produce KA-like nodules [172]. Small KAs, as seen in multiple eruptive KAs, may resemble Darier's disease. Some sebaceous neoplasms in the Muir-Torre syndrome may clinically mimic a KA, with sudden appearance, rapid growth, a central plug, and a heaped-up border [81,167].

Malignant transformation

The KA may be viewed as an "abortive malignancy which only rarely progresses into an invasive squamous cell carcinoma" [1]. The presence of aneuploidy in KAs has been found to be indistinguishable from that of many cutaneous SCCs, supporting the idea that the KA is a true neoplasm rather than a reactive hyperplasia [141]. KAs progressing to SCCs or KA-like SCCs are rare [1,3,132,144,173]. A study of 39 KAs in 35 patients is noteworthy: careful histologic examination revealed six with perineural invasion and one with vascular invasion [133]. During a follow-up period ranging from 4 to 8 years, none of these histologically disturbing findings was associated with metastases, as they may be with cutaneous SCC [174]. However, adequate surgical excision apparently was used in these six patients. Even invasion of medium-sized veins does not suggest malignant transformation [175]. There is evidence that factors other than immunologic ones are responsible for KA regression in humans. In a study of cell-mediated immunity in 11 patients with a solitary KA, no delayed hypersensitivity reaction was observed after intradermal injection of tumor extract [114]. No clinical or histologic finding has been convincingly linked to "malignant transformation." An alternative viewpoint is that malignant transformation does not occur, but rather such a tumor is an SCC from its inception [2], possibly as a malignantly altered clone of keratinocytes initiating proliferation by the same histogenic mechanism as that of a KA.

Immunology of keratoacanthoma

Most patients with a KA have an intact humoral and cellular immune system. Keratin analysis of KA suggests both the characteristics of follicular differentiation and of an SCC [176]. The question is whether regression of KA is immunologically mediated. KA regression may be a cytotoxic immune reaction with a heavy lymphocytic infiltrate composed of CD3+ and CD4+ cells [177]. An alternative theory is that regression is not a result of immune cytotoxicity, but rather of rapidly terminal differentiation stimulated by the immune system [178]. An analysis of lymphocyte subpopulations in a KA was interpreted as displaying a meaningful infiltration of killer T cells and OKT6-positive dendritic cells [179]. Cytotoxic T cells may play a pivotal role in KA regression, but additional mechanisms may also be involved [180]. The role of immunity in spontaneous tumor regression has been argued, noting the following: a halo of erythema around some regressing KAs, tumor regression during febrile illness, increased incidence with advancing age or immunosuppression, dense mononuclear infiltrate and fibroblastic tissue reaction associated with regressing tumors, variable presence of Langerhans cells, and detection of an anti-squamous antibody [67,132,181]. It is possible that a faster activation of CD4$^+$ lymphocytes, via interferon release and cytokine secretion, takes place after imiquimod application, leading to KA regression [182]. Nevertheless, there is growing evidence that the regression of human KAs is not immunologically mediated, implying that it is similar to the pattern of natural regression seen within a normal hair follicle [183–186].

Genetic aberrations have been described in solitary KAs [187]. Evidence shows that microsatellite instability and loss of heterozygosity do not appear to play a significant role in KA development, except in the setting of the Muir-Torre syndrome [188,189]. However, there is a high degree of genetic instability in solitary KAs presumably unrelated to this syndrome [187]. A higher degree of chromosomal instability in SCCs than in KAs was observed. The patterns of recurrent aberrations were also different in the two neoplasms, suggesting different genetic mechanisms involved in their development.

The keratoacanthoma as a marker for internal malignancy

There have been several reports linking KAs to internal malignancy; these have been summarized by Kingman and Callen [28], who concluded there is no evidence relating the solitary KA to internal malignancy in a greater-than-chance association.

However, multiple KAs may be associated with internal malignancy, especially in the Muir-Torre syndrome [81]. In three patients, eruptive KAs were associated with a poorly differentiated laryngeal SCC, an ovarian carcinoma with metastases, and an adenocarcinoma of the fallopian tube plus a stem cell leukemia [78,190]. In addition, a solitary KA may occur as part of a generalized eruption, such as florid cutaneous papillomatosis [88] or the Muir-Torre syndrome [81], both of which are markers for internal malignancy. The KA may also occur with xeroderma pigmentosum, as previously described. Microsatellite instability and immunostaining for MSH2 and MLH1 may be evaluated in KAs to help identify patients with the Muir-Torre syndrome [188].

Diagnosis and treatment

Although KA usually involutes spontaneously, biopsy and treatment are undertaken for several important reasons. Biopsy establishes the diagnosis and serves to rule out SCC. Treatment provides hastened resolution or cure, prevention of rapid enlargement or impingement on important structures, and improvement in overall cosmetic result. Solitary KAs should usually receive complete conservative excision, which also provides an optimal biopsy specimen and in most patients a greater likelihood of a favorable cosmetic outcome than one would anticipate with spontaneous resolution. A fusiform partial excision cut symmetrically through the center so as to include normal lateral tissue and underlying normal fat also provides an adequate specimen to distinguish SCC from KA. If this is done, it is important that the pathologist is informed, so appropriate sections showing the lateral aspects as well as deep margins of the lesions are visualized microscopically. Shave and incisional punch biopsy specimens are not ideal when one is considering the diagnosis of a KA.

Surgical excision is often desirable for the solitary KA [2]. Simple curettage may be used, as may blunt dissection. Curettage is usually employed together with electrodesiccation [191,192]. Radiotherapy with superficial x-ray, orthovoltage radiation, or electron beam may be used primarily, or after the recurrence of a KA following excision or curettage and electrodesiccation [193]. The same tumoricidal doses as those used for an SCC should be employed. Large facial KAs may be treated by radiotherapy with acceptable cosmesis. Laser surgery has also been employed with good success for small solitary KAs in difficult-to-treat locations [194].

Kuflik [195] considers cryosurgery with liquid nitrogen of value, especially for small early KAs. For larger ones, it is usually used as adjunctive therapy to the base after the KA has been removed by excisional biopsy or curettage. The base is frozen completely with at least a 3-mm halo of healthy tissue, after hemostasis has been achieved. Topical podophyllin has been used alone, in combination with curettage and electrodesiccation, or in combination with radiotherapy [196]. Curiously, topical podophyllin may also produce KA formation [115].

Certain anatomic locations may mandate special considerations. Subungual KA sometimes requires amputation of a digit when underlying bone is involved and other options fail [42–45]. Micrographic (Mohs) surgery is an important option in selected patients, as it is tissue sparing, an important factor in critical anatomic locations and for particularly large KAs. Although quantification of KA treatment data is lacking, recurrence of classical KA after excision is a well-known phenomenon, seen in about 4% to 8% of cases [197]. This pattern does not constitute proof that the KA is in any way more malignant than otherwise. Other options may be considered, particularly with multiple KAs, but even in these cases patients must be followed closely, with surgical excision reconsidered if the KA fails to respond within 4 to 6 weeks. The cryosurgical authority E. G. Kuflik estimates that cryosurgery produces a 99% cure rate with a less than 1% KA recurrence rate (personal communication, July 2007).

Additional local therapeutic options

Intralesional and topical 5-fluorouracil (5-FU) therapy for KA, introduced by Klein and associates [198] in 1962, has been widely employed [199–201]. It may be administered by either daily or every-other-day focal injections of 0.1 mL of a 5% solution directly into the base of the KA or by topical application of 5-FU cream or ointment up to five times daily, with or without occlusion. Therapy is continued for about 2.5 weeks. Others used 50 mg/mL of 5-FU injected with a 27- or 30-gauge needle inserted tangentially into the slopes of the KA in three or four sites and 0.1 to 0.3 mL injected circumferentially and 0.1 to 0.2 mL sublesionally [202]. This approach was performed weekly until the KA

size was decreased by 60% to 80%. It took up to 8 weeks, with an average of 3 weeks, for each KA to resolve. Only one of 26 KAs in 14 patients did not respond. This modality provides an excellent therapeutic result and has proven valuable for large KAs in difficult-to-treat locations. It may be ineffective in the KA that is not rapidly proliferating [203]. KA centrifugum marginatum may also be treated with topical 5% 5-FU [33,35]. Giant KA may be successfully handled with intralesional 5-FU [41] or the combined use of ablative erbium-doped yttrium-aluminum-garnet (Er:YAG) laser and topical 5-FU [204].

There are other topical and intralesional options. Intralesional bleomycin, methotrexate, interferon-α-2a, transfer factor, and imiquimod may be employed [205–212]. Imiquimod was applied in a 5% cream every other day for 4 to 12 weeks in four patients with facial KA; in three, it resolved within 4 to 6 weeks. Others have also observed that imiquimod 5% cream applied daily for 8 weeks may lead to or accelerate KA regression [182]. Although out of fashion, intralesional injections of triamcinolone have also been employed with impressive benefit in 10 patients with a total of 17 KAs [213].

Systemic therapy

Systemic chemotherapy has been used for multiple KAs [130,214,215]. A good first choice is often retinoids. Acitretin for 2 months may be effective for multiple KAs, including the multiple eruptive type of Ferguson Smith, the generalized eruptive type of Grzybowski, and KA centrifugum marginatum [33,214,216]. Some have employed relatively toxic chemotherapy with systemic methotrexate [62,217], cyclophosphamide [218], and 5-FU [62], the latter given intravenously. Cryosurgery can be combined with prolonged administration of a retinoid for the multiple eruptive type of Ferguson Smith [215]. A man with multiple KA centrifugum marginatum was successfully treated with methotrexate combined with oral prednisone [219].

The KA occurs most often on sun-exposed sites in light-skinned persons of middle age or older. Thus, minimization of solar exposure should be undertaken. Chemoprevention should be considered for patients with xeroderma pigmentosum, syndromic

Table 6.4 Keratoacanthoma curiosities

In mice, KA developed after topical DMBA (9,10-dimethyl-1, 2-benzanthracene) application only when hair follicles were in telogen or resting phase [222]
Because there are no hair follicles in oral mucosa, KA may develop there from ectopic sebaceous glands [52]
Topical podophyllin is said to induce the formation of a KA on rare occasions [95,115], yet has also been used to treat it [196]

forms of multiple KAs, and possibly transplant recipients. Systemic retinoids and T4 endonuclease V liposome cream have been shown to be chemoprotective in patients with xeroderma pigmentosum [220,221].

The keratoacanthoma: an overview

The KA is a common skin tumor that tends to occur on sun-exposed sites in light-skinned persons of middle age or older. It may be viewed as an aborted SCC that only rarely evolves into a progressively invasive SCC. Sometimes considered a pseudo-malignancy, the KA may in this context merit the alternative designation as pseudo-benignity. It is most likely derived from hair follicle cells. Its etiology is unknown, although ultraviolet light, viruses, and chemical carcinogens have been considered. Its diagnosis should be made by complete conservative excision or by a properly performed fusiform partial excision designed to provide an adequate biopsy specimen to distinguish a KA from an SCC. Some curiosities about KA are noted in Table 6.4.

References

1 Schwartz RA. The keratoacanthoma: a review. J Surg Oncol 1979;12:305–17.
2 Schwartz RA. Keratoacanthoma. J Am Acad Dermatol 1994;30:1–19; quiz 20–2.
3 Schwartz RA. Keratoacanthoma: a clinico-pathologic enigma. Dermatol Surg 2004;30:326–33; discussion 33.
4 Schwartz RA, Blaszczyk M, Jablonska S. Generalized eruptive keratoacanthoma of Grzybowski: follow-up of the original description and 50-year retrospect. Dermatology 2002;205:348–52.
5 Rook A, Whimster I. Keratoacanthoma—a thirty year retrospect. Br J Dermatol 1979;100:41–7.
6 Kwittken J. A histologic chronology of the clinical course of the keratocarcinoma (so-called keratoacanthoma). Mt Sinai J Med 1975;42:127–35.
7 Kwittken J. Dermatologic pseudobenignities. Mt Sinai J Med 1980;47:34–7.
8 Hutchinson J. Morbid growths and tumours. 1. The "crateriform ulcer of the face," a form of acute epithelial cancer. Trans Pathol Soc London 1889;40:275–81.
9 Hutchinson J. A peculiar form of cancer of the skin. Illustrations of clinical surgery consisting of plates, photographs, woodcuts, diagrams, etc illustrating surgical diseases, symptoms and accidents also operative and other methods of treatment with descriptive letterpress. Philadelphia: P. Blakiston & Son; 1888. p. 2, plate 92.
10 Gougerot H. Verrucome avec adenite, a structure epitheliomatifome, curable par le 914. Arch Dermato-Syphililigr Clin Saint-Louis 1929;1:374–85.
11 Rook A, Whimster I. [Kerato-acanthoma]. Arch Belg Dermatol Syphiligr 1950;6:137–46.
12 Ferguson Smith J. A case of multiple primary squamous-celled carcinomata of the skin in a young man, with spontaneous healing. Brit J Dermatol Syphilol 1934;46:267–72.
13 Grzybowski M. A case of peculiar generalized epithelial tumours of the skin. Brit J Dermatol Syphilol 1950;62:310–3.
14 Miedzinski F, Kozakiewicz J. [Keratoacanthoma centrifugum—a special variety of keratoacanthoma]. Hautarzt 1962;13:348–52.
15 Miedzinski F, Dratwinski Z, Brzozowski J, et al. [Nosologic situation of keratoacanthoma centrifugum]. Hautarzt 1973;24:120–3.
16 Miedzinski F. Keratoacanthoma as a pathogenetic and clinico-histological problem, its 40th anniversary. Postepy Dermatol 1990;7:61–70.
17 Dabska M, Madejczykowa A. Rogowiak kolczastokomorkowy—keratoacanthoma (molluscum sebaceum, molluscum psuedocarcinomatosum). Studium patologiczno-kliniczne Nowotwory 1959;9: 1–23.
18 Dabska M. [Keratoacanthoma]. Wiad Lek 1965; 18:1249–50.
19 Ghadially FN, Barton BW, Kerridge DF. The etiology of keratoacanthoma. Cancer 1963;16:603–11.
20 Chuang TY, Reizner GT, Elpern DJ, et al. Keratoacanthoma in Kauai, Hawaii. The first documented

incidence in a defined population. Arch Dermatol 1993;129:317–9.

21 Sullivan JJ. Keratoacanthoma: the Australian experience. Australas J Dermatol 1997;38 Suppl 1: S36–9.

22 Dufresne RG, Marrero GM, Robinson-Bostom L. Seasonal presentation of keratoacanthomas in Rhode Island. Br J Dermatol 1997;136:227–9.

23 Drut R. Solitary keratoacanthoma of the nipple in a male. Case report. J Cutan Pathol 1976;3:195–8.

24 Baer R, Kopf A. Keratoacanthoma. In: Year book of dermatology (1962–1963 series). Chicago: Year Book Medical Publishers;1963. p. 7–41.

25 Schwartz RA. Keratoacanthoma: an abortive squamous cell carcinoma that does not always fail. G Ital Dermatol Venereol 2003;138:355–62.

26 Haas N, Schadendorf D, Henz BM, et al. Nine-year follow-up of a case of Grzybowski type multiple keratoacanthomas and failure to demonstrate human papillomavirus. Br J Dermatol 2002;147:793–6.

27 Bose S, Morgan LJ, Booth DR, et al. The elusive multiple self-healing squamous epithelioma (MSSE) gene: further mapping, analysis of candidates, and loss of heterozygosity. Oncogene 2006;25:806–12.

28 Kingman J, Callen JP. Keratoacanthoma. A clinical study. Arch Dermatol 1984;120:736–40.

29 Stevanovic DV. Keratoacanthoma dyskeratoticum and segregans. Arch Dermatol 1965;92:666–9.

30 Sardana K, Sarkar R, Garg VK, et al. Multinodular keratoacanthoma: a rare but definite entity. Int J Dermatol 2002;41:905–7.

31 Gonul M, Cakmak SK, Kilic A, et al. A case of multiple keratoacanthomas associated with keratoacanthoma centrifugum marginatum. Acta Derm Venereol 2006;86:169–70.

32 Attili S, Attili VR. Keratoacanthoma centrifugum marginatum arising in vitiligo: a case report. Dermatol Online J 2006;12:18.

33 Yuge S, Godoy DA, Melo MC, et al. Keratoacanthoma centrifugum marginatum: response to topical 5-fluorouracil. J Am Acad Dermatol 2006;54:S218–9.

34 Grinspan Bozza NO, Totaro II, Pocovi M, et al. [Keratoacanthoma centrifugum of Miedzinski and Kozakiewicz]. Med Cutan Ibero Lat Am 1989;17:234–8.

35 Divers AK, Correale D, Lee JB. Keratoacanthoma centrifugum marginatum: a diagnostic and therapeutic challenge. Cutis 2004;73:257–62.

36 Kato N, Ito K, Kimura K, et al. Ferguson Smith type multiple keratoacanthomas and a keratoacanthoma centrifugum marginatum in a woman from Japan. J Am Acad Dermatol 2003;49:741–6.

37 Kurschat P, Hess S, Hunzelmann N, et al. Keratoacanthoma centrifugum marginatum accompanied by extensive granulomatous foreign body reaction. Dermatol Online J 2005;11:16.

38 Parvanescu H, Mogoanta L, Foarfa C, et al. Giant keratoacanthoma of the hand. Rom J Morphol Embryol 2005;46:235–8.

39 Giesecke LM, Reid CM, James CL, et al. Giant keratoacanthoma arising in hypertrophic lichen planus. Australas J Dermatol 2003;44:267–9.

40 Saito M, Sasaki Y, Yamazaki N, et al. Self-involution of giant keratoacanthoma on the tip of the nose. Plast Reconstr Surg 2003;111:1561–2.

41 Leonard AL, Hanke CW. Treatment of giant keratoacanthoma with intralesional 5-fluorouracil. J Drugs Dermatol 2006;5:454–6.

42 Bui-Mansfield LT, Pulcini JP, Rose S. Subungual squamous cell carcinoma of the finger. AJR Am J Roentgenol 2005;185:174–5.

43 Sinha A, Marsh R, Langtry J. Spontaneous regression of subungual keratoacanthoma with reossification of underlying distal lytic phalynx. Clin Exp Dermatol 2005;30:20–2.

44 Baran R, Goettmann S. Distal digital keratoacanthoma: a report of 12 cases and a review of the literature. Br J Dermatol 1998;139:512–5.

45 Baran R, Tosti A, De Berker D. Periungual keratoacanthoma preceded by a wart and followed by a verrucous carcinoma at the same site. Acta Derm Venereol 2003;83:232–3.

46 Choi JH, Shin DH, Shin DS, et al. Subungual keratoacanthoma: ultrasound and magnetic resonance imaging findings. Skeletal Radiol 2007;36:769–72.

47 Oliwiecki S, Peachey RD, Bradfield JW, et al. Subungual keratoacanthoma—a report of four cases and review of the literature. Clin Exp Dermatol 1994;19:230–5.

48 Janette A, Pecaro B, Lonergan M, et al. Solitary intraoral keratoacanthoma: report of a case. J Oral Maxillofac Surg 1996;54:1026–30.

49 Habel G, O'Regan B, Eissing A, et al. Intra-oral keratoacanthoma: an eruptive variant and review of the literature. Br Dent J 1991;170:336–9.

50 Ozkan F, Bilgic R, Cesur S. Vulvar keratoacanthoma. APMIS 2006;114:562–655.

51 Leibovitch I, Huilgol SC, James CL, et al. Periocular keratoacanthoma: can we always rely on the clinical diagnosis? Br J Ophthalmol 2005;89:1201–4.

52 Svirsky JA, Freedman PD, Lumerman H. Solitary intraoral keratoacanthoma. Oral Surg Oral Med Oral Pathol 1977;43:116–22.

53 Chen W, Koenig C. Vulvar keratoacanthoma: a report of two cases. Int J Gynecol Pathol 2004;23:284–6.

54 Chowdhury RK, Padhi T, Das GS. Keratoacanthoma of the conjunctiva complicating xeroderma pigmentosum. Indian J Dermatol Venereol Leprol 2005;71:430–1.

55 Perdigao FB, Pierre-Filho Pde T, Natalino RJ, et al. Conjunctival keratoacanthoma. Rev Hosp Clin Fac Med Sao Paulo 2004;59:135–7.

56 Maruani A, Michenet P, Lagasse JP, et al. [Keratoacanthoma of the anal margin]. Gastroenterol Clin Biol 2004;28:906–8.

57 Dauenhauer MA, Wacker D, Neuburg M. Perineural invasion of a Ferguson-Smith-type keratoacanthoma. Dermatol Surg 2006;32:862–3.

58 Ferguson-Smith MA, Wallace DC, James ZH, et al. Multiple self-healing squamous epithelioma. Birth Defects Orig Artic Ser 1971;7:157–63.

59 Puente Duany N. [Spinous cell pseudoepithelioma (keratoacanthoma) of the skin of the anterior face of the thorax: a new multiple, massive & localized clinical variety]. Arch Cuba Cancerol 1959;18:1–14.

60 Green WS, Underwood LJ, Green R. Multiple keratoacanthomas on upper extremities [proceedings]. Arch Dermatol 1977;113:512–3.

61 Richards FM, Goudie DR, Cooper WN, et al. Mapping the multiple self-healing squamous epithelioma (MSSE) gene and investigation of xeroderma pigmentosum group A (XPA) and PATCHED (PTCH) as candidate genes. Hum Genet 1997;101:317–22.

62 Agarwal M, Chander R, Karmakar S, et al. Multiple familial keratoacanthoma of Witten and Zak—a report of three siblings. Dermatology 1999;198:396–9.

63 Boateng B, Hornstein OP, von den Driesch P, et al. [Multiple keratoacanthomas (Witten-Zak type) in prurigo simplex subacuta]. Hautarzt 1995;46:114–7.

64 Witten VH, Zak FG. Multiple, primary, self-healing prickle-cell epithelioma of the skin. Cancer 1952;5:539–50.

65 Reid BJ, Cheesbrough MJ. Multiple keratoacanthomata. A unique case and review of the current classification. Acta Derm Venereol 1978;58:169–73.

66 Friedman RP, Morales A, Burnham TK. Multiple cutaneous and conjunctival keratoacanthomata. Arch Dermatol 1965;92:162–5.

67 Higuchi M, Tanikawa E, Nomura H, et al. Multiple keratoacanthomas with peculiar manifestations and course. J Am Acad Dermatol 1990;23:389–92.

68 Schwartz RA. Multiple persistent keratoacanthomas. Oncology 1979;36:281–5.

69 Pillsbury DM, Beerman H. Multiple keratoacanthoma. Am J Med Sci 1958;236:614–24.

70 Oakley A, Ng S. Grzybowski's generalized eruptive keratoacanthoma: remission with cyclophosphamide. Australas J Dermatol 2005;46:118–23.

71 Chu DH, Hale EK, Robins P. Generalized eruptive keratoacanthoma of Grzybowski. J Drugs Dermatol 2003;2:318–9.

72 Consigli JE, Gonzalez ME, Morsino R, et al. Generalized eruptive keratoacanthoma (Grzybowski variant). Br J Dermatol 2000;142:800–3.

73 Kopf AW, Bart RS. Development of more keratoacanthomas following skin testing with nitrogen mustard in a patient with the multiple keratoacanthoma syndrome. J Dermatol Surg Oncol 1979;5:450–1.

74 Lloyd KM, Madsen DK, Lin PY. Grzybowski's eruptive keratoacanthoma. J Am Acad Dermatol 1989;21:1023–4.

75 Jaber PW, Cooper PH, Greer KE. Generalized eruptive keratoacanthoma of Grzybowski. J Am Acad Dermatol 1993;29:299–304.

76 Sterry W, Steigleder GK, Pullmann H, et al. [Eruptive keratoacanthoma]. Hautarzt 1981;32:119–25.

77 Muir EG, Bell AJ, Barlow KA. Multiple primary carcinomata of the colon, duodenum, and larynx associated with kerato-acanthomata of the face. Br J Surg 1967;54:191–5.

78 Chapman RS, Finn OA. Carcinoma of the larynx in two patients with keratoacanthoma. Br J Dermatol 1974;90:685–8.

79 Schwartz RA, Flieger DN, Saied NK. The Torre syndrome with gastrointestinal polyposis. Arch Dermatol 1980;116:312–4.

80 Schwartz RA, Goldberg DJ, Mahmood F, et al. The Muir-Torre syndrome: a disease of sebaceous and colonic neoplasms. Dermatologica 1989;178:23–8.

81 Schwartz RA, Torre DP. The Muir-Torre syndrome: a 25-year retrospect. J Am Acad Dermatol 1995;33:90–104.

82 Rothenberg J, Lambert WC, Vail JT Jr, et al. The Muir-Torre (Torre's) syndrome: the significance of a solitary sebaceous tumor. J Am Acad Dermatol 1990;23:638–40.

83 Schwartz RA, Whitworth JM, Janniger CK, et al. The Muir-Torre syndrome. Chron Dermatol (Roma) 1996;6:845–52.

84 Ponti G, Losi L, Pedroni M, et al. Value of MLH1 and MSH2 mutations in the appearance of Muir-Torre syndrome phenotype in HNPCC patients presenting sebaceous gland tumors or keratoacanthomas. J Invest Dermatol 2006;126:2158–9.

85 Ponti G, Losi L, Di Gregorio C, et al. Identification of Muir-Torre syndrome among patients with sebaceous tumors and keratoacanthomas: role of clinical features, microsatellite instability, and immunohistochemistry. Cancer 2005;103:1018–25.

86 Bhutto AM, Shaikh A, Nonaka S. Incidence of xeroderma pigmentosum in Larkana, Pakistan: a 7-year study. Br J Dermatol 2005;152:545–51.

87 Gheeraert P, Goens J, Schwartz RA, et al. Florid cutaneous papillomatosis, malignant acanthosis nigricans, and pulmonary squamous cell carcinoma. Int J Dermatol 1991;30:193–7.

88 Schwartz RA, Burgess GH. Florid cutaneous papillomatosis. Arch Dermatol 1978;114:1803–6.

89 Beer GM, Widder W, Cierpka K, et al. Malignant tumors associated with nevus sebaceous: therapeutic consequences. Aesthetic Plast Surg 1999;23:224–7.

90 Buescher L, DeSpain JD, Diaz-Arias AA, et al. Keratoacanthoma arising in an organoid nevus during childhood: case report and literature review. Pediatr Dermatol 1991;8:117–9.

91 Wilkinson SM, Tan CY, Smith AG. Keratoacanthoma arising within organoid naevi. Clin Exp Dermatol 1991;16:58–60.

92 Ujiie H, Kato N, Natsuga K, et al. Keratoacanthoma developing on nevus sebaceous in a child. J Am Acad Dermatol 2007;56:S57–8.

93 Mehregan AH, Pinkus H. Life history of organoid nevi. Special reference to nevus sebaceus of Jadassohn. Arch Dermatol 1965;91:574–88.

94 Shaw JC, Storrs FJ, Everts E. Multiple keratoacanthomas after megavoltage radiation therapy. J Am Acad Dermatol 1990;23:1009–11.

95 Nelson LM. Self-healing pseudocancers of the skin. Calif Med 1959;90:49–54.

96 Stevanovic DV. [Recurrence of keratoacanthoma: change, exacerbation, regrowth, kerathoacanthoma duplex]. Ann Dermatol Syphiligr (Paris) 1969;96:415–20.

97 Hendricks WM. Sudden appearance of multiple keratoacanthomas three weeks after thermal burns. Cutis 1991;47:410–2.

98 Pattee SF, Silvis NG. Keratoacanthoma developing in sites of previous trauma: a report of two cases and review of the literature. J Am Acad Dermatol 2003;48:S35–8.

99 Janik JP, Bang RH. Traumatic keratoacanthoma arising in a 15-year-old boy following a motor vehicle accident. Pediatr Dermatol 2006;23:448–50.

100 Kimyai-Asadi A, Shaffer C, Levine VJ, et al. Keratoacanthoma arising from an excisional surgery scar. J Drugs Dermatol 2004;3:193–4.

101 Goldberg LH, Silapunt S, Beyrau KK, et al. Keratoacanthoma as a postoperative complication of skin cancer excision. J Am Acad Dermatol 2004;50:753–8.

102 Maydan E, Nootheti PK, Goldman MP. Development of a keratoacanthoma after topical photodynamic therapy with 5-aminolevulinic acid. J Drugs Dermatol 2006;5:804–6.

103 Brazzelli V, Barbagallo T, Prestinari F, et al. Keratoacanthoma in vitiligo lesion after UVB narrowband phototherapy. Photodermatol Photoimmunol Photomed 2006;22:211–3.

104 Cox S. Rapid development of keratoacanthomas after a body peel. Dermatol Surg 2003;29:201–3.

105 Daldon PE, Macedo de Souza E, Cintra ML. Hypertrophic lupus erythematosus: a clinicopathological study of 14 cases. J Cutan Pathol 2003;30:443–8.

106 Fanti PA, Tosti A, Peluso AM, et al. Multiple keratoacanthoma in discoid lupus erythematosus. J Am Acad Dermatol 1989;21:809–10.

107 Stevanovic D. [Keratoacanthoma after folliculitis barbae]. Hautarzt 1962;13:286.

108 De Moragas JM. Multiple keratoacanthomas. Relation to Jamarsan therapy of pemphigus foliaceus. Arch Dermatol 1966;93:679–83.

109 Hsu S, Hill AN, Conrad N, et al. Reactive multiple keratoacanthoma in a patient with chronic renal insufficiency. Br J Dermatol 2003;148:1270–1.

110 Kaptanoglu AF, Kutluay L. Keratoacanthoma developing in previous cryotherapy site for solar keratosis. J Eur Acad Dermatol Venereol 2006;20:197–8.

111 Craddock KJ, Rao J, Lauzon GJ, et al. Multiple keratoacanthomas arising post-UVB therapy. J Cutan Med Surg 2004;8:239–43.

112 Letzel S, Drexler H. Occupationally related tumors in tar refinery workers. J Am Acad Dermatol 1998;39:712–20.

113 Ghadially FN. The experimental production of keratoacanthomas in the hamster and the mouse. J Pathol Bacteriol 1959;77:277–82.

114 Ramselaar CG, van der Meer JB. The spontaneous regression of keratoacanthoma in man. Acta Derm Venereol 1976;56:245–51.

115 Maxwell TB, Lamb JH. Unusual reaction to application podophyllum resin. AMA Arch Dermatol Syphilol 1954;70:510–1.

116 Bordea C, Wojnarowska F, Millard PR, et al. Skin cancers in renal-transplant recipients occur more

frequently than previously recognized in a temperate climate. Transplantation 2004;77:574–9.

117 Ghadially FN. The role of the hair follicle in the origin and evolution of some cutaneous neoplasms of man and experimental animals. Cancer 1961;14:801–16.

118 Heslop JH. The histogenesis of experimental molluscum sebaceum. Br J Cancer 1958;12:553–60.

119 Ghadially FN. A comparative morphological study of the kerato-acanthoma of man and similar experimentally produced lesions in the rabbit. J Pathol Bacteriol 1958;75:441–53.

120 Yamagiwa K, Ichikawa K. Experimental study of the pathogenesis of carcinoma. J Cancer Res 1918;3:1–29.

121 Leibowitz E, Janniger CK, Schwartz RA, et al. Xeroderma pigmentosum. Cutis 1997;60:75–7, 81–4.

122 Batinac T, Zamolo G, Jonjic N, et al. p53 protein expression and cell proliferation in non-neoplastic and neoplastic proliferative skin diseases. Tumori 2004;90:120–7.

123 Vickers CF, Ghadially FN. Keratoacanthomata associated with psoriasis. Br J Dermatol 1961;73:120–4.

124 Lain EL, Markus RF. Early and explosive development of nodular basal cell carcinoma and multiple keratoacanthomas in psoriasis patients treated with cyclosporine. J Drugs Dermatol 2004;3:680–2.

125 Chuang TY, Heinrich LA, Schultz MD, et al. PUVA and skin cancer. A historical cohort study on 492 patients. J Am Acad Dermatol 1992;26:173–7.

126 Miot HA, Miot LD, da Costa AL, et al. Association between solitary keratoacanthoma and cigarette smoking: a case-control study. Dermatol Online J 2006;12:2.

127 Gassenmaier A, Pfister H, Hornstein OP. Human papillomavirus 25-related DNA in solitary keratoacanthoma. Arch Dermatol Res 1986;279:73–6.

128 Viviano E, Sorce M, Mantegna M. Solitary keratoacanthomas in immunocompetent patients: no detection of papillomavirus DNA by polymerase chain reaction. New Microbiol 2001;24:295–7.

129 Saftic M, Batinac T, Zamolo G, et al. HPV 6-positive giant keratoacanthoma in an immunocompetent patient. Tumori 2006;92:79–82.

130 Cribier B, Asch P, Grosshans E. Differentiating squamous cell carcinoma from keratoacanthoma using histopathological criteria. Is it possible? A study of 296 cases. Dermatology 1999;199:208–12.

131 Schwartz RA, Tarlow MM, Lambert WC. Keratoacanthoma-like squamous cell carcinoma within the fibroepithelial polyp. Dermatol Surg 2004;30:349–50.

132 Lawrence N, Reed RJ. Actinic keratoacanthoma. Speculations on the nature of the lesion and the role of cellular immunity in its evolution. Am J Dermatopathol 1990;12:517–33.

133 Janecka IP, Wolff M, Crikelair GF, et al. Aggressive histological features of keratoacanthoma. J Cutan Pathol 1977;4:342–8.

134 Zalewska-Kubicka L, Mikulska D, Nowak A. The ultrastructure of squamous cell carcinoma and keratoacanthoma with morphological characterization of the mast cells. Dermatol Klin Zab (Wroclaw) 2001;3:182.

135 Miracco C, De Santi MM, Lio R, et al. Quantitatively evaluated ultrastructural findings can add to the differential diagnosis between keratoacanthoma and well differentiated squamous cell carcinoma. J Submicrosc Cytol Pathol 1992;24:315–21.

136 Van De Staak WJ, Bergers AM. Intranuclear particles in keratoacanthoma: possible association with malignant degeneration. Dermatologica 1979;158:413–6.

137 Binder M, Steiner A, Mossbacher U, et al. Estimation of the volume-weighted mean nuclear volume discriminates keratoacanthoma from squamous cell carcinoma. Am J Dermatopathol 1998;20:453–8.

138 Ichikawa E, Ohnishi T, Watanabe S. Expression of keratin and involucrin in keratoacanthoma: an immunohistochemical aid to diagnosis. J Dermatol Sci 2004;34:115–7.

139 Phillips P, Helm KF. Proliferating cell nuclear antigen distribution in keratoacanthoma and squamous cell carcinoma. J Cutan Pathol 1993;20:424–8.

140 Herzberg AJ, Kerns BJ, Pollack SV, et al. DNA image cytometry of keratoacanthoma and squamous cell carcinoma. J Invest Dermatol 1991;97:495–500.

141 Seidman JD, Berman JJ, Moore GW, et al. Multiparameter DNA flow cytometry of keratoacanthoma. Anal Quant Cytol Histol 1992;14:113–9.

142 Graham JH. Selected precancerous skin and mucocutaneous lesions. In: Neoplasms of the skin and malignant melanoma. Chicago: Year Book Medical Publishers;1976. p. 69–121.

143 Jackson IT. Diagnostic problem of keratoacanthoma. Lancet 1969;1:490–2.

144 Hodak E, Jones RE, Ackerman AB. Solitary keratoacanthoma is a squamous-cell carcinoma: three examples with metastases. Am J Dermatopathol 1993;15:332–42; discussion 43–52.

145 Popkin GL, Brodie SJ, Hyman AB, et al. A technique of biopsy recommended for keratoacanthomas. Arch Dermatol 1966;94:191–3.

146 Chalet MD, Connors RC, Ackerman AB. Squamous cell carcinoma vs. keratoacanthoma: criteria for histologic differentiation. J Dermatol Surg 1975;1: 16–7.

147 Ohashi A, Ishizaki M, Kawana S, et al. Mechanism of transepithelial elimination of elastic fibers in keratoacanthoma. Pathol Int 2004;54:585–94.

148 Batinac T, Zamolo G, Coklo M, et al. Expression of cell cycle and apoptosis regulatory proteins in keratoacanthoma and squamous cell carcinoma. Pathol Res Pract 2006;202:599–607.

149 Kannon G, Park HK. Utility of peanut agglutinin (PNA) in the diagnosis of squamous cell carcinoma and keratoacanthoma. Am J Dermatopathol 1990;12:31–6.

150 Kanitakis J, Hoyo E, Hermier C, et al. Nucleolar organizer region enumeration in keratoacanthomas and squamous cell carcinomas of the skin. Cancer 1992;69:2937–41.

151 Tsuji T. Keratoacanthoma and squamous cell carcinoma: study of PCNA and Le(Y) expression. J Cutan Pathol 1997;24:409–15.

152 Klein-Szanto AJ, Barr RJ, Reiners JJ Jr, et al. Filaggrin distribution in keratoacanthomas and squamous cell carcinoma. Arch Pathol Lab Med 1984;108:888–90.

153 Kane CL, Keehn CA, Smithberger E, et al. Histopathology of cutaneous squamous cell carcinoma and its variants. Semin Cutan Med Surg 2004;23:54–61.

154 Lowes MA, Bishop GA, Cooke BE, et al. Keratoacanthomas have an immunosuppressive cytokine environment of increased IL-10 and decreased GM-CSF compared to squamous cell carcinomas. Br J Cancer 1999;80:1501–5.

155 Ho T, Horn T, Finzi E. Transforming growth factor alpha expression helps to distinguish keratoacanthomas from squamous cell carcinomas. Arch Dermatol 1991;127:1167–71.

156 Shuster S. A pseudo-malignant oncogene for skin cancer. Clin Exp Dermatol 2005;30:316–7.

157 Sleater JP, Beers BB, Stephens CA, et al. Keratoacanthoma: a deficient squamous cell carcinoma? Study of bcl-2 expression. J Cutan Pathol 1994;21:514–9.

158 Hu W, Cook T, Oh CW, et al. Expression of the cyclin-dependent kinase inhibitor p27 in keratoacanthoma. J Am Acad Dermatol 2000;42:473–5.

159 Papadavid E, Pignatelli M, Zakynthinos S, et al. The potential role of abnormal E-cadherin and alpha-, beta- and gamma-catenin immunoreactivity in the determination of the biological behaviour of keratoacanthoma. Br J Dermatol 2001;145:582–9.

160 Slater M, Barden JA. Differentiating keratoacanthoma from squamous cell carcinoma by the use of apoptotic and cell adhesion markers. Histopathology 2005;47:170–8.

161 Basta-Juzbasic A, Klenkar S, Jakic-Razumovic J, et al. Cytokeratin 10 and Ki-67 nuclear marker expression in keratoacanthoma and squamous cell carcinoma. Acta Dermatovenerol Croat 2004;12:251–6.

162 Krunic AL, Garrod DR, Madani S, et al. Immunohistochemical staining for desmogleins 1 and 2 in keratinocytic neoplasms with squamous phenotype: actinic keratosis, keratoacanthoma and squamous cell carcinoma of the skin. Br J Cancer 1998;77:1275–9.

163 Fernandez-Flores A. Apoptotic markers in the differential diagnosis of keratoacanthoma versus squamous cell carcinoma. Histopathology 2007;50:284–5.

164 Schwartz RA, Nemanic MK, Elias PM. Identification of basal cell carcinomas by fluorescent lectin staining of a tumor-specific disaccharide. Clin Res 1981;29:285A.

165 Pilch H, Weiss J, Heubner C, et al. Differential diagnosis of keratoacanthomas and squamous cell carcinomas: diagnostic value of DNA image cytometry and p53 expression. J Cutan Pathol 1994;21:507–13.

166 LeBoit PE. Can we understand keratoacanthoma? Am J Dermatopathol 2002;24:166–8.

167 Burgdorf WH, Pitha J, Fahmy A. Muir-Torre syndrome. Histologic spectrum of sebaceous proliferations. Am J Dermatopathol 1986;8:202–8.

168 Morris SR, deSousa JL, Barrett AW, et al. Benign fibrous histiocytoma of the eyelid mimicking keratoacanthoma. Ophthal Plast Reconstr Surg 2007;23:73–5.

169 Mooney MA, Meine J, Li H, et al. Exophytic pilomatricoma, clinically resembling keratoacanthoma, with peri-pilar differentiation: peripilomatricoma. J Cutan Pathol 1999;26:466.

170 Reich A, Kobierzycka M, Wozniak Z, et al. Keratoacanthoma-like cutaneous metastasis of lung cancer: a learning point. Acta Derm Venereol 2006;86:459–60.

171 Janniger CK, Kapila R, Schwartz RA, et al. Histoid lepromas of lepromatous leprosy. Int J Dermatol 1990;29:494–6.

172 Vassallo C, Brazzelli V, Ardigo M, et al. Multiple, keratoacanthoma-like nodules on a 47-year-old man: a rare presentation of cutaneous lupus erythematosus. Int J Dermatol 2003;42:950–2.

173 Poleksic S, Yeung KY. Rapid development of keratoacanthoma and accelerated transformation into squamous cell carcinoma of the skin: a mutagenic effect

of polychemotherapy in a patient with Hodgkin's disease? Cancer 1978;41:12–6.

174 Godbolt AM, Sullivan JJ, Weedon D. Keratoacanthoma with perineural invasion: a report of 40 cases. Australas J Dermatol 2001;42:168–71.

175 Cooper PH, Wolfe JT 3rd. Perioral keratoacanthomas with extensive perineural invasion and intravenous growth. Arch Dermatol 1988;124:1397–401.

176 Yoshikawa K, Katagata Y, Kondo S. Relative amounts of keratin 17 are higher than those of keratin 16 in hair-follicle-derived tumors in comparison with non-follicular epithelial skin tumors. J Invest Dermatol 1995;104:396–400.

177 Patel A, Halliday GM, Cooke BE, et al. Evidence that regression in keratoacanthoma is immunologically mediated: a comparison with squamous cell carcinoma. Br J Dermatol 1994;131:789–98.

178 Prehn RT. The paradoxical association of regression with a poor prognosis in melanoma contrasted with a good prognosis in keratoacanthoma. Cancer Res 1996;56:937–40.

179 Morita H, Sagami S. Analysis of lymphocyte subpopulations using monoclonal antibodies in a case of keratoacanthomas. Acta Dermatol (Kyoto) 1985;80:209–11.

180 Bayer-Garner IB, Ivan D, Schwartz MR, et al. The immunopathology of regression in benign lichenoid keratosis, keratoacanthoma and halo nevus. Clin Med Res 2004;2:89–97.

181 Korenberg R, Penneys NS, Kowalczyk A, et al. Quantitation of S100 protein-positive cells in inflamed and non-inflamed keratoacanthoma and squamous cell carcinoma. J Cutan Pathol 1988;15:104–8.

182 Di Lernia V, Ricci C, Albertini G. Spontaneous regression of keratoacanthoma can be promoted by topical treatment with imiquimod cream. J Eur Acad Dermatol Venereol 2004;18:626–9.

183 Stone OJ. Non-immunologic enhancement and regression of self-healing squamous cell carcinoma (keratoacanthoma)—ground substance and inflammation. Med Hypotheses 1988;26:113–7.

184 Flannery GR, Muller HK. Immune response to human keratoacanthoma. Br J Dermatol 1979;101:625–32.

185 Ramselaar CG, van der Meer JB. Non-immunological regression of dimethylbenz(A) anthracene-induced experimental keratoacanthomas in the rabbit. Dermatologica 1979;158:142–51.

186 Ramselaar CG, Ruitenberg EJ, Kruizinga W. Regression of induced keratoacanthomas in anagen (hair growth phase) skin grafts in mice. Cancer Res 1980;40:1668–73.

187 Clausen OP, Aass HC, Beigi M, et al. Are keratoacanthomas variants of squamous cell carcinomas? A comparison of chromosomal aberrations by comparative genomic hybridization. J Invest Dermatol 2006; 126:2308–15.

188 Machin P, Catasus L, Pons C, et al. Microsatellite instability and immunostaining for MSH-2 and MLH-1 in cutaneous and internal tumors from patients with the Muir-Torre syndrome. J Cutan Pathol 2002;29:415–20.

189 Langenbach N, Kroiss MM, Ruschoff J, et al. Assessment of microsatellite instability and loss of heterozygosity in sporadic keratoacanthomas. Arch Dermatol Res 1999;291:1–5.

190 Snider BL, Benjamin DR. Eruptive keratoacanthoma with an internal malignant neoplasm. Arch Dermatol 1981;117:788–90.

191 Sheridan AT, Dawber RP. Curettage, electrosurgery and skin cancer. Australas J Dermatol 2000;41:19–30.

192 Nedwich JA. Evaluation of curettage and electrodesiccation in treatment of keratoacanthoma. Australas J Dermatol 1991;32:137–41.

193 Goldschmidt H, Sherwin WK. Radiation therapy of giant aggressive keratoacanthomas. Arch Dermatol 1993;129:1162–5.

194 Neumann RA, Knobler RM. Argon laser treatment of small keratoacanthomas in difficult locations. Int J Dermatol 1990;29:733–6.

195 Kuflik EG. Cryosurgery updated. J Am Acad Dermatol 1994;31:925–44; quiz 44–6.

196 Cipollaro VA. The use of podophyllin in the treatment of keratoacanthoma. Int J Dermatol 1983;22:436–40.

197 Stevanovic D, Krunic A. Keratoacanthoma: a dangerous trap. In: Dermatology in Europe. Proceedings of the 1st Congress of the European Academy of Dermatology and Venereology; 1989 Sept 25–28; Florence, Italy; Oxford, UK: Blackwell; 1991. p. 390–2.

198 Klein E, Helm F, Milgrom H, et al. Tumors of the skin. II. Keratoacanthoma; local effect of 5-fluorouracil. Skin (Los Angeles) 1962;1:153–6.

199 de Visscher JG, van der Wal KG, Blanken R, et al. Treatment of giant keratoacanthoma of the skin of the lower lip with intralesional methotrexate: a case report. J Oral Maxillofac Surg 2002;60:93–5.

200 Gray RJ, Meland NB. Topical 5-fluorouracil as primary therapy for keratoacanthoma. Ann Plast Surg 2000;44:82–5.

201 Starzycki Z. Zastosowanie masci Efudix w lecze-niu rogowiaka kolczystokomorkowego (keratoacan-thoma). I. Kliniczna ocena wynikow leczenia. Przegl Dermatol 1980;67:470–4.

202 Odom RB, Goette DK. Treatment of keratoacan-thomas with intralesional fluorouracil. Arch Derma-tol 1978;114:1779–83.

203 Parker CM, Hanke CW. Large keratoacanthomas in difficult locations treated with intralesional 5-fluorouracil. J Am Acad Dermatol 1986;14:770–7.

204 Thiele JJ, Ziemer M, Fuchs S, et al. Combined 5-fluorouracil and Er:YAG laser treatment in a case of recurrent giant keratoacanthoma of the lower leg. Dermatol Surg 2004;30:1556–60.

205 Andreassi A, Pianigiani E, Taddeucci P, et al. Guess what! Keratoacanthoma treated with intralesional bleomycin. Eur J Dermatol 1999;9:403–5.

206 Remling R, Mempel M, Schnopp N, et al. [In-tralesional methotrexate injection: an effective time and cost saving therapy alternative in keratoacan-thomas that are difficult to treat surgically]. Hautarzt 2000;51:612–4.

207 Somlai B, Hollo P. [Use of interferon-alpha (IFN-alpha) in the treatment of keratoacanthoma]. Hautarzt 2000;51:173–5.

208 Oh CK, Son HS, Lee JB, et al. Intralesional interferon alfa-2b treatment of keratoacanthomas. J Am Acad Dermatol 2004;51:S177–80.

209 Cohen PR, Schulze KE, Teller CF, et al. Intralesional methotrexate for keratoacanthoma of the nose. Skin-med 2005;4:393–5.

210 Spieth K, Gille J, Kaufmann R. Intralesional methotrexate as effective treatment in solitary gi-ant keratoacanthoma of the lower lip. Dermatology 2000;200:317–9.

211 Dendorfer M, Oppel T, Wollenberg A, et al. Topi-cal treatment with imiquimod may induce regression of facial keratoacanthoma. Eur J Dermatol 2003;13:80–2.

212 Spitler LE, Levin AS, Fudenberg HH. Transfer fac-tor II: results of therapy. Birth Defects Orig Artic Ser 1975;11:449–56.

213 McNairy DJ. Intradermal triamcinolone therapy of keratoacanthomas. Arch Dermatol 1964;89:136–40.

214 Street ML, White JW Jr, Gibson LE. Multiple kera-toacanthomas treated with oral retinoids. J Am Acad Dermatol 1990;23:862–6.

215 Kazmierowski M, Bowszyc-Dmochowska M. Multi-ple keratoacanthomas treated with cryosurgery and retinoids. Postepy Dermatol (Poznan) 1997;14:397–402.

216 Ogasawara Y, Kinoshita E, Ishida T, et al. A case of multiple keratoacanthoma centrifugum margina-tum: response to oral etretinate. J Am Acad Dermatol 2003;48:282–5.

217 Szepietowski J, Wasik F. Keratoacanthoma treated with systemic methotrexate. Report of five cases with a short literature review of treatment modalities. Nouv Dermatol 1996;15:559–63.

218 Grine RC, Hendrix JD, Greer KE. Generalized erup-tive keratoacanthoma of Grzybowski: response to cy-clophosphamide. J Am Acad Dermatol 1997;36:786–7.

219 Mangas C, Bielsa I, Ribera M, et al. A case of multiple keratoacanthoma centrifugum marginatum. Derma-tol Surg 2004;30:803–6.

220 Yarosh D, Klein J, O'Connor A, et al. Effect of topi-cally applied T4 endonuclease V in liposomes on skin cancer in xeroderma pigmentosum: a randomised study. Xeroderma Pigmentosum Study Group. Lancet 2001;357:926–9.

221 Wright TI, Spencer JM, Flowers FP. Chemoprevention of nonmelanoma skin cancer. J Am Acad Dermatol 2006;54:933–46; quiz 47–50.

222 Borum K. The role of the mouse hair cycle in epi-dermal carcinogenesis. Acta Pathol Microbiol Scand 1954;34:542–53.

CHAPTER 7
Basal cell carcinoma

Robert A. Schwartz

Basal cell carcinoma (BCC) is the most common type of skin cancer in light-complexioned individuals. Two centuries of fair-skinned Europeans migrating to sunnier lands have boosted its presence. The risk for the development of BCC is increased in light-complexioned people, particularly those who always burn with no tan during exposure to sunlight, and who often have had severe and painful sunburns [1]. In general, its incidence is high in fair-skinned people and low in blacks, with intermediate pigmentation groups such as Polynesians falling in between. Multivariate analysis in a recent BCC study emphasized skin types I, II, and III; high sun exposure during beach holidays; and actinic keratosis as significant risk factors [2]. Unlike melanoma and squamous cell carcinoma (SCC), BCC only rarely metastasizes; rather, it is a local infiltrator, which, if neglected, may invade and destroy its underlying structures. The BCC is derived from incompletely differentiated immature keratinocytes of the epidermis or cutaneous appendages. As such, it has been viewed by some as a locally aggressive hamartoma. This view is supported by the general lack of cellular dysplasia but is contradicted by BCC's rare metastatic behavior. In general, the BCC does not derive from an identifiable precursor lesion.

Incidence and etiology

Indeed, BCC may be the most common human malignancy, affecting 750,000 Americans each year [3]. Its incidence correlates with geographic latitude and cumulative sun exposure [4], with most BCCs arising on sun-exposed body sites. The age-adjusted BCC incidence per 100,000 for non-Hispanic whites was 1269 in men and 692 in women in Arizona

in 1996, as compared with a rate in New Hampshire of 310 and 166 and in North Queensland of 2058 and 1195, all from that same year [5]. In all of America for 1994, the incidence was 407 and 212. In Australia, the age-standardized rate per 100,000 population for all nonmelanoma skin cancers was 1170; for BCC, 884; and for SCC, 387 [6].

The major etiologic pattern of SCC is chronic long-term exposure, whereas the model for BCC appears to be different, with short-term burning episodes being more important [7]. A strong association between actinic damage and BCC suggests that cumulative solar exposure, whether long-term or intense intermittent, is the main risk factor for BCC [8]. A large number of actinic keratoses conferred a greater than threefold risk for BCCs of both the head and the trunk in a recent Australian study. Many lentigines were associated with a greater than threefold risk of truncal BCC compared with a 50% increased risk of BCC of the head. Acute intense solar exposures sufficient to cause sunburn among people whose ability to tan makes the skin of their face generally less susceptible may produce this difference. A common BCC may rarely derive from an actinic keratosis [9].

Although ultraviolet light exposure is the most frequent carcinogenic agent, x-rays may also produce BCCs, especially if they are superficial so that dermal structures are left intact [10,11]. Like SCCs and melanomas, BCCs may develop in thermal and other scars. Unusual settings for BCCs have also been noted, including within chickenpox and vaccination scars, venipuncture sites, leishmanial scars, and burn scars; in an area of chronic otitis media; and within tattoos [12–14]. However, unlike the SCC, the BCC tends to develop on sun-exposed sites that do not entirely correspond to maximal solar exposure, such as in the inner canthus [7]. BCC is seen in excess among Japanese atomic bomb survivors [15].

Chemical carcinogens may produce BCC in animal models such as the mouse and rat; however, the role of arsenic as a possible carcinogen in humans is unclear [16]. Some feel that arsenic produces multiple superficial-type BCCs in humans. The BCC may also develop beside or within melanocytic nevi, actinic keratoses, or seborrheic keratoses, sometimes as a presumably coincidental "collision" event or one stimulated by carcinogenic factors such as irradiation.

Basic work on the biology of BCC has been slow because of the lack of a suitable animal or tissue culture model. The BCC exhibits a remarkable stromal dependence; attempts to transplant BCCs without stroma have been unsuccessful. Much effort has been expended in analyzing the stromal environment of BCCs [17]. BCCs have distinct epithelial–stromal–inflammatory patterns that correlate with BCC subtype and tumor progression. Presumably, diminishing host response and gain of permissive tissue environment facilitates neoplastic evolution from low to high risk for local recurrence of BCC and implicates a histologic continuum of dynamic host–BCC interactions. BCC cells have properties different from those of normal keratinocytes, as demonstrated by a number of lectins, monoclonal antibodies, and autoantibodies [18]. The high molecular weight polysaccharide hyaluronan is a major component of the extracellular matrix between the vital cells of human epidermis. The levels of hyaluronan, and those of the hyaluronan receptor CD44 and the hyaluronan-binding proteoglycan versican, correlate with the aggressiveness of different human carcinomas of epithelial origin. Histochemical and immunocytochemical analysis of BCC subtypes shows promise, employing new technologies, including monoclonal antibodies. Matrix metalloproteinases (MMPs) with collagenolytic and gelatinolytic activities are up-regulated in BCC. An interaction of interstitial fibroblasts with high molecular weight fragments of type I collagen leading to increased MMP production has been demonstrated [19].

BCCs tend to be more aggressive in immunosuppressed patients; both cell-mediated and humoral immunity are probably important defenses against this common skin cancer [20]. BCCs are associated with *PTCH* and/or *p53* tumor suppressor gene alterations [15]. Alteration of both genes may play a role in BCC carcinogenesis. Indeed, mutations associated with its pathogenesis—those known to activate hedgehog (Hh) signaling pathway genes, including *PATCHED* (*PTCH*), sonic hedgehog (*Shh*) and smoothened (*Smo*)—have been studied extensively [3]. In skin, this Shh pathway is crucial for maintaining stem cell population, regulating hair follicle and sebaceous gland development, and activation in many neoplasms. The occasional association with metastatic BCC and AIDS has been noted but does not seem to foreshadow an additional dimension to the AIDS story. Whether chemopreventive effects of oral synthetic retinoids or nonsteroidal anti-inflammatory agents will be useful is still under evaluation [21]. Indeed, development of pathogenesis-based therapies, such as retinoids, cyclooxygenase inhibitors, topical immunomodulators, and inhibitors of the Shh signaling pathway, is intriguing [22].

Historical aspects

The first description of BCC has been credited to the Irish ophthalmologist Arthur Jacob [23] in 1827. He described "a destructive ulceration of peculiar character which I have observed to attack the eyelids, and extend to the eye-ball, orbit and face. The characteristic features of the disease are, the extraordinary slowness of its progress; the peculiar condition of the edges and surface of the ulcer . . . ." He argued that it should not be "confounded with genuine carcinoma." It was known for many years as Jacob's ulcer. Other terms used include *chancroid ulcer, ulcus exedens, benign skin cancer, rodent ulcer,* and *basal cell epithelioma.* The latter is still used today and is equally acceptable.

A number of foreign-language synonyms, including *basalzellenkrebse* and later *basalioma,* have been used since the early 20th century [24]. One still occasionally sees the term *basalioma* used in the English literature.

Table 7.1 Major clinical types of BCC

Noduloulcerative
Superficial
Sclerosing
Pigmented
Cystic

Clinical features

There are five main types of BCC (Table 7.1): typical noduloulcerative, pigmented, cystic, superficial, and sclerosing. All these types tend to be situated on the face, with the exception of superficial BCC, which is more likely on the trunk. However, BCC may occur at any site, including the vulva, where it accounts for 2% to 3% of all vulvar cancers [25,26]; scrotum [27–29]; palms [30]; soles [31]; and the nail bed, where it usually resembles an ulcer, chronic dermatitis, or chronic paronychia [32,33]. Occasionally, BCCs may develop within tattoos, burns, chronic leg ulcers, chickenpox scars, vaccination scars, and colostomy sites [12–14].

Noduloulcerative BCC

Noduloulcerative BCC, the most common form, is classically evident as a pearly dome-shaped nodule with central umbilication and border telangiectasia (Fig. 7.1). In Australia, the age-standardized incidence rates for nodular BCC were 727 per 100,000 men and 411 for women, which is about twice as common as multifocal superficial BCC [34]. Telangiectasia may be evident, with fine ectatic blood vessels transversing the papule or nodule. When evaluating small BCCs, one screens for coloration, because a yellowish hue makes one consider benign sebaceous hyperplasia and the rare BCC with sebaceous differentiation, also known as sebaceous epithelioma. A 1- to 3-mm papular BCC is usually rather regular and smooth. As it expands, a more dome-shaped morphology is apparent, often with a central umbilication and a tendency to be friable after minor trauma. The noduloulcerative BCC is usually nonpigmented, although flecks of brown pigment are not rare.

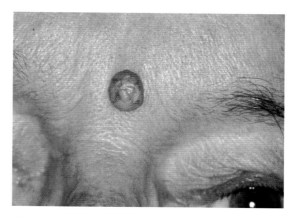

Fig. 7.1 Basal cell carcinoma of the forehead, showing a translucent nodule with central umbilication and border telangiectasia in a light-complexioned man. (Reprinted with permission from Klein E, Schwartz RA. Cancer and the skin. In: Holland JF, Frei S 3rd, editors. Cancer medicine. 2nd ed. Philadelphia: Lea & Febiger; 1982. p. 2057–108.)

Pigmented BCC

Pigmented BCC may display a uniformly dark pigmentation resembling that of a melanoma; however, its biologic behavior is that of the typical noduloulcerative BCC (Fig. 7.2). Occasionally, the cystic BCC may also have a considerable amount of pigmentation, although it is more likely to clinically resemble a benign appendageal tumor than a melanoma [35]. Pigmented BCCs may also rarely occur as giant pedunculated tumors. A nodular BCC may show a "speckled appearance" of brown-black pigmentation within and/or at its border, a helpful clinical sign [36]. Longitudinal melanonychia may rarely represent a subungual BCC [37].

Cystic BCC

Cystic BCC is distinctly uncommon. It may appear as a blue-gray cystic nodule suggestive of an apocrine hidrocystoma [35]. Cystic BCCs may be divided into two clinical types. One is a small cyst of light bluish gray coloration (Fig. 7.3); the other is variable in size and may be quite large. Both are often mistaken for benign cutaneous cysts.

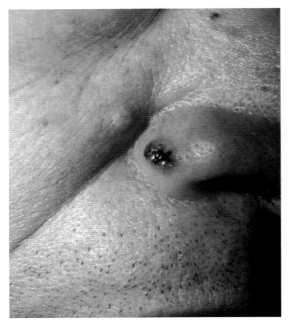

Fig. 7.2 Pigmented BCC on the nose of a Chinese man. The lesion is not translucent and resembles a common melanocytic nevus (mole).

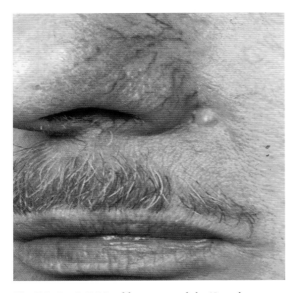

Fig. 7.3 Cystic BCC, a blue-gray nodule. Note the evidence of chronic solar damage, including prominent telangiectasia on the nose. (Reprinted with permission from Martinelli et al. [32].)

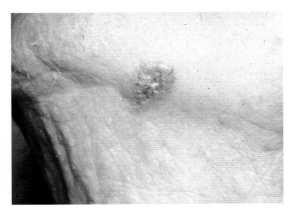

Fig. 7.4 Enlarging superficial BCCs on the chin developing a nodular quality with central atrophy and focal crusting and ulceration.

Superficial BCC

The superficial BCC appears as a flat plaque with a thin threadlike border of pearly translucency (Fig. 7.4). This border facilitates distinction from a plaque of Bowen's disease or of psoriasis. The central part of this usually oval plaque may be somewhat atrophic, at times with focal crusting and ulceration. Spotty pigmentation may be evident. As it enlarges, a more impressive nodular quality may develop. The most common site of the superficial BCC is the trunk, although it may occur elsewhere. Multiple superficial BCCs on the trunk should alert the clinician to the possibility of the basal cell nevus syndrome [38]. A superficial BCC on the scalp may be misdiagnosed and treated as seborrheic dermatitis because of its appearance as an erythematous plaque [39]. Dermoscopic examination of superficial BCC may be of value [40] (see Chapter 12).

Sclerosing BCC

The sclerosing or morphea-like form of BCC is usually evident as an infiltrating plaque, most commonly on the face. It represents about 9% to 11% of BCCs and is also commonly found on the trunk or limbs [39]. There seems to be a more equal distribution of superficial BCCs on face, trunk, and limbs than with nodular BCC [34,41]. Because it is asymptomatic and may not arouse suspicion, it

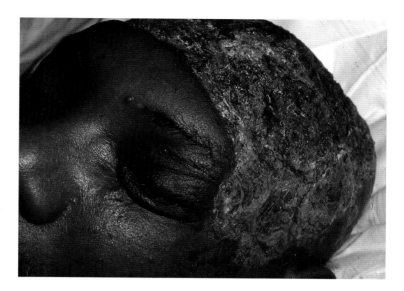

Fig. 7.5 Sclerosing infiltrating BCC involving much of the scalp in a black man who also had BCC metastatic to the bone marrow, producing a myelophthisic anemia. (Reprinted with permission from Schwartz et al. [115].)

may be present for a long time before being evaluated. Its scar-like appearance may be an ominous sign, because sclerosing BCC tends to be deeply invasive. The sclerosing BCC tends to develop at a younger age compared with other BCCs, sometimes during adolescence. At times, the sclerosing component may be less evident than the infiltrating one. Some distinguish a sclerosing BCC from an infiltrative BCC [42], possibly a useful clinicopathologic distinction (Fig. 7.5). A typical nodular BCC may be associated with sclerosing components, which infiltrate deeply.

and histologic pattern of a typical BCC, with erosion. Some believe that the FEP more closely resembles trichoblastoma than BCC [46]. Dermoscopic examination may be of value [47].

The "wild-fire" type of BCC is characterized by a rapidly expanding plaque with crusting, ulceration, and scarring [48]. One can usually appreciate components of both the noduloulcerative BCC and the sclerosing type with peripheral expansion, which prompt urgent recognition.

The giant pore type of BCC is evident on the face as a 2- to 10-mm orifice, usually skin colored

Rare clinical types of BCC

The rare types of BCC are listed in Table 7.2. Although unusual, these variants merit comment. BCC may evolve in a premalignant fibroepithelioma of Pinkus (FEP), or fibroepithelioma, as described by Pinkus [43] in 1953. Clinically, these tumors appear as papillomas or "fleshy" sessile fibromas. They may be broad-based flat plaques or pedunculated, tending to be smooth surfaced with a pink or reddish coloration, and characteristically appear on the lower back. They may be pigmented [44]. They may follow many years after local x-ray therapy [45]. The fibroepithelioma gradually evolves into the clinical

Table 7.2 Rare clinical types of BCC

Fibroepithelioma
"Wild-fire" BCC
Giant pore BCC
Angiomatous BCC
Lipoma-like BCC
Giant exophytic BCC
Keratoproliferative BCC (Kuflik tumor)
Blue-gray cystic BCC
Cystic BCC
Intraoral BCC
Sebaceous epithelioma
Metatypical carcinoma

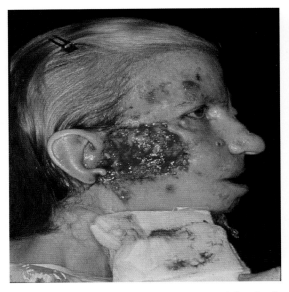

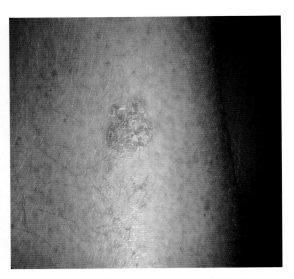

Fig. 7.7 Keratoproliferative (hyperkeratotic) BCC. (Courtesy of E. Kuflik, MD.)

Fig. 7.6 Giant exophytic BCC in a patient with basal cell nevus syndrome.

and without apparent evidence of tumor formation, such as nodularity, translucency, or telangiectasia. It could represent a localized follicular abnormality. Follicular abnormalities are seen in the follicular atrophoderma with BCC syndrome as described by Bazex, which will be discussed shortly.

The angiomatous BCC appears clinically as a bluish or violaceous nodule with a somewhat cystic quality and is exceedingly rare. The lipoma-like BCC, also exceedingly rare, displays a remarkable clinical resemblance to the lipoma [49]. More common of the rare types of BCC than the two previously mentioned is the giant exophytic BCC (Fig. 7.6). These tumors often represent neglected BCCs. They may be seen in the basal cell nevus syndrome [38]. Often the translucent quality of a BCC is missing, and one clinically suspects it may be either a cutaneous lymphoma or an SCC. These large neglected BCCs are the ones that tend to occasionally metastasize [50].

The hyperkeratotic BCC displays prominent hyperkeratotic components clinically, to the extent that it may have the morphology of a cutaneous horn [51]. More commonly, the BCC may show firm, thick adherent scale to suggest other clinical entities. The keratotic component may be especially prominent on the lower extremities, where neovascularization may add to the dull reddish coloration clinically. Labeled "kerato-purpuric" by Kuflik [52], it might better be called the keratoproliferative type of BCC (Fig. 7.7).

The intraoral BCC is a controversial entity. Its clinical features are variable. Many patients reported with it probably had an ameloblastoma or a salivary gland tumor instead. The intraoral BCC may present as a sessile gingival swelling [53], although it may also appear as an exophytic nodule or as an oral ulceration [54].

Metatypical carcinoma (MTC) , an important entity, was first described in 1910 [55,56]. MacKee and Cipollaro [57] in 1937 referred to it as basal-squamous-cell epithelioma and noted that it was known by the French as *épithéliome metatypique*, *épithéliome mixte*, or *épithéliome pavimenteux et intermédaire* and had been described previously by a number of authors. MacKee and Cipollaro [57] commented, "It has been known for many years that about 10 or 15 per cent of clinical basal-cell epitheliomas contain prickle or squamous epithelial cells." Montgomery [24] found characteristics of MTC in 12.6% of a series of 119 cases of clinical BCC. This type of neoplasm was noted then and has been observed since to be clinically indistinguishable from BCC, but with a course more likely to be rapid, with metastases and death [55]. MTC has thus been widely recognized for a long time as a specific entity, defined as a neoplasm with the features of a BCC with foci of squamous differentiation and spindle cell areas. MTC is generally considered more aggressive than the common BCC or the sun-induced cutaneous SCC.

Metatypical carcinoma is not common. In one retrospective study of 2075 skin cancers from pathology records, 31 MTCs were identified in 28 patients with a median age at diagnosis of 68 years (range, 10 to 94 years) [58]. Thus, MTCs constituted 1.5% of the total number of skin cancers. Most were located on the head and neck. MTC may be seen in many settings, including in association with a nevus sebaceous and with xeroderma pigmentosum [59,60]. The clinical diagnosis is difficult and must be confirmed by histologic findings. The course of tumor may be aggressive, with the potential for recurrence and distant metastases. Metastases occur mainly to the lung, bone, lymph node, liver, spleen, and adrenal gland [61]. The aggressive course may be attributed to the immunologic response of the patient, neoplasm size, and degree of anaplasia of the SCC component, which is responsible for the potential of metastasis, because the BCC rarely metastasizes. Therefore, although the dimension of a tumor may play an important role in prognosis, the emphasis should be on the histologic findings, especially the SCC component.

Syndromic BCCs

Basal cell nevus syndrome

The basal cell nevus syndrome (BCNS) is a rare autosomal dominant condition originally described by Nomland [62] in 1932 as "congenital pigmented basal cell nevi." He felt the early skin nodules resembled the common mole clinically; we now know that they are BCCs from their inception. BCNS is caused by mutations of the *PTCH1* gene, which is mapped to chromosome 9q22.3 [63,64]. It is the human homologue of the *Drosophila* segment polarity gene *patched*. Mutations of this gene have been shown

in many but not all pedigrees. In BCNS, developmental abnormalities occur as a result of haploinsufficiency in heterozygotes for the mutated gene, whereas neoplastic complications arise from a classical two-hit tumor suppressor gene model [65]. With dermoscopy, BCCs can be detected in early stages by the presence of blue-gray globules in nodules less than 3 mm in diameter [66]. The acral pits have a characteristic dermoscopic pattern, with red globules that are mainly distributed in parallel lines inside flesh-colored, irregular-shaped, and slightly depressed BCCs.

The syndrome is characterized by combinations of the following [38]:

1 Multiple BCCs, with risk of transformation to aggressive BCCs

2 A positive family history

3 Keratinous cysts of the jaw

4 Epidermal cysts, including milia

5 Visceral hamartomas, such as mesenteric cysts, renal cysts, ovarian fibromas, uterine fibromas, and gastric polyps

6 Visceral malignancies, such as ovarian adenocarcinoma, ovarian fibrosarcoma, fibrosarcoma of the jaw, and ameloblastoma

7 Palmar and/or plantar pits

8 Skeletal abnormalities, including brachymetacarpalism, hypertelorism, and frontal bossing (Fig. 7.8)

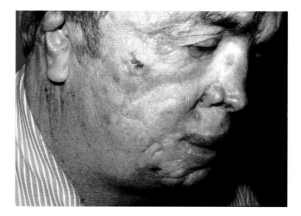

Fig. 7.8 A patient with BCNS displays frontal bossing, multiple BCCs, and extensive scarring as a result of previous treatment of BCCs.

9 Neurologic abnormalities associated with this syndrome, such as epilepsy, meningioma, and medulloblastoma [67–69]
10 Other neoplasms, including leiomyosarcoma, rhabdomyosarcoma, and fibrosarcoma [70–72].

One notable feature of this syndrome is the tendency for BCCs to develop in the patient at an early age, often on regions of the body unexposed to sunlight. In blacks with this syndrome, BCCs are rare and may not manifest themselves until very late in life, up to the age of 70 years [73].

A remarkable feature of this genodermatosis is that ionizing radiation appears to be specifically highly carcinogenic, with a latent period of 0.5 to 3.0 years rather than the usual lag of 20 to 50 years [74]. Chronologic tumor progression from basaloid hyperproliferation to nodular and then infiltrative BCC appears to occur in a stepwise fashion through the accumulation of sequential radiation-induced genetic alterations [75].

There are a number of tumors associated with BCNS, including ameloblastomas, medulloblastomas, meningiomas, and ovarian fibromas [38,73,76]. Probably the most common benign one is the simple epidermal inclusion cyst, which also occurs in Gardner's syndrome. Benign gastric hamartomatous polyps may also be seen in BCNS [38]. I have also seen renal hamartomas. Other benign tumors linked to this syndrome are mesenteric cysts, renal cysts, ovarian fibromas, and uterine fibromas [38,69,73,77,78]. More troubling is the possible tendency to develop ovarian adenocarcinomas and fibrosarcomas [73,79]. Maxillary sinus malignancies, especially fibrosarcomas, have also been observed [38,69,73].

Linear basal cell nevus

The linear unilateral basal cell nevus is a congenital noninherited eruption of closely set BCCs, comedones, epidermal inclusion cysts, and other benign appendageal tumors [80]. It is probably best viewed as a linear systematized nevus. Comedones may be absent. Its most common site is periocular, with half at this anatomic location [81]. This is in essence a type of linear epidermal nevus, so one should carefully evaluate these patients for stigmata of the neurocutaneous syndrome of benign skeletal and central nervous system abnormalities with linear epidermal nevi [82]. It may be significant that the patient reported by Bleiberg and Brodkin [83] had scoliosis. Whereas in the linear unilateral basal cell nevus the BCCs are often present at birth or early in life, there is a parallel disorder in which the BCCs, when and if they evolve, do so after puberty. That hamartoma is called the nevus sebaceus.

The Bazex syndrome

Bazex syndrome or the Bazex-Dupré-Christol syndrome is composed of follicular atrophoderma, evident as "multiple ice pick marks" on the elbow and dorsal hands, with the often early onset of pigmented nevoid BCCs, hypohidrosis, and hypotrichosis [84,85]. Miliaria and follicular atrophoderma may be its first sign [86]. This X-linked dominant disease (gene location: Xp24–q27) that is thought to be a disorder of the hair follicle may be first evident as a scarring scalp folliculitis [87,88]. Scalp hair may show marked twisting and flattening. Keratosis pilaris and pigmentary anomalies may also be seen, as may trichoepitheliomas, a common mimicker of BCC [89].

The Muir-Torre syndrome

The Muir-Torre syndrome (MTS) consists of multiple sebaceous neoplasms and keratoacanthomas in association with multiple internal low-grade malignancies [90,91]. BCCs with sebaceous differentiation, also called sebaceous epitheliomas, are often seen in this syndrome. The sebaceous epithelioma may have a yellowish hue in addition to the usual morphology of a BCC. It usually appears as a small translucent papule or nodule. Recognition of this syndrome is important for a number of reasons:
1 The sebaceous neoplasms with sebaceous epitheliomas or sebaceous carcinomas are slow growing and nonaggressive, whereas some sebaceous carcinomas may be aggressive.
2 The internal malignancies are of low malignant potential, so management may be different. For example, one might resect a solitary pulmonary metastasis in a patient with MTS who has colonic adenocarcinoma.

3 One must evaluate these patients for multiple visceral malignancies and do so at regular intervals, perhaps every 6 months.

4 Because it is probably autosomal dominant, locating one patient mandates investigating the family.

5 The immunohistochemical testing for *MSH2* and *MLH1* of sebaceous adenomas, keratoacanthomas, BCCs, colon polyps, and visceral neoplasms may be useful for rapid identification of an underlying mismatch repair defect and early diagnosis of MTS. Genetic testing may also reveal microsatellite instability in the cutaneous and visceral tumors [92–94].

This syndrome is a model for a defective mismatch repair gene. It is caused by germline mutations in DNA mismatch repair genes, mainly *MLH1* and *MSH2*. Clinical and biomolecular evidence suggests two types of MTS [93]. The germline mutation in one mismatch repair gene is complemented by a second somatic mutation in the contralateral allele, resulting in lack of gene expression and high-grade microsatellite instability due to accumulated mutations in short repetitive DNA sequences (microsatellites) [92]. The most common variant is characterized by defects in mismatch repair genes and early-onset tumors. The second type does not show deficiency in mismatch repair, and has a pathogenesis that remains undefined. There is also a phenotype that has multiple keratoacanthomas and no sebaceous neoplasms [93]. The syndrome may represent a more complete phenotype of the gene responsible for the cancer family syndrome [95]. Families with cutaneous manifestations typical of MTS often show a heritable mutation of the mismatch DNA repair gene *MSH2* and close linkage of that disease to a locus on chromosome 2p [96]. Significant and tight genetic linkage to the D2S123 locus on chromosome 2p was found in some families with MTS, a site also linked to a type of the cancer family syndrome [97]. In addition, a novel genetic defect in DNA replication, microsatellite instability, has been documented in multiple tumors of some MTS patients and others of the cancer family syndrome [93]. This supports the possibility that the subgroup of MTS demonstrating microsatellite instability and cancer family syndrome patients with the same defect may be allelic [93], and further

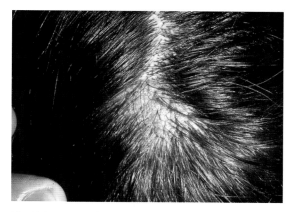

Fig. 7.9 Nevus sebaceus of the scalp, a yellowish nodule with a cobblestoned surface.

upholds the concept of a defective mismatch DNA repair gene accounting for patients with these two syndromes [96,98]. Some patients may represent sporadic cases or fresh mutations; others may be genetically distinct disorders.

Nevus sebaceus with BCC formation

The nevus sebaceus of Jadassohn may be seen at birth as a small, slightly verrucous, yellowish, hairless nodule, which at puberty grows as epidermis and appendageal structures become hyperplasic (Fig. 7.9). In one series of 15 patients, six nevi sebaceus (14%) developed a BCC [99]. Other tumors associated include a host of benign appendageal ones as well as SCC, keratoacanthoma, and rarely apocrine adenocarcinoma [100]. Nevus sebaceus may rarely be extensive and linear.

Congenital and inherited disorders associated with BCC are summarized in Table 7.3.

Table 7.3 Genetic and congenital disorders associated with BCC

Basal cell nevus syndrome
Linear basal cell nevus
Follicular atrophoderma and BCCs (Bazex syndrome)
Muir-Torre syndrome
Xeroderma pigmentosum
Nevus sebaceus with BCC formation

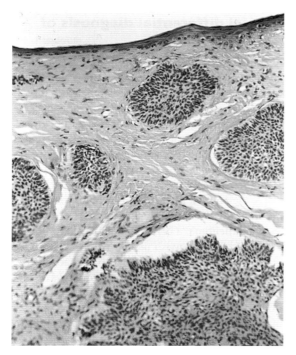

Fig. 7.10 Histologic pattern of common nodular BCC showing normal epidermis with dermal tumor masses. Note the palisading of these cells peripherally and retraction of the tumor within the dermis.

or eccrine glands [120,121]. Rarely, the BCC may display histology resembling that of an ameloblastoma, which is a locally aggressive epidermal tumor of dental origin [96], or other unusual characteristics that will be delineated shortly.

The individual cells of the BCC are usually uniform in appearance, with relatively large nuclei and a strong affinity for basic dyes. Their cytoplasm is scant and basophilic. Individual cell outlines may be indistinct. Desmosomes are less prominent than in the normal stratum basalis, although they may be quite evident in some BCCs. Tumor masses usually appear connected to the epidermis or to an appendageal structure.

The dermis surrounding the tumor masses often displays evidence of interaction. There is a proliferation of young fibroblasts and the appearance of a loose basophilic mucinous connective tissue. During tissue fixation, connective tissue tends to shrink and

retract from the BCC tumor mass, so there may be gaps around the periphery of the tumor. Although the BCC may secrete hyaluronidase, which could reproduce these changes, it is generally agreed that most of the shrinkage is fixation artifact. The basophilic degeneration from solar elastosis may be striking; however, sites of prevalence of BCCs do not entirely correlate with the elastotic patches from solar exposure.

Special types of histological patterns include:
1 Keratotic BCC with parakeratotic stratum corneum
2 Sebaceous differentiation of the sebaceous epithelioma (also called BCC with sebaceous differentiation—a possible marker for MTS of multiple sebaceous neoplasms, keratoacanthomas, and multiple low-grade visceral malignancies) [79]
3 Adenoid histologic-type BCC, with its lace-like pattern of interconnected tumor strands, producing a glandlike structure
4 Sclerosing BCC with abundant dense stroma with multiple islands of compressed tumor cells (Fig. 7.11)
5 Pigmented BCC with histologic evidence of melanocytes with large amounts of melanin
6 Superficial-type BCC with superficial tumor buds that appear to originate at multiple foci from the overlying attached epidermis

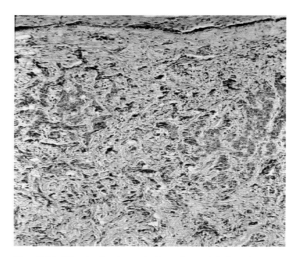

Fig. 7.11 Histologic view of sclerosing BCC showing islands of compressed tumor cells invading deeply.

7 Fibroepithelioma, with its long, thin anastomosing tumor cell strands [44,46,122]

8 Granular cell–type BCC [123,124]

9 Signet-ring–type BCC [125]

10 Clear cell–type BCC [126]

11 Cystic BCC [90,127–129], which may mimic other cysts, including inclusion cysts due to penetrating injury, mucoceles, apocrine hidrocystoma, and necrotic metastatic tumors

12 BCC with eccrine differentiation [120,130]

13 MTC with tumor lobules more irregular and peripheral palisading less pronounced but focally present. Stromal proliferation is more prominent. Often, areas of typical BCC may be seen to merge into a metatypical region. The most important histologic finding that confirms the MTC diagnosis is the absence of a transition zone between the basal cell and squamous cell types. Thus, the MTC is not a collision between a BCC and an SCC.

On occasion, more than one histologic pattern may be evident. For example, cystic changes are common histologically, although they may not be appreciated clinically. A solid-type BCC may be composed of two types of cells: some large and pale, and others dark staining with oval nuclei. More ominously, a solid BCC may show sclerosing components, which tend to infiltrate deeply. It has been suggested that the aggressiveness of an individual BCC be scored based on its depth of growth, degree of palisading, and narrow epithelial strand formation [131].

Therapeutic considerations

There are a number of treatment modalities available for a cutaneous BCC. The goal is to eradicate it with minimal disability and deformity. Each of the standard methods is effective because the BCC characteristically grows in a continuous cellular structure, enlarging by peripheral extension of narrow cellular strands rather than by uniform advancement of an entire tumor border. The four principal therapeutic options are excisional surgery, cryosurgery, curettage and electrodesiccation, and radiotherapy. Each of these techniques cures the BCC if it encompasses the entire tumor. Each BCC should be evaluated individually, and the choice of modality should be based on location, size, extent, clinical and histologic features, metastatic potential, and physician and patient experience with the therapeutic technique. Mohs micrographic surgery has become an important method of surgical excision for selected BCCs.

Small BCCs can be effectively handled with curettage and electrodessication, simple excision, and cryosurgery [132,133]. In certain anatomic locations in elderly persons, radiotherapy may be the treatment of choice. For recurrent BCCs or advanced or poorly defined ones, microscopically controlled excision (Mohs surgery) may be the best option. With superficial BCCs, topical chemotherapy, mainly 5-fluorouracil (5-FU) [134,135] or imiquimod [136,137], may be a useful option. Five percent 5-FU cream is effective and well tolerated, producing a good cosmetic outcome and patient satisfaction [135]. The same may be said for 5% imiquimod cream. Both may be applied daily until clinical resolution for extensive superficial facial BCCs [138]. Both may be beneficial for superficial and small nodular BCCs in BCNS [139]. Local destruction may also be supplemented by topical 5-FU or topical imiquimod.

It is unusual for a BCC to metastasize. When it does, systemic chemotherapy may be a good option [140,141], as may be radiotherapy [142]. Sentinel lymph node biopsy may have a role in treating certain high-risk BCCs [143].

References

1 Maksimovic N, Raznatovic M, Marinkovic J, et al. [Exposure to sun radiation as a risk factor for the occurrence of basal cell carcinoma in the Montenegrin population]. Vojnosanit Pregl 2006;63:643–7.

2 Ruiz Lascano A, Kuznitzky R, Garay I, et al. [Risk factors for basal cell carcinoma. Case-control study in Cordoba]. Medicina (B Aires) 2005;65:495–500.

3 Athar M, Tang X, Lee JL, et al. Hedgehog signalling in skin development and cancer. Exp Dermatol 2006;15:667–77.

4 Madan V, Hoban P, Strange RC, et al. Genetics and risk factors for basal cell carcinoma. Br J Dermatol 2006;154 Suppl 1:5–7.

5 Harris RB, Griffith K, Moon TE. Trends in the incidence of nonmelanoma skin cancers in

southeastern Arizona, 1985–1996. J Am Acad Dermatol 2001;45:528–36.

6 Staples MP, Elwood M, Burton RC, et al. Non-melanoma skin cancer in Australia: the 2002 national survey and trends since 1985. Med J Aust 2006; 184:6–10.

7 MacKie RM. Long-term health risk to the skin of ultraviolet radiation. Prog Biophys Mol Biol 2006; 92:92–6.

8 Neale RE, Davis M, Pandeya N, et al. Basal cell carcinoma on the trunk is associated with excessive sun exposure. J Am Acad Dermatol 2007;56: 380–6.

9 Lambert WC, Schwartz RA. Evidence for origin of basal cell carcinomas in solar (actinic) keratoses. J Cutan Pathol 1988;15:322.

10 Levi F, Moeckli R, Randimbison L, et al. Skin cancer in survivors of childhood and adolescent cancer. Eur J Cancer 2006;42:656–9.

11 Schwartz RA, Klein E. Ultraviolet light-induced carcinogenesis. In: Holland JF, Frei E 3rd, editors. Cancer medicine. Philadelphia: Lea & Febiger; 1982. p. 109–19.

12 Kowal-Vern A, Criswell BK. Burn scar neoplasms: a literature review and statistical analysis. Burns 2005;31:403–13.

13 Gurel MS, Inal L, Ozardali I, et al. Basal cell carcinoma in a leishmanial scar. Clin Exp Dermatol 2005;30:444–5.

14 Durrani AJ, Miller RJ, Davies M. Basal cell carcinoma arising in a laparoscopic port site scar at the umbilicus. Plast Reconstr Surg 2005;116:348–50.

15 Mizuno T, Tokuoka S, Kishikawa M, et al. Molecular basis of basal cell carcinogenesis in the atomic-bomb survivor population: p53 and PTCH gene alterations. Carcinogenesis 2006;27:2286–94.

16 Rossy KM, Janusz CA, Schwartz RA. Cryptic exposure to arsenic. Indian J Dermatol Venereol Leprol 2005;71:230–5.

17 Kaur P, Mulvaney M, Carlson JA. Basal cell carcinoma progression correlates with host immune response and stromal alterations: a histologic analysis. Am J Dermatopathol 2006;28:293–307.

18 Karvinen S, Kosma VM, Tammi MI, et al. Hyaluronan, CD44 and versican in epidermal keratinocyte tumours. Br J Dermatol 2003;148:86–94.

19 Yucel T, Mutnal A, Fay K, et al. Matrix metalloproteinase expression in basal cell carcinoma: relationship between enzyme profile and collagen fragmentation pattern. Exp Mol Pathol 2005;79: 151–60.

20 Synkowski DR, Schuster P, Orlando JC. The immunobiology of basal cell carcinoma: an in situ monoclonal antibody study. Br J Dermatol 1985;113: 441–6.

21 Grau MV, Baron JA, Langholz B, et al. Effect of NSAIDs on the recurrence of nonmelanoma skin cancer. Int J Cancer 2006;119:682–6.

22 Szeimies RM, Karrer S, Backer H. [Therapeutic options for epithelial skin tumors. Actinic keratoses, Bowen disease, squamous cell carcinoma, and basal cell carcinoma]. Hautarzt 2005;56:430–40.

23 Jacob A. An ulcer of peculiar character, which attacks the eye-lids and other parts of the face. Dublin Hosp Rep 1827;4:232–9.

24 Montgomery H. Basal squamous cell epithelioma. Arch Dermatol Syphilol 1928;18:50–73.

25 Pisani C, Poggiali S, De Padova L, et al. Basal cell carcinoma of the vulva. J Eur Acad Dermatol Venereol 2006;20:446–8.

26 de Giorgi V, Salvini C, Massi D, et al. Vulvar basal cell carcinoma: retrospective study and review of literature. Gynecol Oncol 2005;97:192–4.

27 Handa Y, Kato Y, Ishikawa H, et al. Giant superficial basal cell carcinoma of the scrotum. Eur J Dermatol 2005;15:186–8.

28 Kinoshita R, Yamamoto O, Yasuda H, et al. Basal cell carcinoma of the scrotum with lymph node metastasis: report of a case and review of the literature. Int J Dermatol 2005;44:54–6.

29 Ribuffo D, Alfano C, Ferrazzoli PS, et al. Basal cell carcinoma of the penis and scrotum with cutaneous metastases. Scand J Plast Reconstr Surg Hand Surg 2002;36:180–2.

30 Johnson DE. Basal-cell epithelioma of the palm. A report of a case. Arch Dermatol 1960;82:253–6.

31 Hyman AB, Michaelides P. Basal-cell epithelioma of the sole: report of a case with features of the fibroepithelial tumor. Arch Dermatol 1963;87:481–5.

32 Martinelli PT, Cohen PR, Schulze KE, et al. Periungual basal cell carcinoma: case report and literature review. Dermatol Surg 2006;32:320–3.

33 de Giorgi V, Salvini C, Massi D, et al. Ungual basal cell carcinoma on the fifth toe mimicking chronic dermatitis: case study. Dermatol Surg 2005;31: 723–5.

34 Raasch BA, Buettner PG, Garbe C. Basal cell carcinoma: histological classification and body-site distribution. Br J Dermatol 2006;155:401–7.

35 Schwartz RA, Hansen RC, Maize JC. The blue-gray cystic basal cell epithelioma. J Am Acad Dermatol 1980;2:155–60.

36 Goldberg LH, Friedman RH, Silapunt S. Pigmented speckling as a sign of basal cell carcinoma. Dermatol Surg 2004;30:1553–5.

37 Rudolph RI. Subungual basal cell carcinoma presenting as longitudinal melanonychia. J Am Acad Dermatol 1987;16:229–33.

38 Southwick GJ, Schwartz RA. The basal cell nevus syndrome: disasters occurring among a series of 36 patients. Cancer 1979;44:2294–305.

39 Yazici AC, Unal S, Ikizoglu G, et al. Superficial basal cell carcinoma of the scalp mimicking seborrhoeic dermatitis. Scand J Plast Reconstr Surg Hand Surg 2006;40:54–6.

40 Giacomel J, Zalaudek I. Dermoscopy of superficial basal cell carcinoma. Dermatol Surg 2005;31:1710–3.

41 Nadiminti U, Rakkhit T, Washington C. Morpheaform basal cell carcinoma in African Americans. Dermatol Surg 2004;30:1550–2.

42 Siegle RJ, MacMillan J, Pollack SV. Infiltrative basal cell carcinoma: a nonsclerosing subtype. J Dermatol Surg Oncol 1986;12:830–6.

43 Pinkus H. Premalignant fibroepithelial tumors of skin. AMA Arch Dermatol Syphilol 1953;67:598–615.

44 Strauss RM, Edwards S, Stables GI. Pigmented fibroepithelioma of Pinkus. Br J Dermatol 2004;150:1208–9.

45 Colomb D, Brechard JL, Gho A, et al. On five new cases of association of basal cell carcinoma and multiple Pinkus fibroepithelial tumors on the spine following radiation damage to the skin [author's transl]. Ann Dermatol Venereol 1979;106:875–82.

46 Bowen AR, LeBoit PE. Fibroepithelioma of Pinkus is a fenestrated trichoblastoma. Am J Dermatopathol 2005;27:149–54.

47 Zalaudek I, Leinweber B, Ferrara G, et al. Dermoscopy of fibroepithelioma of Pinkus. J Am Acad Dermatol 2005;52:168–9.

48 Kuflik EG. The "field-fire" basal-cell carcinoma: treatment by cryosurgery. J Dermatol Surg Oncol 1980;6:247–9.

49 Sutton RL Jr. Lipoma-like basal cell epithelioma. Arch Dermatol Syphilol 1943;48:176–8.

50 Ionescu DN, Arida M, Jukic DM. Metastatic basal cell carcinoma: four case reports, review of literature, and immunohistochemical evaluation. Arch Pathol Lab Med 2006;130:45–51.

51 Misago N, Satoh T, Narisawa Y. Cornification (keratinization) in basal cell carcinoma: a histopathological and immunohistochemical study of 16 cases. J Dermatol 2004;31:637–50.

52 Kuflik EG. Basal-cell carcinoma: an unusual clinical and histologic variant. J Dermatol Surg Oncol 1980;6:730–2.

53 Andreadis D, Nomikos A, Epivatianos A, et al. Basaloid squamous cell carcinoma versus basal cell adenocarcinoma of the oral cavity. Pathology 2005;37:560–3.

54 Samit AM. Intraoral basal cell carcinoma. J Surg Oncol 1978;10:27–32.

55 MacCormac H. The relationship of rodent ulcer to squamous cell carcinoma of the skin. Arch Meddlesex Hosp 1910;19:172–83.

56 Skroza N, Panetta C, Schwartz RA, et al. Giant metatypical carcinoma: an unusual tumor. Acta Dermatovenerol Croat 2006;14:46–51.

57 MacKee GM, Cipollaro AC. Cutaneous cancer and precancer: a practical monograph. New York: The American Journal of Cancer; 1937. p. 1–222.

58 Martin RC, 2nd, Edwards MJ, Cawte TG, et al. Basosquamous carcinoma: analysis of prognostic factors influencing recurrence. Cancer 2000;88: 1365–9.

59 Sari A, Basterzi Y, Yavuzer R, et al. Linear nevus sebaceus complicated with metatypical carcinoma. Plast Reconstr Surg 2002;109:1466–7.

60 Youssef N, Vabres P, Buisson T, et al. Two unusual tumors in a patient with xeroderma pigmentosum: atypical fibroxanthoma and basosquamous carcinoma. J Cutan Pathol 1999;26: 430–5.

61 Banks ER, Frierson HF Jr, Mills SE, et al. Basaloid squamous cell carcinoma of the head and neck. A clinicopathologic and immunohistochemical study of 40 cases. Am J Surg Pathol 1992;16: 939–46.

62 Nomland R. Multiple basal cell epitheliomas originating from congenital pigmented basal cell nevi. Arch Dermatol 1932;25:1002–8.

63 Panhuysen CI, Karban A, Knodle Manning A, et al. Identification of genetic loci for basal cell nevus syndrome and inflammatory bowel disease in a single large pedigree. Hum Genet 2006;120:31–41.

64 Pruvost-Balland C, Gorry P, Boutet N, et al. [Clinical and genetic study in 22 patients with basal cell nevus syndrome]. Ann Dermatol Venereol 2006;133:117–23.

65 High A, Zedan W. Basal cell nevus syndrome. Curr Opin Oncol 2005;17:160–6.

66 Kolm I, Puig S, Iranzo P, et al. Dermoscopy in Gorlin-Goltz syndrome. Dermatol Surg 2006;32:847–51.

67 Mortimer PS, Geaney DP, Liddell K, et al. Basal cell naevus syndrome and intracranial meningioma. J Neurol Neurosurg Psychiatry 1984;47:210–2.

68 Murphy MJ, Tenser RB. Nevoid basal cell carcinoma syndrome and epilepsy. Ann Neurol 1982;11:372–6.

69 Jackson R, Gardere S. Nevoid basal cell carcinoma syndrome. Can Med Assoc J 1971;105:850 passim.

70 Bhattacharjee P, Leffell D, McNiff JM. Primary cutaneous carcinosarcoma arising in a patient with nevoid basal cell carcinoma syndrome. J Cutan Pathol 2005;32:638–41.

71 Watson J, Depasquale K, Ghaderi M, et al. Nevoid basal cell carcinoma syndrome and fetal rhabdomyoma: a case study. Ear Nose Throat J 2004;83: 716–8.

72 Seracchioli R, Colombo FM, Bagnoli A, et al. Primary ovarian leiomyosarcoma as a new component in the nevoid basal cell carcinoma syndrome: a case report. Am J Obstet Gynecol 2003;188:1093–5.

73 Howell JB. Nevoid basal cell carcinoma syndrome. Profile of genetic and environmental factors in oncogenesis. J Am Acad Dermatol 1984;11:98–104.

74 Bacanli A, Ciftcioglu MA, Savas B, et al. Nevoid basal cell carcinoma syndrome associated with unilateral renal agenesis: acceleration of basal cell carcinomas following radiotherapy. J Eur Acad Dermatol Venereol 2005;19:510–1.

75 Mancuso M, Pazzaglia S, Tanori M, et al. Basal cell carcinoma and its development: insights from radiation-induced tumors in Ptch1-deficient mice. Cancer Res 2004;64:934–41.

76 Rushing EJ, Olsen C, Mena H, et al. Central nervous system meningiomas in the first two decades of life: a clinicopathological analysis of 87 patients. J Neurosurg 2005;103:489–95.

77 Gorlin RJ. Nevoid basal-cell carcinoma syndrome. Medicine (Baltimore) 1987;66:98–113.

78 Johnson AD, Hebert AA, Esterly NB. Nevoid basal cell carcinoma syndrome: bilateral ovarian fibromas in a 3 1/2-year-old girl. J Am Acad Dermatol 1986;14:371–4.

79 Kraemer BB, Silva EG, Sneige N. Fibrosarcoma of ovary. A new component in the nevoid basal-cell carcinoma syndrome. Am J Surg Pathol 1984;8:231–6.

80 Mavrikakis I, Malhotra R, Barlow R, et al. Linear basal cell carcinoma: a distinct clinical entity in the periocular region. Ophthalmology 2006;113:338–42.

81 Lane JE, Allen JH, Lane TN, et al. Unilateral basal cell carcinomas: an unusual entity treated with photodynamic therapy. J Cutan Med Surg 2005;9:336–40.

82 Shumaker PR, Lane K, Harford R. Linear unilateral basal cell nevus: a benign follicular hamartoma simulating multiple basal cell carcinomas. Cutis 2006; 78:122–4.

83 Bleiberg J, Brodkin RH. Linear unilateral basal cell nevus with comedones. Arch Dermatol 1969;100:187–90.

84 Plosila M, Kiistala R, Niemi KM. The Bazex syndrome: follicular atrophoderma with multiple basal cell carcinomas, hypotrichosis and hypohidrosis. Clin Exp Dermatol 1981;6:31–41.

85 Mehta VR, Potdar R. Bazex syndrome. Follicular atrophoderma and basal cell epitheliomas. Int J Dermatol 1985;24:444–6.

86 Beljan G, Metze D. [Miliaria and follicular atrophodermia as an early sign of Bazex-Dupre-Christol syndrome]. J Dtsch Dermatol Ges 2004;2:602–4.

87 Vabres P, Lacombe D, Rabinowitz LG, et al. The gene for Bazex-Dupre-Christol syndrome maps to chromosome Xq. J Invest Dermatol 1995;105:87–91.

88 Gambichler T, Hoffjan S, Altmeyer P, et al. A case of sporadic Bazex-Dupre-Christol syndrome presenting with scarring folliculitis of the scalp. Br J Dermatol 2007;156:184–6.

89 Yung A, Newton-Bishop JA. A case of Bazex-Dupre-Christol syndrome associated with multiple genital trichoepitheliomas. Br J Dermatol 2005;153:682–4.

90 Schwartz RA, Flieger DN, Saied NK. The Torre syndrome with gastrointestinal polyposis. Arch Dermatol 1980;116:312–4.

91 Lambert WC, Kasznica J, Chung HR, et al. Metastasizing basal cell carcinoma developing in a gunshot wound in a black man. J Surg Oncol 1984;27: 97–105.

92 Marazza G, Masouye I, Taylor S, et al. An illustrative case of Muir-Torre syndrome: contribution of immunohistochemical analysis in identifying indicator sebaceous lesions. Arch Dermatol 2006;142:1039–42.

93 Ponti G, Ponz de Leon M, Losi L, et al. Different phenotypes in Muir-Torre syndrome: clinical and biomolecular characterization in two Italian families. Br J Dermatol 2005;152:1335–8.

94 Ollila S, Fitzpatrick R, Sarantaus L, et al. The importance of functional testing in the genetic assessment of Muir-Torre syndrome, a clinical subphenotype of HNPCC. Int J Oncol 2006;28:149–53.

95 Barsky SH, Grossman DA, Bhuta S. Desmoplastic basal cell carcinomas possess unique basement membrane-degrading properties. J Invest Dermatol 1987;88:324–9.

96 Lerchin E, Rahbari H. Adamantinoid basal cell epithelioma. A histological variant. Arch Dermatol 1975;111:586–8.

97 Ono T, Egawa K, Higo J, et al. Basal cell epithelioma with giant tumor cells. J Dermatol 1985;12:344–8.

98 Mrak RE, Baker GF. Granular cell basal cell carcinoma. J Cutan Pathol 1987;14:37–42.

99 Baykal C, Buyukbabani N, Yazganoglu KD, et al. [Tumors associated with nevus sebaceous]. J Dtsch Dermatol Ges 2006;4:28–31.

100 Miller CJ, Ioffreda MD, Billingsley EM. Sebaceous carcinoma, basal cell carcinoma, trichoadenoma, trichoblastoma, and syringocystadenoma papilliferum arising within a nevus sebaceus. Dermatol Surg 2004;30:1546–9.

101 Mohs FE, Lathrop TG. Modes of spread of cancer of skin. AMA Arch Dermatol Syphilol 1952;66:427–39.

102 Farley RL, Manolidis S, Ratner D. Aggressive basal cell carcinoma with invasion of the parotid gland, facial nerve, and temporal bone. Dermatol Surg 2006;32:307–15; discussion 15.

103 Batra RS, Kelley LC. Predictors of extensive subclinical spread in nonmelanoma skin cancer treated with Mohs micrographic surgery. Arch Dermatol 2002;138:1043–51.

104 Bailin PL, Levine HL, Wood BG, et al. Cutaneous carcinoma of the auricular and periauricular region. Arch Otolaryngol 1980;106:692–6.

105 Van Scott EJ, Reinertson RP. The modulating influence of stromal environment on epithelial cells studied in human autotransplants. J Invest Dermatol 1961;36:109–31.

106 Brown CI, Perry AE. Incidence of perineural invasion in histologically aggressive types of basal cell carcinoma. Am J Dermatopathol 2000;22:123–5.

107 Morris JG, Joffe R. Perineural spread of cutaneous basal and squamous cell carcinomas. The clinical appearance of spread into the trigeminal and facial nerves. Arch Neurol 1983;40:424–9.

108 Tomich JM, Wagner RF Jr. Late recurrent basal cell carcinoma presenting as a unilateral exophthalmos. J Dermatol Surg Oncol 1986;12:866–8.

109 Rosen HM. Periorbital basal cell carcinoma requiring ablative craniofacial surgery. Arch Dermatol 1987;123:376–8.

110 Kleinberg C, Penetrante RB, Milgrom H, et al. Metastatic basal cell carcinoma of the skin. Metastasis to the skeletal system producing myelophthisic anemia. J Am Acad Dermatol 1982;7:655–9.

111 Chandler JJ, Lee L. Lymph node metastases from basal cell carcinoma. N Y State J Med 1982;82: 67–9.

112 von Domarus H, Stevens PJ. Metastatic basal cell carcinoma. Report of five cases and review of 170 cases in the literature. J Am Acad Dermatol 1984;10:1043–60.

113 Guillan RA, Johnson RP. Aspiration metastases from basal cell carcinoma: the 92nd known case. Arch Dermatol 1978;114:589–90.

114 Wermuth BM, Fajardo LF. Metastatic basal cell carcinoma. A review. Arch Pathol 1970;90:458–62.

115 Schwartz RA, De Jager RL, Janniger CK, et al. Giant basal cell carcinoma with metastases and myelophthisic anemia. J Surg Oncol 1986;33:223–6.

116 Coletta DF, Haentze FE, Thomas CC. Metastasizing basal cell carcinoma of the skin with myelophthisic anemia. Cancer 1968;22:879–84.

117 Lichtenstein HL, Lee JC. Amyloidosis associated with metastasizing basal cell carcinoma. Cancer 1980;46:2693–6.

118 Wieman TJ, Shively EH, Woodcock TM. Responsiveness of metastatic basal-cell carcinoma to chemotherapy. A case report. Cancer 1983;52:1583–5.

119 Westrom DR, Lapins NA. Merkel cell carcinoma mimicking a basal cell carcinoma. J Assoc Milit Dermatol 1986;12:15–7.

120 Hanke CW, Temofeew RK. Basal cell carcinoma with eccrine differentiation (eccrine epithelioma). J Dermatol Surg Oncol 1986;12:820–4.

121 Sakamoto F, Ito M, Sato S, et al. Basal cell tumor with apocrine differentiation: apocrine epithelioma. J Am Acad Dermatol 1985;13:355–63.

122 Katona TM, Ravis SM, Moores WB, et al. Expression of androgen receptor by fibroepithelioma of Pinkus—evidence supporting classification as a basal cell carcinoma variant. Am J Dermatopathol 2006;28: 230.

123 Kanitakis J, Chouvet B. Granular-cell basal cell carcinoma of the skin. Eur J Dermatol 2005;15:301–3.

124 Dundr P, Stork J, Povysil C, et al. Granular cell basal cell carcinoma. Australas J Dermatol 2004;45: 70–2.

125 Proia AD, Selim MA, Reutter JC, et al. Basal cell-signet-ring squamous cell carcinoma of the eyelid. Arch Pathol Lab Med 2006;130:393–6.

126 Morioka D, Kinoshita Y, Tanabe T, et al. Clear-cell basal cell carcinoma of the upper eyelid: a case report. Ann Plast Surg 1999;43:215–7.

127 Buckel TB, Helm KF, Ioffreda MD. Cystic basal cell carcinoma or hidrocytoma? The use of an excisional biopsy in a histopathologically challenging case. Am J Dermatopathol 2004;26:67–9.

128 Toyoda M, Morohashi M. Infundibulocystic basal cell carcinoma. Eur J Dermatol 1998;8:51–3.

129 Karcioglu ZA, al-Hussain H, Svedberg AH. Cystic basal cell carcinoma of the orbit and eyelids. Ophthal Plast Reconstr Surg 1998;14:134–40.

130 Chang YT, Liu HN, Wong CK. Penile basal cell carcinoma with eccrine differentiation. Clin Exp Dermatol 1995;20:487–9.

131 Afzelius LE, Ehnhage A, Nordgren H. Basal cell carcinoma in the head and neck. The importance of location and histological picture, studied with a new scoring system, in predicting recurrences. Acta Pathol Microbiol Scand [A] 1980;88:5–9.

132 Bath-Hextall F, Perkins W, Bong J, et al. Interventions for basal cell carcinoma of the skin. Cochrane Database Syst Rev 2007:CD003412.

133 Rodriguez-Vigil T, Vazquez-Lopez F, Perez-Oliva N. Recurrence rates of primary basal cell carcinoma in facial risk areas treated with curettage and electrodesiccation. J Am Acad Dermatol 2007;56: 91–5.

134 Klein E, Stoll HL Jr, Milgrom H, et al. Tumors of the skin. IV. Double-blind study on effects of local administration of anti-tumor agents in basal cell carcinoma. J Invest Dermatol 1965;44:351–3.

135 Gross K, Kircik L, Kricorian G. 5% 5-Fluorouracil cream for the treatment of small superficial basal cell carcinoma: efficacy, tolerability, cosmetic outcome, and patient satisfaction. Dermatol Surg 2007;33:433–40.

136 Choontanom R, Thanos S, Busse H, et al. Treatment of basal cell carcinoma of the eyelids with 5% topical imiquimod: a 3-year follow-up study [published online ahead of print on March 8, 2006]. Graefes Arch Clin Exp Ophthalmol. PMID: 17345092.

137 Vanaclocha F, Dauden E, Badia X, et al. Cost-effectiveness of treatment of superficial basal cell carcinoma: surgical excision vs. imiquimod 5% cream. Br J Dermatol 2007;156:769–71.

138 Micali M, Nasca MR, Musumeci ML. Treatment of an extensive superficial basal cell carcinoma of the face with imiquimod 5% cream. Int J Tissue React 2005;27:111–4.

139 Micali G, De Pasquale R, Caltabiano R, et al. Topical imiquimod treatment of superficial and nodular basal cell carcinomas in patients affected by basal cell nevus syndrome: a preliminary report. J Dermatolog Treat 2002;13:123–7.

140 Jefford M, Kiffer JD, Somers G, et al. Metastatic basal cell carcinoma: rapid symptomatic response to cisplatin and paclitaxel. ANZ J Surg 2004;74:704–5.

141 Carneiro BA, Watkin WG, Mehta UK, et al. Metastatic basal cell carcinoma: complete response to chemotherapy and associated pure red cell aplasia. Cancer Invest 2006;24:396–400.

142 Caloglu M, Yurut-Caloglu V, Kocak Z, et al. Metastatic giant basal cell carcinoma and radiotherapy. J Plast Reconstr Aesthet Surg 2006;59:783–4.

143 Harwood M, Wu H, Tanabe K, et al. Metastatic basal cell carcinoma diagnosed by sentinel lymph node biopsy. J Am Acad Dermatol 2005;53:475–8.

CHAPTER 8

Appendageal carcinomas and cutaneous sarcomas

Robert A. Schwartz

There are a number of uncommon skin cancers that are nevertheless noteworthy. This chapter covers cutaneous appendageal tumors and cutaneous sarcomas other than Kaposi's sarcoma. These cutaneous tumors are described histologically in Chapter 19.

Malignant appendageal tumors

Adnexal skin cancers are rare and can be divided by their origin into eccrine, apocrine, and pilosebaceous neoplasms. The histologic features, histogenesis, and classification of sweat gland carcinomas remain controversial [1,2]. These are further subdivided into neoplasms developing de novo and those arising from a precursor, which may be either a benign counterpart or a cutaneous multipotential hamartoma, especially the nevus sebaceus of Jadassohn. Low-grade adnexal carcinoma of the skin with multidirectional (glandular, trichoblastomatous, spiradenocylindromatous) differentiation also occurs [3]. Malignant sweat gland tumors commonly resemble cutaneous metastases from the breast and other sites. At times, there is a lack of correlation between histologic features and biologic behavior.

Eccrine cancers

Malignant eccrine poroma (eccrine porocarcinoma) was first described by Pinkus and Mehregan [4] in 1963 as epidermotropic eccrine carcinoma because of its ability to "parasitize the epidermis," producing a histologic pattern as seen in Paget's disease. It originates from the intraepidermal ductal portion (acrosyringium) of the eccrine gland [5]. It is a rare tumor that mostly affects older persons. It is the commonest eccrine cancer and may be evident as a solitary, sometimes ulcerated, nodule or plaque on the extremities or trunk in middle or old age that has the potential to metastasize widely [6]. It may resemble a cutaneous horn [7]. It may also be evident on the eyelid [8], or may develop within a nevus sebaceus [9]. Intraepidermal malignant eccrine poroma may pose diagnostic difficulties [10]. Regional cutaneous and systemic metastases are rarely observed; when they are, management has been generally unsuccessful [11].

Squamoid eccrine ductal carcinoma should be considered in the differential diagnosis of squamous cell carcinoma (SCC) and other cutaneous adnexal neoplasms showing squamoid and ductal features of differentiation. Mohs micrographic surgery may be a good option sufficient for complete surgical removal of eccrine carcinomas such as squamoid eccrine ductal carcinoma [12]. Clear cell hidradenoma has histopathologic features resembling those of eccrine poroma and eccrine spiradenoma. The biological behavior of the tumor is aggressive, with local recurrences in more than 50% of the surgically treated cases [13].

The Brooke-Spiegler syndrome is autosomal dominant and characterized by cylindromas, trichoepitheliomas, and occasionally spiradenomas [14]. Malignant degeneration of eccrine cylindroma ("turban tumor") is rare; when it occurs, local invasion into bone and brain may be seen [15,16]. Microcystic adnexal carcinoma (also known as syringomatous eccrine carcinoma, malignant

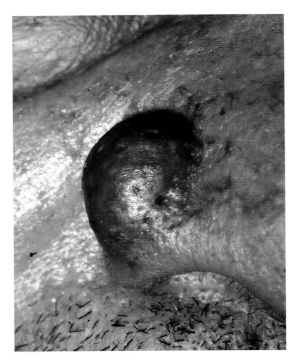

Fig. 8.1 Adenoid cystic carcinoma on the nose of an elderly white man.

syringoma, and sclerosing carcinoma of sweat ducts) tends to appear as a nonspecific slow-growing nodule or infiltrated plaque on the face, scalp, trunk, or extremities [17–19]. Of 15 patients in one review, half were men; the median age at presentation was 56 years [20]. It can occasionally be seen in children too. It may be locally destructive or metastasize widely. Some may be radiotherapy induced [21]. Mohs micrographic surgery is a good therapeutic option for it [22]. Mucinous eccrine carcinoma (primary mucinous carcinoma of skin) usually occurs as a painless, slow-growing nodule on the head and neck of middle-aged men [23], although it may appear anywhere on the body and in children or adults [24]. This neoplasm only rarely metastasizes and must be distinguished from the more common metastatic mucinous carcinoma of the breast and other sites, as well as from carcinoma of the salivary glands, and primary adenoid cystic carcinoma of the skin (Fig. 8.1) [25]. The latter

usually is an indolent locally aggressive nodule that may have regional lymph node metastases [26,27]. It has a high potential for recurrence after local excision [28]. Other rare eccrine tumors include the clear cell eccrine carcinoma, also known as nodular hidradenocarcinoma, which may be locally recurrent and tend to metastasize [29]. Malignant variants of eccrine spiradenomas are rare [30,31]. They may develop de novo or arise in preexisting benign eccrine spiradenoma, the former being most frequent [32]. Spiradenoma is a benign skin adnexal neoplasm that usually appears as a solitary nodule in any area of the body. Malignant transformation of a benign eccrine spiradenoma, first described by Maria Dabska [33] in 1972, has been observed by others [34]. Most cases have originated in a longstanding cutaneous nodule. These tumors may be aggressive; some have led to the patient's death [35]. Benign tumors demonstrating both spiradenomatous and cylindromatous features have been infrequently reported. The term *spiradenocylindrocarcinoma* was proposed to describe malignant tumors with features of both a spiradenoma and a cylindroma [30,36].

Aggressive digital papillary adenocarcinoma is a rare neoplasm of eccrine sweat gland origin that typically is evident as a mass on a finger, a toe, or the adjacent skin. Fewer than 100 cases have been noted. The majority have been in men in their fifth to seventh decade [37,38]. The tumors are locally aggressive, with a 50% local recurrence rate; 14% of them metastasize [39].

Apocrine cancers

Apocrine adenocarcinomas other than breast cancer and extramammary Paget's disease are rare. They usually occur where apocrine glands are located, in the axillae, vulva, and scrotum, although they can be anywhere [40,41]. They develop slowly in elderly people as reddish or violaceous tumors. Apocrine adenocarcinomas of the ocular region have the potential for aggressive biological behavior, including distant metastases [42]. In a series of 10 patients ranging from 25 to 91 years old, the apocrine adenocarcinomas were first evident as single or multinodular rubbery or cystic masses [43]. Ceruminoma and adenocarcinoma of Moll's glands of the eyelid are cancers of specialized apocrine glands of specific anatomic locations, ceruminous glands being confined to the skin lining of the cartilaginous part of the external auditory meatus. These cancers vary in histology and in malignant potential. The ceruminoma begins as a small nodule in the external auditory canal. When metastases occur, the regional lymph nodes are first involved, although lung and bone may become infiltrated. Controversy exists regarding the term *ceruminoma*. This neoplasia should be classified precisely as an adenoma, adenocarcinoma, adenoid cystic carcinoma, or pleomorphic ceruminous adenoma [44]. One should consider the possibility that an apparent apocrine adenocarcinoma of the skin may actually be a metastatic apocrine adenocarcinoma of the breast proper, or of ectopic or residual breast tissue. Primary cutaneous cribriform carcinoma is a rare apocrine tumor occurring in middle-aged people. This neoplasm is often located on the limbs [45].

Apocrine adenocarcinoma may arise from a benign apocrine hidrocystoma or from a nevus sebaceus [46]. Features that favor the diagnosis of a primary apocrine adenocarcinoma include the presence of relatively mature neoplastic glands high in the dermis, and a transitional zone with normal apocrine glands [47]. A positive correlation between tumor differentiation and prognosis has been noted. The distinction between apocrine adenomas and apocrine adenocarcinoma may at times be difficult [43]. Rarely, invasive apocrine adenocarcinoma may arise in a benign apocrine adenoma. Some mucinous carcinoma of the skin may have apocrine-type differentiation [48].

Sebaceous cancers

Sebaceous carcinoma is an unusual, aggressive, malignant tumor derived from the epithelium of sebaceous glands [49]. It may arise in ocular or extraocular sites and is often evident as an ulcerated or intact cystic nodule measuring up to 8 cm in diameter. It may rarely have a morpheaform appearance or appear as a periocular cutaneous horn [50]. A significant number of extraocular sebaceous carcinomas have been associated with metastases and a high mortality rate. True sebaceous carcinomas of the skin need to be distinguished from basal cell carcinomas (BCCs) with partial sebaceous differentiation, sebaceous epitheliomas, SCCs involving the hair follicles (producing malignant squamous masses with sebaceous differentiation), and cutaneous metastases of salivary gland tumors. The true sebaceous carcinoma of the skin is rare. Its malignant potential may vary from low to high. The most common eyelid malignancy in a 2006 study from the Republic of China was BCC (65.1%), followed by SCC (12.6%) and sebaceous cell carcinoma (7.9%) [51]. It tends to appear as a nonspecific slow- or fast-growing, ulcerated, solitary pink to red or yellowish nodule, most commonly on the upper eyelid or elsewhere on the face. Sebaceous carcinoma is known to masquerade clinically and histologically as a variety of periocular conditions, resulting in a delayed diagnosis. Histopathologic diagnosis may be challenging when this tumor has a bowenoid pattern of intraepithelial spread. Initial clinical diagnoses include blepharitis, blepharoconjunctivitis, and cicatrizing conjunctivitis. Many are misdiagnosed as Bowen's disease on the initial biopsy. Sebaceous carcinoma should always be considered in the histologic differential diagnosis of any eyelid lesion that resembles Bowen's disease, particularly if the upper eyelid is involved or if multivacuolated cytoplasmic clear cell changes are seen [52]. The eyelids have abundant sebaceous glands, including meibomian glands on the tarsal plates and glands of Zeis at the lid margin, caruncle, eyebrow, and lid skin. The most common type of sebaceous carcinoma originates in the meibomian glands; it may therefore be misdiagnosed and treated as a chalazion—a potential disaster, because widespread metastases may occur if the diagnosis is delayed. With a more lateral horizontal growth pattern, it may resemble conjunctivitis, blepharitis, or keratitis. In a series of 104 patients with sebaceous carcinoma of the eyelid and ocular adnexa, the average age was 64.5 years, with an age range from 32 to 93 years [53]. Therapeutic radiation to the ocular adnexa may be a predisposing factor. One should be sure that an apparent extraocular sebaceous carcinoma is not actually a metastasis from an eyelid or parotid gland primary cancer.

True sebaceous gland carcinomas, whether or not on the eyelid [54], may also occur as part of the Muir-Torre syndrome, in association with other sebaceous neoplasms (mostly sebaceous adenomas but also BCCs with sebaceous differentiation) [55]. Sebaceous carcinoma may arise in nevus sebaceus [56]. The Muir-Torre syndrome is discussed in Chapter 17. The histologic considerations of sebaceous carcinomas are covered in Chapter 19.

Pilar carcinomas

Pilomatrix carcinoma (or malignant pilomatricoma) is a rare malignancy that tends to be locally aggressive; at least three patients with this tumor have had metastatic disease [57,58]. Most pilomatrix carcinomas occur on the head and neck of elderly individuals, with a 5:1 predilection for males. Recently, a tumor was described arising from the stroma of a trichoblastoma, labeled a trichoblastic sarcoma [59]. Pilomatrix carcinoma is often clinically misdiagnosed as a sebaceous cyst. Surgical wide resection is the recommended treatment to reduce the risk of local recurrence by 50% [60]. Malignant pilomatricoma has a high risk of metastases to bones, lungs, and lymph nodes. No feature is specific to distinguish whether a malignant pilomatricoma has arisen de novo or represents the malignant transformation of a preexisting benign pilomatricoma.

Cutaneous sarcomas

Skin sarcomas are divided into those of vascular, fibrous, fat, muscular, and neural tissue origin. These may arise from the dermis or the subcutis. Their histology is described in Chapter 19. Patients with leiomyosarcomas, clear cell sarcomas, and malignant fibrous histiocytomas had a poorer survival rate, whereas those with fibrosarcomas, liposarcomas, and neurofibrosarcomas fared better [61]. Appropriate imaging, predictive immunologic and genetic studies, improved surgery, and newer methods of adjunctive and neoadjunctive treatment should result in improvements in outcomes for patients with these tumors.

Vascular tissue sarcoma

Malignant vascular tumors of the dermal and subcutaneous tissue include Kaposi's sarcoma, malignant angioendothelioma, and hemangiopericy-

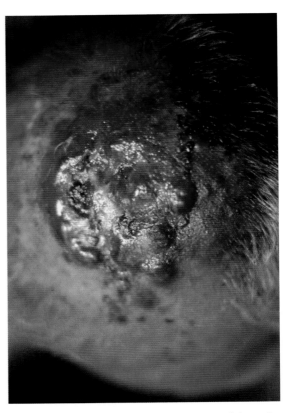

Fig. 8.2 Low-grade cutaneous angiosarcoma of the scalp. (Courtesy of Professor Chull-Wan Ihm, MD, President, Korean Dermatological Association and Chairman, Dermatology, Chonbuk National University, Jeonju.)

toma. Angiosarcomas resembling Kaposi's sarcoma have been described in homosexual men, but distinguishing anaplastic Kaposi's sarcoma from other angiosarcomas may be difficult [62]. Kaposi's sarcoma is the subject of Chapter 9.

Malignant angiosarcoma is clinically distinctive, appearing as a bruise-like plaque or as an erythematous nodule on the scalp, face, or neck in the elderly; it rapidly spreads to become a large colorless or purplish infiltrated plaque, at times displaying regions of erosion and purpura [63] (Fig. 8.2). It usually appears in normal skin, although it may do so in skin affected by discoid lupus erythematosus [64]. Underlying tissue may be infiltrated down to bone. Metastases to regional lymph nodes, lung, liver, and other viscera may occur within months. Three fourths of patients are men [65]. Tumor diameter, depth of invasion, positive margins, metastases, and tumor recurrence are the best predictors of outcome. The overall 5-year survival in one series was 34%. Low-grade angioendotheliomas may rarely complicate the nevus flammeus (port-wine stains) in children [66]. Cutaneous angiosarcoma may occur in patients with xeroderma pigmentosum [67].

The Dąbska tumor is a rare low-grade angiosarcoma also known as malignant endovascular papillary angioendothelioma of childhood [68]. First described by Maria Dąbska [69] in 1969, it primarily affects the skin of children and has a distinctive histologic pattern of anastomosing vascular channels with intravascular papillary outpouchings that project, sometimes in a glomerulus-like pattern, into a lumen lined by atypical columnar endothelial cells.

Another distinctive angiosarcoma, the Stewart-Treves syndrome, occurs on chronically edematous extremities as purplish red nodules [70,71]. It may be seen in congenital or acquired lymphedema, particularly after mastectomy [72]. Satellite areas develop and become confluent. Such lesions may be bullous or become ulcerative, necrotic, or papillomatous. Immunotherapy may be beneficial [73]. Angiosarcoma may also arise in sclerodermatous skin [74], a rare finding.

The development of cutaneous angiosarcoma is a rare but well-recognized complication after radiation therapy [75]. The average time from radiation to cutaneous angiosarcoma was 6 years. Angiosarcoma has also been reported in patients with Maffucci's syndrome of cavernous hemangioma and dyschondroplasia, although chondrosarcomas are a more frequent complication [76].

Proliferating angiomatosis (proliferating systematized angioendotheliomatosis, systemic endotheliomatosis, malignant proliferating angioendotheliomatosis, angioendotheliomatosis proliferans systematisata) may represent an intravascular angiosarcoma, an angiotrophic lymphoma, or a benign vascular hamartoma. This rare disorder has violaceous nodules and plaques that may be widespread across the skin and viscera or be confined to the lower extremities [77]. The lesions may resemble erythema nodosum or leukocytoclastic

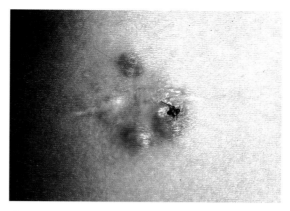

Fig. 8.3 Dermatofibrosarcoma protuberans, morphea-like sclerotic plaque, an early lesion.

vasculitis. Mason's pseudosarcoma (intravascular papillary endothelial hyperplasia) is a localized form appearing as cutaneous or subcutaneous nodules that may simulate benign vascular neoplasms. Histologically, it resembles an angiosarcoma but is benign.

Hemangiopericytomas arise from the pericytes of the capillaries in the skin; subcutaneous and musculoskeletal tissue, especially of the lower extremities and penis; the oral cavity; the mediastinum; and elsewhere [78–80]. Cutaneous malignant hemangiopericytoma tends to be evident as a nonspecific, solitary tumor. This sarcoma may occur congenitally, although it is most commonly acquired in the fifth and sixth decades of life. Median survival was 19 months for patients with hemangiopericytomas in one small series [79].

Fibrous tissue sarcomas

Tumors of the fibrous tissue of the skin include dermatofibrosarcoma protuberans (DFSP), subcutaneous fibrosarcoma, atypical fibroxanthoma, desmoid tumor, and nodular fasciitis. DFSP is an uncommon soft tissue sarcoma with a low to intermediate grade of malignancy that is locally aggressive [81,82]. DFSP is first evident as a small indurated fibrous plaque on the trunk or proximal extremities typically in people between 20 and 40 years old. However, it may occur at any age, including at birth, and may be challenging to diagnose in children [83–85] (Fig. 8.3). Surgical excision with adequate margins is the main treatment, as otherwise it has a high recurrence rate. Mohs surgery is a good option. DFSP may progress to multiple protuberant nodules and may ulcerate; it may have a sclerotic or morphea-like atrophic morphology instead of a protuberant contour [86]. This pattern tends to recur and may require a wider excision than might otherwise appear necessary. Fatal metastases do sometimes occur. Platelet-derived growth factor B is a near-universal translocation partner in chromosomal rearrangements in DFSP, leading to successful therapy targeting platelet-derived growth factor receptors [87]. Patients with locally advanced disease not suitable for wide surgical excision or with metastatic disease can be managed with the platelet-derived growth factor receptor inhibitor imatinib, with a high probability of response.

Subcutaneous fibrosarcomas occur most commonly as nonspecific nodules with normal skin overlying them [88]. This tumor most frequently involves the extremities in adults, characteristically between the ages of 40 and 60 years, and the head and neck in children. In the adult, it tends to recur after local excision. Metastases are much more common in adults than in children, so much so that the childhood form is sometimes considered benign and called aggressive fibromatosis or desmoid tumor. Thus, this tumor is a neoplasm that rarely becomes malignant. It does not metastasize but demonstrates an ability to locally infiltrate tissue. It is characterized by a high risk of recurrence after surgical treatment [89].

Epithelioid sarcoma is a distinctive fibrosarcoma, a tumor at times mistaken for a cutaneous granuloma, synovial sarcoma, angiosarcoma, or SCC [90–92]. It occurs in young adults as a firm, slow-growing, scar-like plaque, often on the extremities. It has a high propensity for locoregional recurrence and distant metastases. Adverse prognostic factors include large size, male sex, older age, necrosis, vascular invasion, rhabdoid cytomorphology, and inadequate excision. Early and vigorous surgery is necessary to avoid recurrences and late metastases.

The atypical fibroxanthoma (AFX) is usually a solitary cutaneous nodule on the extensively sun- or x-ray–damaged faces of elderly people [93,94] (Fig. 8.4). It resembles a vascular nodule with over-

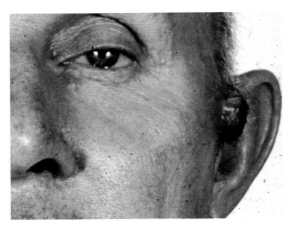

Fig. 8.4 Atypical fibroxanthoma on sun-exposed facial skin preauricularly.

lying skin normal, crusted, or ulcerated, and is suggestive of BCC, SCC, or pyogenic granuloma. Rarely, this tumor may occur on non–sun-exposed areas as a slowly enlarging nodule with normal overlying skin. Microscopically, it appears highly malignant, although only very rarely does it metastasize. Clear cell AFX is a rare variant of AFX, a pleomorphic dermal tumor associated with a good prognosis. Its diagnosis requires the exclusion of other pleomorphic clear cell tumors using a combination of morphology, immunohistochemistry, and electron microscopy [95]. AFXs recur in approximately 10% of cases but only rarely metastasize. Features associated with recurrence are inadequate excision and invasion into fat; those linked with metastasis include recurrence, vascular invasion, deep tissue invasion, and tumor necrosis [96]. This tumor is closely related to the malignant fibrous histiocytoma. The latter is much more likely to recur locally and to metastasize widely. Its benign counterpart, the fibrous histiocytoma, may at times require careful histologic distinction (Fig. 8.5).

The angiomatous malignant fibrous histiocytoma tends to occur in children and young adults as a cystic mass often accompanied by marked bleeding [97]. Myxofibrosarcoma is a subcutaneous, multinodular, or diffusely infiltrative neoplasm usually on the extremities of elderly people [98]. It should be excised radially. Nodular fasciitis is evident as a

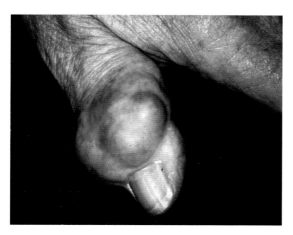

Fig. 8.5 Fibrous histiocytoma of the thumb, often classified as a giant cell tendon tumor.

solitary, rapidly developing, sometimes painful subcutaneous nodule that has been called a pseudosarcoma because of its fulminant growth and sarcoma-like histology [99]. It is most frequent in adults over 40 years of age, usually on the extremities. This not uncommon neoplasm is, fortunately, benign. However, it must be distinguished clinically from another painful deep nodular tumor, the synovial sarcoma [100]. Desmoid tumors are benign, often locally invasive fibrous neoplasms originating from muscle aponeuroses [101,102]. These firm nontender overgrowths of fibrous tissue are also known as "aggressive fibromatosis," tend to recur, and may be part of the autosomal dominant Gardner (familial adenomatosis polyposis) syndrome.

Liposarcomas

Liposarcomas are malignant neoplasms of fat [103,104]. They are seen as bulky, diffuse nodular tumors with normal overlying skin, sometimes attaining a huge size. They are most common on the upper thighs and buttocks, where they appear to arise from intermuscular fascia. They may rarely arise from a lipoma or be seen in patients with neurofibromatosis. Metastases to lungs and liver occur commonly, although microscopically well-differentiated tumors are less likely to metastasize than are more anaplastic ones. Higher age of onset, tumor grade, and tumor size seem to have a neg-

ative influence on survival [105]. Early diagnosis and appropriate therapy should give a high salvage rate. Some liposarcomas display a histologic pattern resembling that of the brown fat of hibernating animals, hence the name *malignant hibernoma*. However, several benign lipomatous tumors, such as benign lipoblastomas, intramuscular lipomas, spindle cell lipomas, and pleomorphic lipomas, may display the histologic criteria of malignancy.

Leiomyosarcoma

Cutaneous leiomyosarcomas are rare tumors originating from the arrector muscle of hair follicles or the smooth muscle of blood vessels that appear as nonspecific slow-growing nodules or an indurated plaque [106–109]. They may be tender and sometimes ulcerate. Metastases occur, particularly to the lymph nodes and lungs. Superficially localized leiomyosarcomas tend to be smaller than deeper-located sarcomas. The most reliable prognostic factor is the depth of tumor invasion. Cutaneous leiomyosarcomas have an indolent biological course if treated by surgical excision with wide margins.

Nerve tissue sarcomas

Tumors arising from neural structures in cutaneous and subcutaneous tissue include those developing from malignant degeneration of neurofibromas in neurofibromatosis, the rare malignant granular cell tumor, malignant neurilemoma, and multiple mucosal neuromas. Neurofibrosarcoma arises from small cutaneous nerves, is locally aggressive, and has a potential for metastasis [110]. It tends to be seen on the extremities of children and young to middle-aged adults as ill-defined cutaneous or subcutaneous nodules, occurring as sporadic neoplasms or in association with neurofibromatosis type 1 (von Recklinghausen's disease; NF-1). In one series of NF-1 patients, neurofibrosarcoma was documented in 1.8% [111]. Neurofibrosarcoma, the main cause of death of NF-1 patients less than 40 years of age, may develop de novo or from sarcomatous degeneration of a preexisting plexiform neurofibroma [112]. It should be suspected in patients with new onset of symptoms or in those with changing symptoms. Imaging shows a large heterogeneous tumor invading adjacent structures. The prognosis of childhood neurofibrosarcoma remains poor, with a high incidence of relapse, particularly in the lungs, suggesting that more aggressive therapy to control both local and distant relapse is needed. Malignant schwannoma also occurs without neurofibromatosis, sometimes at radiation sites, most often as a subcutaneous nodule on the extremities [113]. This rare sarcoma is located mostly on the trunk and extremities; the head and neck are unusual sites for its development. Almost half arise from neurofibromas with or without von Recklinghausen's disease, and most of the remainder develop de novo from peripheral nerve trunks. Malignant neurilemoma is also a rare, aggressive tumor, usually occurring as degeneration of a neurilemoma in a patient with neurofibromatosis [114,115]. The malignant granular cell tumor is a rare neoplasm that usually appears as a nonspecific, slowly growing, poorly defined nodule or mass. Extensive metastases may occur [116].

Other sarcomas

Rarely, one sees cutaneous rhabdomyosarcoma, osteosarcoma, chondrosarcoma, alveolar soft part sarcoma, extraskeletal Ewing's sarcoma, osteogenic sarcoma, or sometimes unclassifiable sarcoma. The clear cell sarcoma is usually best classified as a melanoma. Rhabdomyosarcoma is evident as a rare asymptomatic dermal nodule without distinctive clinical features [117,118]. It originates from the embryonic mesenchymal precursor of striated muscle and is even rarer in adults [119]. Congenital rhabdomyosarcoma is a highly malignant tumor with few if any long-term survivors. Alveolar soft part sarcoma is a rare malignancy of uncertain histogenesis; its two main sites are the lower extremities in adults and the head and neck in children [120]. It may appear as a slow-growing, painful, and pruritic mass in a child [121]. Children with this tumor have a more favorable prognosis than do adults. Tumor size seems to correlate with metastatic disease at onset and is the major factor influencing survival [122]. Surgery is the mainstay of therapy. Extraskeletal Ewing's sarcoma of the skin is rare [123]. Among 37 cases of cutaneous and subcutaneous Ewing's sarcoma, 21 were in girls and 16 in boys. Mean age at diagnosis was 15 years; mean tumor size was 3 cm (range, 1 to 12 cm) [124]. The prognosis for cutaneous Ewing's sarcoma appears more favorable than that of Ewing's sarcoma in bone. Of the 37 patients treated, seven had metastases and two relapsed. Treatment for cutaneous Ewing's sarcoma consists of polychemotherapy associated with surgery and/or radiotherapy. There is considerable overlap between primitive neuroectodermal tumor and extraosseous Ewing's sarcoma, as they may be the same tumor [125]. Some of the soft tissue sarcomas have pluripotential mesenchymal cell derivation or dedifferentiation, so classification may be difficult. Moreover, visceral sarcomas such as leiomyosarcomas, chondrosarcomas, and malignant fibrous histiocytomas may be first evident with cutaneous metastases [126] (see Chapter 16). Langerhans cell sarcoma is a rare proliferation of Langerhans cells with overtly malignant cytologic features diagnosed by CD1a positivity and/or the presence of Birbeck granules and cellular atypia with frequent mitoses. It occurs in skin, lymph nodes, liver, spleen, lung, and bone [127–129]. It may be first evident as a scalp or thigh tumor. It tends to have aggressive clinical behavior and a poor prognosis.

References

1 Urso C, Bondi R, Paglierani M, et al. Carcinomas of sweat glands: report of 60 cases. Arch Pathol Lab Med 2001;125:498–505.

2 Obaidat NA, Alsaad KO, Ghazarian D. Skin adnexal neoplasms—part 2: an approach to tumours of cutaneous sweat glands. J Clin Pathol 2007;60:145–59.

3 Kazakov DV, Kutzner H, Mukensnabl P, et al. Low-grade adnexal carcinoma of the skin with multidirectional (glandular, trichoblastomatous, spiradenocylindromatous) differentiation. Am J Dermatopathol 2006;28:341–5.

4 Pinkus H, Mehregan AH. Epidermotropic eccrine carcinoma. A case combining features of eccrine poroma and Paget's dermatosis. Arch Dermatol 1963;88:597–606.

5 Aydin E, Akdogan V, Akkuzu G, et al. Malignant eccrine poroma invading the parotid gland. Acta Otolaryngol 2006;126:435–7.

6 Goel R, Contos MJ, Wallace ML. Widespread metastatic eccrine porocarcinoma. J Am Acad Dermatol 2003;49:S252–4.

7 Lee YH, Kim SH, Suh MK, et al. Malignant eccrine poroma of the left upper eyelid resembling a cutaneous horn. Korean J Dermatol 2006;44:1469–71.

8 Kim Y, Scolyer RA, Chia EM, et al. Eccrine porocarcinoma of the upper eyelid. Australas J Dermatol 2005;46:278–81.

9 Tarkhan, II, Domingo J. Metastasizing eccrine porocarcinoma developing in a sebaceous nevus of Jadassohn. Report of a case. Arch Dermatol 1985;121:413–5.

10 Aslan F, Demirkesen C, Cagatay P, et al. Expression of cytokeratin subtypes in intraepidermal malignancies: a guide for differentiation. J Cutan Pathol 2006;33:531–8.

11 de Bree E, Volalakis E, Tsetis D, et al. Treatment of advanced malignant eccrine poroma with locoregional chemotherapy. Br J Dermatol 2005;152:1051–5.

12 Kim YJ, Kim AR, Yu DS. Mohs micrographic surgery for squamoid eccrine ductal carcinoma. Dermatol Surg 2005;31:1462–4.

13 Liapakis IE, Korkolis DP, Koutsoumbi A, et al. Malignant hidradenoma: a report of two cases and review of the literature. Anticancer Res 2006;26:2217–20.

14 Szepietowski JC, Wasik F, Szybejko-Machaj G, et al. Brooke-Spiegler syndrome. J Eur Acad Dermatol Venereol 2001;15:346–9.

15 Volter C, Baier G, Schwager K, et al. [Cylindrocarcinoma in a patient with Brooke-Spiegler syndrome]. Laryngorhinootologie 2002;81:243–6.

16 Pizinger K, Michal M. Malignant cylindroma in Brooke-Spiegler syndrome. Dermatology 2000;201:255–7.

17 Fernandez-Figueras MT, Montero MA, Admella J, et al. High (nuclear) grade adnexal carcinoma with microcystic adnexal carcinoma-like structural features. Am J Dermatopathol 2006;28:346–51.

18 Leibovitch I, Huilgol SC, Richards S, et al. Periocular microcystic adnexal carcinoma: management and outcome with Mohs' micrographic surgery. Ophthalmologica 2006;220:109–13.

19 Gabillot-Carre M, Weill F, Mamelle G, et al. Microcystic adnexal carcinoma: report of seven cases including one with lung metastasis. Dermatology 2006;212:221–8.

20 Friedman PM, Friedman RH, Jiang SB, et al. Microcystic adnexal carcinoma: collaborative series review and update. J Am Acad Dermatol 1999;41:225–31.

21 Beer KT, Buhler SS, Mullis P, et al. A microcystic adnexal carcinoma in the auditory canal 15 years after radiotherapy of a 12-year-old boy with nasopharynx carcinoma. Strahlenther Onkol 2005;181:405–10.

22 Lee K, Goo B, Jang JY, et al. Microcystic adnexal carcinoma treated by Mohs' micrographic surgery. Korean J Dermatol 2006;44:1444–7.

23 Antley CA, Carney M, Smoller BR. Microcystic adnexal carcinoma arising in the setting of previous radiation therapy. J Cutan Pathol 1999;26:48–50.

24 Bindra M, Keegan DJ, Guenther T, et al. Primary cutaneous mucinous carcinoma of the eyelid in a young male. Orbit 2005;24:211–4.

25 Schwartz RA, Wiederkehr M, Lambert WC. Secondary mucinous carcinoma of the skin: metastatic breast cancer. Dermatol Surg 2004;30:234–5.

26 Fueston JC, Gloster HM, Mutasim DF. Primary cutaneous adenoid cystic carcinoma: a case report and literature review. Cutis 2006;77:157–60.

27 Doganay L, Bilgi S, Aygit C, et al. Primary cutaneous adenoid cystic carcinoma with lung and lymph node metastases. J Eur Acad Dermatol Venereol 2004;18:383–5.

28 Krunic AL, Kim S, Medenica M, et al. Recurrent adenoid cystic carcinoma of the scalp treated with Mohs micrographic surgery. Dermatol Surg 2003;29:647–9.

29 Ohta M, Hiramoto M, Fujii M, et al. Nodular hidradenocarcinoma on the scalp of a young woman: case report and review of literature. Dermatol Surg 2004;30:1265–8.

30 Mashkevich G, Undavia S, Iacob C, et al. Malignant cylindroma of the external auditory canal. Otol Neurotol 2006;27:97–101.

31 Hantash BM, Chan JL, Egbert BM, et al. De novo malignant eccrine spiradenoma: a case report and review of the literature. Dermatol Surg 2006;32:1189–98.

32 Chou SC, Lin SL, Tseng HH. Malignant eccrine spiradenoma: a case report with pulmonary metastasis. Pathol Int 2004;54:208–12.

33 Dabska M. Malignant transformation of eccrine spiradenoma. Pol Med J 1972;11:388–96.

34 Fernandez-Acenero MJ, Manzarbeitia F, Mestre de Juan MJ, et al. Malignant spiradenoma: report of two cases and literature review. J Am Acad Dermatol 2001;44:395–8.

35 Granter SR, Seeger K, Calonje E, et al. Malignant eccrine spiradenoma (spiradenocarcinoma): a clinicopathologic study of 12 cases. Am J Dermatopathol 2000;22:97–103.

36 Carlsten JR, Lewis MD, Saddler K, et al. Spiradenocylindrocarcinoma: a malignant hybrid tumor. J Cutan Pathol 2005;32:166–71.

37 Bazil MK, Henshaw RM, Werner A, et al. Aggressive digital papillary adenocarcinoma in a 15-year-old female. J Pediatr Hematol Oncol 2006;28:529–30.

38 Mori O, Nakama T, Hashimoto T. Aggressive digital papillary adenocarcinoma arising on the right great toe. Eur J Dermatol 2002;12:491–4.

39 Keramidas EG, Miller G, Revelos K, et al. Aggressive digital papillary adenoma-adenocarcinoma. Scand J Plast Reconstr Surg Hand Surg 2006;40:189–92.

40 Ota Y, Fukasawa I, Shimizu K, et al. A case of T1N0M0 vulvar apocrine gland carcinoma with a positive outcome. Gynecol Oncol 2003;90:601–4.

41 Kiyohara T, Kumakiri M, Kawami K, et al. Apocrine carcinoma of the vulva in a band-like arrangement with inflammatory and telangiectatic metastasis via local lymphatic channels. Int J Dermatol 2003;42:71–4.

42 Shintaku M, Tsuta K, Yoshida H, et al. Apocrine adenocarcinoma of the eyelid with aggressive biological behavior: report of a case. Pathol Int 2002;52:169–73.

43 Warkel RL, Helwig EB. Apocrine gland adenoma and adenocarcinoma of the axilla. Arch Dermatol 1978;114:198–203.

44 Castro MC, Fagundes-Pereyra WJ, Oliveira Filho LN, et al. [Tumor of ceruminous gland with intracranial invasion: case report]. Arq Neuropsiquiatr 2000;58:324–9.

45 Adamski H, Le Lan J, Chevrier S, et al. Primary cutaneous cribriform carcinoma: a rare apocrine tumour. J Cutan Pathol 2005;32:577–80.

46 MacNeill KN, Riddell RH, Ghazarian D. Perianal apocrine adenocarcinoma arising in a benign apocrine adenoma; first case report and review of the literature. J Clin Pathol 2005;58:217–9.

47 Sugita K, Yamamoto O, Hamada T, et al. Primary apocrine adenocarcinoma with neuroendocrine differentiation occurring on the pubic skin. Br J Dermatol 2004;150:371–3.

48 Wako M, Nishimaki K, Kawamura N, et al. Mucinous carcinoma of the skin with apocrine-type differentiation: immunohistochemical studies. Am J Dermatopathol 2003;25:66–70.

49 Innocenzi D, Balzani A, Lupi F, et al. Morpheaform extra-ocular sebaceous carcinoma. J Surg Oncol 2005;92:344–6.

50 Kitagawa H, Mizuno M, Nakamura Y, et al. Cutaneous horn can be a clinical manifestation of underlying sebaceous carcinoma. Br J Dermatol 2007;156:180–2.

51 Lin HY, Cheng CY, Hsu WM, et al. Incidence of eyelid cancers in Taiwan: a 21-year review. Ophthalmology 2006;113:2101–7

52 Leibovitch I, Selva D, Huilgol S, et al. Intraepithelial sebaceous carcinoma of the eyelid misdiagnosed as Bowen's disease. J Cutan Pathol 2006;33:303–8.

53 Rao NA, Hidayat AA, McLean IW, et al. Sebaceous carcinomas of the ocular adnexa: a clinicopathologic study of 104 cases, with five-year follow-up data. Hum Pathol 1982;13:113–22.

54 Demirci H, Nelson CC, Shields CL, et al. Eyelid sebaceous carcinoma associated with Muir-Torre syndrome in two cases. Ophthal Plast Reconstr Surg 2007;23:77–9.

55 Schwartz RA, Torre DP. The Muir-Torre syndrome: a 25-year retrospect. J Am Acad Dermatol 1995;33:90–104.

56 Kazakov DV, Calonje E, Zelger B, et al. Sebaceous carcinoma arising in nevus sebaceus of Jadassohn: a clinicopathological study of five cases. Am J Dermatopathol 2007;29:242–8.

57 Niwa T, Yoshida T, Doiuchi T, et al. Pilomatrix carcinoma of the axilla: CT and MRI features. Br J Radiol 2005;78:257–60.

58 Sable D, Snow SN. Pilomatrix carcinoma of the back treated by Mohs micrographic surgery. Dermatol Surg 2004;30:1174–6.

59 Rosso R, Lucioni M, Savio T, et al. Trichoblastic sarcoma: a high-grade stromal tumor arising in trichoblastoma. Am J Dermatopathol 2007;29:79–83.

60 Petit T, Grossin M, Lefort E, et al. [Pilomatrix carcinoma: histologic and immunohistochemical features. Two studies]. Ann Pathol 2003;23:50–4.

61 Mankin HJ, Hornicek FJ. Diagnosis, classification, and management of soft tissue sarcomas. Cancer Control 2005;12:5–21.

62 Schwartz RA, Kardashian JF, McNutt NS, et al. Cutaneous angiosarcoma resembling anaplastic Kaposi's sarcoma in a homosexual man. Cancer 1983;51:721–6.

63 Chen W, Shih CS, Wang YT, et al. Angiosarcoma with pulmonary metastasis presenting with spontaneous bilateral pneumothorax in an elderly man. J Formos Med Assoc 2006;105:238–41.

64 Sarashi C, Nishioka K, Maeda M, et al. Malignant hemangioendothelioma in discoid lupus erythematosus. J Dermatol 1986;13:45–8.

65 Morgan MB, Swann M, Somach S, et al. Cutaneous angiosarcoma: a case series with prognostic correlation. J Am Acad Dermatol 2004;50:867–74.

66 Girard C, Johnson WC, Graham JH. Cutaneous angiosarcoma. Cancer 1970;26:868–83.

67 Marcon I, Collini P, Casanova M, et al. Cutaneous angiosarcoma in a patient with xeroderma pigmentosum. Pediatr Hematol Oncol 2004;21:23–6.

68 Schwartz RA, Dabski C, Dabska M. The Dabska tumor: a thirty-year retrospect. Dermatology 2000;201:1–5.

69 Dabska M. Malignant endovascular papillary angioendothelioma of the skin in childhood. Clinicopathologic study of 6 cases. Cancer 1969;24:503–10.

70 Ruocco V, Schwartz RA, Ruocco E. Lymphedema: an immunologically vulnerable site for development of neoplasms. J Am Acad Dermatol 2002;47:124–7.

71 Fernández G, Schwartz RA. Stewart-Treves syndrome. eMedicine Dermatology [journal serial online] 2007. Available from: http://emedicine.com/derm/topic898.htm.

72 Shehan JM, Ahmed I. Angiosarcoma arising in a lymphedematous abdominal pannus with histologic features reminiscent of Kaposi's sarcoma: report of a case and review of the literature. Int J Dermatol 2006;45:499–503.

73 Klein E, Schwartz RA, Case RW, et al. Accessible tumors. In: LoBuglio AF, editor. Clinical immunotherapy. New York: Marcel Dekker; 1980. p. 31–71.

74 Puizina-Ivic N, Bezic J, Marasovic D, et al. Angiosarcoma arising in sclerodermatous skin. Acta Dermatovenerol Alp Panonica Adriat 2005;14:20–5.

75 Brenn T, Fletcher CD. Radiation-associated cutaneous atypical vascular lesions and angiosarcoma: clinicopathologic analysis of 42 cases. Am J Surg Pathol 2005;29:983–96.

76 Miyake M, Tateishi U, Maeda T, et al. MR features of angiosarcoma in a patient with Maffucci's syndrome. Radiat Med 2005;23:508–12.

77 Lin BT, Weiss LM, Battifora H. Intravascularly disseminated angiosarcoma: true neoplastic angioendotheliomatosis? Report of two cases. Am J Surg Pathol 1997;21:1138–43.

78 Kim KJ, Jee MS, Koh GJ, et al. Cutaneous malignant hemangiopericytoma with unusual clinical behavior. J Dermatol 2002;29:323–4.

79 Daugaard S, Hultberg BM, Hou-Jensen K, et al. Clinical features of malignant haemangiopericytomas and haemangioendotheliosarcomas. Acta Oncol 1988;27:209–13.

80 Fletcher CD. The evolving classification of soft tissue tumours: an update based on the new WHO classification. Histopathology 2006;48:3–12.

81 Ruiz-Tovar J, Fernandez Guarino M, Reguero Callejas ME, et al. Dermatofibrosarcoma protuberans: review of 20-years experience. Clin Transl Oncol 2006;8:606–10.

82 Fidalgo A, Feio AB, Bajanca R. Congenital dermatofibrosarcoma protuberans. J Eur Acad Dermatol Venereol 2006;20:879–81.

83 Zaraa I, Cherif E, Ferchichi L, et al. [Dermatofibrosarcoma protuberans. About 18 cases]. Tunis Med 2005;83:622–6.

84 Thornton SL, Reid J, Papay FA, et al. Childhood dermatofibrosarcoma protuberans: role of preoperative imaging. J Am Acad Dermatol 2005;53:76–83.

85 Maire G, Fraitag S, Galmiche L, et al. A clinical, histologic, and molecular study of 9 cases of congenital dermatofibrosarcoma protuberans. Arch Dermatol 2007;143:203–10.

86 Lambert WC, Abramovits W, Gonzalez-Sevra A, et al. Dermatofibrosarcoma non-protuberans: description and report of five cases of a morpheaform variant of dermatofibrosarcoma. J Surg Oncol 1985;28:7–11.

87 McArthur GA. Dermatofibrosarcoma protuberans: a surgical disease with a molecular savior. Curr Opin Oncol 2006;18:341–6.

88 Nakayama H, Kamiji I, Naruse K, et al. Well differentiated adult-type fibrosarcoma arising from the occipital subcutaneous tissue in a 17-year-old man: case report with immunohistochemical study. Jpn J Clin Oncol 1998;28:511–6.

89 Ferenc T, Sygut J, Kopczynski J, et al. Aggressive fibromatosis (desmoid tumors): definition, occurrence, pathology, diagnostic problems, clinical behavior, genetic background. Pol J Pathol 2006;57:5–15.

90 de Visscher SA, van Ginkel RJ, Wobbes T, et al. Epithelioid sarcoma: still an only surgically curable disease. Cancer 2006;107:606–12.

91 Fisher C. Epithelioid sarcoma of Enzinger. Adv Anat Pathol 2006;13:114–21.

92 Casanova M, Ferrari A, Collini P, et al. Epithelioid sarcoma in children and adolescents: a report from the Italian Soft Tissue Sarcoma Committee. Cancer 2006;106:708–17.

93 Carson JW, Schwartz RA, McCandless CM Jr, et al. Atypical fibroxanthoma of the skin. Report of a case with Langerhans-like granules. Arch Dermatol 1984;120:234–9.

94 Seavolt M, McCall M. Atypical fibroxanthoma: review of the literature and summary of 13 patients treated with Mohs micrographic surgery. Dermatol Surg 2006;32:435–41; discussion 9–41.

95 Murali R, Palfreeman S. Clear cell atypical fibroxanthoma—report of a case with review of the literature. J Cutan Pathol 2006;33:343–8.

96 Dettrick A, Strutton G. Atypical fibroxanthoma with perineural or intraneural invasion: report of two cases. J Cutan Pathol 2006;33:318–22.

97 Yamamoto Y, Arata J, Yonezawa S. Angiomatoid malignant fibrous histiocytoma associated with marked bleeding arising in chronic radiodermatitis. Arch Dermatol 1985;121:275–6.

98 Stepanova A, Marsch WC, Stadie V. [A rare low-grade malignant scalp tumor. Atypical fibroxanthoma]. Hautarzt 2005;56:679–82.

99 Choi MH, Jeon J, Son SW, et al. A case of recurrent nodular fasciitis. Korean J Dermatol 2006;44:1457–9.

100 Flieder DB, Moran CA. Primary cutaneous synovial sarcoma: a case report. Am J Dermatopathol 1998;20:509–12.

101 Schwartz RA, Trovato MJ, Lambert PC. Desmoid tumor: a locally aggressive neoplasm. Cesko-Slovenská Dermatol 2007;82:34–8.

102 Schwartz RA, Trovato MJ, Lambert PC. Desmoid tumor. eMedicine Dermatology [journal serial online] 2007. Available from: http://emedicine.com/derm/topic778.htm.

103 Sharma PK, Janniger CK, Schwartz RA, et al. The treatment of atypical lipoma with liposuction. J Dermatol Surg Oncol 1991;17:332–4.

104 Mentzel T. Cutaneous lipomatous neoplasms. Semin Diagn Pathol 2001;18:250–7.

105 Ten Heuvel SE, Hoekstra HJ, van Ginkel RJ, et al. Clinicopathologic prognostic factors in myxoid liposarcoma: a retrospective study of 49 patients with long-term follow-up. Ann Surg Oncol 2007;14:222–9.

106 Kuflik JH, Schwartz RA, Rothenberg J. Dermal leiomyosarcoma. J Am Acad Dermatol 2003;48:S51–3.

107 Bellezza G, Sidoni A, Cavaliere A, et al. Primary cutaneous leiomyosarcoma: a clinicopathological and immunohistochemical study of 7 cases. Int J Surg Pathol 2004;12:39–44.

108 Berzal-Cantalejo F, Sabater-Marco V, Perez-Valles A, et al. Desmoplastic cutaneous leiomyosarcoma: case report and review of the literature. J Cutan Pathol 2006;33 Suppl 2:29–31.

109 Utikal J, Haus G, Poenitz N, et al. Cutaneous leiomyosarcoma with myxoid alteration arising in a setting of multiple cutaneous smooth muscle neoplasms. J Cutan Pathol 2006;33 Suppl 2:20–3.

110 Neville H, Corpron C, Blakely ML, et al. Pediatric neurofibrosarcoma. J Pediatr Surg 2003;38:343–6.

111 Boulanger JM, Larbrisseau A. Neurofibromatosis type 1 in a pediatric population: Ste-Justine's experience. Can J Neurol Sci 2005;32:225–31.

112 Jacques C, Dietemann JL. [Imaging features of neurofibromatosis type 1]. J Neuroradiol 2005;32:180–97.

113 Demir Y, Tokyol C. Superficial malignant schwannoma of the scalp. Dermatol Surg 2003;29:879–81.

114 Garcia-Alvarez Garcia FE, Garcia-Alvarez Garcia I, Castiella T, et al. [Forearm malignant epithelioid schwannoma associated with melanoma]. An Med Interna 2003;20:195–7.

115 Kikuchi A, Akiyama M, Han-Yaku H, et al. Solitary cutaneous malignant schwannoma. Immunohistochemical and ultrastructural studies. Am J Dermatopathol 1993;15:15–9.

116 Haustein UF. Malignant granular cell tumour with generalized metastases and polymyositis. Acta Derm Venereol 2001;81:307–8.

117 Tari AS, Amoli FA, Rajabi MT, et al. Cutaneous embryonal rhabdomyosarcoma presenting as a nodule on cheek; a case report and review of literature. Orbit 2006;25:235–8.

118 Brecher AR, Reyes-Mugica M, Kamino H, et al. Congenital primary cutaneous rhabdomyosarcoma in a neonate. Pediatr Dermatol 2003;20:335–8.

119 Setterfield J, Sciot R, Debiec-Rychter M, et al. Primary cutaneous epidermotropic alveolar rhabdomyosarcoma with t(2;13) in an elderly woman: case report and review of the literature. Am J Surg Pathol 2002;26:938–44.

120 Charrier JB, Esnault O, Brette MD, et al. Alveolar soft-part sarcoma of the cheek. Br J Oral Maxillofac Surg 2001;39:394–7.

121 Yilmaz T, Kamani T, Sungur A. Alveolar soft part sarcoma on the glabella. Int J Pediatr Otorhinolaryngol 2004;68:569–71.

122 Casanova M, Ferrari A, Bisogno G, et al. Alveolar soft part sarcoma in children and adolescents: a report from the Soft-Tissue Sarcoma Italian Cooperative Group. Ann Oncol 2000;11:1445–9.

123 Santos-Juanes J, Galache C, Miralles M, et al. Primary cutaneous extraskeletal osteosarcoma under a previous electrodessicated actinic keratosis. J Am Acad Dermatol 2004;51:S166–8.

124 Kourda M, Chatti S, Sfia M, et al. [Primary cutaneous extraskeletal Ewing's sarcoma]. Ann Dermatol Venereol 2005;132:986–9.

125 Somers GR, Shago M, Zielenska M, et al. Primary subcutaneous primitive neuroectodermal tumor with aggressive behavior and an unusual karyotype: case report. Pediatr Dev Pathol 2004;7:538–45.

126 Arce FP, Pinto J, Portero I, et al. Cutaneous metastases as initial manifestation of dedifferentiated chondrosarcoma of bone. An autopsy case with review of the literature. J Cutan Pathol 2000;27: 262–7.

127 Ferringer T, Banks PM, Metcalf JS. Langerhans cell sarcoma. Am J Dermatopathol 2006;28:36–9.

128 Bohn OL, Ruiz-Arguelles G, Navarro L, et al. Cutaneous langerhans cell sarcoma: a case report and review of the literature. Int J Hematol 2007;85:116–20.

129 Kawase T, Hamazaki M, Ogura M, et al. CD56/NCAM-positive Langerhans cell sarcoma: a clinicopathologic study of 4 cases. Int J Hematol 2005;81:323–9.

CHAPTER 9
Kaposi's sarcoma

Robert A. Schwartz

In 1872, Moriz Kaposi [1] first described *idiopathisches multiples Pigmentsarkom der Haut*, which has become known as Kaposi's sarcoma (KS) [1–8]. His original 1872 description of five patients resembles more the KS seen in AIDS (KS-AIDS) than the classic form of KS expected today in elderly men of Italian, Jewish, or Mediterranean linkage, in whom the disease behavior is usually benign. Kaposi's original five patients had a uniformly fatal outcome within 2 to 3 years. "According to our experience, this disease seems to be incurable and lethal from the very beginning," Kaposi wrote [9]. The disease that he described displayed brownish red to bluish red nodules in the skin and similar ones of the mucosa, especially of the larynx, trachea, stomach, liver, and colon. Although one had tended to view classic Kaposi's sarcoma as an indolent, slowly growing cancer in middle-aged Americans—that a patient died *with* rather than *of*—the aggressive course originally noted by Kaposi has become part of the devastation of AIDS, especially among homosexuals.

For most of the 20th century, classic KS in Europe and America was typically an indolent neoplasm [10–12]. American AIDS was identified in 1981 in three reports of KS as an original defining element of AIDS, two from New York City and one from San Francisco [5,13,14]. KS was initially seen in about one third of those with early AIDS, often as the presenting sign, a pattern markedly reduced in recent times since the introduction of highly active antiretroviral therapy (HAART) [15]. Homosexuals with AIDS exhibited KS much more commonly than did others with AIDS, with the exception of small foci of homosexuals in isolated communities in the American Midwest. The explanation came in 1994, when human herpesvirus type

8 (HHV-8), also known as KS-associated herpesvirus (KSHV), was identified using representational difference analysis by Moore and Chang [15,16]. It has been shown that HHV-8 is necessary but not sufficient for the development of all types of KS. Moore believes that we should use the term *KSHV* instead of *HHV-8*, as most of these herpesviruses are called by name rather than number (personal communication to author, 2005).

The ability to readily and accurately diagnose KSHV, or HHV-8, infection in individuals is challenging because the sensitivities and specificities of available diagnostic methods range widely, with many inadequate for large-scale screening studies [17]. Accurate determination of infection has been hindered by the lack of a "gold standard" for comparison of serologic assays used to estimate KSHV prevalence in serosurveys conducted in different settings. A 2007 study found commercially available enzyme-linked immunosorbent assay (ELISA)-based tests yielded the lowest specificities [18]. HHV-8 has a low prevalence in the general population of the United States and United Kingdom, with an intermediate rate in Italy and Greece and a high one in Uganda. In Italy, hot spots include the Po River Valley, Sardinia, and southern Italy, including Sicily, possibly related to a high density of blood-sucking insects [17,19,20]. Seropositive mothers may use their infected saliva to relieve the pruritus of insect bites in their children, thereby transmitting HHV-8 [21]. Nevertheless, questions remain, such as whether KS is a hyperplasia or a neoplasm, why there is a large male predominance with classic KS, whether KS is multicentric or metastatic [2] or at times both, the role of lymphedema [22], and whether different subtypes

Table 9.1 Groups predisposed to Kaposi's sarcoma

Elderly men of Mediterranean (especially Greek and Italian) and Jewish lineage

African blacks, particularly those in Uganda, Zambia, and the Democratic Republic of the Congo

Patients with AIDS

---

of HHV-8 may produce varied clinical patterns of KS [23].

Kaposi's sarcoma has a remarkable epidemiology that may provide insight into the pathogenesis, prophylaxis, and rational therapy for cancer in general (Table 9.1).

Incidence and epidemiology

"Traditional" Kaposi's sarcoma

Kaposi's sarcoma traditionally is an uncommon disease usually afflicting middle-aged and elderly men of Mediterranean or Jewish lineage [10,24]. In one American study, 51% of patients were Italian and 38% of Jewish lineage, and 93% were in the fifth decade or older, confirming earlier epidemiologic reports [10]. Classic KS has an overwhelming male predominance, with a male-to-female ratio of approximately 10 to 15:1. A similar focus of KS exists in the same age and gender groups in parts of Africa [25,26]. KS incidence in the Mediterranean had been up to 10-fold higher than in the rest of Europe and the United States. Classic KS occurs as a rare and indolent form in elderly Mediterranean men, with particularly high incidence in Italy, Greece, Turkey, and Israel [20,25]. Classic KS of middle-aged and older American men of Mediterranean and Eastern European (Ashkenazi) Jewish lineage represents about 0.2% of cancer cases in the United States. The incidence of classic KS in the United States has been estimated to be 0.34 for men and 0.08 for women per 100,000 population per year. In Israel, rates of classic KS of 2.07 in men and 0.75 in women per 100,000 were calculated [24]. Interestingly, the highest rates in Israel were in Jewish men of North African lineage, correlating with high levels of anti–HHV-8 antibodies. Crudely calculated

data have suggested that KS may be common among Arabians as well [27]. Other areas of high incidence include Iceland and the Faeroe Islands [28]. Classic KS has been found to be common in Peru, with sporadic cases found throughout the country and some clustering in the coastal region [29].

The incidence of classic KS in Italy has been estimated to be 1.0 for men and 0.4 for women per 100,000 population per year. But it varied between 0.3 in Umbria and 4.7 in Sassari for men, and between 0.1 in Parma and 1.7 in Sassari for women [30]. In another study, the annual KS incidence rates for men in Malta, Ragusa (Sicily), and northeastern Sardinia have been estimated at 2.2, 6.2, and 8.8 per 100,000 per year, with women's rates being 1.8, 2.5, and 2.1, respectively [31]. A cross-sectional study was conducted in the provinces of Sassari (northern Sardinia) and Cagliari (southern Sardinia) to estimate the prevalence of infection with HHV-8 and the incidence of classic KS among HHV-8–infected individuals [19]. Of tested individuals, 32.0% had antibodies against HHV-8 in Sassari and 30.0% in Cagliari. Although the overall prevalence of HHV-8 seemed similar in Sassari and in Cagliari, the risk of KS was higher in Sassari, suggesting different cofactor(s) or a different distribution of the same cofactor(s) between the two provinces of Sardinia. The incidence of KS estimated in the region around Venice, Italy, resembled that of the rest of Italy, but with rates higher in the coastal and alpine valleys [32], also implying a cofactor.

In Greece, classic KS has an estimated annual incidence of 0.47 new cases per 100,000 population (men, 0.62; women, 0.32). Classic KS in Greece exhibits some special characteristics, including older age of onset; lower male-to-female ratio; endemic clustering; disseminated skin disease at diagnosis, often accompanied by lymphedema; more common visceral or lymph node involvement; and a more frequent association with second malignancies. There is a focus described in the Peloponnese region of Greece, with an estimated rate of 0.8 per 100,000, but with a dense clustering in southern Peloponnese raising it markedly [33,34]. Peloponnese, like Sardinia, is an isolated volcanic region with silicaceous volcanic clay, a feature also noted in endemic African regions [35].

Possible risk factors for classic KS are evident in Italy. In addition to previously mentioned siliceous volcanic soil and abundant blood-sucking insects, old age is an important risk factor. One work showed the risk of having classic KS was significantly increased in subjects farming cereals, whereas a previous history of malaria did not influence the risk of developing classic KS [36]. Extensive epidemiologic studies in Italy demonstrate a strong influence of ethnogeography on HHV-8 seropositivity and KS incidence, with a marked gradient increasing from the north to the south.

The rarity of familial cases of KS, even in the areas considered endemic, is of interest. Familial KS was described in a cluster of five Israeli cases [37] and in a family of Lebanese descent in Australia [38]. Their scarcity is noteworthy.

AIDS-associated Kaposi's sarcoma

Kaposi's sarcoma has been the most frequent neoplasm in homosexual and bisexual men with AIDS [20]. In the AIDS grouping, KS originally accounted for as many as 35% of patients, an incidence that has been declining with the use of HAART for HIV disease [3], although KS prevalence may not be as reduced [39]. In Italy, KS-AIDS has produced notable epidemiologic changes. A doubling of KS incidence rates was noted in Italian men younger than 50 years from 1976 to 1984 to 1985 to 1990; however, no change, or possibly a decline, was observed in older men. The incidence of KS as an AIDS-defining cancer in Italy dropped significantly from 1986 to 1998 [40]. During the mid-1990s, KS incidence declined sharply, particularly in San Francisco, where KS rates among white men had risen from 0.5 per 100,000 people per year in 1973 to between 31.1 and 33.3 from 1987 through 1991 and then declined to 2.8 in 1998 [41]. In Sardinia, where classic KS is endemic, the arrival of AIDS has altered the ratio of male-to-female cases, which has dropped from 10:1 to 3:1 [36,42].

Human herpesvirus type 8 was found to be highly prevalent in the homosexual population before the AIDS epidemic. In San Francisco, in the first 6 months of 1978, the prevalence of HHV-8 was 24.9%, with a concurrent HIV-1 prevalence of only 1.8% [43]. Amazingly, the HHV-8 infection rate has remained steady while the HIV rate rose strikingly then dropped substantially, implying that "safe sex" practices do not protect against HHV-8 infection, probably because of spread via saliva. In the HAART therapy era, the incidence of KS has declined markedly, documented in one survey from 30 per 1000 patient-years before 1995 to 0.03 per 1000 patient-years in 2001 [44]. In a study from London University, the current incidence of KS among European HIV patients was found to be less than 10% of that reported in 1994 [45]. The proportion of AIDS diagnoses made on the basis of KS diagnoses was about 6%. Most individuals who developed KS while on HAART began with low CD4 cell counts and developed KS within 6 months of the initiation of HAART. Thus, there continues to be an increased incidence of KS among homosexual men yet a greatly reduced incidence of KS among patients with higher CD4 counts.

An increased prevalence of HHV-8 among injection drug users (IDUs) has been observed, suggesting that HHV-8 may be transmitted through blood-borne or other exposures common in this population. KS incidence in IDUs and non-IDUs with AIDS in the United States was evaluated. KS incidence was highest among homosexual men (5.7 per 100 person-years), substantially lower among heterosexual men (0.7 per 100 person-years), and lowest among women (0.4 per 100 person-years) [46]. After adjustment for age, race, registry location, and year of AIDS onset, relative risks for KS associated with injection drug use were 1.3 (0.9 to 1.8) among women, 1.1 (0.7 to 1.6) among heterosexual men, and 0.9 (0.8 to 0.9) among homosexual men. It was concluded that injection drug use was not associated with an increased risk of AIDS-related KS.

Iatrogenic Kaposi's sarcoma

The clinical course of iatrogenic KS varies from chronicity to rapid progression [11,12]. Its induction by immunosuppressive therapy and its subsequent regression on removal of immunosuppression provided some of the earliest clinical recognition of the reversibility of KS. The incidence of KS in transplant recipients is 400 to 500 times greater than that in the general population [47].

Iatrogenic KS shows ethnogeographic associations, occurring in only about 0.4% of transplant patients in the United States and Western Europe [48] but in about 4.0% to 5.3% of renal transplant patients in Arabia [27]. A male-to-female ratio of 1.5:1 also was evident among renal transplant recipients in Arabia [49]. KS represents 87.5% of posttransplantation neoplasia in Saudi Arabia and 80% of posttransplantation cancers in Turkey [50]. The high frequency of iatrogenic KS in Saudi Arabia reflects the 7% endemic seroprevalence of HHV-8 in healthy Arabians [27,49]. There is also a propensity in those with iatrogenically induced KS in America and Canada to be middle-aged and elderly American and European men of Mediterranean or Jewish lineage [51], a finding not noted among persons in the KS-AIDS group.

The incidence of KS among American renal transplant recipients is approximately 0.4% [52] but is 10 times higher in Saudi Arabia [27]. In a Sardinian study, 23% of patients who were HHV-8 positive before transplantation developed KS [53]. The incidence of KS among renal transplant recipients may be 3.6% or higher in regions endemic for KS, which is significantly more than the 0.4% incidence among renal transplant recipients in the United States and Western Europe [54]. In a small series in Sudan, 13.3% developed KS [55].

Differences in immunosuppressive therapy may favor HHV-8 reactivation in transplant recipients [56,57]. KS may develop after immunosuppressive therapy with prednisone or other immunosuppressives in settings other than that of transplantation [57]. KS has been seen more often in patients whose treatment includes cyclosporine [58], a drug that may reactivate HHV-8 from latency to lytic replication in tissue culture [59]. Remission of iatrogenic KS on cessation of immunosuppression is the norm [50]. Using sirolimus instead of another immunosuppressant may prevent or reduce the incidence of KS in these predisposed individuals [60,61].

A great deal of data support the inference that most iatrogenic KS patients are HHV-8 positive before transplantation, suggesting that reactivation of latent viral infection leads to disease. Although less frequent, seroconversion following transplantation does occur, suggesting infection from the donated organ [62,63]. Fatal disseminated KS following HHV-8 primary infection in liver transplant recipients has been described [57].

African Kaposi's sarcoma

Endemic African KS has accounted for 10% of cancers in central Africa, with a male-to-female ratio near unity in childhood KS cases, rising in puberty to 15:1 [64–68]. The seroprevalence of HHV-8 in Uganda was 79% in those with KS as compared with 50% in those without it; the risk of the KS rose with increasing anti-KSHV antibody titers [69]. The risk of KS is clearly linked to antibody status for HHV-8, with other factors in Uganda also important. More recently, in those under 15 years of age, the median age was 4 years, the male-to-female ratio was 1.7:1, and 78% tested HIV positive. The Kampala Cancer Registry has shown a significant alteration in the incidence of KS in the era of AIDS. In Uganda, KS has caused almost one half (48.9%) of the cancer cases in men and 17.9% in women. The incidence in men (30.1 cases per 100,000) represents a more than 10-fold rise in men since the 1950s and is approximately three times the incidence found in women (11 cases per 100,000). The incidence in boys and girls was approximately the same in childhood (birth to 14 years), with small peaks in girls younger than 5 years and boys aged 5 to 9 years. Subsequently, a progressive rise in incidence peaked in women aged 25 to 29 years and in men aged 35 to 39 years. Lymphadenopathic KS affected 12% of total cases; 42% of childhood cases were of this type.

In neighboring Zambia, the disorder was particularly aggressive among children, more than 80% of whom were HIV seropositive [46]. Of a total of 915 cases of KS analyzed in Zambia, 85 (9.25%) were in children under 14 years of age. The age ranged from 7 months to 14 years (average: 5.6 years). KS was found to represent as much as 25% of childhood cancers. The average male-to-female ratio was 1.76:1, with male predominance higher in children older than 5 years (2.5:1 ratio) than in children younger than 5 years (1.4:1 ratio).

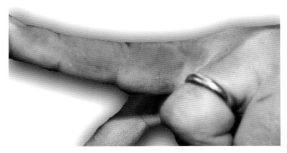

Fig. 9.1 Patch stage classical KS in a middle-aged man of Italian ancestry.

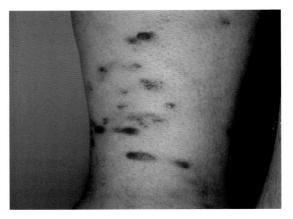

Fig. 9.2 Typical violaceous nodules in an elderly American of Armenian ancestry with classical KS.

Clinical features

Kaposi's sarcoma is a multicentric neoplasm that often manifests with multiple vascular nodules in the skin and other organs. The pattern of KS is variable, with a course ranging from indolent, with only skin manifestations, to fulminant, with extensive cutaneous and visceral involvement. With AIDS, KS is commonly first evident with multiple nodules on the upper body, head, and neck, and tends to evolve rapidly on skin and in viscera, with dissemination leading to organ dysfunction and high mortality. Regardless of AIDS, KS may also be evident on a wide variety of cutaneous and mucosal sites, including the face, genitalia, pinna, and external auditory canal [70]. KS also may arise primarily in the oral mucosa, lymph nodes, and/or viscera without cutaneous findings. KS may be first evident in any organ of the body. Chronic lymphedema may precede KS; it may rarely be first evident as generalized lymphedema [22,71].

Kaposi's sarcoma usually occurs in one of many morphologic variants, the most common being localized nodular, locally aggressive, and generalized lymphadenopathic:

1 Patch stage (Fig. 9.1)
2 Localized (nondestructive) nodular KS (Fig. 9.2)
3 Exophytic KS (Fig. 9.3)
4 Infiltrative KS
5 Generalized lymphadenopathic KS (Fig. 9.4) (often with widespread cutaneous nodules)
6 Disseminated cutaneous and visceral KS
7 Telangiectatic (Fig. 9.5)
8 Keloidal
9 Ecchymotic
10 Cavernous KS
11 Lymphangioma-like

Cutaneous KS usually begins as discrete red or purple patches that are bilaterally symmetric (Fig. 9.1) and initially tend to involve the lower extremities [72]. In Sardinia, 155 of 200 KS patients had initial lower extremity KS [73]. Patches become elevated, evolving into plaques and nodules (Fig. 9.2). Nodules may be spongy to the touch. Early KS as violaceous patches (patch stage KS) may resemble large junctional melanocytic nevi or may appear as irregular-shaped patches similar to the

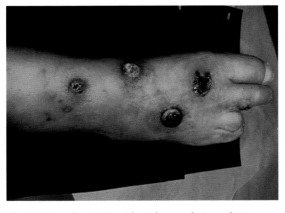

Fig. 9.3 Exophytic KS with widespread visceral KS.

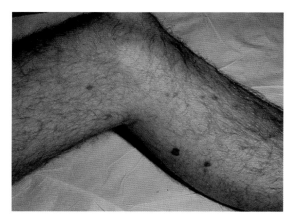

Fig. 9.4 Young homosexual man with small patches of KS and lymphadenopathy. His partner had squamous cell carcinoma of the tongue.

nevus flammeus. More commonly, KS is seen as violaceous plaques or nodules on the lower extremities. The nodules tend to enlarge into dome-shaped tumors. Cutaneous KS rarely may be infiltrative or exophytic [74]. Infiltrative KS has not been described outside of Africa. Exophytic KS is also endophytic, as it may erode downward into bone.

Lymphadenopathic KS may be evident as small pityriasis rosea–like macules (Fig. 9.4) or as more typical nodules. KS also occurs as a large infiltrating mass or as multiple cone-shaped friable tumors. In locally aggressive KS, nodules or tumors

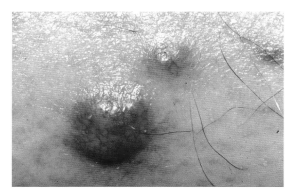

Fig. 9.5 Telangiectatic KS in an elderly man of Greek lineage with thymoma, myasthenia gravis, and chronic immunosuppressive therapy.

may adhere firmly to underlying anatomic structures including bone. Lymphadenopathic KS may occur in an indolent form in which visceral involvement is minimal, although such a pattern is distinctly unusual [75]. There may be no evidence of progression of KS, even without therapy. Localized lymphadenopathic KS is best viewed as a type of localized nodular KS. However, among Ugandan children in the AIDS era, two lymphadenopathic patterns were observed: orofacial dominant (79%) and inguinal–genital dominant (13%) [76].

Telangiectatic KS is an eruption of pink translucent nodules with prominent telangiectasia (Fig. 9.5) [77]. Ecchymotic KS is an apt description, often periorbital in location [78]. Keloidal KS is evident as somewhat brown to violaceous keloidal nodules [79]. Cavernous KS is a rare type of locally aggressive KS [74]. Lymphangioma-like or cavernous KS has dilated vascular spaces producing a bullous-appearing eruption, typically on the lower legs. It is easily compressible, may appear clinically as fluid-filled cysts [77,80], and is sometimes described as cystic KS [81].

Postirradiation primary KS of the head and neck occurring after radiotherapy of a brain tumor has been described [82], as it has in other areas of trauma [83,84], probably best viewed as a manifestation covered under Professor Vincenzo Ruocco's term *isotopic response* in which KS occurs at the site of unrelated skin diseases or trauma [84].

Conjunctival, oral, and genital KS may be noteworthy (Fig. 9.6) [85,86]. Although primary penile KS is uncommon in HIV-negative men, one should consider this possibility when treating nonspecific penile lesions [87]. A small penile nodule without distinctive clinical features may be the exclusive manifestation of KS. In addition, it may appear as a skin-colored nodule suggestive of a primary squamous cell carcinoma [88]. Clearly, histologic evaluation would be mandated to establish the diagnosis. In a study of 279 patients with classic KS, 36 had mucosal involvement, with two having them only in the mouth and four only on the genitalia [85]. Mucosal KS was seen together with cutaneous KS on the conjunctivae in nine and on the male genitalia in eight of the 36 patients. Involvement of the vulva may be evident [34]. Oral nodules may be

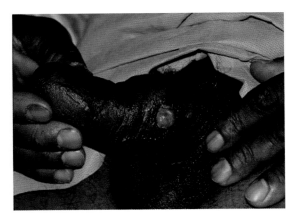

Fig. 9.6 Kaposi's sarcoma of the penis in an HIV-negative man from Haiti.

the first and only sign of KS. They have long been observed when examining the skin and accessible oral mucosa. A prospective study of 279 Sardinian patients with classic KS from 1977 to 2001 found 36 had mucosal KS on first examination, with most having both oral and skin KS [85]. Oral KS is seen as patches and nodules, especially of the palate.

Extracutaneous Kaposi's sarcoma

Visceral KS is most evident in gut and lymph nodes [10,89–92]. The frequency of visceral involvement in classic American KS is about one third, well below the almost uniform systemic involvement seen in the outbreak in homosexuals and others with AIDS-related KS. In one series of patients with AIDS-associated KS, the most common visceral involvement sites were the gastrointestinal tract (50%), lymph nodes (50%), and lung (37%) [91]. An endoscopic upper gastrointestinal tract evaluation of 87 Greek classic KS patients showed 71 (81.6%) had gastrointestinal lesions [92]. All had KS of the stomach. KS was also detected in the esophagus in 19 patients and in the proximal duodenum in eight patients, whereas additional involvement in both the esophagus and duodenum was identified in two patients. It may appear as small rectal nodules.

The gastrointestinal tract is the most common extracutaneous affected site, followed by liver, lungs, abdominal lymph nodes, and heart [67,89,91].

Pancreas, brain, spleen, testes, adrenals, tonsils, kidneys, seminal vesicles, urinary bladder, thyroid, and other organs may be involved [67]. Amazingly, gut involvement tends to be asymptomatic in classic KS, but in homosexuals and in post–renal transplantation patients with KS, hemorrhage may occur and, in fact, may be massive [93]. Classic and other KS patients may have gastrointestinal involvement such that they are first seen clinically with protein-losing enteropathy and/or an intractable diarrhea mimicking colitis [94]. Other complications include intussusception [95], perforation [96], and obstruction [97]. Pulmonary KS in the era of HAART remains an ominous sign [98]. AIDS-related KS pulmonary parenchymal disease is characterized by multiple, bilateral flame-shaped or nodular lesions with ill-defined margins distributed along bronchovascular bundles. Pulmonary KS may also be associated with pleural effusions and involvement of the sternum, ribs, or thoracic spine [99,100].

Ultrasound, computed tomography, positron emission tomography, and various endoscopic techniques have been employed to evaluate extracutaneous KS [101,102]. Certain scintigraphic procedures may be valuable in diagnosis, staging, and differential diagnosis of KS, particularly in the latter case in differentiating KS from lymphoma and opportunistic infection [99]. A technetium Tc 99m–hexakis-2-methoxy isobutyl isonitrile (^{99m}Tc-MIBI) scan was found to demonstrate cutaneous and subcutaneous KS of the extremities with 73.53% sensitivity, 96.91% specificity, and 91.31% accuracy and was more sensitive in detecting abnormal lymph nodes and lymphedema than was clinical assessment [102]. This ^{99m}Tc-MIBI imaging can provide precise staging and therapeutic planning and may be useful as a predictive test or follow-up of response of KS to treatment.

Differential diagnoses

Disorders that may require distinction include bacillary angiomatosis, blue rubber bleb nevus syndrome, pyogenic granuloma, tufted angioma, melanocytic nevi, melanoma, cavernous hemangioma, angiokeratoma, Stewart-Treves syndrome,

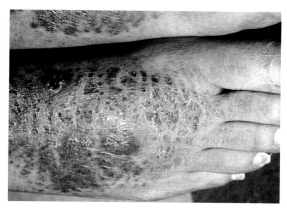

Fig. 9.7 Violaceous plaques and tumors of pseudo-KS.

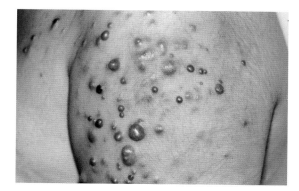

Fig. 9.8 Violaceous tumors of bacillary angiomatosis.

carcinoma cutis (especially renal cell carcinoma), nodal angiomatosis, nodal myofibromatoma, interstitial granuloma annulare, spindle cell hemangioendothelioma, arteriovenous malformations (pseudo-KS), severe stasis dermatitis (pseudo-KS), and the Dabska tumor [103–113]. Histologic criteria often used to differentiate between pyogenic granuloma and KS are not always helpful; the only distinguishing feature may be the presence or absence of HHV-8 latent nuclear antigen-1 (LNA-1) staining. The presence of HHV-8 LNA-1 staining seems to be a specific marker for KS when comparing pyogenic granuloma and pyogenic granuloma–like KS [114], and when comparing lymphangioma-like KS variants with lymphangiomas [115]. Iron and HHV-8 staining in combination may be reliable markers for KS compared with interstitial granuloma annulare [113]. Pseudo-KS and bacillary angiomatosis merit special consideration.

Pseudo-KS or acral angiodermatitis is a benign angiomatous proliferation of the extremities associated with chronic venous stasis or with acquired or congenital arteriovenous malformations (Fig. 9.7). Sometimes violaceous tumors are produced; their clinical and histologic pattern may closely resemble KS. Histologically, there may be a proliferation of capillaries and fibroblasts, extravasated red blood cells, and hemosiderin deposition similar to true KS, but usually lacking the narrow vascular slits. Such lesions remain localized. Expression of the CD34 antigen may distinguish KS from pseudo-KS his-

tologically [109]. Radiologic techniques, including digital subtraction angiography, may also be useful [116].

Bacillary angiomatosis may resemble KS both clinically and histologically [104,105] (Fig. 9.8). Bacillary angiomatosis is usually evident as a violaceous angiomatous tumor resembling KS or a nodule resembling a pyogenic granuloma. Subcutaneous nodules, with or without ulceration, may sometimes be seen. Bacillary angiomatosis is a type of bartonellosis that may also be first noted with systemic involvement, such as a destructive bone mass, lymphadenopathy, or liver dysfunction, without skin involvement. Histologically, a pattern resembling KS may be seen in affected skin, oral mucosa, lymph nodes, liver, spleen, bone marrow, larynx, gastrointestinal tract, peritoneum, diaphragm, bronchial mucosa, and brain. The Grocott-methenamine silver stain and the Warthin-Starry stain at pH 3.2 show the bacterial etiologic agent to good advantage, although these bacteria may also be evident employing the hematoxylin-eosin, periodic acid-Schiff and alcian blue stains. To complicate matters, a combination of KS and bacillary angiomatosis may occur. Although treatable and presumably curable with common antibiotics, bacillary angiomatosis may be life threatening if untreated. Thus, it is critical that this entity be distinguished from KS. A proliferating angioplasia resembling KS is evident histologically in the eruptive cutaneous and subcutaneous nodes of another type of bartonellosis—verruga peruana—a disorder limited to a certain part of Peru where its insect vector resides [117].

Kaposi's sarcoma of the lymph nodes may resemble a benign vascular transformation of the sinuses called nodal angiomatosis [118]. This condition may be the result of venous obstruction and is characterized by a vascularized sinusoidal fibrosis of the node.

Laboratory studies

Serum glucose levels may reflect an increased incidence of diabetes mellitus with classic KS [10]. Ketoacidosis is unusual in these patients. Hemograms in nonimmunosuppressed patients with KS tend to be within normal limits, but occasionally monocytosis or eosinophilia has been noted. Eosinophilia is seen especially in African patients and patients who are homosexual, in whom parasitosis may be common. In KS-AIDS, cytopenia of one or more cell lines is frequent. Anemia, if present, may result from gastrointestinal bleeding or may be associated with an autoimmune hemolytic anemia or a hematologic malignancy. Findings of immunologic studies of classic KS patients are usually normal with localized KS, but may be reduced with generalized KS [119–121]. Cutaneous skin testing for anergy in Uganda may correlate with generalized KS and an unfavorable prognosis [67]. The evolution of classic KS from early stages to the more advanced KS may be associated with a gradual decrease in the number of total and B lymphocytes [122]. Assays for HHV-8 have been challenging. At present, no universally accepted method exists. The polymerase chain reaction (PCR) assay often is used but may have false-positive results because of its high susceptibility to contamination. Methods based on both lytic- and latent-phase viral antigens remain promising [123,124]. Antibodies against HHV-8 glycoprotein K8.1 may correlate more than the HHV-8 seropositive rate with the risk of KS [125]. The prevalence of antibodies to the HHV-8–lytic gene ORF73 between KS-negative and -positive men who were seropositive for both HIV and HHV-8 was found to be higher in the patients who developed KS than in those who did not [126].

It remains unclear whether KS is a monoclonal cell proliferation or a polyclonal, hyperplastic, reactive process [127]. KS cytogenetics are few and restricted to late-stage disease and cell lines. Clonal loss of chromosome Y was detected in all early male KS, with additional chromosomal aberrations appearing during development to late KS. This increase in chromosomal abnormalities during tumor growth suggests genetic instability and the selection of survival cell clones establishing late, aggressive sarcoma growth. These data support the view that KS begins as a hyperplastic reactive cell proliferation that develops into a clonal tumor.

Associated disorders

There are a number of diseases associated with KS [7,11,12,128]. In addition to diabetes mellitus [10], leukemia, and lymphoma, one may find innumerable disorders associated in those with KS-AIDS. KS coexists with Hodgkin's and non-Hodgkin's lymphomas in a greater-than-chance association [10,129–131]. These non-Hodgkin's lymphomas include myeloma, angioimmunoblastic lymphadenopathy, B cell immunoblastic lymphoma, autoimmune hemolytic anemia, and hairy cell leukemia. Castleman's disease (giant lymph node hyperplasia) is also linked to both KS and HHV-8 infection [15,125]. In patients with classic KS, there is also an increased incidence of non-Hodgkin's lymphoma; they may occur simultaneously. In a study of Greek patients with classic KS, five of 66 also had a reticuloendothelial cancer [34]. The most common complications include secondary malignancy and secondary infections. In particular, secondary infection occurs with the KS-AIDS group of patients. A relatively common clinical concern is to distinguish pulmonary KS from opportunistic infection and lymphoma.

Histopathology

Kaposi's sarcoma usually shows a normal epidermis, but a dermis with increased spindle cells and vascular structures in a network of collagen and reticular fibers (Figs. 9.9 and 9.10). The vascular component tends to appear as clefts between spindle cells or as delicate capillaries. Extravasated erythrocytes and hemosiderin-laden macrophages are often evident.

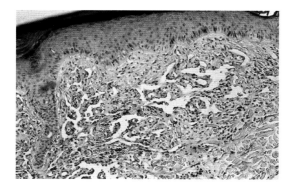

Fig. 9.9 Histopathologic view of patch stage KS.

Spindle cells may show nuclear pleomorphism. KS seen in lymph nodes and viscera resembles that in skin.

Four main histopathologic patterns may be evident. A mixed-cell type with a variable proportion of spindle cells, vascular clefts, and well-formed capillaries is relatively common, as is the mononuclear pattern with prominent proliferation of one cell type, usually spindle cells. An anaplastic form demonstrates cellular pleomorphism and numerous mitotic figures [74,132,133]. Subtle early KS resembles granulation tissue and consists of areas of capillary and small vessel-like proliferation [72]. Glomerulus-like vascular formations may be seen. Angioneoplasia may occur in clinically uninvolved perilesional KS skin [134,135]. Early KS may resemble a dermatofibroma.

Kaposi's sarcoma variants should be noted as well. Ecchymotic KS shows a large amount of extravasated red blood cells, no evidence of amyloidosis, and a dermis containing foci of proliferating moderately atypical spindle cells, vascular slits, erythrophagocytosis, and other features of KS [78]. Keloidal KS demonstrates a keloidal component [79]. Cavernous KS may resemble a cavernous hemangioma, but with endothelial cells and their nuclei being large and prominent, bulging into the cavity [74]. Lymphangioma-like KS has dilated vascular spaces that produce a bullous-appearing eruption, typically on the lower legs [80,81]. The vascular channels are lined by banal-appearing endothelial cells permeating the dermis in the absence of spindle cell proliferation.

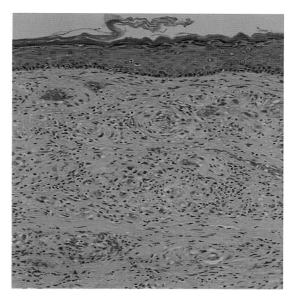

Fig. 9.10 Histology of typical KS.

Kaposi's sarcoma tends to evolve from the early inflammatory or patch stage to the nodular and then late proliferative stage. The glomerulus-like vascular formations in early patch stage KS and in some more advanced lesions may reflect the histogenesis of KS (Fig. 9.9) [72]. These early skin findings may be subtle, with newly formed vessels dilated and sometimes encircled by oval endothelial cells. Areas of dermal hemorrhage, hemosiderin deposition, and a polymorphic inflammatory cell infiltration with a prominent plasma cell component are often seen.

As KS progresses, nodules of distorted, endothelialized vessels and nonendothelialized, slit-like spaces may become evident (Fig. 9.10). The vessels are cuffed by the same oval and spindle cells that appear as single cells infiltrating the dermal collagen bundles. These slit-like spaces often contain erythrocytes, which may extravasate. The inflammatory cell component is unaltered. The later plaques show diffuse dermal involvement, exhibiting the same histologic features seen in the nodular stage. These may either resolve, with involution of the vascular components and formation of scar tissue, or become extremely pleomorphic, invading the deeper tissues. Anaplastic progression is unusual [132,133]. A nodule may enlarge rapidly, sometimes with osteolytic change in underlying bone. The undifferentiated spindle cells are strongly positive for factor VII–related antigen and CD34 antigen. Histologic characterization of progressive regression in KS-AIDS includes spindle cell proliferation and expression of HHV-8 latency genes, latency-associated nuclear antigen-1 (*LANA-1*), and cyclin-D1 [136,137]. *LANA-1* expression is a highly sensitive and specific marker of KS in both the general population and HIV-positive patients, whereas HHV-8 PCR is positive in a small subset of non-KS vascular tumors, most likely as the result of detection of HHV-8 within intratumoral blood mononuclear cells by the highly sensitive real-time PCR technique. Thus, LANA-1 immunostaining is preferable to HHV-8 PCR for the evaluation of problematic vascular proliferations in HIV-positive individuals [138].

Lymphadenopathy present in KS shows different patterns:
1 Marked follicular hyperplasia and hypervascularity
2 Nonspecific inflammation in regional lymph nodes that drain ulcerated cutaneous KS
3 Development of lymphomas in patients with KS
4 Development of bacillary angiomatosis in patients with KS
5 Actual involvement of lymph nodes by KS, with or without classic cutaneous involvement
6 A combination of KS and lymphoma or bacillary angiomatosis [104,139]
More than one of these processes may occur in the same node. KS in nodes shows typical proliferation of spindle cells separated by slit-like spaces containing red blood cells, accompanied by marked follicular hyperplasia and plasmacytic infiltration [140]. The first changes begin in the subcapsular and trabecular sinuses, but eventually there is involvement of the entire node and extension into the perinodal tissues. These alterations may be discrete or widespread within a given lymph node. The degree of lymphocytic, plasmacytic, and immunoblastic proliferation may be sufficient to simulate a lymphoma.

The electron microscopic and immunohistochemical features of KS are remarkable [134,135]. Staining with CD34, factor VII–related antigen, the lectin *Ulex europaeus* I, LANA-1, and human leukocyte antigen DR (HLA-DR) may support or confirm the diagnosis of KS [109]. Ultrastructural and immunohistochemical testing favors the endothelial cell, probably of lymphatic lineage, as the cell of origin for KS [141]. Most of the spindle cells in both early and late KS express the lymphatic markers lymphatic vessel endothelial receptor 1 (LYVE-1), D2-40, and vascular endothelial growth factor receptor 3 (VEGFR-3); the blood vascular endothelial/endothelial precursor cell marker CD34; and endothelial stem cell marker VEGFR-2. The presence of factor VII–related antigen, HLA-DR, von Willebrand factor, and the lectin *Ulex europaeus* I (which all are markers for endothelial cells) is suggestive. Reactivity with two monoclonal antibodies (EN4 and PAL E) implies that KS is derived from endothelium of lymphatic origin; however, KS spindle cells express CD34 antigen, a glycoprotein expressed by endothelial cells of small blood vessels (but not those of lymphatic origin). A monoclonal antibody to VEGFR-3, a tyrosine kinase receptor expressed almost exclusively by lymphatic endothelium in the adult, reacts with a small number of cases of KS and cutaneous lymphangiomas [142].

However, alternative interpretations exist, including that KS cells represent a proliferation of a special subset of macrophages with endothelial features, the sinus-lining cells of the spleen and lymph nodes [31]. In addition, in both early- and late-stage KS, approximately 18% of the spindle cells were CD34+/LANA-/LYVE-1 and could represent newly recruited endothelial precursor cells that become infected and eventually undergo a phenotype switch [141]. Expression of VEGFR-3 is a sensitive marker of KS and kaposiform and Dabska-type hemangioendotheliomas, suggesting that all show at least partial lymphatic endothelial differentiation. Expression of VEGFR-3 does not reliably distinguish KS from other angiosarcomas [142].

Staging

Staging this multicentric disorder has been a challenge [8,143–148]. The value of each scheme is limited.

The AIDS Clinical Trials Group classification by Krown and colleagues [149] uses the following three categories, with a tumor/immune/system/systemic (TIS) illness grading method:

• Tumor (T): Good or bad risk signs (good when KS is confined to skin and/or lymph nodes and/or demonstrates minimal oral disease)
• Immune system (I): CD4 cell levels equal to or greater than $150/mm^3$ (good risk) versus less than $150/mm^3$ (poor risk)
• Systemic illness (S): Good or poor risk

Another classification by Mitsuyasu [146] divides KS into four stages:

• Stage I: Localized nodular KS in elderly men in North America and Europe
• Stage II: Localized, invasive, and aggressive KS (mostly seen in Africa)
• Stage III: Disseminated mucocutaneous KS in African children and patients who are homosexual
• Stage IV: Stage III with visceral involvement

Schwartz and associates [8] originally proposed and currently prefer the following classification system (with new modifications):

• Stage I: Localized nodular KS, with fewer than 15 cutaneous lesions or involvement restricted to one bilateral anatomic site, and few, if any, gut nodules
• Stage II: Includes both exophytic destructive KS and locally infiltrative cutaneous lesions as locally aggressive KS or nodular KS, with more than 15 cutaneous lesions or involvement of more than one bilateral anatomic site, and few or many gut nodules
• Stage III (generalized lymphadenopathic KS): Widespread lymph node involvement with or without cutaneous KS, but with limited if any visceral involvement
• Stage IV (disseminated visceral KS): Widespread KS, usually progressing from stage II or stage III, with involvement of multiple visceral organs, with or without cutaneous KS

The authors modify each stage as follows:

• A: Associated opportunistic infection(s) is (are) evident
• B: Patient is HIV-1 seropositive
• C: Cutaneous anergy or other evidence of severe immunodeficiency is present

There are other staging ideas as well, including thoughtful ones by Cottoni and Montesu [150] and by Brambilla and colleagues [144]. Assessment of the AIDS Clinical Trials Group Staging System in the HAART era is under way, as refinements are needed [143]. For example, the CD4 level does not seem to provide useful prognostic information.

Therapy

Therapeutic options for KS are often based on disease stage, progression pattern, anatomic distribution, and KS clinical form [151–154]. Because the natural history of KS is variable, assessment of therapy may be difficult. Treatment usually is based on the extent of disease and the patient's immune status. The challenge is to treat KS effectively without immunocompromising the patient, and if possible, with reconstitution of the immune system if impaired. Management modalities for KS include nonintervention; surgical removal of skin nodules or severely affected areas, such as intussuscepted gut; laser surgery; conventional and megavoltage radiotherapy; chemotherapy; immunotherapy; antiviral drugs; and cessation of immunosuppressive therapy or switching to sirolimus in iatrogenically immunosuppressed patients. The incidence of KS, especially visceral KS, has fallen sharply since the advent of potent combined antiretroviral treatment [155]. This effect is probably the result of immune restoration rather than of a specific effect on the tumoral process. Remission from KS on HAART appears associated with suppression of HIV replication [156].

Localized Kaposi's sarcoma

Indolent skin tumors in elderly patients may not require specific therapy; however, systemic vinblastine (or other chemotherapy) attacks both cutaneous and visceral lesions. Localized nodular disease may respond well to surgical excision, radiotherapy, the Food and Drug Administration (FDA)-approved topical retinoid alitretinoin 0.1% gel (discussed later), and intralesional and outpatient low-dose vinblastine chemotherapy. The latter combination of local and systemic regimens may be preferable. Patients should be informed that KS is a multicentric disease with silent gut or other visceral involvement that also may regress with a systemic approach.

Radiotherapy often produces good therapeutic results with classic nodular KS but tends to be only palliative in patients with KS-AIDS [157,158]. Electron-beam radiotherapy, which has limited penetration beyond the dermis, may be a good modality for superficial nodules [159]. Deeper or unresponsive KS may be treated using standard non–electron-beam radiation or other options. Initial response to radiotherapy usually is complete or demonstrates marked regression of the nodules. The more extensive the involvement, the less responsive it tends to be. Radiotherapy may be more effective on new, rather than chronic, lesions and may provide local KS control in patients with KS-AIDS. Scintigraphic procedures may be valuable in detecting occult KS infiltration in the subcutaneous and muscular tissues and draining lymph nodes, allowing improved efficiency of large-field radiotherapy [116]. Solitary KS may be excised surgically or destroyed by laser surgery. Intralesional chemotherapy [151], surgical destruction [7], radiotherapy, or laser therapies [160,161] are often used with early-stage disease confined to skin or mucosa. Immunomodulators such as imiquimod may also be beneficial [162].

One excellent approach is the Klein regimen of weekly outpatient intravenous vinblastine titered against white cell count levels to avoid falling below $4000/mm^3$ [151]. Intralesional injections of vinblastine may be provided for persistent cutaneous nodules; intra-arterial vinblastine may be valuable in certain settings for locally aggressive KS. Systemic vinblastine (3.5 to 10 mg intravenously [IV] weekly with, at times, one intralesional injection of 0.1 mg) usually is best for both the patient with classic KS and, occasionally, patients with KS-AIDS.

Generalized, systemic, and AIDS-related Kaposi's sarcoma

Despite the concept of skin and gut being together and mandating systemic therapy, systemic cytotoxic drugs are often reserved for patients with disseminated disease [11,12]. Chemotherapeutic agents inhibit KS cell growth and proliferation. Vinblastine is an important vinca alkaloid, the salt of a common flowering herb: the periwinkle (*Vinca rosea*). The usual adult dosage is 4 to 6 mg IV weekly

and intralesional injections of 0.1 mg [151]. Although low-dose vinblastine may be good therapy in KS patients, in many settings combined with other modalities, a number of other chemotherapeutic agents or combinations may also be effective [163]. These include interferon-α and chemotherapy such as pegylated-liposomal anthracyclines and paclitaxel. However, the systemic medications approved by the United States FDA for systemic administration are liposomal daunorubicin, liposomal doxorubicin, paclitaxel, and interferon-α [164].

Anthracyclines are probably the most effective cytotoxic agents against KS, especially with encapsulation in pegylated liposomes to improve drug diffusion [165–167]. They have anti-KS activity comparable to that of commonly used combination chemotherapy, but are less toxic. Liposomal anthracyclines are now standard therapy for advanced AIDS-related KS. Liposomal anthracyclines with potential utility in KS include pegylated liposomal doxorubicin (PLD), daunorubicin citrate liposome (DNX), and nonpegylated liposomal doxorubicin (NPLD). Preclinical data showed that pegylated liposomes accumulate preferentially in highly vascularized KS. If they or multiple chemotherapy agents fail, paclitaxel should be considered, as it has been shown to be effective [168]. Etoposide alone in low dosages may be safe and effective for refractory or progressing AIDS-related KS after use of liposomal anthracyclines and paclitaxel [169].

All these therapies (except low-dose vinblastine) are significantly immunosuppressive and, theoretically, risk accelerating the disease. Combining chemotherapy for KS with chemotherapy for HIV is an attractive option. Interferon also may be used in this way. Thus, the combination of zidovudine, interferon, and low-dose intravenous vinblastine may be employed for patients with KS-AIDS. However, chemotherapy alone for HIV may also be considered. In resource-limited settings, intravenous vincristine, oral etoposide, or intramuscular bleomycin may be suitable options [170].

Highly Active Antiretroviral Therapy

Impressive evidence is accumulating that anti-HIV HAART containing at least one inhibitor of the HIV protease or a non-nucleoside reverse transcriptase inhibitor can reduce the incidence or induce the regression of KS, as well as of other AIDS-associated tumors [44,171,172]. In some patients, KS-AIDS may resolve clinically with the use of HAART. KS exhibits a less aggressive onset in patients already receiving HAART compared with patients who are naive to HAART at KS diagnosis. However, the natural history and outcome do not appear to be influenced by the initiation of HAART before development of KS [171]. Regimens based on non-nucleoside reverse transcriptase inhibitors or protease inhibitors have been equally effective in preventing KS, with the incidence of KS steeply declining [44]. Interferon-α-2b with protease inhibitor–based antiretroviral therapy in patients with AIDS-associated KS is being assessed [173].

Immunotherapy

Experimental treatments for KS infections are myriad. Many come under the rubric of immunotherapy, pioneered for KS by Klein in the early 1960s [151]. Interferon-α-2a is a protein product manufactured by recombinant DNA technology [165,174]. Its mechanisms of antitumor activity may be by direct antiproliferative effects against KS cells and by modulation of host immune response. Low well-tolerated dosing of interferon may be effective in combination with antiretroviral therapy [174]. The value of recombinant interferon-α and other modalities may depend on the pretreatment immune status of the patient as the best predictor of response.

In addition to interferon, other agents used for immunomodulation include bovine-thymic extracts, thymosin, IMREG-1, thalidomide, imiquimod, endothelial growth factor inhibitor (SU5416), human chorionic gonadotropin, isoprinosine, thymopoietin, monoclonal antibodies to T-suppressor (T8) cells, bacille Calmette-Guérin (BCG) vaccine, and cord factor. New matrix metalloproteinase-2 inhibitors, such as COL-3 [175], are in clinical trials for the treatment of KS. Immunologic agents may also be anti-angiogenic compounds such as IM862 and TNP-470 peptides [176–178], retinoic acids [176], the VEGFR-2 inhibitor SU5416 [179], interferon, and thalidomide [180,181]. Interleukin-12 (IL-12), which enhances Th1-type T cell responses and exerts anti-angiogenic effects, has substantial activity when given subcutaneously against AIDS-related KS, with acceptable toxicity [182].

In iatrogenic KS, cessation of immunosuppressive therapy, sometimes combined with chemotherapy, may be the most effective treatment, particularly with limited disease [183]. Patients on immunosuppressive therapy, specifically corticosteroids and cytotoxic drugs, may have partial or complete regression when therapy is discontinued. One need be concerned about medications stimulating or facilitating HIV and/or HHV-8 infection(s) or KS tumor proliferation [184]. If possible, immunosuppressive medication dosages should be reduced or discontinued before beginning specific therapy for iatrogenic KS. Sirolimus, a new immunosuppressive agent, may be substituted for calcineurin inhibitors. Sirolimus inhibits tumor growth, whereas calcineurin inhibitors promote it. Thus, sirolimus may constitute effective KS therapy. Moreover, sirolimus inhibits the progression of dermal Kaposi's sarcoma in kidney transplant recipients while providing effective immunosuppression [60,185].

Retinoids

Retinoids decrease the cohesiveness of abnormal hyperproliferative keratinocytes and may reduce their potential for malignant degeneration. They modulate keratinocyte differentiation and have been shown to reduce the risk of skin cancer formation in renal transplant patients. Alitretinoin 0.1% gel is FDA-approved for topical treatment for cutaneous KS [186]. This naturally occurring endogenous retinoid inhibits growth of KS by binding to retinoid receptors. It is applied generously to affected cutaneous lesions twice a day initially and increased up to four times a day as tolerated. Oral 9-*cis*-retinoic acid in capsule form has shown moderate activity in AIDS-related KS patients, but its toxic effects limit its value [187]. Intravenous liposomal tretinoin remains another option [188].

HHV-8 medication

Anti-herpesvirus drugs are also promising. Foscarnet and ganciclovir may decrease the risk of developing KS [189,190]. Unfortunately, acyclovir has shown no benefit. Agents such as foscarnet and ganciclovir may not sufficiently reduce the risk of KS or regularly induce KS regression because they block productive but not latent HHV-8 infection [191,192]. Antiviral therapy with foscarnet may not only reduce progression of KS in patients, but may lower its occurrence substantially in patients with HIV disease. Abatement of cutaneous KS associated with cidofovir treatment has been described, but a pilot study with this anti-herpesvirus agent was not impressive [193]. Antiviral agents active against HHV-8 represent an important potential intervention and prevention option [194].

Prevention

Reducing the HHV-8 infection rate lowers the number of people who develop KS. Accordingly, an anti-herpetic agent should be considered. Screening transplant recipients and blood donors for HHV-8 infection may be beneficial. It may also be of value to evaluate donors for HHV-8 [63]. In addition, use of the anti-HIV therapy HAART reduces the risk of developing new KS significantly. As mentioned, HAART regimens reduce the incidence of KS as an AIDS-defining disease [45]. The use of ritonavir in the prevention of AIDS-related KS was found to confer no advantages as compared with other regimens, presumably because KS regression is mediated by improved immune function rather than by the effects of specific antiretroviral agents [195].

Human herpesvirus type 8 encodes a G protein–coupled receptor (vGPCR) implicated in the initiation of KS, identifying vGPCR as an attractive target for preventing KS in an animal model [196]. However, only a small fraction of cells in advanced KS express vGPCR. Surprisingly, despite the expression of HHV-8–latent genes in the vast majority of tumor cells, specifically targeting only the few vGPCR-expressing cells in established tumors resulted in tumor regression. vGPCR may play a key role in KS progression and provide experimental justification for developing molecular-based therapies specifically targeting vGPCR and its effectors.

Prognosis

Clinical classification of KS may be the best prognosticator, comparing localized nodular disease, locally aggressive disease, and generalized KS. Cutaneous skin testing for anergy may correlate with clinical disease type and prognosis [67,197]. Prognosis appears to correlate with the degree of immunosuppression and older age among classic KS patients [198]. Localized nodular KS has the best prognosis, with few deaths directly attributable to it. Locally aggressive KS has an intermediate prognosis. The 1975 Ugandan data showing a 3-year survival rate of 64% with locally aggressive KS match that of today with KS patients on HAART therapy [66,171]. Patients in Uganda with generalized KS, the form seen most commonly in patients with KS-AIDS, had a 3-year survival rate closer to 0% without therapy. American and European patients with advanced KS and AIDS usually succumb either to disseminated KS or to an intervening opportunistic infection within 3 years of diagnosis, regardless of the form of therapy. In Uganda, the median survival was less than 3.5 months [197]. Protease inhibitor–based HAART was associated with a median survival of 31 months (range, 1.8 to 48) in HIV-associated advanced KS patients treated with chemotherapy as compared with only 7 months (range, 1 to 28) in those without HAART [172]. Additionally, 81% were alive at 18 months from start of chemotherapy as compared with only 12% in the non-HAART group. KS remains an ominous diagnosis in the era of HAART, with a median survival of just 1.6 years [98].

Patients with traditional KS tend to die with KS rather than of KS. Patients with KS-AIDS tend to die from associated opportunistic infections or from disseminated visceral KS [172]. The mean survival of patients with KS-AIDS has been approximately 15 to 24 months, although the introduction into the United States of apparent immune system reconstitution using HAART may extend survival in some patients. However, another analysis showed that when KS develops in patients on HAART, it seems to exhibit a less aggressive clinical pattern in patients already receiving HAART as compared with those naive to this treatment, but the natural history and outcome are not altered [143,171]. The 3-year survival rate was 64% for KS-HAART patients as compared with 78% for those without HAART. KS may be fatal as a result of gut perforation, cardiac tamponade, massive pulmonary obstruction or, rarely, brain metastases. In Kaposi's original description, death usually ensued within 3 years and was linked to fever, diarrhea, and hemoptysis. Inanition may be an important factor. Patients with AIDS-related KS often have widespread visceral KS, although KS limited to the skin also is common. Iatrogenic KS usually responds to reduction of immunosuppression or to the substitution of sirolimus for another immunosuppressant [60].

References

1 Kaposi M. Idiopathisches multiples pigmentsarkom der Haut. Arch Dermatol Syphilol (Prague) 1872;4: 265–73.

2 Schwartz RA. Kaposi's sarcoma: an update. J Surg Oncol 2004;87:146–51.

3 Schwartz RA. Kaposi's sarcoma: advances and perspectives. J Am Acad Dermatol 1996;34:804–14.

4 Borkovic SP, Schwartz RA. Kaposi's sarcoma. Am Fam Physician 1982;26:133–7.

5 Borkovic SP, Schwartz RA. Kaposi's sarcoma presenting in the homosexual man – a new and striking phenomenon! Ariz Med 1981;38:902–4.

6 Kaposi M. Pathology and treatment of diseases of the skin for practitioners and students. Translation of the last German edition under the supervision of James C. Johnston. New York: William Wood; 1895.

7 Schwartz RA, Lambert WC. Kaposi's sarcoma. eMedicine Dermatology [Journal serial online] 2007. Available from: http://emedicine.com/derm/topic203.htm.

8 Schwartz RA, Volpe JA, Lambert MW, et al. Kaposi's sarcoma. Semin Dermatol 1984;3:303–15.

9 Richter F, Hill GJ, Schwartz RA. Professor Kaposi's original concepts of Kaposi's sarcoma. J Cancer Educ 1995;10:113–6.

10 Laor Y, Schwartz RA. Epidemiologic aspects of American Kaposi's sarcoma. J Surg Oncol 1979;12:299–303.

11 Hengge UR, Ruzicka T, Tyring SK, et al. Update on Kaposi's sarcoma and other HHV8 associated diseases. Part 1: epidemiology, environmental predispositions, clinical manifestations, and therapy. Lancet Infect Dis 2002;2:281–92.

12 Hengge UR, Ruzicka T, Tyring SK, et al. Update on Kaposi's sarcoma and other HHV8 associated diseases. Part 2: pathogenesis, Castleman's disease, and pleural effusion lymphoma. Lancet Infect Dis 2002;2:344–52.

13 Friedman-Kien AE. Disseminated Kaposi's sarcoma syndrome in young homosexual men. J Am Acad Dermatol 1981;5:468–71.

14 Gottlieb GJ, Ragaz A, Vogel JV, et al. A preliminary communication on extensively disseminated Kaposi's sarcoma in young homosexual men. Am J Dermatopathol 1981;3:111–4.

15 Moore PS, Chang Y. Kaposi's sarcoma (KS), KS-associated herpesvirus, and the criteria for causality in the age of molecular biology. Am J Epidemiol 1998;147:217–21.

16 Chang Y, Cesarman E, Pessin MS, et al. Identification of herpesvirus-like DNA sequences in AIDS-associated Kaposi's sarcoma. Science 1994;266:1865–9.

17 Laney AS, Peters JS, Manzi SM, et al. Use of a multi-antigen detection algorithm for diagnosis of Kaposi's sarcoma-associated herpesvirus infection. J Clin Microbiol 2006;44:3734–41.

18 Nascimento MC, de Souza VA, Sumita LM, et al. Comparative study of Kaposi's sarcoma-associated herpesvirus serological assays using clinically and serologically defined reference standards and latent class analysis. J Clin Microbiol 2007;45:715–20.

19 Serraino D, Cerimele D, Piselli P, et al. Infection with human herpesvirus type 8 and Kaposi's sarcoma in Sardinia. Infection 2006;34:39–42.

20 Dourmishev LA, Dourmishev AL, Palmeri D, et al. Molecular genetics of Kaposi's sarcoma-associated herpesvirus (human herpesvirus-8) epidemiology and pathogenesis. Microbiol Mol Biol Rev 2003; 67:175–212.

21 Ascoli V, Facchinelli L, Valerio L, et al. Distribution of mosquito species in areas with high and low incidence of classic Kaposi's sarcoma and seroprevalence for HHV-8. Med Vet Entomol 2006;20:198–208.

22 Ruocco V, Schwartz RA, Ruocco E. Lymphedema: an immunologically vulnerable site for development of neoplasms. J Am Acad Dermatol 2002;47:124–7.

23 Serwin AB, Mysliwiec H, Wilder N, et al. Three cases of classic Kaposi's sarcoma with different subtypes of Kaposi's sarcoma-associated herpesvirus. Int J Dermatol 2006;45:843–6.

24 Guttman-Yassky E, Bar-Chana M, Yukelson A, et al. Epidemiology of classic Kaposi's sarcoma in the

Israeli Jewish population between 1960 and 1998. Br J Cancer 2003;89:1657–60.

25 Iscovich J, Boffetta P, Franceschi S, et al. Classic kaposi sarcoma: epidemiology and risk factors. Cancer 2000;88:500–17.

26 Grossman Z, Iscovich J, Schwartz F, et al. Absence of Kaposi sarcoma among Ethiopian immigrants to Israel despite high seroprevalence of human herpesvirus 8. Mayo Clin Proc 2002;77:905–9.

27 Qunibi W, Al-Furayh O, Almeshari K, et al. Serologic association of human herpesvirus eight with post-transplant Kaposi's sarcoma in Saudi Arabia. Transplantation 1998;65:583–5.

28 Hjalgrim H, Tulinius H, Dalberg J, et al. High incidence of classical Kaposi's sarcoma in Iceland and the Faroe Islands. Br J Cancer 1998;77:1190–3.

29 Mohanna S, Ferrufino JC, Sanchez J, et al. Epidemiological and clinical characteristics of classic Kaposi's sarcoma in Peru. J Am Acad Dermatol 2005;53:435–41.

30 Dal Maso L, Polesel J, Ascoli V, et al. Classic Kaposi's sarcoma in Italy, 1985–1998. Br J Cancer 2005; 92:188–93.

31 Vitale F, Briffa DV, Whitby D, et al. Kaposi's sarcoma herpes virus and Kaposi's sarcoma in the elderly populations of 3 Mediterranean islands. Int J Cancer 2001;91:588–91.

32 Ascoli V, Zambon P, Manno D, et al. Variability in the incidence of classic Kaposi's sarcoma in the Veneto region, Northern Italy. Tumori 2003;89:122–4.

33 Stratigos JD, Katoulis AC, Stavrianeas NG. An overview of classic Kaposi's sarcoma in Greece. Adv Exp Med Biol 1999;455:503–6.

34 Stratigos JD, Potouridou I, Katoulis AC, et al. Classic Kaposi's sarcoma in Greece: a clinico-epidemiological profile. Int J Dermatol 1997;36:735–40.

35 Montesu MA, De Marco R, Cottoni F. Soil silicates and Kaposi's sarcoma in Sardinia. Lancet 1995;346:1436–7.

36 Cottoni F, Masala MV, Budroni M, et al. The role of occupation and a past history of malaria in the etiology of classic Kaposi's sarcoma: a case-control study in north-east Sardinia. Br J Cancer 1997;76: 1518–20.

37 Weissmann-Brenner A, Friedman-Birnbaum R, Brenner B. Familial Kaposi's sarcoma: a cluster of five Israeli cases. Clin Oncol (R Coll Radiol) 2004; 16:125–8.

38 Hale LR, Kelly JW. Familial Kaposi's sarcoma and Paget's disease of bone. Australas J Dermatol 1998; 39:241–3.

39 Buonaguro FM, Tomesello ML, Buonaguro L, et al. Kaposi's sarcoma: aetiopathogenesis, histology and clinical features. J Eur Acad Dermatol Venereol 2003;17:138–54.

40 Franceschi S, Dal Maso L, Pezzotti P, et al. Incidence of AIDS-defining cancers after AIDS diagnosis among people with AIDS in Italy, 1986–1998. J Acquir Immune Defic Syndr 2003;34:84–90.

41 Eltom MA, Jemal A, Mbulaiteye SM, et al. Trends in Kaposi's sarcoma and non-Hodgkin's lymphoma incidence in the United States from 1973 through 1998. J Natl Cancer Inst 2002;94:1204–10.

42 Santarelli R, De Marco R, Masala MV, et al. Direct correlation between human herpesvirus-8 seroprevalence and classic Kaposi's sarcoma incidence in Northern Sardinia. J Med Virol 2001;65:368–72.

43 Osmond DH, Buchbinder S, Cheng A, et al. Prevalence of Kaposi sarcoma-associated herpesvirus infection in homosexual men at beginning of and during the HIV epidemic. JAMA 2002;287:221–5.

44 Portsmouth S, Stebbing J, Gill J, et al. A comparison of regimens based on non-nucleoside reverse transcriptase inhibitors or protease inhibitors in preventing Kaposi's sarcoma. AIDS 2003;17:F17–22.

45 Mocroft A, Kirk O, Clumeck N, et al. The changing pattern of Kaposi sarcoma in patients with HIV, 1994–2003: the EuroSIDA Study. Cancer 2004;100:2644–54.

46 Athale UH, Patil PS, Chintu C, et al. Influence of HIV epidemic on the incidence of Kaposi's sarcoma in Zambian children. J Acquir Immune Defic Syndr Hum Retrovirol 1995;8:96–100.

47 Atkinson JO, Biggar RJ, Goedert JJ, et al. The incidence of Kaposi sarcoma among injection drug users with AIDS in the United States. J Acquir Immune Defic Syndr 2004;37:1282–7.

48 Penn I. Kaposi's sarcoma in transplant recipients. Transplantation 1997;64:669–73.

49 Almuneef M, Nimjee S, Khoshnood K, et al. Prevalence of antibodies to human herpesvirus 8 (HHV-8) in Saudi Arabian patients with and without renal failure. Transplantation 2001;71:1120–4.

50 Duman S, Toz H, Asci G, et al. Successful treatment of post-transplant Kaposi's sarcoma by reduction of immunosuppression. Nephrol Dial Transplant 2002;17:892–6.

51 Stribling J, Weitzner S, Smith GV. Kaposi's sarcoma in renal allograft recipients. Cancer 1978;42:442–6.

52 Khan MY, Khanum H, Koneru B, et al. Kaposi's sarcoma in a liver transplantation series. J Med 1999; 30:185–90.

53 Cattani P, Capuano M, Graffeo R, et al. Kaposi's sarcoma associated with previous human herpesvirus 8 infection in kidney transplant recipients. J Clin Microbiol 2001;39:506–8.

54 Lesnoni La Parola I, Masini C, Nanni G, et al. Kaposi's sarcoma in renal-transplant recipients: experience at the Catholic University in Rome, 1988–1996. Dermatology 1997;194:229–33.

55 Sabeel AI, Qunibi WY, Alfurayh OA, et al. Kaposi's sarcoma in Sudanese renal transplant recipients: a report from a single center. J Nephrol 2003;16:412–6.

56 Nagy S, Gyulai R, Kemeny L, et al. Iatrogenic Kaposi's sarcoma: HHV8 positivity persists but the tumors regress almost completely without immunosuppressive therapy. Transplantation 2000;69:2230–1.

57 Hoshaw RA, Schwartz RA. Kaposi's sarcoma after immunosuppressive therapy with prednisone. Arch Dermatol 1980;116:1280–2.

58 El-Agroudy AE, El-Baz MA, Ismail AM, et al. Clinical features and course of Kaposi's sarcoma in Egyptian kidney transplant recipients. Am J Transplant 2003;3:1595–9.

59 Cattaneo D, Gotti E, Perico N, et al. Cyclosporine formulation and Kaposi's sarcoma after renal transplantation. Transplantation 2005;80:743–8.

60 Gutierrez-Dalmau A, Sanchez-Fructuoso A, Sanz-Guajardo A, et al. Efficacy of conversion to sirolimus in posttransplantation Kaposi's sarcoma. Transplant Proc 2005;37:3836–8.

61 Paghdal KV, Schwartz RA. Sirolimus (rapamycin): from the soil of Easter Island to a bright future [published online ahead of print on June 19, 2007]. J Am Acad Dermatol. PMID: 17583372.

62 Parravicini C, Olsen SJ, Capra M, et al. Risk of Kaposi's sarcoma-associated herpes virus transmission from donor allografts among Italian posttransplant Kaposi's sarcoma patients. Blood 1997;90:2826–9.

63 Marcelin AG, Roque-Afonso AM, Hurtova M, et al. Fatal disseminated Kaposi's sarcoma following human herpesvirus 8 primary infections in liver-transplant recipients. Liver Transpl 2004;10:295–300.

64 Lothe F. Kaposi's sarcoma in Uganda Africans. Acta Pathol Microbiol Scand Suppl 1963;Suppl 161:1+.

65 Ziegler JL, Templeton AC, Vogel CL. Kaposi's sarcoma: a comparison of classical, endemic, and epidemic forms. Semin Oncol 1984;11:47–52.

66 Templeton AC, Bhana D. Prognosis in Kaposi's sarcoma. J Natl Cancer Inst 1975;55:1301–4.

67 Templeton AC. Kaposi's sarcoma. Pathol Annu 1981;16:315–36.

68 Onunu AN, Okoduwa C, Eze EU, et al. Kaposi's sarcoma in Nigeria. Int J Dermatol 2007;46:264–7.

69 Ziegler J, Newton R, Bourboulia D, et al. Risk factors for Kaposi's sarcoma: a case-control study of HIV-seronegative people in Uganda. Int J Cancer 2003;103:233–40.

70 Nervi SJ, Benson B, Gounder S, et al. Pathology quiz case 2. Kaposi sarcoma (KS) of the pinna and external auditory canal. Arch Otolaryngol Head Neck Surg 2006;132:555, 557–8.

71 Frans E, Blockmans D, Peetermans W, et al. Kaposi's sarcoma presenting as generalized lymphedema. Acta Clin Belg 1994;49:19–22.

72 Schwartz RA, Burgess GH, Hoshaw RA. Patch stage Kaposi's sarcoma. J Am Acad Dermatol 1980;2:509–12.

73 Montesu MA, Rosella M, Cottoni F. Le sedi nel sarcoma di Kaposi classico. Studio su una casistica di 200 pazienti. G Ital Dermatol Venereol 1998;133:247–50.

74 Schwartz RA, Kardashian JF, McNutt NS, et al. Cutaneous angiosarcoma resembling anaplastic Kaposi's sarcoma in a homosexual man. Cancer 1983;51:721–6.

75 Schwartz RA, Brenden LD, Breeden JH, et al. Indolent lymphadenopathic Kaposi's sarcoma. J Surg Oncol 1987;34:243–7.

76 Ziegler JL, Katongole-Mbidde E. Kaposi's sarcoma in childhood: an analysis of 100 cases from Uganda and relationship to HIV infection. Int J Cancer 1996;65:200–3.

77 Snyder RA, Schwartz RA. Telangiectatic Kaposi's sarcoma. Occurrence in a patient with thymoma and myasthenia gravis receiving long-term immunosuppressive therapy. Arch Dermatol 1982;118:1020–1.

78 Schwartz RA, Spicer MS, Thomas I, et al. Ecchymotic Kaposi's sarcoma. Cutis 1995;56:104–6.

79 Schwartz RA, Spicer MS, Janniger CK, et al. Keloidal Kaposi's sarcoma: report of three patients. Dermatology 1994;189:271–4.

80 Kalambokis G, Kitsanou M, Stergiopoulou C, et al. Lymphangioma-like Kaposi's sarcoma with gastric involvement in a patient with lung cancer. J Eur Acad Dermatol Venereol 2005;19:653–4.

81 Katona I, Török L, Sérenyi P. Cystic Kaposi's sarcoma. Acta Dermatovenerol Alp Panonica Adriat 1995;4:63–6.

82 De Pasquale R, Nasca MR, Micali G. Postirradiation primary Kaposi's sarcoma of the head and neck. J Am Acad Dermatol 1999;40:312–4.

83 Maral T. The Koebner phenomenon in immuno-suppression-related Kaposi's sarcoma. Ann Plast Surg 2000;44:646–8.

84 Wolf R, Lotti T, Ruocco V. Isomorphic versus isotopic response: data and hypotheses. J Eur Acad Dermatol Venereol 2003;17:123–5.

85 Cottoni F, Masala MV, Piras P, et al. Mucosal involvement in classic Kaposi's sarcoma. Br J Dermatol 2003;148:1273–4.

86 Ruszczak Z, Stadler R, Schwartz RA. Kaposi's sarcoma limited to penis treated with cobalt-60 radiotherapy. J Med 1996;27:211–20.

87 Micali G, Nasca MR, De Pasquale R, et al. Primary classic Kaposi's sarcoma of the penis: report of a case and review. J Eur Acad Dermatol Venereol 2003;17: 320–3.

88 Schwartz RA, Cohen JB, Watson RA, et al. Penile Kaposi's sarcoma preceded by chronic penile lymphoedema. Br J Dermatol 2000;142:153–6.

89 Templeton AC. Studies in Kaposi's sarcoma. Postmortem findings and disease patterns in women. Cancer 1972;30:854–67.

90 Rosella M, Masotti A, Cottoni F. Endoscopic examination in Kaposi's sarcoma. J Eur Acad Dermatol Venereol 2000;14:225–6.

91 Lemlich G, Schwam L, Lebwohl M. Kaposi's sarcoma and acquired immunodeficiency syndrome. Postmortem findings in twenty-four cases. J Am Acad Dermatol 1987;16:319–25.

92 Kolios G, Kaloterakis A, Filiotou A, et al. Gastroscopic findings in Mediterranean Kaposi's sarcoma (non-AIDS). Gastrointest Endosc 1995;42:336–9.

93 Neff R, Kremer S, Voutsinas L, et al. Primary Kaposi's sarcoma of the ileum presenting as massive rectal bleeding. Am J Gastroenterol 1987;82:276–7.

94 Bouhnik Y, Chaussade S, Robin P, et al. [Protein-losing enteropathy syndrome caused by a localization of Kaposi's sarcoma in AIDS]. Gastroenterol Clin Biol 1989;13:838–40.

95 Wang NC, Chang FY, Chou YY, et al. Intussusception as the initial manifestation of AIDS associated with primary Kaposi's sarcoma: a case report. J Formos Med Assoc 2002;101:585–7.

96 Yoshida EM, Chan NH, Chan-Yan C, et al. Perforation of the jejunum secondary to AIDS-related gastrointestinal Kaposi's sarcoma. Can J Gastroenterol 1997;11:38–40.

97 Wheeler DW, Baigrie RJ. Palliative surgery for acute bowel obstruction caused by Kaposi's sarcoma in a patient with AIDS. Int J Clin Pract 2003;57: 347–8.

98 Palmieri C, Dhillon T, Thirlwell C, et al. Pulmonary Kaposi sarcoma in the era of highly active antiretroviral therapy. HIV Med 2006;7:291–3.

99 Restrepo CS, Martinez S, Lemos JA, et al. Imaging manifestations of Kaposi sarcoma. Radiographics 2006;26:1169–85.

100 Wolff SD, Kuhlman JE, Fishman EK. Thoracic Kaposi sarcoma in AIDS: CT findings. J Comput Assist Tomogr 1993;17:60–2.

101 Kulasegaram R, Saunders K, Bradbeer CS, et al. Is there a role for positron emission tomography scanning in HIV-positive patients with Kaposi's sarcoma and lymphadenopathy: two case reports. Int J STD AIDS 1997;8:709–12.

102 Peer FI, Pui MH, Mosam A, et al. 99mTc-MIBI imaging of cutaneous AIDS-associated Kaposi's sarcoma. Int J Dermatol 2007;46:166–71.

103 Schwartz RA, Dabski C, Dabska M. The Dabska tumor: a thirty-year retrospect. Dermatology 2000; 201:1–5.

104 Schwartz RA, Nychay SG, Janniger CK, et al. Bacillary angiomatosis: presentation of six patients, some with unusual features. Br J Dermatol 1997;136:60–5.

105 Schwartz RA, Gallardo MA, Kapila R, et al. Bacillary angiomatosis in an HIV seronegative patient on systemic steroid therapy. Br J Dermatol 1996;135:982–7.

106 Schwartz RA. Cutaneous metastatic disease. J Am Acad Dermatol 1995;33:161–82; quiz 183–6.

107 Schwartz RA. Histopathologic aspects of cutaneous metastatic disease. J Am Acad Dermatol 1995; 33:649–57.

108 Fernández G, Schwartz RA. Stewart-Treves syndrome. eMedicine Dermatology [Journal serial online] 2006. Available from: http://emedicine.com/derm/topic898.htm.

109 Kanitakis J, Narvaez D, Claudy A. Expression of the CD34 antigen distinguishes Kaposi's sarcoma from pseudo-Kaposi's sarcoma (acroangiodermatitis). Br J Dermatol 1996;134:44–6.

110 Lin RL, Janniger CK. Pyogenic granuloma. Cutis 2004;74:229–33.

111 Sbano P, Miracco C, Risulo M, et al. Acroangiodermatitis (pseudo-Kaposi sarcoma) associated with verrucous hyperplasia induced by suction-socket lower limb prosthesis. J Cutan Pathol 2005;32:429–32.

112 Korber A, Dissemond J. Pseudo-Kaposi sarcoma. Intern Med J 2006;36:535.

113 Wada DA, Perkins SL, Tripp S, et al. Human herpesvirus 8 and iron staining are useful in differentiating kaposi sarcoma from interstitial granuloma annulare. Am J Clin Pathol 2007;127:1–8.

114 Urquhart JL, Uzieblo A, Kohler S. Detection of HHV-8 in pyogenic granuloma-like kaposi sarcoma. Am J Dermatopathol 2006;28:317–21.

115 Ramirez JA, Laskin WB, Guitart J. Lymphangioma-like Kaposi sarcoma. J Cutan Pathol 2005;32:286–92.

116 Spanu A, Madeddu G, Cottoni F, et al. Usefulness of 99mTc-tetrofosmin scintigraphy in different variants of Kaposi's sarcoma. Oncology 2003;65:295–305.

117 Caceres-Rios H, Rodriguez-Tafur J, Bravo-Puccio F, et al. Verruga peruana: an infectious endemic angiomatosis. Crit Rev Oncog 1995;6:47–56.

118 Bedrosian SA, Goldman RL. Nodal angiomatosis: relationship to vascular transformation of lymph nodes. Arch Pathol Lab Med 1984;108:864–5.

119 Della Bella S, Nicola S, Brambilla L, et al. Quantitative and functional defects of dendritic cells in classic Kaposi's sarcoma. Clin Immunol 2006;119:317–29.

120 Yoshii N, Kanekura T, Eizuru Y, et al. Transcripts of the human herpesvirus 8 genome in skin lesions and peripheral blood mononuclear cells of a patient with classic Kaposi's sarcoma. Clin Exp Dermatol 2006;31:125–7.

121 Brown EE, Whitby D, Vitale F, et al. Virologic, hematologic, and immunologic risk factors for classic Kaposi sarcoma. Cancer 2006;107:2282–90.

122 Stratigos AJ, Malanos D, Touloumi G, et al. Association of clinical progression in classic Kaposi's sarcoma with reduction of peripheral B lymphocytes and partial increase in serum immune activation markers. Arch Dermatol 2005;141:1421–6.

123 Hong A, Davies S, Lee CS. Immunohistochemical detection of the human herpes virus 8 (HHV8) latent nuclear antigen-1 in Kaposi's sarcoma. Pathology 2003;35:448–50.

124 Kazakov DV, Schmid M, Adams V, et al. HHV-8 DNA sequences in the peripheral blood and skin lesions of an HIV-negative patient with multiple eruptive dermatofibromas: implications for the detection of HHV-8 as a diagnostic marker for Kaposi's sarcoma. Dermatology 2003;206:217–21.

125 Engels EA, Pittaluga S, Whitby D, et al. Immunoblastic lymphoma in persons with AIDS-associated Kaposi's sarcoma: a role for Kaposi's sarcoma-associated herpesvirus. Mod Pathol 2003;16:424–9.

126 Inoue N, Spira T, Lam L, et al. Comparison of serologic responses between Kaposi's sarcoma-positive and -negative men who were seropositive for both human herpesvirus 8 and human immunodeficiency virus. J Med Virol 2004;74:202–6.

127 Pyakurel P, Montag U, Castanos-Velez E, et al. CGH of microdissected Kaposi's sarcoma lesions reveals recurrent loss of chromosome Y in early and additional chromosomal changes in late tumour stages. AIDS 2006;20:1805–12.

128 Cottoni F, Masia IM, Cossu S, et al. Classical Kaposi's sarcoma and chronic lymphocytic leukaemia in the same skin biopsy. Report of two cases. Br J Dermatol 1998;139:753–4.

129 Liu W, Lacouture ME, Jiang J, et al. KSHV/HHV8-associated primary cutaneous plasmablastic lymphoma in a patient with Castleman's disease and Kaposi's sarcoma. J Cutan Pathol 2006;33 Suppl 2:46–51.

130 Carbone A. KSHV/HHV-8 associated Kaposi's sarcoma in lymph nodes concurrent with Epstein-Barr virus associated Hodgkin lymphoma. J Clin Pathol 2005;58:626–8.

131 Carbone A, Gloghini A, Vaccher E, et al. Kaposi's sarcoma-associated herpesvirus/human herpesvirus type 8-positive solid lymphomas: a tissue-based variant of primary effusion lymphoma. J Mol Diagn 2005;7:17–27.

132 Cerimele D, Carlesimo F, Fadda G, et al. Anaplastic progression of classic Kaposi's sarcoma. Dermatology 1997;194:287–9.

133 Satta R, Cossu S, Massarelli G, et al. Anaplastic transformation of classic Kaposi's sarcoma: clinicopathological study of five cases. Br J Dermatol 2001;145:847–9.

134 Ruszczak Z, Mayer da Silva A, Orfanos CE. Kaposi's sarcoma in AIDS. Multicentric angioneoplasia in early skin lesions. Am J Dermatopathol 1987;9:388–98.

135 Ruszczak Z, Mayer da Silva A, Orfanos CE. Angioproliferative changes in clinically noninvolved, perilesional skin in AIDS-associated Kaposi's sarcoma. Dermatologica 1987;175:270–9.

136 Pantanowitz L, Dezube BJ, Pinkus GS, et al. Histological characterization of regression in acquired immunodeficiency syndrome-related Kaposi's sarcoma. J Cutan Pathol 2004;31:26–34.

137 Matsumura S, Fujita Y, Gomez E, et al. Activation of the Kaposi's sarcoma-associated herpesvirus major latency locus by the lytic switch protein RTA (ORF50). J Virol 2005;79:8493–505.

138 Hammock L, Reisenauer A, Wang W, et al. Latency-associated nuclear antigen expression and human herpesvirus-8 polymerase chain reaction in the evaluation of Kaposi sarcoma and other vascular tumors in HIV-positive patients. Mod Pathol 2005;18:463–8.

139 Ngan KW, Kuo TT. Simultaneous occurrence of Hodgkin's lymphoma and Kaposi's sarcoma within

the same lymph nodes of a non-AIDS patient. Int J Surg Pathol 2006;14:85–8.

140 O'Connell KM. Kaposi's sarcoma in lymph nodes: histological study of lesions from 16 cases in Malawi. J Clin Pathol 1977;30:696–703.

141 Pyakurel P, Pak F, Mwakigonja AR, et al. Lymphatic and vascular origin of Kaposi's sarcoma spindle cells during tumor development. Int J Cancer 2006;119:1262–7.

142 Folpe AL, Veikkola T, Valtola R, et al. Vascular endothelial growth factor receptor-3 (VEGFR-3): a marker of vascular tumors with presumed lymphatic differentiation, including Kaposi's sarcoma, kaposiform and Dabska-type hemangioendotheliomas, and a subset of angiosarcomas. Mod Pathol 2000;13:180–5.

143 Nasti G, Talamini R, Antinori A, et al. AIDS-related Kaposi's Sarcoma: evaluation of potential new prognostic factors and assessment of the AIDS Clinical Trial Group Staging System in the Haart Era—the Italian Cooperative Group on AIDS and Tumors and the Italian Cohort of Patients Naive From Antiretrovirals. J Clin Oncol 2003;21:2876–82.

144 Brambilla L, Boneschi V, Taglioni M, et al. Staging of classic Kaposi's sarcoma: a useful tool for therapeutic choices. Eur J Dermatol 2003;13:83–6.

145 Krown SE, Testa MA, Huang J. AIDS-related Kaposi's sarcoma: prospective validation of the AIDS Clinical Trials Group staging classification. AIDS Clinical Trials Group Oncology Committee. J Clin Oncol 1997;15:3085–92.

146 Mitsuyasu RT. Clinical variants and staging of Kaposi's sarcoma. Semin Oncol 1987;14:13–8.

147 Krigel RL, Laubenstein LJ, Muggia FM. Kaposi's sarcoma: a new staging classification. Cancer Treat Rep 1983;67:531–4.

148 Volberding PA. Moving towards a uniform staging for human immunodeficiency virus-associated Kaposi's sarcoma. J Clin Oncol 1989;7:1184–5.

149 Krown SE, Metroka C, Wernz JC. Kaposi's sarcoma in the acquired immune deficiency syndrome: a proposal for uniform evaluation, response, and staging criteria. AIDS Clinical Trials Group Oncology Committee. J Clin Oncol 1989;7:1201–7.

150 Cottoni F, Montesu MA. Kaposi's sarcoma classification: a problem not yet defined. Int J Dermatol 1996;35:480–3.

151 Klein E, Schwartz RA, Laor Y, et al. Treatment of Kaposi's sarcoma with vinblastine. Cancer 1980;45:427–31.

152 Gascon P, Schwartz RA. Kaposi's sarcoma. New treatment modalities. Dermatol Clin 2000;18:169–75, x.

153 Gascon P, Schwartz RA. Treatment of Kaposi's sarcoma. Dermatol Clin 1994;12:451–6.

154 Masia IM, Satta R, Rosella M, et al. Terapia del sarcoma di Kaposi classico. G Ital Dermatol Venereol 2000;135:569–78.

155 Grabar S, Abraham B, Mahamat A, et al. Differential impact of combination antiretroviral therapy in preventing Kaposi's sarcoma with and without visceral involvement. J Clin Oncol 2006;24:3408–14.

156 Martinez V, Caumes E, Gambotti L, et al. Remission from Kaposi's sarcoma on HAART is associated with suppression of HIV replication and is independent of protease inhibitor therapy. Br J Cancer 2006;94:1000–6.

157 Becker G, Bottke D. Radiotherapy in the management of Kaposi's sarcoma. Onkologie 2006;29:329–33.

158 Yildiz F, Genc M, Akyurek S, et al. Radiotherapy in the management of Kaposi's sarcoma: comparison of 8 Gy versus 6 Gy. J Natl Med Assoc 2006;98:1136–9.

159 Ekmekci TR, Kendirci M, Kizilkaya O, et al. Sildenafil citrate-aided radiotherapy for the treatment of Kaposi's sarcoma of the penis. J Eur Acad Dermatol Venereol 2005;19:603–4.

160 Tardivo JP, Del Giglio A, Paschoal LH, et al. New photodynamic therapy protocol to treat AIDS-related Kaposi's sarcoma. Photomed Laser Surg 2006;24:528–31.

161 Szeimies RM, Lorenzen T, Karrer S, et al. [Photochemotherapy of cutaneous AIDS-associated Kaposi sarcoma with indocyanine green and laser light]. Hautarzt 2001;52:322–6.

162 Rosen T. Limited extent AIDS-related cutaneous Kaposi's sarcoma responsive to imiquimod 5% cream. Int J Dermatol 2006;45:854–6.

163 Brambilla L, Miedico A, Ferrucci S, et al. Combination of vinblastine and bleomycin as first line therapy in advanced classic Kaposi's sarcoma. J Eur Acad Dermatol Venereol 2006;20:1090–4.

164 Dezube BJ, Pantanowitz L, Aboulafia DM. Management of AIDS-related Kaposi sarcoma: advances in target discovery and treatment. AIDS Read 2004;14:236–8, 243–4, 251–3.

165 Kreuter A, Rasokat H, Klouche M, et al. Liposomal pegylated doxorubicin versus low-dose recombinant interferon Alfa-2a in the treatment of advanced classic Kaposi's sarcoma; retrospective analysis of three German centers. Cancer Invest 2005;23:653–9.

166 Cattel L, Ceruti M, Dosio F. From conventional to stealth liposomes: a new frontier in cancer chemotherapy. Tumori 2003;89:237–49.

167 Cooley T, Henry D, Tonda M, et al. A randomized, double-blind study of pegylated liposomal doxorubicin for the treatment of AIDS-related Kaposi's sarcoma. Oncologist 2007;12:114–23.

168 Dhillon T, Stebbing J, Bower M. Paclitaxel for AIDS-associated Kaposi's sarcoma. Expert Rev Anticancer Ther 2005;5:215–9.

169 Evans SR, Krown SE, Testa MA, et al. Phase II evaluation of low-dose oral etoposide for the treatment of relapsed or progressive AIDS-related Kaposi's sarcoma: an AIDS Clinical Trials Group clinical study. J Clin Oncol 2002;20:3236–41.

170 Aldenhoven M, Barlo NP, Sanders CJ. Therapeutic strategies for epidemic Kaposi's sarcoma. Int J STD AIDS 2006;17:571–8.

171 Nasti G, Martellotta F, Berretta M, et al. Impact of highly active antiretroviral therapy on the presenting features and outcome of patients with acquired immunodeficiency syndrome-related Kaposi sarcoma. Cancer 2003;98:2440–6.

172 Leitch H, Trudeau M, Routy JP. Effect of protease inhibitor-based highly active antiretroviral therapy on survival in HIV-associated advanced Kaposi's sarcoma patients treated with chemotherapy. HIV Clin Trials 2003;4:107–14.

173 Krown SE, Lee JY, Lin L, et al. Interferon-alpha2b with protease inhibitor-based antiretroviral therapy in patients with AIDS-associated Kaposi sarcoma: an AIDS malignancy consortium phase I trial. J Acquir Immune Defic Syndr 2006;41:149–53.

174 Krown SE, Li P, Von Roenn JH, et al. Efficacy of low-dose interferon with antiretroviral therapy in Kaposi's sarcoma: a randomized phase II AIDS clinical trials group study. J Interferon Cytokine Res 2002;22:295–303.

175 Dezube BJ, Krown SE, Lee JY, et al. Randomized phase II trial of matrix metalloproteinase inhibitor COL-3 in AIDS-related Kaposi's sarcoma: an AIDS Malignancy Consortium Study. J Clin Oncol 2006;24:1389–94.

176 Levine AM, Tulpule A. Clinical aspects and management of AIDS-related Kaposi's sarcoma. Eur J Cancer 2001;37:1288–95.

177 Tulpule A, Scadden DT, Espina BM, et al. Results of a randomized study of IM862 nasal solution in the treatment of AIDS-related Kaposi's sarcoma. J Clin Oncol 2000;18:716–23.

178 Kruger EA, Figg WD. TNP-470: an angiogenesis inhibitor in clinical development for cancer. Expert Opin Investig Drugs 2000;9:1383–96.

179 Noy A, von Roenn J, Politsmakher A, et al. Fatal hepatorenal failure and thrombocytopenia with SU5416, a vascular endothelial growth factor Flk-1 receptor inhibitor, in AIDS-Kaposi's sarcoma. AIDS 2007;21:113–5.

180 Krown SE. Therapy of AIDS-associated Kaposi's sarcoma: targeting pathogenetic mechanisms. Hematol Oncol Clin North Am 2003;17:763–83.

181 Paghdal KV, Schwartz RA. Thalidomide and its dermatologic uses. Acta Derm Venerol Croatica 2007;15:34–9.

182 Little RF, Pluda JM, Wyvill KM, et al. Activity of subcutaneous interleukin-12 in AIDS-related Kaposi sarcoma. Blood 2006;107:4650–7.

183 Moray G, Basaran O, Yagmurdur MC, et al. Immunosuppressive therapy and Kaposi's sarcoma after kidney transplantation. Transplant Proc 2004;36:168–70.

184 Stallone G, Schena A, Infante B, et al. Sirolimus for Kaposi's sarcoma in renal-transplant recipients. N Engl J Med 2005;352:1317–23.

185 Yilmaz R, Akoglu H, Kirkpantur A, et al. A novel immunosuppressive agent, sirolimus, in the treatment of Kaposi's sarcoma in a renal transplant recipient. Ren Fail 2007;29:103–5.

186 Bodsworth NJ, Bloch M, Bower M, et al. Phase III vehicle-controlled, multi-centered study of topical alitretinoin gel 0.1% in cutaneous AIDS-related Kaposi's sarcoma. Am J Clin Dermatol 2001;2:77–87.

187 Miles SA, Dezube BJ, Lee JY, et al. Antitumor activity of oral 9-cis-retinoic acid in HIV-associated Kaposi's sarcoma. AIDS 2002;16:421–9.

188 Bernstein ZP, Chanan-Khan A, Miller KC, et al. A multicenter phase II study of the intravenous administration of liposomal tretinoin in patients with acquired immunodeficiency syndrome-associated Kaposi's sarcoma. Cancer 2002;95:2555–61.

189 Mocroft A, Youle M, Gazzard B, et al. Anti-herpesvirus treatment and risk of Kaposi's sarcoma in HIV infection. Royal Free/Chelsea and Westminster Hospitals Collaborative Group. AIDS 1996;10:1101–5.

190 Glesby MJ, Hoover DR, Weng S, et al. Use of anti-herpes drugs and the risk of Kaposi's sarcoma: data from the Multicenter AIDS Cohort Study. J Infect Dis 1996;173:1477–80.

191 Bossini N, Sandrini S, Setti G, et al. [Successful treatment with liposomal doxorubicin and foscarnet in a patient with widespread Kaposi's sarcoma and human herpes virus 8-related, serious hemophagocytic syndrome, after renal transplantation]. G Ital Nefrol 2005;22:281–6.

192 Verucchi G, Calza L, Trevisani F, et al. Human herpesvirus-8-related Kaposi's sarcoma after liver transplantation successfully treated with cidofovir and liposomal daunorubicin. Transpl Infect Dis 2005; 7:34–7.

193 Little RF, Merced-Galindez F, Staskus K, et al. A pilot study of cidofovir in patients with Kaposi sarcoma. J Infect Dis 2003;187:149–53.

194 Casper C, Wald A. The use of antiviral drugs in the prevention and treatment of Kaposi sarcoma, multicentric Castleman disease and primary effusion lymphoma. Curr Top Microbiol Immunol 2007; 312:289–307.

195 Stebbing J, Portsmouth S, Nelson M, et al. The efficacy of ritonavir in the prevention of AIDS-related Kaposi's sarcoma. Int J Cancer 2004;108: 631–3.

196 Montaner S, Sodhi A, Ramsdell AK, et al. The Kaposi's sarcoma–associated herpesvirus G protein-coupled receptor as a therapeutic target for the treatment of Kaposi's sarcoma. Cancer Res 2006;66:168–74.

197 Morgan D, Malamba SS, Orem J, et al. Survival by AIDS defining condition in rural Uganda. Sex Transm Infect 2000;76:193–7.

198 Brenner B, Weissmann-Brenner A, Rakowsky E, et al. Classical Kaposi sarcoma: prognostic factor analysis of 248 patients. Cancer 2002;95:1982–7.

CHAPTER 10

Dysplastic nevus and dysplastic nevus syndrome

Christopher J. Steen, Philip J. Cohen, and Robert A. Schwartz

The dysplastic nevus is a special kind of atypical melanocytic nevus, with clinical and histologic features suggestive of an intermediate form between the common acquired melanocytic nevus and melanoma. Dysplastic nevi are important markers for both familial and nonfamilial melanoma. As many as 50% of patients with "sporadic" melanoma have been observed to have dysplastic nevi [1–3]. The incidence of dysplastic nevi in the general population has been estimated to be 1.8% to 10% and possibly as high as 19% [4–11].

The presence of dysplastic nevi has been established as an independent risk factor for melanoma, along with several other cutaneous traits, including red or blonde hair, solar lentigines, skin type 1 or 2, and increased numbers of common acquired melanocytic nevi [12–14]. One study found the adjusted relative risk of melanoma to be 2 for a single dysplastic nevus and 12 for 10 or more dysplastic nevi [14]. Another found a relative risk of 1.6 when one to four dysplastic nevi were counted and 6.1 for five or more dysplastic nevi [12]. The risk of melanoma attributable to dysplastic nevi may be further exacerbated by the coexistence of other melanoma risk factors, such as skin type 1 or 2 [15].

The increased risk for melanoma is particularly true in the setting of the dysplastic nevus syndrome (DNS). DNS encompasses individuals with multiple dysplastic nevi arising sporadically or in a setting of a family history of dysplastic nevi or melanoma. DNS has been divided into a number of forms [16] (Table 10.1). Type A is sporadic dysplastic nevus without melanoma; type B is familial dysplastic nevus without melanoma; type C is sporadic dysplastic nevus with a personal history of melanoma; type D-l is familial dysplastic nevus with one family member with melanoma; and type D-2 is familial dysplastic nevus with two or more family members with melanoma. Meticulous screening of family members may demonstrate that presumptive cases of sporadic DNS are actually familial.

All patients with DNS have an increased risk for developing melanoma, although the magnitude of the risk varies among the DNS types. A study by Marghoob and colleagues [17] found an overall relative risk of melanoma in DNS of 60 and a 10-year cumulative risk of 10.7%. The relative risk of melanoma is least in patients with DNS types A and B, and has been estimated to be 7 with a cumulative lifetime risk of 6% [3]. The relative risk of melanoma in type D-2 patients may be as high as 1000 or greater compared with the general population [15,18,19]. Individuals with DNS also appear to be at an increased risk for multiple primary cutaneous melanomas. One study found a 35.5% cumulative 10-year risk of developing a second melanoma in those with DNS and a history of melanoma as compared with a 17% 10-year risk of developing a second melanoma in those with a history of melanoma but without DNS [20]. Patients with DNS may also be at increased risk of conjunctival and intraocular melanoma [21–24]. The recognition of DNS may allow early detection of melanoma and identification of those at risk and provide the opportunity for the initiation of preventive measures.

A great deal of discussion has centered on the validity of the dysplastic nevus as a distinct entity and its potential for progression to melanoma. Much

Table 10.1 Forms of dysplastic nevus syndrome

Type	Definition
A	Sporadic dysplastic nevi without personal or family history of melanoma
B	Familial dysplastic nevi without personal or family history of melanoma
C	Sporadic dysplastic nevi with personal history of melanoma
D-1	Familial dysplastic nevi with one family member with melanoma
D-2	Familial dysplastic nevi with two or more family members with melanoma

disagreement over its nature stems from a lack of uniform clinical and histologic criteria to define it. In fact, even the term *dysplastic nevus* has contributed to the controversy. Strictly speaking, the term *dysplastic* is a histologic one. The purist may object to the clinical description of a melanocytic nevus as "dysplastic-looking." Dysplastic nevi generally demonstrate both clinical and histologic evidence of distorted and disordered architecture. A statement by the National Institutes of Health (NIH) Consensus Conference in 1992 sought to eliminate the variability in nomenclature and recommended that the term *dysplastic nevus* be replaced with *atypical mole* and the histologic diagnosis be termed *nevi with architectural disorder* along with a description of the degree of melanocytic atypia [25]. A 2004 survey revealed that the term *dysplastic nevus* remains commonplace [26]. It is the term that we, too, prefer.

History of the dysplastic nevus syndrome

Melanoma arising in a familial context and in association with multiple, often unusual-appearing nevi, was first reported by Norris [27] in 1820. In 1974, Munro [28] described atypical, "active" junctional nevi in a patient with a family history of melanoma. The significance of such nevi was not emphasized until 1976 when Clark and associates [1] described

the atypical melanocytic nevi in familial melanoma patients. The observation was confirmed in 1977 by Frichot and Lynch [29]. In 1978, Clark and colleagues [1] named the disorder the "B-K mole syndrome" after the last initials of the group's first two affected families. The original B-K mole series consisted of 37 patients from six families followed for up to 6 years. Two dysplastic nevi in this group were photographically demonstrated to progress to histologically confirmed melanoma [1]. The same year, Lynch and associates [30] reported a family with "familial atypical multiple mole-melanoma syndrome" (FAMMM), a term that was felt to better describe this genodermatosis. In a family followed for 10 years, the biopsy of a large irregular nevus in one member showed "junctional activity." Two years later, the remainder had become a level 4 melanoma [19]. These cases inspired intensive clinical and histopathologic studies of these melanocytic nevi.

The initial description of dysplastic nevus in the most severely affected cases (B-K mole syndrome patients) emphasized the following characteristics [1]:

1 Outline: Irregular
2 Color: Haphazard, with some pink and some depigmented areas
3 Size: Frequently 5 to 10 mm or larger
4 Number: Less than 10 to greater than 100
5 Distribution: Mainly on the upper trunk and extremities, but also found on the lower extremities and bathing suit areas
6 Histology: Disordered nests of melanocytes, lentiginous proliferation of individual melanocytes, and occasional atypical melanocytes. A dermal nevus component was often found centrally and showed uniform maturation without unusual features. A delicate lamellar fibroplasia, prominent vessels, and a sparse patchy lymphocytic infiltrate were commonly present in the papillary dermis.

The B-K mole syndrome and FAMMM, corresponding with DNS type D-2, associated familial aggregations of melanomas and the unusual nevi noted in the affected patients and close relatives. The concept was extended by Elder and coworkers [31] to include both familial and sporadic forms and was termed the dysplastic nevus syndrome, in which these unusual nevi were associated with sporadically occurring melanoma. Rahbari and Mehregan [32] further described sporadic cases of atypical melanocytic nevi in the absence of a family history of melanoma. Fusaro and colleagues [33] responded that because family history may be notoriously inaccurate, patients with the phenotypic expression of FAMMM should be closely followed, as some may develop melanoma or transmit the genotype to progeny. The 1992 NIH Consensus Statement on the diagnosis and treatment of early melanoma recommended that the syndrome for melanoma-prone families with atypical moles be called familial atypical mole and melanoma syndrome (FAMM) [25]. The consensus statement defined FAMM as follows: (1) occurrence of melanoma in one or more first- or second-degree relatives; (2) large numbers of moles (often >50), some of which are atypical and often variable in size; and (3) moles that demonstrate certain distinct histologic features [25].

Pathogenesis of dysplastic nevus syndrome

Dysplastic nevus syndrome has an autosomal dominant inheritance pattern with incomplete penetrance and variable expressivity. Although considerable progress has been made to elucidate the genetics involved in the pathogenesis of familial melanoma, the genetic defects involved in DNS remain uncertain. Melanoma susceptibility genes can be found at multiple chromosomal loci, including 1p36, 9p21, and 12q14 [34]. Most investigation into these loci has focused on 9p21, where a tumor-suppressor gene, *p16*, has been identified. Also known as cyclin-dependent kinase 2A (*CDKN2A*), this gene functions as a cell cycle regulator at the G1 checkpoint, and when mutated, may result in uncontrolled cell division [35–37]. Mutations in several other genes, including *CDK4*, *PTEN*, *ARF*, and *BRAF*, have been associated with melanoma. Although mutations in particular genes, including *CDKN2A* and *CDK4*, have been identified in some families with dysplastic nevi and melanoma, studies to identify the genetic basis for DNS have been inconsistent [38–40]. A recent analysis failed to find evidence of the aforementioned genetic defects

among 28 probands with DNS [41]. Variation in the number and anatomic distribution of dysplastic nevi in individuals with DNS may be attributed to incomplete penetrance of the gene and/or effects of ultraviolet (UV) radiation on the genome. Cytogenetic studies have demonstrated increased frequencies of cells with chromosomal rearrangements in patients with DNS, a finding that suggests DNS may involve chromosomal instability [42,43]. Multiple studies have found an increased sensitivity to UV-induced DNA damage in individuals with DNS or familial melanoma [44–49]. Further research is needed to better define the genetic basis for DNS.

Clinical recognition of dysplastic nevi

Dysplastic nevi do not follow an evolutionary pattern of either persistence with stability or differentiation in the direction of ultimate regression, as seen in common acquired melanocytic nevi [50]. Rather, dysplastic nevi demonstrate a persistent and disordered growth, evident both clinically and histologically. The clinical recognition of dysplastic nevi focuses on several characteristics that help distinguish them from common acquired melanocytic nevi: shape, border, color, diameter, and topography (Fig. 10.1, Table 10.2). Many of these features may also be seen in melanoma, although often to a greater degree.

1 Shape: The shape may be round or oval, like the common acquired nevus, although asymmetric notching and/or outgrowth of pseudopodia are usually observed in lesions over 3 to 4 mm in diameter.

2 Border: The boundary may be irregular with slightly indiscrete to frankly hazy or fuzzy areas, with traces of pink or brownish pigment spilling into surrounding normal skin.

3 Color: The coloration of dysplastic nevi is often variegated, with irregular speckling with tan/brown colors and sometimes including foci of tan/brown/dark brown hues or black pigment. Erythema may be seen as a component of dysplastic nevi but is not normally seen in common acquired melanocytic nevi. This is manifest as a pink background color, the intensity of which may vary from trace to slight to moderate. Sometimes only a focal

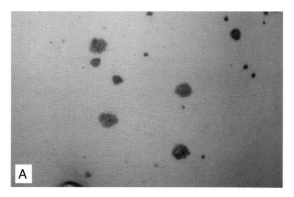
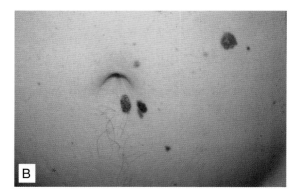

Fig. 10.1 *A* and *B*: Dysplastic nevi demonstrating irregular border, asymmetry, and variegated color.

area of pink or a subtle pink hue at the periphery may be seen. The erythema does not blanch readily; the degree of erythema varies considerably from lesion to lesion and from patient to patient.

4 Diameter: Dysplastic nevi are most easily recognized when larger than 5 mm in diameter. The Clark group's [1] initial description of dysplastic nevi in B-K mole syndrome patients had emphasized that they were frequently 5 to 10 mm or larger, and that size was an important clue in identifying dysplastic nevi. Large size, however, is not a prerequisite for the diagnosis of dysplastic nevi.

5 Topography: The topography within any given dysplastic nevus may include macular and papular components. A minimal elevation to tangential lighting is noted in most of them. The skin surface markings may be suggestive of early lichen simplex chronicus, showing subtle elevation and

Table 10.2 Screening criteria for the clinical diagnosis of dysplastic nevi

Criteria	Common Acquired Nevi	Dysplastic Nevi
Shape[a]	Approximately round or oval	May be irregular in shape with asymmetric notching or pseudopodia
Border[a]	Sharp and well defined	May be irregular with slightly indiscrete to frankly hazy or fuzzy areas
Color[b]	Uniformly tan, brown, or flesh colored	Tan/brown/dark brown hues or bluish black pigment with variegation and/or irregular speckling; may have erythema manifest as pinkish background color
Diameter[a,c]	Usually smaller than 5 mm	Often larger than 5 mm
Topography[a]	Overall uniformity	Macular component is usual; flat or mildly dome-shaped papular component common; pebbly contour to surface highly suggestive

[a] Helpful if present, not exclusionary if absent.
[b] Irregular bluish black color (like a lead pencil–injury tattoo) should raise the suspicion of early melanoma.
[c] Dysplastic nevi smaller than 5 mm usually require an experienced physician's examination for diagnosis.

coarsening. Scale is only infrequently noted. Erosion is not seen in the nontraumatized dysplastic nevus.

The clinical presentation of patients with dysplastic nevi seems as varied as the morphology of individual dysplastic nevi. The classical type D-2 phenotype may be first evident with numerous distinctly large, irregular, variegate nevi, mostly concentrated on the trunk and less numerous on the head, neck, and lower extremities. More commonly, however, dysplastic nevi are not strikingly large. From several to a dozen dysplastic nevi may be mixed among several to several dozen common acquired melanocytic nevi. In patients with a solitary dysplastic nevus, it may be located anywhere.

Technique for examination of patients for dysplastic nevi

The entire cutaneous surface of each patient should be examined, including the scalp and interdigital web spaces. A total skin examination of all new patients may reveal dysplastic nevi and unsuspected melanoma. Unlike basal cell carcinoma, which has an overwhelming predilection for sun-exposed areas, dysplastic nevi and melanoma are far more likely to occur on normally nonexposed surfaces, including the scalp, buttocks, or female breasts [51–54]. The first presentation of familial dysplastic nevi in prepubertal children may be atypical-appearing scalp nevi, frequently overlooked on cursory examination [53,54]. Because ocular melanomas may be part of DNS [21–24], it may be desirable to carefully inspect the iris, fundus, and conjunctivae of each patient.

Good lighting is an invaluable aid in proper diagnosis. A strong incandescent light, preferably a quartz-halogen light source, applied closely and tangentially to the skin reveals the subtleties of coloration that may clarify the diagnosis. Overhead fluorescent lighting is inadequate, because the greenish hues of the fluorescent light may obscure the pink hues of dysplastic nevi, causing them to appear grayish. Each melanocytic nevus is best studied with gentle stretching between the examiner's fingers to reveal its salient clinical features.

Clinical differential diagnosis of dysplastic nevi

The subtle changes that characterize the mildly and moderately dysplastic nevus may be confused most frequently with nevoid lentigines, as the junctional melanocytes proliferate and start to form intradermal nests. Compound nevi with lateral junctional hyperplasia, as may be seen following sunburn stimulation, often have a scalloped, slightly hazy outline. These may have a reddish brown pigmentation that may be confused with the pinker hue of the base coloration of dysplastic nevi. Benign lentigines may be difficult to distinguish from dysplastic nevi of the lentiginous type. Focal dysplastic changes in compound nevi may resemble folliculitis. Some irritated seborrheic keratoses resemble dysplastic nevi, as may pigmented basal cell carcinomas and pigmented actinic keratoses. Occasionally, dermatofibromas, blue nevi, or melanocytic nevi with regressive changes may resemble dysplastic nevi.

Histopathology of dysplastic nevi

Considerable discussion has arisen among dermatopathologists regarding the nomenclature and histopathologic features of dysplastic nevi, including questioning of the term *dysplastic* [55,56]. Although some are of the opinion that dysplastic nevi do not exist as a separate entity and are merely part of the spectrum of benign melanocytic nevi [55,57], others believe that dysplastic nevi represent distinct nevi with aberrant melanocytic differentiation [58]. Unfortunately, much of the disagreement stems from a lack of universally accepted criteria for the reproducible diagnosis of dysplastic nevi. Among those who feel that dysplastic nevi are a unique entity, histopathologic diagnosis requires examination of both architectural and cytologic features of a given melanocytic nevus.

Architectural features of dysplastic nevi suggest a disordered hyperplasia. They are often poorly circumscribed and may display asymmetry. Lentiginous melanocytic proliferation almost always is seen in conjunction with elongation of the rete ridges (Fig. 10.2). Nests of melanocytes tend to form horizontal bridging between the tips of adjacent rete

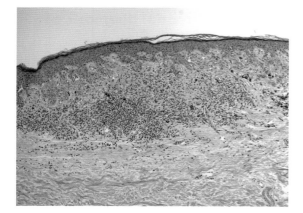

Fig. 10.2 Compound dysplastic nevus demonstrating elongation of rete ridges, bridging of adjacent rete ridges, and moderate dermal lymphocytic infiltrate.

ridges (Fig. 10.3). Often, the "dysplastic" changes are found confined to the melanocytic nests of the epidermis, whereas the deeper cells show the histologic appearance of a common melanocytic nevus, with nevus cells demonstrating an orderly maturation. Junctional melanocytes may be seen singly or in nests extending several rete ridges away from the

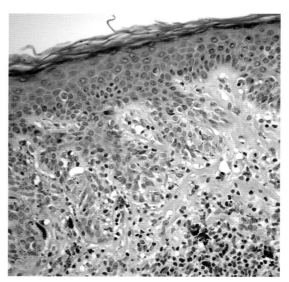

Fig. 10.4 Concentric eosinophilic fibrosis surrounding rete ridges.

main dermal component, a phenomenon known as "shouldering." Concentric eosinophilic fibrosis and lamellar fibroplasia also are frequently seen (Fig. 10.4). A lymphocytic host response, sometimes in a perivascular or lichenoid pattern, may be present, but is not a reliable diagnostic sign. The essential architectural features of dysplastic nevi are summarized in Table 10.3.

The degree of cytologic atypia varies greatly within dysplastic nevi, with some demonstrating only a few atypical cells and others composed almost entirely of atypical cells. The melanocytes of dysplastic nevi may exhibit a spectrum of cytologic aberrancy, from mild nuclear pleomorphism to frank cellular atypia, often with entrapment of

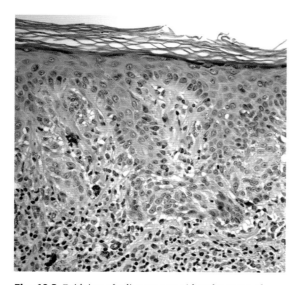

Fig. 10.3 Bridging of adjacent rete ridges by nests of melanocytes.

Table 10.3 Histologic architectural features of dysplastic nevi

Hypertrophy and/or elongation of tips of rete ridges
Horizontal melanocytic bridging of rete ridges
Concentric fibroplasia
Lamellar fibroplasia
Perivascular or lichenoid lymphocytic host response

atypical nevus cell nests in the dense collagen. Hyperchromatism, nuclear enlargement, and prominent nucleoli are sometimes observed. Mitotic figures are rarely seen.

Management and follow-up

Once diagnosed, patients with DNS require regular lifelong follow-up with complete skin examinations to identify potential melanomas as early as possible when they are the thinnest and have the best prognosis. Recommended follow-up intervals range from 3 to 12 months, depending on risk factors, and should be more frequent in individuals with a personal or family history of melanoma. New atypical nevi may appear throughout a patient's lifetime; there may be times when nevi undergo rapid growth without apparent cause. During these periods, skin evaluations every 3 months may be advisable. Phenotypic DNS patients who become immunosuppressed, whether because of an illness such as HIV or immunosuppressive therapy, should be considered at increased risk for melanoma [59–61]. It would seem advisable to follow such patients at 3-month intervals and to excise their atypical nevi at early stages of development.

Patients with DNS should be encouraged to have annual ophthalmologic examinations, as multiple dysplastic nevi have been associated with an increased incidence of ocular melanoma [62–64]. In addition to melanoma, patients with DNS may be at elevated risk for developing visceral malignancies, particularly pancreatic cancer [65–68]. As such, routine medical follow-up with complete physical examination and age-appropriate cancer screening is recommended.

Regular self–skin examination should be encouraged among patients with DNS. Preliminary studies indicate that self–skin examination may allow for earlier detection of melanoma with a subsequent reduction in overall mortality [69–71]. Patients should be educated about the warning signs of melanoma and advised to examine their skin monthly. They should be further encouraged to seek medical attention in a timely manner once a suspicious lesion is detected.

Dysplastic nevus syndrome patients need to be aware that solar exposure may promote the development of more and larger dysplastic nevi and has been implicated as an important factor in the pathogenesis of melanoma. They should be counseled on sun avoidance and sun protection in addition to broad-spectrum UV-A and UV-B sunscreen and sun block use. Because there is insufficient evidence to prove that sunscreen use alone prevents melanoma, patients should be advised that sunscreen is merely an adjunct protective measure to be used when sun exposure is unavoidable.

Recognizing subtle changes in nevi in patients with many dysplastic nevi may be challenging. Baseline photographs of the entire body and/or specific lesions may be useful in these patients. By allowing comparison of the appearance of nevi at subsequent visits, subtle changes of early melanoma can be detected and a more timely diagnosis and treatment offered when prognosis is better [72,73]. Photographs may also prevent unnecessary biopsies by verifying a lack of change in clinically dysplastic nevi [72,73]. Examination of nevi with conventional handheld or digital epiluminescence microscopy (dermatoscopy) may also aid in the detection of melanoma when used by experienced practitioners [74–77]. A recent study concluded that there are so far no digital dermoscopic criteria that can clearly distinguish dysplastic nevi from in situ melanomas [78]. Dermoscopy is the subject of Chapter 12.

Given the genetic link in DNS, cutaneous screening should be recommended in first- and second-degree relatives of patients with DNS. This may aid in clarifying the type of DNS as well as the potential melanoma risk. Screening of family members may also help identify DNS and melanoma in affected relatives.

Surgical removal of melanocytic nevi in patients with DNS has been another source of controversy. Although previously viewed as precursors to melanoma, dysplastic nevi are now primarily regarded as markers for increased melanoma risk. Several studies have examined the efficacy of prophylactic removal of dysplastic nevi to detect and prevent melanoma. A cohort study of 278 adults with multiple dysplastic nevi identified 20 melanomas among 16 patients during the study period [73]. Of the melanomas identified, only three arose from preexisting dysplastic nevi whereas 13 arose de novo. The authors estimated that had they removed all dysplastic nevi on patients in the study (almost 6000 lesions), they would only have prevented three melanomas [73]. They further concluded that the potential cost and morbidity of removing all dysplastic nevi are not justified by the decrease in melanoma risk [73]. Because the majority of melanomas arise de novo and not from preexisting dysplastic nevi, the primary role for removal of an individual dysplastic nevus is to rule out melanoma.

In general, suspicious pigmented lesions should be removed in entirety by excision down to subcutaneous fat to provide the dermatopathologist with optimal tissue for diagnosis. The 1992 NIH consensus guidelines state, "a biopsy should be a total removal by punch, saucerization, or elliptical excision to include a portion of underlying subcutaneous fat" [25]. Recent studies have addressed the use of shave excisions for removal of dysplastic nevi [79,80]. Shave excision of macular melanocytic nevi resulted in their complete removal in 88% of cases [80]. These authors concluded that deep razor blade excision is a highly useful and inexpensive technique for the removal and histologic diagnosis of macular, melanocytic nevi; is potentially less scarring than traditional excision; and may be particularly useful in patients with multiple nevi, such as those with DNS [80].

Multiple medications have been applied to dysplastic nevi in an effort to identify agents with the potential for melanoma chemoprevention without the associated morbidity and scarring of traditional excisional surgery. Studies of topical tretinoin, 5-fluorouracil, and imiquimod have shown variable results, with some reports of minor histologic improvements in atypia [81–85]. Although some of these agents may warrant further controlled study with proper histopathologic controls, we do not recommend the treatment of dysplastic nevi with any of these agents, as there is currently no convincing evidence of effective melanoma chemoprophylaxis with their use.

Conclusion

The recognition of DNS may allow for identification of those at increased risk for melanoma, facilitate the early detection of melanoma, and provide the opportunity for the initiation of preventive measures. In the presence of a family history of melanoma, there is little question that the presence of dysplastic nevi identifies family members at greatest risk. In this selected population, dysplastic nevi are identified in half or more of the cases. We suspect that with more rigorous family screening, a large portion of DNS cases classified as sporadic will be reclassified as familial.

Far less clear, however, is the significance of the truly sporadic dysplastic nevi discovered on routine screening of an unselected population. What positive predictive value do dysplastic nevi have in estimating the risk of melanoma? Several studies have cited a risk attributable to dysplastic nevi that approximates the risk associated with sunburn or increased numbers of nevi. The quantification of the relative risk associated with dysplastic nevi in an unselected population awaits further study.

References

1 Clark WH Jr, Reimer RR, Greene M, et al. Origin of familial malignant melanomas from heritable melanocytic lesions. 'The B-K mole syndrome.' Arch Dermatol 1978;114:732–8.

2 Holly EA, Kelly JW, Shpall SN, et al. Number of melanocytic nevi as a major risk factor for malignant melanoma. J Am Acad Dermatol 1987;17:459–68.

3 Kraemer KH, Tucker M, Tarone R, et al. Risk of cutaneous melanoma in dysplastic nevus syndrome types A and B. N Engl J Med 1986;315:1615–6.

4 Crutcher WA, Sagebiel RW. Prevalence of dysplastic naevi in a community practice. Lancet 1984;1:729.

5 Nordlund JJ, Kirkwood J, Forget BM, et al. Demographic study of clinically atypical (dysplastic) nevi in patients with melanoma and comparison subjects. Cancer Res 1985;45:1855–61.

6 Augustsson A, Stierner U, Suurkula M, et al. Prevalence of common and dysplastic naevi in a Swedish population. Br J Dermatol 1991;124:152–6.

7 Cooke KR, Spears GF, Elder DE, et al. Dysplastic naevi in a population-based survey. Cancer 1989;63: 1240–4.

8 Grulich AE, Bataille V, Swerdlow AJ, et al. Naevi and pigmentary characteristics as risk factors for melanoma in a high-risk population: a case-control study in New South Wales, Australia. Int J Cancer 1996;67:485–91.

9 Karlsson P, Stenberg B, Rosdahl I. Prevalence of pigmented naevi in a Swedish population living close to the Arctic Circle. Acta Derm Venereol 2000;80:335–9.

10 Titus-Ernstoff L, Ding J, Perry AE, et al. Factors associated with atypical moles in New Hampshire, USA. Acta Derm Venereol 2007;87:43–8.

11 Slade J, Marghoob AA, Salopek TG, et al. Atypical mole syndrome: risk factor for cutaneous malignant melanoma and implications for management. J Am Acad Dermatol 1995;32:479–94.

12 Garbe C, Buttner P, Weiss J, et al. Associated factors in the prevalence of more than 50 common melanocytic nevi, atypical melanocytic nevi, and actinic lentigines: multicenter case-control study of the Central Malignant Melanoma Registry of the German Dermatological Society. J Invest Dermatol 1994;102:700–5.

13 Garbe C, Buttner P, Weiss J, et al. Risk factors for developing cutaneous melanoma and criteria for identifying persons at risk: multicenter case-control study of the Central Malignant Melanoma Registry of the German Dermatological Society. J Invest Dermatol 1994;102:695–9.

14 Tucker MA, Halpern A, Holly EA, et al. Clinically recognized dysplastic nevi. A central risk factor for cutaneous melanoma. JAMA 1997;277:1439–44.

15 Kraemer KH, Greene MH. Dysplastic nevus syndrome. Familial and sporadic precursors of cutaneous melanoma. Dermatol Clin 1985;3:225–37.

16 Greene MH, Clark WH Jr, Tucker MA, et al. Acquired precursors of cutaneous malignant melanoma. The familial dysplastic nevus syndrome. N Engl J Med 1985;312:91–7.

17 Marghoob AA, Kopf AW, Rigel DS, et al. Risk of cutaneous malignant melanoma in patients with 'classic' atypical-mole syndrome. A case-control study. Arch Dermatol 1994;130:993–8.

18 Marghoob AA. The dangers of atypical mole (dysplastic nevus) syndrome. Teaching at-risk patients to protect themselves from melanoma. Postgrad Med 1999;105:147–8, 151–2, 154 passim.

19 Kraemer KH, Greene MH, Tarone R, et al. Dysplastic naevi and cutaneous melanoma risk. Lancet 1983;2:1076–7.

20 Marghoob AA, Slade J, Kopf AW, et al. Risk of developing multiple primary cutaneous melanomas in patients with the classic atypical-mole syndrome: a case-control study. Br J Dermatol 1996;135:704–11.

21 Friedman RJ, Rodriguez-Sains R, Jakobiec F. Ophthalmologic oncology: conjunctival malignant melanoma in association with sporadic dysplastic nevus syndrome. J Dermatol Surg Oncol 1987;13:31–4.

22 McCarthy JM, Rootman J, Horsman D, et al. Conjunctival and uveal melanoma in the dysplastic nevus syndrome. Surv Ophthalmol 1993;37:377–86.

23 Singh AD, Wang MX, Donoso LA, et al. Genetic aspects of uveal melanoma: a brief review. Semin Oncol 1996;23:768–72.

24 Toth-Molnar E, Olah J, Dobozy A, et al. Ocular pigmented findings in patients with dysplastic naevus syndrome. Melanoma Res 2004;14:43–7.

25 Diagnosis and treatment of early melanoma. NIH Consensus Development Conference. January 27–29, 1992. Consens Statement 1992;10:1–25.

26 Shapiro M, Chren MM, Levy RM, et al. Variability in nomenclature used for nevi with architectural disorder and cytologic atypia (microscopically dysplastic nevi) by dermatologists and dermatopathologists. J Cutan Pathol 2004;31:523–30.

27 Norris W. A case of fungoid disease. Edinburgh Med Surg J 1820;16:562–5.

28 Munro DD. Multiple active junctional naevi with family history of malignant melanoma. Proc R Soc Med 1974;67:594–5.

29 Frichot BC 3rd, Lynch HT, Guirgis HA, et al. New cutaneous phenotype in familial malignant melanoma. Lancet 1977;1:864–5.

30 Lynch HT, Frichot BC 3rd, Lynch JF. Familial atypical multiple mole–melanoma syndrome. J Med Genet 1978;15:352–6.

31 Elder DE, Goldman LI, Goldman SC, et al. Dysplastic nevus syndrome: a phenotypic association of sporadic cutaneous melanoma. Cancer 1980;46:1787–94.

32 Rahbari H, Mehregan AH. Sporadic atypical mole syndrome. A report of five nonfamilial B-K mole syndrome–like cases and histopathologic findings. Arch Dermatol 1981;117:329–31.

33 Fusaro RM, Lynch HT, Kimberling WJ. Familial atypical multiple mole melanoma syndrome (FAMMM). Arch Dermatol 1983;119:2–3.

34 Greene MH. The genetics of hereditary melanoma and nevi. 1998 update. Cancer 1999;86:2464–77.

35 Quelle DE, Ashmun RA, Hannon GJ, et al. Cloning and characterization of murine p16INK4a and p15INK4b genes. Oncogene 1995;11:635–45.

36 Ranade K, Hussussian CJ, Sikorski RS, et al. Mutations associated with familial melanoma impair p16INK4 function. Nat Genet 1995;10:114–6.

37 Serrano M, Hannon GJ, Beach D. A new regulatory motif in cell-cycle control causing specific inhibition of cyclin D/CDK4. Nature 1993;366:704–7.

38 Molven A, Grimstvedt MB, Steine SJ, et al. A large Norwegian family with inherited malignant melanoma, multiple atypical nevi, and CDK4 mutation. Genes Chromosomes Cancer 2005;44:10–8.

39 Papp T, Pemsel H, Rollwitz I, et al. Mutational analysis of N-ras, p53, CDKN2A (p16(INK4a)), p14(ARF), CDK4, and MC1R genes in human dysplastic melanocytic naevi. J Med Genet 2003;40: E14.

40 Rulyak SJ, Brentnall TA, Lynch HT, et al. Characterization of the neoplastic phenotype in the familial atypical multiple-mole melanoma-pancreatic carcinoma syndrome. Cancer 2003;98:798–804.

41 Celebi JT, Ward KM, Wanner M, et al. Evaluation of germline CDKN2A, ARF, CDK4, PTEN, and BRAF alterations in atypical mole syndrome. Clin Exp Dermatol 2005;30:68–70.

42 Caporaso N, Greene MH, Tsai S, et al. Cytogenetics in hereditary malignant melanoma and dysplastic nevus syndrome: is dysplastic nevus syndrome a chromosome instability disorder? Cancer Genet Cytogenet 1987;24:299–314.

43 Lynch HT, Fusaro RM, Sandberg AA, et al. Chromosome instability and the FAMMM syndrome. Cancer Genet Cytogenet 1993;71:27–39.

44 Abrahams PJ, Houweling A, Cornelissen-Steijger PD, et al. Impaired DNA repair capacity in skin fibroblasts from various hereditary cancer-prone syndromes. Mutat Res 1998;407:189–201.

45 Jung EG, Bohnert E, Boonen H. Dysplastic nevus syndrome: ultraviolet hypermutability confirmed in vitro by elevated sister chromatid exchanges. Dermatologica 1986;173:297–300.

46 Moriwaki SI, Tarone RE, Tucker MA, et al. Hypermutability of UV-treated plasmids in dysplastic nevus/familial melanoma cell lines. Cancer Res 1997;57:4637–41.

47 Noz KC, Bauwens M, van Buul PP, et al. Comet assay demonstrates a higher ultraviolet B sensitivity to DNA damage in dysplastic nevus cells than in common melanocytic nevus cells and foreskin melanocytes. J Invest Dermatol 1996;106:1198–202.

48 Ramsay RG, Chen P, Imray FP, et al. Familial melanoma associated with dominant ultraviolet radiation sensitivity. Cancer Res 1982;42:2909–12.

49 Smith PJ, Greene MH, Devlin DA, et al. Abnormal sensitivity to UV-radiation in cultured skin fibroblasts from patients with hereditary cutaneous malignant melanoma and dysplastic nevus syndrome. Int J Cancer 1982;30:39–45.

50 Rhodes AR, Harrist TJ, Day CL, et al. Dysplastic melanocytic nevi in histologic association with 234 primary cutaneous melanomas. J Am Acad Dermatol 1983;9:563–74.

51 Reimer RR, Clark WH Jr, Greene MH, et al. Precursor lesions in familial melanoma. A new genetic preneoplastic syndrome. JAMA 1978;239:744–6.

52 Rigel DS, Friedman RJ, Kopf AW, et al. Importance of complete cutaneous examination for the detection of malignant melanoma. J Am Acad Dermatol 1986;14:857–60.

53 Tucker MA, Greene MH, Clark WH Jr, et al. Dysplastic nevi on the scalp of prepubertal children from melanoma-prone families. J Pediatr 1983;103:65–9.

54 Fernandez M, Raimer SS, Sanchez RL. Dysplastic nevi of the scalp and forehead in children. Pediatr Dermatol 2001;18:5–8.

55 Roth ME, Grant-Kels JM, Ackerman AB, et al. The histopathology of dysplastic nevi. Continued controversy. Am J Dermatopathol 1991;13:38–51.

56 Shapiro PE. Making sense of the dysplastic nevus controversy. A unifying perspective. Am J Dermatopathol 1992;14:350–6.

57 Ackerman AB. Dysplastic nevus. Am J Surg Pathol 2000;24:757–8.

58 Hussein MR. Melanocytic dysplastic naevi occupy the middle ground between benign melanocytic naevi and cutaneous malignant melanomas: emerging clues. J Clin Pathol 2005;58:453–6.

59 Le Mire L, Hollowood K, Gray D, et al. Melanomas in renal transplant recipients. Br J Dermatol 2006;154:472–7.

60 Leveque L, Dalac S, Dompmartin A, et al. [Melanoma in organ transplant patients]. Ann Dermatol Venereol 2000;127:160–5.

61 Pantanowitz L, Schlecht HP, Dezube BJ. The growing problem of non-AIDS-defining malignancies in HIV. Curr Opin Oncol 2006;18:469–78.

62 Hungerford JL. Surgical treatment of ocular melanoma. Melanoma Res 1993;3:305–12.

63 Richtig E, Langmann G, Mullner K, et al. Ocular melanoma: epidemiology, clinical presentation and relationship with dysplastic nevi. Ophthalmologica 2004;218:111–4.

64 Vink J, Crijns MB, Mooy CM, et al. Ocular melanoma in families with dysplastic nevus syndrome. J Am Acad Dermatol 1990;23:858–62.

65 Cowgill SM, Muscarella P. The genetics of pancreatic cancer. Am J Surg 2003;186:279–86.

66 Lynch HT, Fusaro RM. Pancreatic cancer and the familial atypical multiple mole melanoma (FAMMM) syndrome. Pancreas 1991;6:127–31.

67 Rieder H, Bartsch DK. Familial pancreatic cancer. Fam Cancer 2004;3:69–74.

68 Vasen HF, Gruis NA, Frants RR, et al. Risk of developing pancreatic cancer in families with familial atypical multiple mole melanoma associated with a specific 19 deletion of p16 (p16-Leiden). Int J Cancer 2000;87:809–11.

69 Berwick M, Begg CB, Fine JA, et al. Screening for cutaneous melanoma by skin self-examination. J Natl Cancer Inst 1996;88:17–23.

70 Carli P, De Giorgi V, Palli D, et al. Dermatologist detection and skin self-examination are associated with thinner melanomas: results from a survey of the Italian Multidisciplinary Group on Melanoma. Arch Dermatol 2003;139:607–12.

71 Munoz C, Vazquez-Botet M. Melanoma in situ in Puerto Rico: clinical characteristics and detection patterns. P R Health Sci J 2004;23:179–82.

72 Feit NE, Dusza SW, Marghoob AA. Melanomas detected with the aid of total cutaneous photography. Br J Dermatol 2004;150:706–14.

73 Kelly JW, Yeatman JM, Regalia C, et al. A high incidence of melanoma found in patients with multiple dysplastic naevi by photographic surveillance. Med J Aust 1997;167:191–4.

74 Banky JP, Kelly JW, English DR, et al. Incidence of new and changed nevi and melanomas detected using baseline images and dermoscopy in patients at high risk for melanoma. Arch Dermatol 2005;141:998–1006.

75 Haenssle HA, Krueger U, Vente C, et al. Results from an observational trial: digital epiluminescence microscopy follow-up of atypical nevi increases the sensitivity and the chance of success of conventional dermoscopy in detecting melanoma. J Invest Dermatol 2006;126:980–5.

76 Salopek TG, Kopf AW, Stefanato CM, et al. Differentiation of atypical moles (dysplastic nevi) from early melanomas by dermoscopy. Dermatol Clin 2001;19:337–45.

77 Wang SQ, Kopf AW, Koenig K, et al. Detection of melanomas in patients followed up with total cutaneous examinations, total cutaneous photography, and dermoscopy. J Am Acad Dermatol 2004;50:15–20.

78 Burroni M, Sbano P, Cevenini G, et al. Dysplastic naevus vs. in situ melanoma: digital dermoscopy analysis. Br J Dermatol 2005;152:679–84.

79 Armour K, Mann S, Lee S. Dysplastic naevi: to shave, or not to shave? A retrospective study of the use of the shave biopsy technique in the initial management of dysplastic naevi. Australas J Dermatol 2005;46:70–5.

80 Gambichler T, Senger E, Rapp S, et al. Deep shave excision of macular melanocytic nevi with the razor blade biopsy technique. Dermatol Surg 2000;26:662–6.

81 Bondi EE, Clark WH Jr, Elder D, et al. Topical chemotherapy of dysplastic melanocytic nevi with 5% fluorouracil. Arch Dermatol 1981;117:89–92.

82 Dusza SW, Delgado R, Busam KJ, et al. Treatment of dysplastic nevi with 5% imiquimod cream, a pilot study. J Drugs Dermatol 2006;5:56–62.

83 Edwards L, Jaffe P. The effect of topical tretinoin on dysplastic nevi. A preliminary trial. Arch Dermatol 1990;126:494–9.

84 Halpern AC, Schuchter LM, Elder DE, et al. Effects of topical tretinoin on dysplastic nevi. J Clin Oncol 1994;12:1028–35.

85 Meyskens FL Jr, Edwards L, Levine NS. Role of topical tretinoin in melanoma and dysplastic nevi. J Am Acad Dermatol 1986;15:822–5.

CHAPTER 11
Melanoma

Philip J. Cohen, Maja A. Hofmann, Wolfram Sterry, and Robert A. Schwartz

The earliest description of melanoma is generally attributed to Hippocrates in the 5th century BC. It has also been noted in Inca mummies of comparable antiquity [1]. The term *melanoma* was first proposed by Carswell [2] in 1838. As late as the 1950s, however, this disease was known by numerous designations, including melanosarcoma, melanocarcinoma, and nevocarcinoma [3,4]. It is now well understood that this malignancy of the pigment-producing cell arises from neural crest–derived tissue. During early gestation, melanocytes migrate from the neural crest to the skin and mucous membranes, uveal tract, and meninges, so they normally appear in the epidermis, hair bulb, leptomeninges, and retina. Most melanomas occur in the skin.

Melanocytes also undergo migration to soft tissues, such as the esophagus, parotids, gallbladder, adrenals, prostate, lungs, and tendon aponeuroses, possibly accounting for the rare primary melanomas arising at these sites [5–8]. The development of melanoma depends on the presence of melanocytes, not necessarily melanogenesis, as is illustrated by the occurrence of amelanotic melanoma in albinos [9,10].

The terms *melanoma* and *malignant melanoma* are, by convention, used interchangeably. Both are acceptable. The latter term is redundant, though, because all melanomas are malignant, one of the most malignant of all cancers. Yet with early recognition, it is almost always curable. Fortunately, primary melanoma is usually cutaneous and thus accessible to direct observation. In Australia, where light-complexioned people of British Isles origin reside in more tropical latitudes, the incidence of melanoma is among the highest in the world [11]. There, increased public awareness about this malignancy has resulted in significant reductions in mortality due to earlier recognition [12]. Given the lethal potential of melanoma and its high probability for cure with timely intervention, all physicians should maintain a heightened index of suspicion for this malignancy and proficiency in its early recognition.

Epidemiology

The cumulative lifetime risk for invasive melanoma in the United States has been estimated at one in 59 persons [13]. In the United States, the overall incidence of melanoma increased from 4.2 per 100,000 for the period 1969 to 1971 to 18.2 per 100,000 for the period 2000 to 2003 [14–18]. Incidence by age and sex were essentially stable for the period 1974 to 1994 [19]. It has been reliably predicted that 59,940 new cases of invasive melanoma and 48,290 cases of in situ melanoma would be diagnosed in 2007, whereas 8110 deaths would be attributed to this neoplasm [13]. Melanoma is responsible for three out of every four deaths caused by skin cancer—a striking statistic, considering that more than a million cases of basal cell and squamous cell carcinoma will be diagnosed in 2007 [13]. The epidemiologic data for the United States, summarized in Table 11.1, illustrate trends that are evident worldwide in developed countries:

1 The incidence of melanoma continues to increase [13–17,19–25]

2 The dramatic increase is seen among whites, with an overall male predominance

3 The incidence in blacks is low and shows no increase

In the 25-year period from the mid-1950s to the late 1970s, the incidence of melanoma increased three

Table 11.1 Age-adjusted incidence per 100,000 of invasive melanoma in the United States

Race and Sex	1969–1971[a]	1973–1977[b]	1977–1981[b]	2000–2003[c]
Overall	4.2	6.4	8.0	18.2
White males	4.6	8.0	9.7	26.5
White females	4.4	6.2	8.4	17.3
Black males	0.9	1.1	1.0	1.1
Black females	0.7	1.2	–	0.9

[a]*Source:* Cutler et al. [15].
[b]*Source:* Horm et al. [16].
[c]*Source:* National Cancer Institute [18].

to five times in all Nordic countries [26]. A Hawaiian study found the incidence tripled in whites from 1960 to 1977, with whites also representing about 80% of cases overall. No increase was observed for nonwhites [27]. During the 1990s, incidence rates were by far the highest in northern and western Europe, whereas mortality was higher among males in eastern and southern Europe [22]. The most recently reported incidences for Australia were 36.1 per 100,000 males and 28.0 per 100,000 females [23]. Worldwide, the highest yearly incidence was reported in New Zealand, with 77.7 per 100,000 [24]. The incidence of melanoma, rare in childhood, increases steadily with age (Table 11.2). In the United States from 2000 to 2003, the median age at diagnosis for cutaneous melanoma was 58 years, with approximately 0.9% diagnosed under the age of 20 and 19.1% diagnosed between 45 and 54 [13].

There is abundant evidence that the phenotypes at greatest risk for melanoma are those with fair skin, fair or red hair, a tendency to freckle, and a tendency to burn rather than tan [25,28]. One study reported the presence of more than 100 facial freckles to be the strongest single risk factor for melanoma, associated with a 20-fold increase in risk [29]. The ability to tan appears protective [28,29]. An increased susceptibility of more light-complexioned phenotypes is suggested by the differential incidence of melanoma seen in various ethnicities (Table 11.3).

Table 11.2 Age-specific incidence per 100,000 of invasive melanoma in the United States

Age, years	1973–1977[a]	1977–1981[a]	2000–2003[b]
0–4	0.0	0.1	0.1
5–9	0.1	0.1	0.1
10–14	0.2	0.2	0.3
15–19	1.1	1.2	1.7
20–24	3.0	3.3	4.0
25–29	5.5	6.2	6.9
30–34	6.6	9.0	9.5
35–39	8.5	10.9	12.3
40–44	9.8	12.9	18.0
45–49	12.4	14.6	21.6
50–54	13.1	15.8	27.6
55–59	13.0	16.9	34.6
60–64	13.4	19.1	41.1
65–69	14.8	18.3	49.3
70–74	13.6	19.8	60.7
75–79	17.0	20.4	65.9
80–84	18.9	20.2	70.5
85+	22.1	24.7	63.7

[a]*Source:* Horm et al. [16].
[b]*Source:* National Cancer Institute [18].

In 18th century Europe, moles, natural or as appliqués, were viewed as a sign of beauty and inspired admiration. It is now recognized that an increased number of common acquired melanocytic nevi correlates with an increased risk of melanoma, an association repeatedly confirmed [28–34] (Table 11.4).

Table 11.3 Incidence per 100,000 of invasive melanoma by ethnic origin in the United States, 2000–2003

Race/Ethnicity	Total	Male	Female
All races	18.2	23.2	14.7
White non-Hispanic	24.1	30.2	19.8
White Hispanic	4.3	4.4	4.4
Black	1.0	1.1	0.9
Asian/Pacific Islander	1.4	1.6	1.2
American Indian/Alaska Native	2.7	–	–

Source: National Cancer Institute [18].

The number of *palpable* common melanocytic nevi on the *arms* was found to be a strong risk factor for melanoma in one study [28]. The presence of *any* melanocytic nevus on the *arms* increased risk by 30-fold in another [35]. The number of palpable common melanocytic nevi over the *entire body* also emerged as a significant risk factor [36,37]. Notably, a greater number of common melanocytic nevi correlates with fair complexion (as measured by burning/tanning ability), with fair eye and hair color, and with an increased freckling tendency [37]. Moreover, a specific kind of melanocytic nevus, the dysplastic nevus, has been shown to be a significant risk factor for melanoma and is the subject of Chapter 10. Dysplastic nevi may enlarge and increase in number upon sun exposure [38].

The epidemiology of most melanomas is intertwined with ultraviolet (UV) light carcinogenesis, combined with a variety of genetic factors. Based on data from the Connecticut Tumor Registry accumulated over 40 years, the rising incidence of melanoma has followed a cyclic pattern, each new

Table 11.4 Number of acquired melanocytic nevi as a risk factor for melanoma

Reference	Location	How Defined	Number	Relative Risk
Holly et al. [31]	California	Observation of melanocytic nevi ≥2 mm	0–10	1.0
			11–25	1.6
			26–50	4.4
			51–100	5.4
			>100	9.8
Swerdlow et al. [30]	England	Observation of melanocytic nevi ≥2 mm	0	1.0
			10–24	6.7
			25–49	10.7
			≥50	53.9
Dubin et al. [29]	New York	Patient self-assessment by comparison with diagrams	0	0.18
			1–25	1.0
			26–100	1.98
			>100	3.43
Holman & Armstrong [28]	Australia	Observation of palpable melanocytic nevi on arms	0	1.0
			1–4	2.0
			5–9	4.0
			>9	11.3
Naldi et al. [33]	Italy	Observation of melanocytic nevi ≥2 mm	0–5	1.0
			6–15	1.7
			16–30	2.2
			31–45	2.8
			>45	9.5

successive peak in incidence following sunspot activity [39]. In the past several years, two major genes conferring a 10-fold higher susceptibility to melanoma have been identified in high-risk families: *CDKN2A* (also known as *p16* and *MTS1*) and *CDK4* [40]. *CDKN2A* encodes a cell-cycle regulator that inhibits the activities of cdk4 and cdk6, two protein kinases that phosphorylate the retinoblastoma protein. Mutation at this locus results in uncontrolled melanocyte proliferation. Differential risk factors for melanomas arising on surfaces with and without chronic sun exposure suggest different pathways for these tumors [41]. Indeed, distinct patterns of genetic alterations have been identified in melanomas with and without chronic sun exposure [42].

Most melanomas occur on surfaces either intermittently or chronically exposed to the sun. Lentigo maligna melanoma (LMM) arises in areas of chronic sun exposure, as in an occupational setting, whereas both superficial spreading melanoma (SSM) and nodular melanoma (NM) are associated with acute sunburn of nontanned skin, as may occur during vacation exposures, SSM showing the stronger association [43]. Overall, intermittent sun exposure is more highly associated with melanoma risk than chronic high levels of sun exposure [44]. Sun exposure appears to be a risk factor for intraocular melanoma [45]. However, the apparent increased risk of cutaneous melanoma among ocular melanoma patients may be largely attributable to the greater skin cancer surveillance of these patients [46]. Physical protection from sunlight is generally accepted as one of the most important elements in melanoma prevention [43,47].

Some melanomas arise on regions that receive little or no solar exposure, such as the esophagus, genitalia, and volar surfaces. Among blacks, Japanese, and Chinese, melanomas occur most frequently on the foot [48]. Nonsolar risk factors for development of melanoma are the subject of much controversy. These include fluorescent lighting, hormonal factors in women, diet, tobacco, arsenic, and antioxidant vitamins. None has been strongly correlated as a risk factor for cutaneous melanoma in light-complexioned persons. Fluorescent light has been thoroughly investigated. The data have not affirmed any significant association with melanoma risk [49,50].

Classification of primary cutaneous melanoma

The current system of classification of primary cutaneous melanoma is based on the pioneering work of Clark and colleagues [51] and McGovern [52]. The overwhelming majority of melanomas fall within five clinicopathologic subsets:

1 LMM
2 SSM
3 NM
4 Acral lentiginous melanoma (ALM)
5 Mucosal melanoma (MCM)

In instances when neither clinical presentation nor histology permits classification, the tumor is designated as indeterminate or unclassifiable [53].

With rare exceptions, cutaneous and mucosal melanomas arise from atypical melanocytes situated along the dermal–epidermal junction. Melanoma in situ is confined to the epidermis, where there is no vasculature and thus no conduit for metastases. Invasive melanoma breaches the dermal–epidermal junction, gaining access to blood vessels and lymphatic channels.

Of these five major varieties of melanoma, four (LMM, SSM, ALM, and MCM) are characterized by a biphasic growth pattern, in which a slower "radial growth phase" is succeeded by a more rapid, invasive "vertical growth phase" [54]. During the radial growth phase, the primary melanoma undergoes centrifugal enlargement. Melanomas in their radial growth phase tend to be relatively flat. Their outlines may be irregular, but the overall shape is circular to oval. This period of radial growth may persist for years, during which time the melanoma develops little, if any, tendency to metastasize. Surgery performed during the radial growth phase is generally curative.

The vertical growth phase, which subsequently appears as a focal nodularity within an otherwise flat lesion, appears to represent a new and distinct clone of tumor cells [55–58]. The dome-shaped nodule grows rapidly. During this invasive growth phase, the neoplasm penetrates the underlying

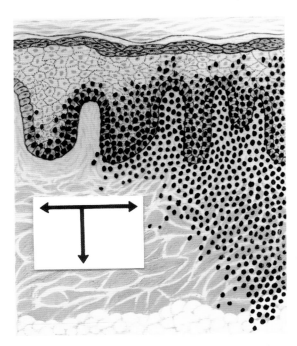

Fig. 11.1 Schematic representation of biphasic growth pattern. In the radial growth phase, atypical melanocytes proliferate along the dermal – epidermal junction along a horizontal plane. Individual cells may show "shotgunning" through the epidermis or spread through the papillary dermis along a horizontal plane. In the vertical growth phase, atypical melanocytes penetrate toward deeper tissue levels.

connective tissue, gaining access to blood and lymph vessels, resulting in metastases.

Nodular melanoma exhibits a monophasic growth pattern, with the melanoma apparently in a vertical growth phase from the outset. Whether the radial growth phase is absent or abbreviated is debated [59]. However, the nodule appears to arise on otherwise normal skin, with no indolent radial growth phase clinically observed. The two growth phases are schematically represented in Fig. 11.1.

Lentigo maligna melanoma

Lentigo maligna melanoma represents about 10% of melanomas among whites [54] and about 8.0% among Japanese [60], and is rarely seen in blacks [61]. The incidence of this subtype may be increas-

ing among whites. Data from Stanford University showed that in northern California from 1990 to 2000, LMM and its in situ form, lentigo maligna (LM), increased at a higher rate than all other subtypes of melanoma among patients aged 45 and older [62]. Indeed, LMM and LM were the only subtypes that increased in incidence. Thus, for men 45 years and older, at least 75% of all in situ melanomas were LM. For men 65 years and older, at least 27% of all invasive melanomas were LMM.

Lentigo maligna melanoma is preceded by a prolonged in situ phase of radial growth, during which it is known as lentigo maligna or by its earlier designation, melanotic freckle of Hutchinson. LM typically occurs in elderly individuals on sun-exposed surfaces, especially the head, neck, and face, but may involve extracranial and extrafacial sites in 17.5% of cases—the trunk in 68% of men and the lower legs in 80% of women [63].

Lentigo maligna appears as a tan to brown patch, speckled with minute brown or black flecks (Fig. 11.2). It is characteristically impalpable, as is a common lentigo. LM and LMM occur in the same areas as solar lentigines, or "age spots," and LM may appear to be an age spot. With the availability of over-the-counter depigmenting creams, the mistaken use of topical hydroquinone for melanoma is a potential danger. This is illustrated by the report of a woman who treated an enlarging LM of the face with a hydroquinone cream for 1 year, allowing it to grow

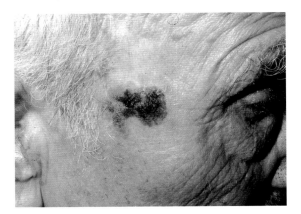

Fig. 11.2 Lentigo maligna on the face: a persistent, slowly enlarging patch with irregular pigmentation.

to considerable size (4.5 cm) and delaying medical attention. Despite its rapid growth, the patient had persisted in self-treatment, encouraged by successful depigmentation [64].

Histologically, the proliferation of atypical melanocytes in LM is confined to the epidermis, as occurs with typical melanocytes of the common lentigo. The LM may slowly increase in size over years. Uneven spread along the circumference plus partial regression in some areas may contribute to an irregular outline, with projections and notches. Regression is indicated clinically by the presence of shades of white or gray. LM may attain a size of 4 to 7 cm before the onset of the vertical growth phase. Progression into an invasive LMM is evident clinically with the development of one or more blue-to-black nodules or an area of induration.

The estimated lifetime risk of LM progressing to LMM is 5% [65]. The median age at diagnosis of LMM is 65 years, with a slight female predilection [54]. The 5-year survival rate for patients with localized cutaneous disease (stage I or II) is the same as for those with any other melanoma of the same thickness.

Superficial spreading melanoma

Superficial spreading melanoma is the most common subtype among whites, accounting for about 70% of melanomas [54], in contrast with about 17.5% of melanomas among Japanese [60]. Like LMM, SSM exhibits a slight female predilection, but typically occurs at a younger age than does LMM; the median age at diagnosis is 44 years [54]. SSM develops on both sun-exposed and non–sun-exposed surfaces and shows a predilection for the lower legs in women and upper back in men—areas prone toward intermittent, rather than chronic, sun exposure. It tends to have an arciform contour and an irregular, indefinite border (Figs. 11.3 and 11.4). Notching, a sign of focal tumor regression, may be prominent and helpful in diagnosis. Other signs of regression include central hypopigmentation or an asymmetrical halo of hypopigmentation. In contrast with the flat LMM, SSM often has a hyperkeratotic surface and distinctly palpable margins. It may be multicolored, displaying a mosaic of black, brown, tan, blue, red, and white. Admixtures of these col-

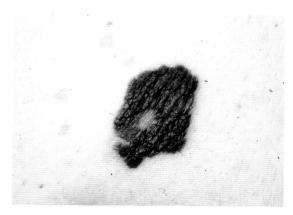

Fig. 11.3 Superficial spreading melanoma, showing notching and an area of regression.

ors may produce a spectrum of intermediate shades, including purple, pink, and gray. The radial growth phase of SSM may persist from a few months to 12 years, most commonly 4 to 5 years, attaining a diameter of about 2.5 cm before the development of focal nodules or papules, signifying invasion by progression into the vertical growth phase.

Some morphologic differences between LMM and SSM may be understood in terms of their respective histologies. During its radial growth phase, LMM spreads along the dermal–epidermal junction in a "lentiginous" pattern, with the atypical

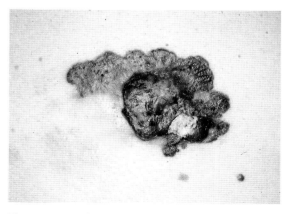

Fig. 11.4 Superficial spreading melanoma with a scalloped, arcuate border; regression; and marked nodularity.

spindle-shaped melanocytes oriented parallel to the basement membrane. In its radial growth phase, LMM is essentially intraepidermal, producing a flat, nonpalpable lesion. During the radial growth phase of SSM, the atypical melanocytes also spread along the dermal–epidermal junction, but also in a pagetoid pattern, with atypical cells "shotgunned" throughout the epidermis as individual cells and in nests; invasion of the papillary dermis may occur as well. This dermal component produces the elevated surface and palpable margins characteristic of SSM. The dermal component also adds to the richer spectrum of colors. In addition to the expected melanin-derived hues of black, brown, and tan, SSM may display red, white, and blue. Red indicates hyperemia associated with an inflammatory response. Whitish hues reflect immunologically mediated tumor regression. Blue results from the Tyndall light-scattering effect, as light is reflected from dermal pigment through the colloidal medium of the dermis. Blue may be the most ominous, as it suggests deeper tumor invasion. The 5-year survival rate for patients with localized cutaneous disease (stages I and II) is the same as for those with any other melanoma of the same thickness [66].

Nodular melanoma

Nodular melanoma has the most aggressive clinical course from its first appearance. Among whites, NM comprises approximately 10% of cutaneous melanomas [54], whereas among the Japanese it accounts for about 25% of melanomas [60]. The median age at diagnosis among whites is 53 years, with men more commonly affected by a ratio of 60:40. The most frequently affected sites are the back, head, neck, arms, and legs [54].

Typically, the patient is first seen with a rapidly growing pigmented nodule. The gross morphology is usually hemispherical with a smooth or ulcerated surface. Less commonly, the surface may appear plaque-like. As it evolves over months, the tumor often exhibits a uniform color, usually dark, but may be black, blue, red, gray, or hypopigmented (amelanotic) (Fig. 11.5). For amelanotic NM, close inspection with a hand lens under good lighting may reveal blue to black flecks.

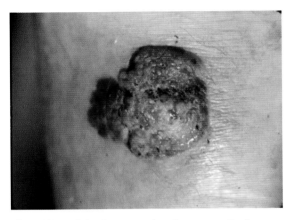

Fig. 11.5 Nodular (verrucous) melanoma on the leg. Note the verrucous surface. (Reprinted with permission from Schwartz et al. [259].)

At the time of clinical detection, it has usually deeply invaded the underlying connective tissue, accounting for the worse prognosis for this type. Polypoid melanoma is a rare variant of NM. It frequently ulcerates and may be amelanotic. It may resemble a pyogenic granuloma, pedunculated melanocytic nevus, seborrheic keratosis, pedunculated fibroma, or other benign-appearing pedunculated tumor. Although the polypoidal morphology has been associated with a poor prognosis, the dominant prognostic variable appears to be primary tumor thickness and not morphology [67,68].

Acral melanoma (palmar–plantar–subungual melanoma)

By the early 1970s, the classification scheme of melanoma contained the three categories discussed so far: SSM, LMM, and NM [52,69]. As it became apparent that melanomas occurring on the palms, soles, and mucous membranes—non–hair-bearing areas with minimal exposure to the sun—were different in their clinical character, several new categories were introduced, including "plantar lentiginous melanoma" and "melanoma of the palmar–plantar–subungual–mucosal type" [70–72]. ALM has become the more widely recognized designation for this clinically aggressive variety of melanoma, which displays certain histologic similarities to LMM in its radial component. However, although many cases fit into this category [54,73–75], not all melanomas in the volar and subungual areas are ALM [54,72]. Some show a mixed histology of LMM and SSM; others display a picture consistent with SSM and NM; some defy classification [54,74–76]. In Japan, for example, where acral melanomas predominate, about 80% of these are ALM, 15% are NM, and 3% are SSM [77]. We suggest that the term *acral melanoma* be used clinically.

The incidence of acral melanomas for all races is similar [72]. On a percentage basis, however, acral melanomas are far more common in Asians and blacks than in whites [48]. In Japan, acral melanoma comprises approximately 49% of melanoma [60,77]. Among the Chinese of Hong Kong, acral melanoma accounts for about 75% [73]. In Taiwan, ALM accounted for 58% of melanomas [78]. Nearly all acral melanoma in blacks has been reported to be ALM [54,61]. In a series of 13 American blacks, plantar melanoma accounted for about 70%, in agreement with 65% seen in Uganda [79] and in conformity with a retrospective review of 27 melanomas in black patients, which found plantar melanoma in 67% [61]. The sole is the most common site for acral melanomas, with about half of these occurring on the heel [72,74,80,81].

Acral lentiginous melanoma, the most common clinicohistologic type of acral melanoma, shares some histologic features with LMM but differs from LMM in its younger age at onset, its anatomic site, the absence of chronic sun exposure, and the greater depth of penetration at diagnosis [72]. Even an indolent-appearing, flat ALM may prove deeply invasive. The colors may form a mosaic of tan, dark brown, and black. The border is irregular and ill defined. As the tumor advances, its borders become more highly irregular and notched. Although the radial growth phase may persist up to 10 years, a shorter one is common. When the vertical growth phase supervenes, a characteristic nodule may appear and may exhibit a verrucous surface or shallow ulceration (Fig. 11.6).

A less common but distinctive variant of acral melanoma is subungual melanoma, which comprises about 1% to 3% of all cases among whites, but about 10% of all melanomas among Japanese and about 25% of melanomas among the Chinese

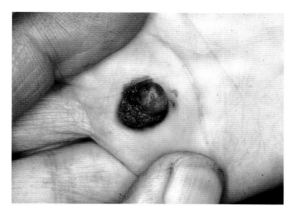

Fig. 11.6 Acral lentiginous melanoma on the hand, with central amelanotic nodulation.

of Hong Kong [75,77,82–85]. The great toe and thumb are most often affected, with these sites accounting for 75% to 90% of subungual melanomas. For whites, subungual melanomas of the upper extremity have been seen almost exclusively in men [74,82,86]. Among the Japanese, three quarters of subungual melanomas in both sexes occur on the upper extremity, in contrast to nonsubungual acral melanomas, which occur predominately on the feet [74,75].

Subungual melanoma may be first evident as a split nail, a swelling of part of the nail bed, an ulceration with a bloody crust, or a longitudinal black or brown streak in the nail bed (Fig. 11.7). Variegated colors within a subungual streak should arouse suspicion. The diffusion of black-brown pigment to the periungual nail fold is Hutchinson's sign and must be regarded as melanoma until proven otherwise [72,86–88] (Fig. 11.8). Subungual melanomas may be amelanotic. Unfortunately, subungual melanoma may resemble paronychia or a traumatic subungual hematoma and as Hutchinson [88] observed in 1886, is often erroneously attributed to injury, delaying diagnosis. To further confound the diagnosis, a history of trauma, including evulsion and laceration with subsequent infection, may precede the onset of subungual melanoma. Hutchinson's sign is seen in only a minority of subungual melanomas and may reflect benign disorders as well as Bowen's disease of the

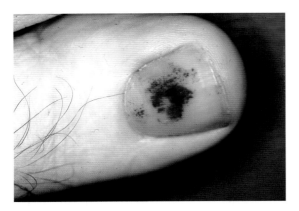

Fig. 11.7 Subungual melanoma on the thumb showing the diffusion of pigment onto the proximal nail fold (Hutchinson's sign). (Courtesy of Roger H. Brodkin, MD.)

nail unit [89]. In a suspected subungual melanoma, an index of suspicion must be maintained even if an initial biopsy should fail to demonstrate the melanoma [90,91].

The median age at diagnosis of ALM in a recent French study was 63 years [72]. There was a slight female predilection; 28% of these ALMs were unpigmented. The 5-year survival rate was 76%. The median disease-free survival was 10.1 years. Multivariate analysis showed that greater Breslow tumor thickness, male gender, and amelanosis were significantly associated with a poorer prognosis.

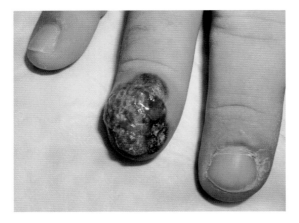

Fig. 11.8 Melanoma on distal finger with hyperpigmentation of the nail folds.

The clinical features of the most common types of melanoma are summarized in Table 11.5. The differential diagnoses of volar and subungual melanomas are presented in Table 11.6.

Mucosal melanoma

Primary melanomas arising on the conjunctiva, upper respiratory tract, lips, oral mucosa, genitalia, or anorectal mucosa are uncommon, with an incidence of approximately 7.6% of all melanomas [92].

Conjunctival melanoma

Ocular melanoma accounts for 70% to 80% of all extracutaneous melanomas, with the uveal tract as the most common site of origin (85%); conjunctival melanoma is far less common, comprising 2% of all ocular melanomas [93–95]. Conjunctival melanoma arises in the bulbar conjunctiva and may first appear as a brown-to-black macule that slowly enlarges for many years before developing one or more invasive nodules. Alternatively, a black nodule may appear de novo. It is difficult to ascertain whether conjunctival melanoma has arisen from a precursor melanocytic nevus, because the precursor lesion that the patient recalls may have represented the radial growth phase, which may last for years [96]. Conjunctival melanoma arising in association with sporadic dysplastic nevus syndrome has been noted [97]. Conjunctival melanoma in childhood is exceedingly rare and when suspected, usually turns out to be the benign spindle and epithelioid nevus of Spitz. A conjunctival melanoma with desmoplastic histology may simulate a chalazion [98].

The diagnosis and classification of conjunctival melanomas are hampered because the specimens are often small. Moreover, because the conjunctival substantia propria lacks the histologic stratification of the dermis, the tissues are not analogous. Two types of conjunctival melanomas are recognized: (1) a focal nodular tumor arising de novo and (2) primary acquired melanosis (PAM), in which a flat radial in situ component precedes the appearance of invasive melanoma [99]. A study of conjunctival melanomas in 37 white patients found 43% to develop from PAM [100]. Rarely, a cellular blue nevus of the conjunctiva may give rise to a melanoma

Table 11.5 Clinical features of the most common types of primary cutaneous melanoma

Clinical Feature	LMM	SSM	NM	ALM
Frequency in whites[a]	~ 10%	~ 70%	~ 10%	~ 5%
Site	Exposed surfaces: especially face & temporal areas	All surfaces: head & neck M > F; trunk M > F; lower legs F > M	All surfaces: head & neck M > F; back M > F; arms, legs	Volar surfaces, especially soles; subungual, esp. great toe & thumb
Median age at dx	65 years	44 years	53 years	65 years
Sex predilection	F > M (slight)	F > M (slight)	M > F (60:40)	F > M (slight)
Margin	Flat	Distinctly palpable	Palpable: spheroid	Flat
Color	Black, brown, tan; gray & white areas signifying regression	Mosaic of brown, black, tan; red, white, & blue may be present; pink & gray common	Uniform bluish black; gray & pink in early tumor; occasional depigmented halo	Black, brown, tan; little variegation of color
Size	4–7 cm	2.5 cm	1–2 cm	3 cm
Growth pattern	Biphasic—radial phase: lentiginous spread 5–20 years; vertical phase: rapid invasion of dermis over weeks to months	Biphasic—radial phase: pagetoid spread 1–12 years; vertical phase: rapid invasion of dermis over weeks to months	Monophasic—vertical phase from the outset; tumor present months to 2 years at time of dx	Biphasic—radial phase: 1–10 years, of various histology; rapid invasion of dermis over weeks to months

[a] Approximately 5% are rare forms or unclassifiable.
dx, diagnosis; F, female; M, male.

[101]. Clinically, it is difficult to identify PAM at high risk for progression to melanoma. PAM with cytologic atypia has a 50% chance of progressing to melanoma [99]. The prognosis for conjunctival melanoma was found closely related to its specific anatomic location and depth of invasion, with thin tumors less commonly metastasizing. Exenteration does not always prevent metastases, and a high rate

Table 11.6 Differential diagnosis of volar, subungual, and amelanotic melanomas

Volar Melanoma	Subungual Melanoma	Amelanotic Melanoma
Verruca vulgaris	Glomus tumor	Bowen's disease
Lentigo	Infection	Pyogenic granuloma
Clavus vasculare	Hemorrhage	Verruca vulgaris
Black heel	Kaposi's sarcoma	Dermatitis
Melanoacanthoma	Melanocytic nevus	Seborrheic keratosis
Tattoo	Foreign body granuloma	Extramammary Paget's disease
Kaposi's sarcoma	Bowen's disease	Basal cell carcinoma
Targetoid hemosiderotic nevus	Keratoacanthoma	Kaposi's sarcoma
	Pyogenic granuloma	

of recurrence may follow local excisional biopsy of PAM [100]. Rarely, metastasis to the conjunctiva may be the presenting sign of disseminated cutaneous melanoma [102].

Several nonmalignant conditions may produce acquired conjunctival pigmentation as the result of increased production of melanin without any abnormality of the melanocytes, analogous to a freckle. These may occur idiopathically in black patients or may be secondary to Addison's disease, x-ray exposure, or arsenic poisoning. The current ophthalmologic terminology for such pigmented lesions is *benign epithelial melanosis*.

Anogenital melanoma

The vulva is the most common site for MCM. Vulvar melanoma represents less than 1% of all melanomas, but is the second most common vulvar malignancy, representing between 3.4% and 10% of vulvar neoplasms [92,103]. Among 203 published cases of vulvar melanoma in the United States, the data revealed an incidence of 0.108 per 100,000, a 5-year survival rate of 50%, and an average age at diagnosis of 66 years [104]. The most common presenting complaints were an enlarging mole, pruritus, and bleeding. Vulvar melanoma may be evident as a macule, plaque, or nodule, brown to blue-black in color. In a study of 20 cases, the histologic subtypes were superficial spreading (45%), mucosal lentiginous (30%), unclassified (15%), and nodular (10%) [103]. Survival correlated with tumor thickness, ulceration, and lymph node involvement.

A few cases of melanoma of the penis and male urethra have been reported, including one with histologic features resembling desmoplastic melanoma [105–107]. This neoplasm may be present for years, evident as pain, intermittent bleeding, or an enlarging black ulcerated nodule. The glans is the most common site, seen in two thirds of penile melanoma, with the prepuce the second most frequent. Risk factors for penile melanoma appear to be melanosis and a preexisting melanocytic nevus. Delayed diagnosis tends to result in histologically thick melanomas being identifed, accounting for the usually poor prognosis. All too often, metastatic melanoma is already present at the time of diagnosis [108]. Genital melanosis and nodules should be considered for histologic analysis [105].

Anorectal melanoma is rare, representing about 1% of all melanomas, and is much less common than squamous cell carcinoma in this site [109,110]. The usual presenting symptoms are pain, bleeding, and a mass that may mimic a hemorrhoid. Often, because it is detected late, the prognosis is poor, with a 5-year survival rate of 10% [109]. Most patients already have distant metastases when first seen. In a series of 24 patients, 19 had positive lymph node involvement; the mean disease-free survival in these patients was 10.3 months. Disease-free survival among the five patients who were node negative was 26.5 months. A rising trend in the overall incidence of anorectal melanoma has been noted among young men in the San Francisco area over the last two decades, implicating HIV infection as a potential risk factor [111].

Clinical variants of melanoma

The common variants of primary cutaneous melanoma outlined above (LMM, SSM, NM, ALM, and MCM) account for about 95% of all clinical presentations. However, cutaneous melanoma may have unusual morphology or be seen in distinctive clinical settings. Variations in the presentation of melanoma are described below and summarized in Table 11.7.

Melanoma arising within the dermis

In almost every instance, melanoma begins with junctional activity, arising from atypical melanocytes situated at the dermal–epidermal junction. However, melanoma may at times arise from melanocytes of dermal origin, found within a blue nevus or within the dermal component of a congenital melanocytic nevus (CMN) [112,113]. This constitutes a distinct and rare subtype of melanoma. A primary melanoma of the dermis, when confined to the dermis and/or subcutaneous fat, may histologically resemble a metastasis but is associated with an unexpectedly prolonged survival [114].

Table 11.7 Clinical variations of melanoma

Primary Melanoma with Special Morphology
Verrucous melanoma
Polypoidal melanoma
Amelanotic melanoma[a]
Melanoma with vitiligo[a]

Primary Melanoma with Special Origin or Clinical Setting
Arising in childhood with a CMN
Arising in childhood with NCM
Arising congenitally with CMN or NCM
Arising within a blue nevus
Familial predisposition to melanoma: dysplastic nevus
  syndrome
Familial predisposition to melanoma: xeroderma
  pigmentosum
Familial predisposition to melanoma: red-headed frecklers
Familial predisposition to melanoma: multiple primary
  melanoma

Noncutaneous or Nonprimary Melanoma
Melanoma arising in a visceral site (gallbladder, lung,
  esophagus, etc.)
Satellite melanomas and in-transit metastases
Late metastases following regression of melanoma
Metastatic melanoma without a demonstrable primary
Melanoma with vitiligo[a]
Amelanotic melanoma[a]
Disseminated melanoma with melanosis, melanuria, and
  melanoptysis

---

[a] May be seen in the setting of primary, recurrent, or metastatic disease.
NCM, neurocutaneous melanosis.

Arising within blue nevus

The malignant blue nevus is a rare condition, usually arising within a cellular blue nevus [115]. In contrast to the cellular blue nevus, the common blue nevus is not known to undergo malignant change. Malignant blue nevus usually appears as a solitary firm blue nodule. The surface may be ulcerated. When arising in a cellular blue nevus, the malignant blue nevus may closely resemble it, occurring in similar sites: the scalp, neck, chest, buttocks, and dorsa of the hands and feet. Further confusion may arise from the propensity of the benign cellular blue nevus to spread to the regional lymph nodes, thus mimicking a malignant process. Lambert and

Brodkin [116] described a woman who underwent extensive surgery, with considerable morbidity, for a presumed metastatic melanoma. On review, it was a cellular blue nevus on the dorsum of the foot, a characteristic location, in association with a cellular blue nevus in the inguinal lymph nodes. It was termed a "pseudometastasizing pseudomelanoma."

The malignant blue nevus may also arise in the nevus of Ota [117–119]. The nevus of Ota usually appears on the forehead, periorbital region, malar area, or nose and is usually unilateral, consisting of a brown and slate-blue patch. The nevus of Ota may be present at birth or may appear during adolescence. It often involves the ipsilateral eye, producing a bluish discoloration of the sclera.

We consider the malignant blue nevus to be melanoma, as do others [120]. When a malignant blue nevus appears to arise de novo in the absence of a precursor, an alternate diagnosis should be considered [121].

Arising with a congenital melanocytic nevus

Congenital melanocytic nevi are apparent at birth or within a few days of birth and tend to spare the palms, soles, and genitalia. Thus, they appear to develop independently of UV light. They have been shown to be genetically distinct from common melanocytic nevi that develop later [122]. The incidence of CMN among newborn babies is between 0.2% and 2.1% [123]. Giant CMN, especially the "bathing trunk" or "garment" type, are well recognized as precursors to melanoma. At birth, the nevus is usually light to dark brown and impalpable, with increased skin markings (Fig. 11.9). With time, it nearly always develops a pronounced hairy component and a verrucous surface (Fig. 11.10). Often it has satellite nevi. It tends to increase in size, stabilizing after puberty. When the scalp and neck are involved, there may be associated neurocutaneous melanocytosis with leptomeningeal involvement. The reported frequency of melanomas has ranged between 0.05% and 10.7%, with the higher numbers from smaller studies [124]. Most agree that CMN over 20 cm in diameter pose a significant risk as a melanoma precursor [125], but exactly what size they must attain to present substantial risk of

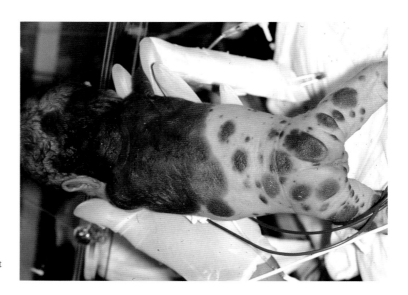

Fig. 11.9 Giant congenital (bathing trunk) melanocytic nevus in an infant with neurocutaneous melanosis.

transformation to melanoma is not known. The risk of malignant transformation of large CMN appears to be very high in the first decade of life. Melanomas usually develop before the age of 20 [126]. In one study of 205 patients with large CMN, 71% had 10 or more satellite nevi; there was a significant association between greater numbers of satellite nevi and the occurrence of melanoma [127]. For large CMN, the use of the tissue expander may facilitate primary excision with one-stage closure and good cosmesis [125,128,129].

The risk of melanoma arising in small CMN appears less than previously believed [125,126]. Some studies have failed to detect any melanomas arising in small and medium-sized CMN, including a study of 265 patients in which no melanomas were detected at any anatomic location over a median follow-up period of 25 years [130–132]. Small CMN often resemble a café-au-lait macule at birth, but may be distinguished by their increased surface markings. Commonly, dark brown speckling of pigment may be present at the periphery of a small congenital melanocytic nevus. With maturation, most small CMN develop coarse dark hairs, a darker color, and a coarsely verrucous or finely beaded surface. Although melanoma arising within nevus spilus is rare, the risk is substantially heightened if the

nevus spilus was present since birth and is large [132].

The classification of CMN by size was originally based on a pragmatic consideration—whether it was so large that it could not be excised and the defect closed primarily in a single surgical procedure. Kopf and colleagues [133] suggested the arbitrary classification of CMN as small (<1.5 cm), medium (1.5 to <20 cm), and large (≥20 cm), measured at the largest diameter. Some division by size appears to have clinical significance, differentiating melanocytic nevi that vary in their histologic depth and behavior as melanoma precursors [126]. The vast majority of CMN are small [124,126]. The absolute number of CMN may have independent prognostic significance. An American study found that a child with three or more CMN, regardless of size, carried a 6.7% lifetime risk of melanoma [127], which contrasted with a lifetime risk of 2% for males and 1.4% for females in the general U.S. population [18]. A study of 23,354 male military conscripts from southern Italy found a 0.67% prevalence of CMN, in agreement with the rates reported in other European countries [134]. No diagnosis or history of melanoma was found. Until more definitive data are available, therapy of medium-sized congenital nevi should be individualized, with consideration given

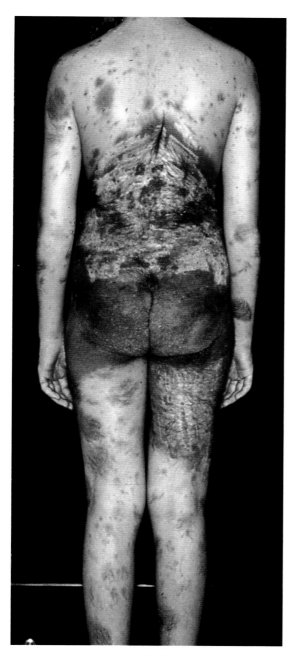

Fig. 11.10 Giant congenital (bathing trunk) melanocytic nevus in a 17-year-old girl, with a history of two melanomas developing within the nevus.

to additional melanoma risk factors [125]. Size may also influence the decision to perform surgery early in the patient's life or postpone it until he or she is closer to puberty.

The differential diagnosis of pigmented melanocytic nevi in newborns includes common and uncommon entities such as lentigo, café-au-lait macule, nevus sebaceus, postinflammatory hyperpigmentation, mongolian spot, nevus of Ota, solitary mastocytoma, and epithelial nevus [113,135]. The histology of CMN is discussed below.

Congenital melanoma
Congenital melanoma may occur in association with a giant congenital melanocytic nevus. If present, congenital melanoma may metastasize within the fetus or to the placenta. Melanoma may rarely metastasize transplacentally from a mother with disseminated melanoma [136,137].

Neurocutaneous melanosis
A rare syndrome of giant, often multiple CMN on the trunk and extremities and leptomeningeal pigmentation or melanocytic nodules is known as neurocutaneous melanosis (NCM) (Fig. 11.9). Although survival past the age of 20 had generally been considered uncommon [138], a study of 1072 patients with CMN reported that of those with truncal large CMN, about 5% developed symptomatic NCM [139]. Of the small number with multiple CMN without a giant nevus, 71% developed symptomatic NCM and 41% died of it. These children may develop seizures, hydrocephalus, and melanoma. When a giant congenital melanocytic nevus is on the head or neck, or when large numbers of satellite nevi are present, leptomeningeal involvement is more likely [140].

Malignant change occurs as multifocal cerebral invasion or localized tumor formation, with other areas showing a benign melanocytic picture [113]. These melanocytic brain nodules have features of both cellular blue nevi and spindle cell melanomas [141]. Whether these tumors are true melanomas is unanswered. Meningeal melanocytosis with benign histologic features may occur in patients without accompanying skin signs, sometimes as an incidental finding at autopsy [142].

Melanoma in children and adolescents

Overall, melanoma in childhood (<20 years of age) is unusual [143]. In the United States, approximately 2% (1% to 4%) of all melanomas occur in children [136,143–145]. Childhood melanoma often has atypical clinical features (e.g., amelanotic or exophytic) as well as a nodular histologic architecture and may be thick at diagnosis. In one study of 33 cases from Italy, half of childhood melanomas were amelanotic [145]. Childhood melanoma may resemble a pyogenic granuloma [146]. In boys, the predominant sites are the head, neck, and trunk. In girls, the arms and legs are most commonly affected. Melanoma in children is seven times more frequent in the second decade of life than in the first decade [144,147].

The most important benign nevus that may mimic melanoma in children is the spindle and epithelioid nevus of Spitz [148]. Formerly, it was believed to be a malignancy with an unusually benign course and was known as juvenile melanoma, a misleading and obsolete term (discussed further under "Differential Diagnosis"). Histologic features of a spitzoid melanoma may make the distinction between spitzoid melanoma and Spitz's nevus problematic [149].

The role of CMN in childhood melanoma has been discussed. Melanoma in children with xeroderma pigmentosum is discussed below.

Familial melanoma

Certain familial syndromes appear to predispose to a higher incidence of melanoma: dysplastic nevus syndrome, xeroderma pigmentosum, and red-headed frecklers. Dysplastic nevus syndrome may be familial or sporadic. This syndrome may affect 5% to 20% of the general population and increases the risk of melanoma. This subject is presented in Chapter 10. Xeroderma pigmentosum is a rare recessively transmitted disorder characterized by impaired DNA repair following UV light damage [150]. The genetics may be complex, with multiple genes involved [151,152]. These patients display a high incidence of excessive freckling, actinic keratoses, basal cell carcinomas, squamous cell carcinomas, keratoacanthomas, and melanomas. A detailed review of this subject is presented in Chapter 3. Red-headed frecklers seem to be at high risk for

melanoma [153]. One study found heavy freckling (defined as >100 facial freckles in summer) to be a significant risk factor for melanoma, with a 20-fold increased risk [29].

Surprisingly, melanoma in association with oculocutaneous albinism is rare, although one might expect it more frequently [154]. In a series of 350 black albinos from Tanzania, the overwhelming majority of skin cancers were squamous cell carcinomas, with a few basal cell carcinomas and only one melanoma [155].

Where there is a family history of melanoma, the age at diagnosis is considerably younger, and the incidence of multiple primary melanomas is higher [156]. In first-degree relatives of patients with melanoma, there is an increased risk of melanoma; prostate, breast, and colon cancer; non-Hodgkin's lymphoma; and multiple myeloma. In second-degree relatives, an increased risk for melanoma, prostate cancer, and multiple myeloma has also been identified. These observations suggest heritable cancer syndromes [157]. Individuals with a family history of melanoma should strictly adhere to recommended screenings for all cancers.

Mutations in two loci encoding cell-cycle regulatory proteins have been identified in familial melanoma. The tumor-suppressor gene *p16*, also known as cyclin-dependent kinase 2A (*CDKN2A*), is a high-penetrance, low-prevalence gene located on chromosome 9p21. About 20% of melanoma-prone families were found to have a mutation in the *CDKN2A* locus [158]. One study found strikingly different mutations in *CDKN2A* in different geographic areas. There was little evidence for an association between *CDKN2A* mutations in these patients and either neural system tumors or uveal melanomas [159,160]. A second, much less common, high-penetrance melanoma susceptibility gene, the cyclin-dependent kinase (*CDK4*) on 12q13, has been linked to melanoma in only three families worldwide [160].

Germline mutations in the *CDKN2A* gene predispose to melanoma. A study of 20 melanoma-prone French families found penetrance of the *CDKN2A* gene to be significantly influenced by host factors (nevus phenotypes and sunburn) and by variants of the *MC1R* gene (RHC [red hair color] variants), which are consistently associated with red hair and fair skin. RHC variants and dysplastic nevi were identified as the most important modulators of melanoma risk in *CDKN2A* mutation carriers [153]. Such results may improve the prediction of melanoma risk in families and identify those for whom preventive measures and enhanced surveillance are prudent. Multiple primary melanoma patients should be considered for *CDKN2A* mutational screening to improve early detection of melanoma in this subset of high-risk patients and improve phenotypic characterization.

Verrucous melanoma

In 1967, Clark [161] reported that at times an LMM or SSM may be grossly hyperkeratotic and clinically almost indistinguishable from a large seborrheic keratosis (Fig. 11.5). He suggested "verrucous malignant melanoma" as a distinct fourth type, in addition to LMM, SSM, and NM. He reviewed 17 cases of verrucous melanomas and found the histologic pattern most consistent with that of SSM. Subsequently, Clark deemphasized verrucous melanoma as a fourth distinct variant [51]. A study of 101 verrucous melanomas found 75% occurring in women, with about 70% arising on the extremities [162]. Thirty-six percent of these were classifiable as SSM and 25% were LMM, whereas 28% exhibited a distinctive clinicopathogic presentation, which the authors termed *verrucous melanoma in sensu stricto*. These were all uniformly black or brown with other coloration. Their histology resembled ALM. None was found to ulcerate. The prognosis did not differ from that of other melanomas of the same thickness. It is important to recognize this unusual variant of melanoma, as it may be confused both clinically and pathologically with benign neoplasms [163].

Melanoma with halo nevi and vitiligo

Halo nevi are benign melanocytic nevi surrounded by a rim of vitiligo-like depigmentation. They are common in children, adolescents, and pregnant women. The mechanism of depigmentation appears to be a cell-mediated immune response with the secondary formation of antimelanocyte antibodies [164]. When immunologically mediated regression occurs in melanoma, common melanocytic nevi as

well as normally pigmented skin may be secondarily affected. Vitiligo-like depigmentation was found in 15 (1.3%) of 1130 unselected melanoma patients with stage I or II disease [165]. Thus, halo nevi and vitiligo, although usually benign in etiology, may also be an alerting sign to melanoma elsewhere. As halo nevi are symmetrical, halo asymmetry warrants careful scrutiny for melanoma.

Amelanotic melanoma

Although melanomas may appear clinically devoid of pigment, truly histologically amelanotic primary melanoma is rare [51,166,167]. Rapid melanoma growth is associated with atypical clinical features, including amelanosis [168]. The reported incidence of clinically amelanotic melanoma generally ranges from 2% to 8% [51,52,166,169,170]. Many amelanotic melanomas are recurrent, visceral, or metastatic [170–173]. The incidence of metastatic amelanotic melanoma of unknown primary has been reported to be between 12% and 29%, in contrast with the 4% incidence for pigmented metastatic melanomas [166,174]. Pigmented primary melanomas may have amelanotic metastases [166,175]. Melanoma in children is more likely to be amelanotic than in adults and may resemble a pyogenic granuloma [176].

Amelanotic melanoma is difficult to diagnose clinically; several presentations may occur. Amelanotic NM is likely to simulate pyogenic granuloma or basal cell carcinoma. Close inspection under good lighting may reveal a gray hue and minute blue or black flecks at the base. Recurrent LMM may be amelanotic and may resemble a dermatitis at the prior excision site [171]. Plaque-like amelanotic melanomas have been described, simulating Bowen's disease [177], squamous cell carcinoma [178], extramammary Paget's disease [179], and verruca plantaris [180]. Amelanotic melanoma may be evident as a nonhealing, nonpigmented, pruritic, or scaly patch, or appear in a scar [181]. In a subungual location, amelanotic melanoma may be mistaken for an ingrown toenail, a simple split nail, an infection, or an inflammatory process [74,182,183]. Subungual melanoma should be considered in the differential diagnosis of all persistent abnormalities of the nail bed, pigmented or nonpigmented. The differential diagnosis of amelanotic melanoma is presented in Table 11.6.

Primary melanoma arising in a visceral site

The incidence of noncutaneous primary melanoma is approximately one sixth that of cutaneous melanoma; approximately 80% are intraocular, mainly involving the choroid [92]. When primary melanomas appear in unusual sites, it may be difficult to rule out the possibility that the visceral involvement is metastatic from a regressed cutaneous primary melanoma. Primary melanomas are known to arise in the upper respiratory tract, esophagus, rectum, gallbladder, ovaries, cervix, vagina, genitourinary tract, and leptomeninges. The prognosis is poor [104,106,109,142,184–193].

Multiple primary melanoma

An American study of 354 cases showed that within 2 years of diagnosis of an initial primary melanoma, 8% developed a second primary melanoma, 6% of these occurring within the first year after diagnosis [194]. Among 5250 Australian cases of primary invasive melanoma, the prevalence of multiple primary melanoma in this group was 5.6%. Double primary melanoma occurred in 88.6%, triple melanoma occurred in 8.7%, and three to five melanomas occurred in 2.7%. Only 26.2% of patients had multiple melanomas synchronously [195]. In this series, those with three or more primary tumors survived longer than expected, whereas those with two primary tumors survived as anticipated. The incidence of multiple primary melanomas is higher in patients for whom there is a family history of melanoma or of atypical moles. Some patients with multiple primary melanomas, but without a family history of melanoma, may have germ cell mutations of the *CDKN2A* gene [196,197].

The challenge in diagnosing multiple primary melanomas is to establish that the multiple tumors are truly primary. Several criteria that can help differentiate between a primary melanoma and intraepidermal (epidermotrophic) metastasis are described below and summarized in Table 11.8. The prognosis is best reflected by the thickness of the most advanced primary tumor and the presence or

Table 11.8 Differentiation of primary melanoma and intraepidermal metastases

	Primary Melanoma	Intraepidermal Metastases
Clinical	Mosaic of color Margins irregular Likely melanotic	Uniform color Smooth surface Likely amelanotic
Histologic	≥Two cell morphologies	One cell type
		"Indian-filing" of dermal tumor cells Invasion of vascular spaces
		Absence of radial intraepidermal spread beyond bulk of tumor mass

absence of nodal metastases, rather than multiplicity per se.

Metastatic melanoma arising without a demonstrable cutaneous primary

The occurrence of metastases with no apparent primary melanoma occurs in approximately 2% to 4% of all cases of melanoma [92,198,199]. In a series of 2485 melanoma patients seen in a Boston teaching hospital, 2.6% had an unknown primary. The median age at diagnosis was 54 years, and 63% were male. In this series, 46% had lymph node metastases, 18% had cutaneous or subcutaneous metastases, and 35% had visceral metastases. More than half the cases involved the axillary nodes.

In evaluating a patient with melanoma of the lymph nodes and no apparent primary cutaneous neoplasm, careful history taking may disclose that a birthmark or skin blemish was previously removed or that a pigmented lesion had simply disappeared. Wood's UV light examination may demonstrate residual depigmentation (vitiliginous change) at the former site. The cutaneous region drained by the involved node deserves particular scrutiny, and even a vaguely suspicious lesion deserves biopsy. A thorough physical examination is required to ascertain whether the melanoma has spread beyond the regional nodes; an ophthalmologic evaluation is necessary to rule out a primary ocular melanoma, metastatic to skin [200].

The most probable explanation for melanoma with an unknown primary is spontaneous regression of a cutaneous melanoma so that it becomes inapparent [201]. Partial regression of primary cutaneous melanoma is a common finding and occurs in 10% to 35% of cases [202]. Complete regression of primary cutaneous malignant melanoma is a rare occurrence, with only 34 well-documented cases in the indexed English-language literature [203].

Late metastases of cutaneous melanoma

The overwhelming majority of recurrences occur within 5 years after treatment. However, melanoma may remain clinically occult for decades before regional or distant recurrence becomes evident. This protracted melanoma-free interval makes a "cure" for melanoma difficult to pronounce [204]. A disease-free interval of 26 years has been documented [205].

Analysis of data from 6298 patients with cutaneous melanoma seen in Munich between 1977 and 1998 showed 31 patients (0.5%) who first experienced metastatic disease 10 or more years after surgical treatment of a primary melanoma [206]. In more than half, metastases were at distant sites, such as lungs, liver, stomach, and bone marrow, with the remainder of tumors being local, in transit, or in regional lymph nodes [204]. Survival after late melanoma recurrence appears to correlate with site of recurrence, rather than length of disease-free survival [204,206]. Long-term spontaneous regression of melanoma does occur; even metastatic melanoma may undergo regression [87,203, 207].

Satellite melanomas and in-transit metastases

Nodules within 2 cm of a primary melanoma are arbitrarily labeled satellites, and those beyond 2 cm in a lymphatic draining pattern are called in-transit metastases. Both findings signify melanoma cell dissemination through local lymphatic channels and are foreboding [208]. Performing a sentinel node biopsy in patients with cutaneous melanoma treated by wide local excision does not seem to increase the incidence of in-transit metastasis [209].

Disseminated melanoma with melanosis, melanuria, and melanoptysis

Generalized melanosis is a rare feature of disseminated melanoma in which melanin pigment is deposited extensively throughout the dermis and viscera. Clinically, the skin and mucous membranes show a diffuse slate-blue discoloration and, in most of the cases, melanuria. This particular skin coloration is imparted by the Tyndall light-scattering effect from melanin pigment within the dermis [210–212]. Melanin is also found diffusely in the visceral organs and is highly concentrated within the reticuloendothelial system [213,214].

Melanuria, which occurs in disseminated melanoma, is a misnomer, as melanin is not itself excreted in the urine. Rather, colorless phenol and indole metabolites of melanin precursors are excreted into the urine. Left to stand for several hours, these undergo subsequent oxidation and blacken [212,215]. Melanoptysis may contain frank tumor or result from the presence of melanin granules in alveolar macrophages [214].

Dermoscopy

Dermoscopy (epiluminescence microscopy, dermatoscopy, skin-surface microscopy, incident light microscopy) has been established in the last two decades as a noninvasive method for improving accuracy in diagnosing malignant melanoma [216]. Diagnostic accuracy is heavily dependent on operator experience. In experienced hands, dermoscopy may improve diagnostic accuracy by 5% to 30% [216,217]. Dermoscopy uses recognition of surface structures, pigment patterns, and blood vessel patterns as an aid in diagnosis. Various diagnostic algorithms, such as the ABCD dermoscopic rule [218], Menzies' method [219], seven-point check list [220], modified ABC-point list [221], and the CASH (color, architecture, symmetry, and homogeneity) algorithm [222], may serve as valuable guidelines. (See Chapter 12.)

Histology

The histologic diagnosis of melanoma is often difficult, requiring considerable expertise. Criteria for the diagnosis of melanoma include both the architectural pattern and cytologic features. Architectural clues include:

1 An increased number of atypical melanocytes, singly and/or in nests, within the epidermis
2 Atypical melanocytes at all levels of the epidermis
3 Lateral extension of atypical melanocytes along the dermal–epidermal junction, beyond the bulk of the neoplasm
4 Failure of nuclei to show maturation (normally, the nuclei appear smaller with progressive descent into the dermis)
5 Extension of atypical melanocytes along the epithelia of adnexal structures
6 Confluence of nests of atypical melanocytes
7 Variation in size and shape of nests of atypical melanocytes
8 Asymmetry of the overall lesion (appreciated in low-power viewing).

Cytologic features include:

1 Large nuclei, often with prominent nucleoli that are usually a striking magenta color on routine hematoxylin-eosin staining
2 Irregular shape of the nucleus
3 Variable hyperchromatism
4 Pleomorphism, which may be present or, particularly in SSM, completely absent
5 Peripheral chromatin deposition in a rim pattern along the nuclear membrane
6 Mitotic figures with bizarre mitoses in some areas deep in the dermis.

Some special considerations in the histology of melanoma are discussed in Chapter 19.

With the rare exception of melanoma arising from a blue nevus or from the intradermal component of a congenital melanocytic nevus, cutaneous melanomas originate from melanocytes proliferating at the dermal–epidermal junction. Although melanomas are classified into several histologic patterns, they appear to have little prognostic significance, with the possible exception of minimal deviation melanoma and borderline melanoma, described below.

About one third of melanomas have histologic evidence of nonmalignant benign melanocytes, which may have been part of a precursor lesion. A recent study of 8593 patients demonstrated that, based on the patient's history, 42% of melanomas developed from a preexisting nevus, 34% arose de novo, and in almost a quarter, the historical origin could not be determined. It is speculative whether melanomas arising in a preexisting nevus have a greater Breslow thickness at diagnosis and, hence, a worse prognosis [223]. One study found dysplastic nevi histologically in continuity with about half of melanomas in a small series of excised acquired nonfamilial melanomas [224].

Rarely, primary melanoma may consist entirely of atypical melanocytes arranged in a well-structured glandular pattern [225] or with numerous signet-ring cells [226]. These unusual variants highlight the importance of immunohistochemical staining with markers such as S-100 and HMB-45 to confirm melanocytic differentiation.

Histology of lentigo maligna melanoma

Lentigo maligna (Hutchinson's melanotic freckle) is an in situ melanoma that tends to first display a few heavily pigmented spindle-shaped melanocytes at the basal layer. The melanocytes themselves appear somewhat atypical and usually pleomorphic, arranged randomly, and having enlarged hyperchromatic nuclei. Similar melanocytes may also be seen along the basal layer of hair follicles. Some nesting may become evident as the tumor progresses. The dermis may show a lymphohistiocytic inflammatory infiltrate, moderate to large amounts of "dropped" pigment held within macrophages (melanophages), and changes of solar or x-ray damage. LM may display single atypical melanocytes in the superficial dermis, a finding that may be obscured by dermal fibrosis or an inflammatory infiltrate [227]. At times, vacuolar changes at the basal layer may be the most striking alteration appreciated for LM. This vacuolar change is a shrinkage artifact that occurs during processing of the specimen, because proliferating melanocytes lack desmosomes. The unwary pathologist may mistake this shrinkage artifact for the basal vacuolar changes seen in inflammatory diseases, such as lupus erythematosus. In such a case, the presence of a lymphocytic dermal infiltrate and solar elastosis may further confuse the diagnosis.

In time, LM develops a focal extension into the dermis, at which point it becomes LMM. Invasion is evident as a downward proliferation into the dermis by melanocytes either in nests or strands. In an apparent LM, careful examination of multiple step sections is necessary to avoid overlooking an invasive component.

Histology of superficial spreading melanoma

In addition to their congregation near the dermal–epidermal junction, the atypical melanocytes of SSM may also appear dispersed singly and in nests throughout all levels of the epidermis. This "shotgunning" or "buckshotting" of malignant cells throughout the epidermis is the characteristic feature of SSM known as pagetoid spread (Fig. 11.11). The halo lacunae that surround these melanocytes occur as a processing artifact, because these cells do not have desmosomes. Individual melanocytes are atypical with hyperchromatic nuclei, but pleomorphism is frequently absent.

The pagetoid pattern of the SSM may require distinction from other epidermotropic neoplasms, including metastatic melanoma, mycosis fungoides, mammary or extramammary Paget's disease, pagetoid Bowen's disease, and metastatic mesothelioma [228]. The distinction may be challenging in Bowen's disease and extramammary Paget's disease when melanin phagocytosed from tissues is contained within the cytoplasm of pagetoid cells. Architectural features are helpful. Melanoma tends to show a characteristic nesting of some cells at the dermal–epidermal junction, with shotgunning throughout the epidermis sometimes seen, whereas the pagetoid cells of extramammary or mammary Paget's disease tend to spare this interface and lie within or above the basal layer, leaving a narrow rim of basal cell cytoplasm beneath. Pagetoid Bowen's disease may also involve the basal layer, sparing the dermal–epidermal interface. Desmosomes connecting markedly atypical cells are observed in Bowen's disease. A few very large atypical Bowen's cells may be present.

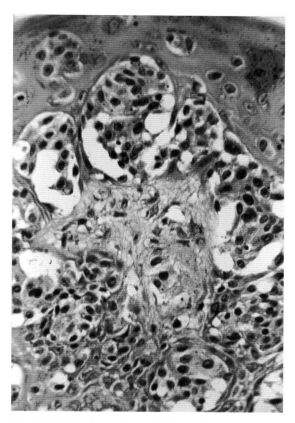

Fig. 11.11 Histology of superficial spreading melanoma, with multiple irregularly sized and shaped nests of atypical cells at the dermal–epidermal interface and extending into the epidermis and dermis (×99).

The differentiation of pagetoid melanoma, mammary Paget's disease, and extramammary Paget's disease may at times be difficult. Immunohistologic staining may help distinguish these tumors. Pagetoid melanoma cells are almost always S-100 positive and negative for carcinoembryonic antigen (CEA), cytokeratin, and keratin. Mammary and extramammary Paget's disease is S-100 negative, strongly positive for CEA and cytokeratin, and variably positive for keratin. Bowen's disease shows no reactivity for S-100 and CEA, variable positivity for cytokeratin, and strong positivity for keratin. As junctional melanoma cells may express a lesser amount of S-100 antigen, a negative S-100 reaction does not exclude the diagnosis of melanoma.

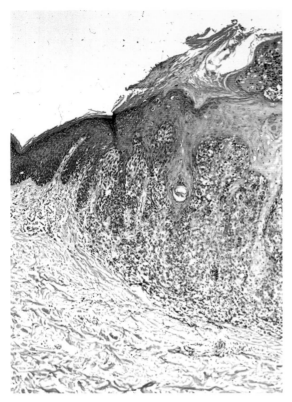

Fig. 11.12 Histology of nodular melanoma showing a mass of poorly differentiated melanocytic cells destroying normal architecture. In contrast to most other types of melanoma, the edge is well defined (×14.5).

Melanoma also shows positivity for the vimentin antigen, which is negative in carcinomas. For further discussion, see Chapter 19.

Histology of nodular melanoma

Nodular melanoma is an invasive melanoma lacking the lateral epidermal component (Fig. 11.12). The atypical melanocytes may be streaming downward from the epidermis or may be scattered in neuroid or other patterns. As with most melanomas, the tumor cells tend to proliferate along the dermal–epidermal interface at the edge of the lesion; when severe, this process causes destruction of the epidermis. Sometimes the diagnosis is obvious. At other times, it is difficult to recognize, as in the case of balloon cell

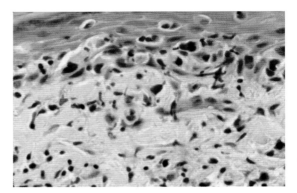

Fig. 11.13 Histology of acral lentiginous melanoma, with atypical dendritic melanocytic cells at the dermal–epidermal interface and extending insidiously into the epidermis and dermis, giving a false impression of benignity (×39).

melanoma, which often has a deceptively benign-appearing histology.

Histology of acral lentiginous melanoma

Acral melanomas may have a variety of histologies, but the special pattern most associated with acral melanoma, the so-called lentiginous pattern, is often difficult to diagnose, as early ALM may show only focal melanocytic hyperplasia and atypia. More fully developed ALM may have a spindle cell pattern similar to that of LMM (Fig. 11.13). ALM and LMM may exhibit both dendritic cells and pagetoid cells, but with certain distinctions. The dendritic cell of ALM tends to have multiple dendritic processes projecting in all directions, as in a starburst pattern; the dendritic processes of LMM tend to be bipolar, projecting in two directions. Pagetoid features may be seen in both ALM and LMM, but these are less commonly seen in ALM. The pagetoid cells of ALM, when present, tend to be concentrated focally; that is, ALM may exhibit an area of pagetoid cells within the tumor. In LMM, pagetoid cells tend to be interspersed diffusely throughout the tumor.

Acral melanomas in blacks and mucosal melanomas are overwhelmingly of this "acral lentiginous" histologic pattern [54,67]. In neoplasms of the volar and subungual surfaces, whether benign or malignant, the morphology of the melanocytes tends to be dendritic. Thus, benign tumors, such as a subungual melanocytic nevus, may be confused with ALM [229].

Histology of malignant blue nevus

The malignant blue nevus, a rare type of melanoma, histologically lacks junctional activity. Nuclear pleomorphism is evident. The nests of atypical cells may display a variety of histologies, appearing as nests of dysplastic cuboidal cells, dendritic cells, and rounded cells. A spindle cell component containing melanin granules is characteristic. Multiple mitoses and tumor cell necrosis are seen [121].

Histology of cellular blue nevus

The cellular blue nevus tends to show two cell types: (1) large epithelioid to spindle-shaped cells with oval nuclei showing a tendency to form nests and (2) more dendritic, fusiform cells with elongated, darkly staining nuclei, displaying a tendency to lie between these nests. Few mitoses without atypia may be present. Hyperchromatic nuclei and necrosis are not features of the cellular blue nevus.

Histology of congenital melanocytic nevus

Melanoma may evolve from a congenital melanocytic nevus, especially when it is very large. Histologically, CMN can be distinguished from acquired melanocytic nevi by their increased size and the presence of nevus cells deep within the dermis, dermal appendages, and neurovascular structures [113]. The presence of nevus cells within the lower two thirds of the reticular dermis and the piloerector muscle is quite sensitive and specific for the diagnosis of a congenital melanocytic nevus; the presence of nevus cells within appendageal structures, perineural sheaths, and blood or lymphatic vessel walls is a highly specific finding [230]. CMN have been documented to have high numbers of estrogen- and progesterone-binding sites, a property they share with melanomas and dysplastic nevi, but not acquired melanocytic nevi [231].

Melanomas may arise from the junctional or dermal component of a giant congenital melanocytic nevus. When deriving from the dermal component, the malignancy often develops deep in the reticu-

lar dermis and consists of variably sized cuboidal to spindle-shaped cells, devoid of melanin and with multiple mitotic figures. In smaller congenital melanocytic nevi, melanomas tend to arise junctionally [126].

Histology of minimal deviation melanoma and borderline melanoma

Minimal deviation melanoma (MDM) is characterized by a mass proliferation of atypical nevoid melanocytes in the papillary dermis with extension into the reticular dermis and mitotic figures deep in the dermis. The latter feature is particularly helpful in diagnosing MDM [232]. The borderline melanoma has a similar vertical growth pattern, but only extends as far as the papillary dermis [229,233]. In both borderline melanona and MDM, the individual melanocytes display only a minimal degree of cytologic atypica. These tumors are not as biologically aggressive as other melanomas and seem to have a better prognosis [234]. MDM and borderline melanoma tend to develop before the age of 40, though they may arise in middle to late life [229]. Frequently, both MDM and borderline melanoma may show histologic resemblance to a spindle and epithelioid nevus of Spitz [67] usually seen in childhood. Thus, the appearance in an adult of an apparent spindle and epithelioid nevus should alert the physician to the possibility of MDM or borderline melanoma. Both are relatively rare.

Histology of desmoplastic melanoma

Desmoplastic melanoma is a rare variant characterized by the proliferation of amelanotic spindle cells in a fibrotic stroma and most commonly develops in the lentiginous radial component of ALM and LMM [235–237]. The spindle cells display large bizarre and hyperchromatic nuclei and mitoses and are arranged in fascicles within a collagenized dermal matrix [237]. The fibrotic stroma may obscure the epithelial nature of this neoplasm. Tumor cells may not be appreciated as melanocytes on conventional microscopy; electron microscopic demonstration of melanosomes may be necessary to establish the correct diagnosis. The fibrotic component is produced by the dedifferentiated tumor cells, rather than reactive fibroblasts. The tumor tends to be deeply invasive and has a poor prognosis. Desmoplastic melanoma must be differentiated from fibrosarcoma, fibromatosis, spindle cell squamous cell carcinoma, and fibrohistiocytic tumors. This type of melanoma has a higher local recurrence rate than other melanomas.

In recurrences, a neurotropic pattern may be seen, with invasion of the cutaneous nerves [235,237–239]. The tumor cells often have a distinctive neuroid or schwannian cell differentiation. Recurrent tumors tend to be amelanotic and evident as scarred and indurated plaques with palpably ill-defined margins [181]. Neurotropism complicates clinical management, as the margins are difficult to evaluate. The dermal pattern is often deceptively bland and may be mistaken for a neurofibroma, a blue nevus, or reactive fibroplasia. Moreover, the blue nevus shares features of neurotropism, desmoplasia, and fasciculation. It is hypothesized that trauma may play a role in the transformation of a desmoplastic melanoma into a neurotropic variant.

Desmoplastic melanoma may be difficult to diagnose [236]. Immunohistochemical studies may be useful in clarifying the cell of origin. S-100 protein is positive in most melanomas, including the desmoplastic and neurotropic variety, but S-100 has been demonstrated in Schwann cells and Langerhans cells as well. Neuron-specific enolase is expressed by melanoma cells, including those of desmoplastic and neurotropic melanoma, as well as a wide range of neuroendocrine tumors, but has not been found in Schwann cells [237]. Thus, despite possible anomalous situations, these markers may clarify the cell of origin. Melanoma cells are also characteristically DOPA (3,4-dihydroxy-phenylalanine) positive, the demonstration of which requires unfixed, frozen tissue. For further discussion of desmoplastic melanoma see Chapter 19.

Histology of balloon cell melanoma

Any melanoma or melanocytic nevus may display balloon cell morphology. The balloon cell melanoma may be deceptively benign appearing, consisting of a mass of clear foam cells with little atypia and rare mitotic figures [240]. The presence of a transition zone of spindle or epithelioid tumor cells adjacent to the balloon cells can clarify the diagnosis. In the absence of a transition zone, balloon cell melanoma may be difficult to distinguish from a balloon cell nevus, xanthoma, granular cell tumor, liposarcoma, or metastatic hypernephroma.

Histology of metastatic melanoma

Melanomas metastatic to skin tend to lack an epidermal component, being either within the dermis or within the subcutaneous tissue [200,228]. However, involvement of the epidermis may occur with junctional activity, and epidermotropic metastatic melanoma may simulate primary melanoma. Certain features may help clarify metastatic origin (Table 11.8). "Indian-filing" of dermal tumor cells, such that individual cells are lined up along collagen bundles in a single-file arrangement, may point to metastatic origin [241]. The presence of atypical melanocytes within vascular spaces suggests metastatic origin. The absence of a zone of radial intraepidermal spread beyond the bulk of tumor mass, by itself, might imply either metastatic melanoma or nodular melanoma. However, metastatic melanoma tends to be confined to the papillary dermis, whereas the tumor mass of nodular melanoma tends to produce more strikingly deep invasion.

Histology of pseudomelanoma

Kornberg and Ackerman [242] delineated changes seen in a recurrent melanocytic nevus following its partial surgical removal or electrodessication. Such "pseudomelanomas" tend to be sharply circumscribed without lateral spread of individual melanocytes at the periphery and show confinement of atypical melanocytes to epidermis. There is dermal fibrosis and few, if any, melanocytes in mitosis. The fibrosis results from surgical trauma. *It is, however, important to remember that melanomas may also recur.* Pseudomelanoma has been described after shave excision followed by intralesional injection of triamcinolone acetonide [243], Solcoderm therapy [244], dermabrasion [245], and laser therapy [246].

Differential diagnosis

Melanoma must be distinguished from a variety of cutaneous and mucosal lesions, pigmented and

Table 11.9 Clinical diagnosis of melanoma: sensitivity and specificity

Reference	Sensitivity, %	Specificity, %
Becker [3]	48	42
McMullan & Hubener [314]	51	38
Swerdlow [315]	59	28
Kopf et al. [316]	77	80
Bono et al. [317]	43	91

nonpigmented, benign and malignant. As Table 11.9 suggests, clinical misdiagnosis is common. Becker's [3] classic study remains instructive today. Of 169 lesions diagnosed clinically as melanoma, 43% were confirmed microscopically (i.e., 57% were false positives). Of 151 specimens diagnosed microscopically, 48% were diagnosed clinically (i.e., 52% were false negatives).

Among the most common simulators of melanoma are the ephelis (common freckle), lentigo, melanocytic nevus (common mole), dermatofibroma, and subungual hemorrhage. Basal cell carcinoma, squamous cell carcinoma, and seborrheic keratosis may be difficult to separate clinically from melanoma, especially when deeply pigmented. A melanocytic nevus in which thrombosis develops may present a striking simulation of the rapidly developing tumor nodule in a vertical growth phase. Although it is an accepted practice to destroy seborrheic keratoses without histopathologic confirmation, melanoma may not only mimic a seborrheic keratosis, but may arise within a seborrheic keratosis [247]. Tables 11.6 and 11.10 present lesions that may simulate melanoma.

Melanocytic lesions in the differential diagnosis of melanoma

In Becker's [3] series, the most common error in the underdiagnosis or overdiagnosis of melanoma involved benign melanocytic lesions. Of 169 cases diagnosed clinically as melanoma, 25% proved histologically to be common acquired melanocytic nevi, blue nevi, or lentigines. Of 151 cases diagnosed histologically as melanoma, 28% had

Table 11.10 The differential diagnosis of melanoma

I. Melanocytic lesions
  A. Ephelis (common freckle)
  B. Lentigines
    1. Lentigo simplex
    2. Solar lentigo
  C. Acquired melanocytic nevi[a]
    1. Common acquired nevi (junctional, compound, intradermal)
    2. Blue nevus
    3. Cellular blue nevus
    4. Spindle & epithelioid nevus of Spitz
    5. Halo nevus
    6. Dysplastic nevus

II. Tumors[b]
  A. Actinic keratosis
  B. Angiokeratoma
  C. Basal cell carcinoma
  D. Bowen's disease/ squamous cell carcinoma
  E. Apocrine hidrocystoma
  F. Dermatofibroma
  G. Keratoacanthoma
  H. Kaposi's sarcoma
  I. Melanoacanthoma
  J. Paget's disease
  K. Seborrheic keratosis
  L. Verruca vulgaris

III. Vascular lesions[a]
  A. Pyogenic granuloma
  B. Hemangioma
    1. Capillary hemangioma (strawberry nevus)
    2. Senile hemangioma (cherry angioma)
  C. Capillary aneurysm
  D. Glomus tumor

IV. Inflammatory lesions
  A. Dermatitis
  B. Subungual infection
  C. Subungual foreign body granuloma

V. Traumatic lesions
  A. Black heel
  B. Clavus vasculare
  C. Targetoid hemosiderotic nevus
  D. Subungual hematoma
  E. Tattoo (asphalt, graphite, metal)

[a] Especially when thrombosed.
[b] Especially when deeply pigmented.

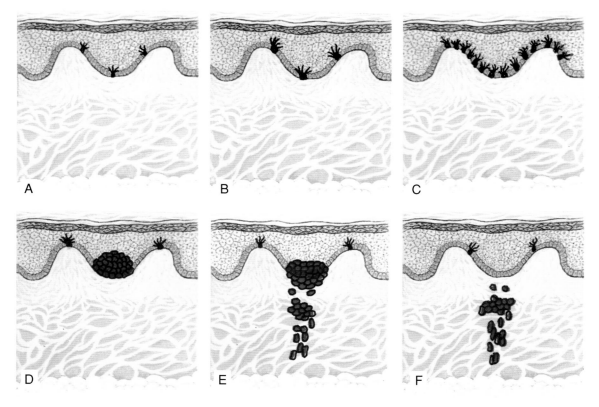

Fig. 11.14 Comparative histology of the most common benign pigmented lesions. *A*, Normal skin: dendritic melanocytes along the dermal–epidermal junction. *B*, Ephelis: increase in size but not density of melanocytes; increased melanin production. *C*, Lentigo: increased density of melanocytes along the dermal–epidermal junction. *D*, Junctional nevus: nests of rounded melanocytes above the basement membrane. *E*, Compound nevus: nests of melanocytes with junctional and intradermal components. *F*, Intradermal nevus: nests of intradermal melanocytes, minimal to absent junctional component.

been judged clinically to be benign melanocytic lesions.

Ephelis (freckle)

Ephelides, or common freckles, are tan to brown macules occurring on sun-exposed surfaces. Histologically, they demonstrate increased melanin, with larger individual melanocytes but no increase in the number of melanocytes (Fig. 11.14). Freckles appear early in childhood. They darken in the summer in response to UV irradiation and lighten in the winter. LM develops irregularities of color, margins, and surface characteristics and enlarges progressively, unlike a common freckle.

Lentigo

Benign lentigines are usually tan to brown, flat, and oval, measuring 5 to 10 mm in diameter. Lentigines, whether benign or LM, do not fade when shielded from light. Histologically, they are characterized by an increased number of normal dendritic melanocytes along the dermal–epidermal junction (Fig. 11.14) and have two main subtypes: lentigo simplex and solar lentigo. Lentigo simplex may appear on any cutaneous or mucosal surface. These pigmented, circular to ovoid macules commonly arise in childhood and darken little, if at all, in response to sunlight. On volar surfaces, a lentigo may appear as a streak with somewhat indistinct borders and may be clinically indistinguishable from acral melanoma. The solar lentigo (also known by the less accurate terms *lentigo senilis* and *liver spot*) appears on sun-exposed surfaces during middle to late life, in common with LM, and may closely resemble LM. However, lentigo senilis does not progressively enlarge or develop irregularities of color and margins.

Common acquired melanocytic nevus (common mole)

In Becker's [3] series, common acquired melanocytic nevi were most frequently implicated in the underdiagnosis or overdiagnosis of melanoma. Common melanocytic nevi are hamartomas that arise during the first years of life and puberty, usually distributed above the waist. Their de novo occurrence after the third decade of life is unusual and even suspicious. It is characteristic that common melanocytic nevi enlarge and darken during puberty and pregnancy. This change is not alarming, especially when the maturation of all such nevi is synchronous. Disproportionate change of a single pigmented nevus, however, should arouse suspicion. The common melanocytic nevus has three patterns: junctional, compound, and intradermal.

The junctional melanocytic nevus is the common mole of childhood, when it is acquired. All melanocytes are found above the basement membrane and occur in nests (Fig. 11.14). Clinically, it is light to dark brown, flat, circular, and hairless. It may occur on any cutaneous or mucosal surface. Pigmented nevi of the palms, soles, and genitalia are almost always junctional. The color of the nevus is uniform, not variegated. The margin may be somewhat indistinct but does not appear notched or indented. The common junctional nevus has little tendency to undergo malignant transformation; most evolve into compound nevi.

The compound melanocytic nevus is the most common nevus of adults. Nevus cells are found in both the epidermis and dermis (Fig. 11.14). Clinically, it is tan to brown and resembles the junctional nevus, with the addition of some degree of elevation, produced by its intradermal component. The slow evolution toward nodularity differs from the rapid vertical growth phase of melanoma. The compound nevus infrequently develops into melanoma but more commonly matures into an intradermal nevus.

The intradermal melanocytic nevus is the common hairy mole of adults. Histologically, nevus cells are found only in the dermis (Fig. 11.14). It may appear on most surfaces, especially on the scalp, face, and neck, but is not known to occur on palms, soles, and genitalia. The color varies from darkly pigmented to flesh colored. The surface may be dome-shaped, polypoid, or even verrucous but is regular and symmetrical. Intradermal nevi on the face tend to persist and even enlarge throughout life. In other locations, they usually slowly regress after the third decade of life. The clinical characteristics and comparative histology of the above common pigmented lesions are summarized in Table 11.11 and Fig. 11.14.

The normal number of moles varies through the life cycle. A British study of 432 healthy white subjects found an average total body mole count of three for females and two for males in the first decade of life, rising to 23 for women and 18 for men in the second decade, and peaking at 33 and 22, respectively, in the third decade. Thereafter, numbers of moles slowly decrease until in the eighth decade, they approximate the levels seen in prepubertal children [248]. A New Zealand study of 349 adolescents found similar second-decade total body mole counts [249]. A Lithuanian study of 484 children aged 1 to 15 years found a median number for all common acquired melanocytic nevi of 12 in boys and 11 in girls; the number of nevi increased with age [250].

There are several features that can aid in distinguishing the common melanocytic nevus from melanoma. The "ABCD" rule, which has been expanded to the "ABCDE" rule, provides a helpful aid in the diagnosis of pigmented lesions [250–254]:

A = Asymmetry
B = Border irregularity
C = Color variegation
D = Diameter greater than 6 mm
E = Elevation

Generally, the common mole displays a regularity of color, margins, and topography. The color of a

Table 11.11 Clinical presentation of the most common benign melanocytic lesions

Lesion	Size, mm	Appearance	Site	History
Ephelis (freckle)	2–3	Tan to brown macule	Sun-exposed surfaces	Appears early childhood; darkens on sun exposure, fades without sun exposure
Lentigo simplex	3–5	Tan to brown oval macule	All surfaces	Arises in childhood; does not fade
Lentigo senilis	4–10	Tan to brown oval macule	Sun-exposed surfaces	Arises middle to late years; does not fade
Junctional nevus[a]	2–4	Dark brown to black; smooth, flat, hairless; skin markings preserved	All surfaces	Almost all nevi in children are junctional; may evolve into compound nevus
Compound nevus[a]	2–5	Dark brown to tan; domed, polypoid, or verrucous; ± coarse hairs	All surfaces	Most common mole in adults; may evolve into intradermal nevus
Intradermal nevus[a]	2–5	Dark brown to tan to flesh colored; domed, polypoid, or verrucous; ± coarse hairs	Usually scalp, face, neck; not on palms, soles, genitalia	Common hairy mole of adults; may involute

[a] Common acquired nevi usually appear above the waist, arise during the first years of life and at puberty, are unusual after the third decade of life; and enlarge during puberty and pregnancy.
±, with or without.

benign melanocytic nevus, whether black, brown, tan, or flesh colored, is uniform. A melanocytic nevus may exhibit a fine black stippling, but this is evenly distributed (Fig. 11.15). To the naked eye, the border may appear sharply demarcated; however, closer examination with a hand lens may reveal a "haziness" of the border, present uniformly throughout the border. Melanoma, in contrast, is best characterized by its irregularity and asymmetry. An uneven border with notching or irregular angulations suggests a malignant process. The color tends to be variegated; various shades of melanin pigment (tan to brown to black) may be splayed in an uneven mosaic. Admixtures of red, white, and/or blue may be present. A diameter greater than 6 mm is suspect for melanoma, although many moles, especially dysplastic nevi, are 6 mm or more in diameter. An uneven topography or, more ominously, the development of focal nodularity, suggests malignancy.

Blue nevus and cellular blue nevus
The blue nevus is a dark blue or black, hairless, dome-shaped nodule, ranging in diameter from a

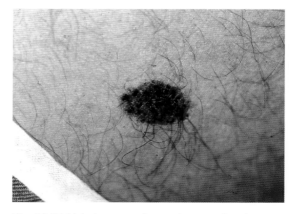

Fig. 11.15 Light brown melanocytic nevus showing uniform darkly pigmented stippling throughout the tumor.

few millimeters to several centimeters, but usually measuring about 5 mm. Its color results from the Tyndall light-scattering effect of light reflected from deeply placed dermal pigment through the colloidal medium of the dermis. It most commonly occurs on the head and neck, dorsum of the hands and feet, and buttocks. There is a female predilection. It may be seen at birth or develop at any age. Once present, it remains stable throughout life. The cellular blue nevus is usually larger, up to several centimeters in diameter, occurring in a distribution similar to that of the blue nevus. The cellular blue nevus may occasionally be found in lymph nodes, where it may be mistaken for melanoma [116].

Spindle and epithelioid nevus of Spitz

The spindle and epithelioid nevus of Spitz has several alternative designations, based on historical precedent or the dominant histologic component. These include spindle cell nevus, epithelioid cell nevus, spindle and/or epithelioid nevus, compound nevus of Spitz, and benign juvenile melanoma. The latter term is inaccurate and should be avoided, because there are no benign melanomas. Although first described as a kind of melanoma by Spitz in 1948 [255] and separated from melanoma in 1953 [256], this benign tumor continues to pose a differential diagnostic challenge. It most commonly occurs in prepubescent children or at puberty and may appear on any body surface, most commonly the cheek. The sudden appearance of this rapidly growing neoplasm may be alarming. It is usually dome-shaped but may be soft or hard, sessile or pedunculated. It is usually pink to red but may be brown or flesh colored. In contrast to melanoma, the patient can usually pinpoint the onset of the tumor. The nevus may persist but more commonly evolves into an intradermal melanocytic nevus. Histologically, the spindle and epithelioid nevus is characterized by a cellular uniformity, as opposed to the pleomorphism that characterizes malignancy. The development of an apparent spindle and epithelioid nevus after puberty should be regarded with concern [148,257].

Halo nevus

The halo nevus (leukoderma acquisitum centrifugum) is usually seen in children, adolescents, and women during pregnancy. These most frequently occur on the back and may be solitary or multiple. Most commonly, a compound or intradermal nevus becomes surrounded by a symmetrical ring of hypopigmentation. With time, most halo nevi undergo spontaneous involution, leaving a flat, hypopigmented macule, which may persist or resolve to normal-appearing skin. The halo surrounding the halo nevus is symmetrical. In contrast, the presence of an asymmetrical or partial halo in association with a pigmented lesion is suspicious for a halo melanoma. Histologically, melanocyte disappearance in a regressing halo nevus occurs in the absence of fibrosis, whereas regressing melanomas show fibrosis [258].

Dysplastic nevus

The dysplastic nevus syndrome is the subject of Chapter 10.

Tumors

The actinic keratosis occurs on exposed surfaces, particularly in light-complexioned persons with a history of excessive sun exposure. It usually occurs as a scaling papule, with a characteristic rough surface. When pigmented, it may resemble LMM or SSM. The actinic keratosis, an indolent precursor of squamous cell carcinoma, is the subject of Chapter 2. Pigmented squamous cell carcinoma may resemble LMM or SSM.

The pigmented seborrheic keratosis may resemble verrucous melanoma, SSM, or LMM. When dome shaped and black, it may simulate NM. Seborrheic keratoses often appear on the face, neck, and trunk, and may occur singly or in large numbers. The color ranges from yellow or tan to dark brown or black. The surface is often waxy and verrucous, but may be dry or flat. The most characteristic feature is its "stuck-on" appearance. Small pieces may dislodge with minor trauma. In contrast, melanoma may be a firmly embedded nodule or may be friable. Verrucous melanoma may closely resemble a hyperplastic seborrheic keratosis [259].

The dermatofibroma (fibrous histiocytoma, sclerosing hemangioma) is a small, firm nodule, less than 1 cm in diameter, smooth and hairless, with a regular outline. Pigmentation is uniform and may appear yellow, tan, pink, red, brown, or dark blue. This common benign neoplasm is most often seen on the legs of middle-aged women and may resemble NM. The "dimple sign" helps distinguish it: when compressed laterally between the thumb and index finger, the dermatofibroma becomes indented. NM, in contrast, will protrude above the skin [260].

The pigmented basal cell carcinoma may resemble SSM or NM. The pigment is usually unevenly distributed, favoring the periphery. Red, white, and bluish hues may predominate, with the absence of black or brown, because this tumor often lacks epidermal melanin. Careful examination usually reveals telangiectasias and an annular rim with a translucent quality, neither of which occurs in melanoma.

The apocrine hidrocystoma (apocrine cystadenoma, black hidrocystoma) is an uncommon benign appendageal tumor with a predilection for the scalp, face, and ears [261,262]. These are usually solitary, dome shaped, and smooth surfaced, and may range in color from gray to blue-black. The tumor is filled with a fluid, which may be black, brown, or colorless. Transillumination of the cyst helps to clarify the diagnosis. However, a cystic basal cell carcinoma may mimic this benign neoplasm [263].

The melanoacanthoma is a rare benign proliferation of melanocytes and keratinocytes [264]. In this tumor, melanin is restricted almost entirely to the melanocytes, leaving keratinocytes devoid of melanin, in contrast to the melanin-bearing keratinocytes of the pigmented seborrheic keratosis. The tumor most often occurs on the head and neck, but may arise on the trunk or extremities. The color is brown to black, the surface papillomatous or verrucous, and the diameter up to 10 cm. It may involute. Melanoacanthomas of the oral mucosa and lip display extensive dendritic differentiation and, thus, may mimic the histology of ALM [229,264].

The keratoacanthoma, in common with the spindle and epithelioid nevus of Spitz, may produce the sudden onset of a rapidly growing pigmented nodule, a presentation similar to that of NM. Several vascular lesions, including pyogenic granuloma, thrombosed hemangioma, and capillary aneurysm, may also produce similar findings and are discussed below.

Angiokeratomas are not true angiomas, but rather ectasias of preexisting vessels, covered by a rough, hyperkeratotic epidermis. Of six clinical variants, two merit discussion here: solitary angiokeratoma and angiokeratoma circumscriptum. Solitary angiokeratoma appears as an indented blue-black nodule occurring on the lower extremity. When thrombosis develops, the resulting enlarging, firm nodule closely simulates NM. Angiokeratoma circumscriptum consists of a rough irregular plaque, usually found on the lower extremity. When thrombosed, it may closely resemble SSM in its vertical growth phase [265].

Kaposi's sarcoma is an affliction predominantly of men [266]. An indolent form occurs in middle-aged men of Mediterranean and Ashkenazic Jewish origin, whereas an aggressive variant is seen in young African males and in patients with AIDS. Kaposi's sarcoma usually appears as multiple violaceous plaques or nodules on the lower extremity. Older tumors tend to assume a reddish brown hue, a pigmentation produced by extravasated red blood cells, and may regress as new ones appear. Ulceration and hemorrhage are frequently seen. Edema of the affected extremity is a common finding and may precede the appearance of these tumors. Kaposi's sarcoma is the subject of Chapter 9.

The pyogenic granuloma is a benign tumor that can be likened to an exuberant proliferation of granulation tissue [267,268]. It is most commonly seen in children, young adults, and pregnant women. When solitary, it may have a pink or dark red to purple hue and may be sessile or pedunculated. The tumor nodule ranges from 5 to 20 mm in diameter and may closely mimic amelanotic or pigmented NM (Fig. 11.8). The surface of a pyogenic granuloma is frequently eroded, a finding that would be ominous when occurring in melanoma. The tumor may bleed after trauma, also suggestive of an advanced NM. A helpful differentiating sign is the presence of blue-black flecks at the base of an amelanotic NM, a finding that is absent in pyogenic granuloma.

Unusual plaque-like amelanotic melanomas have been described, simulating Bowen's disease [177], extramammary Paget's disease [179], and verruca plantaris [269]. Pigmented Paget's disease may resemble melanoma [167].

Vascular neoplasms

Hemangiomas are benign neoplasms composed of mature blood vessels [270,271]. The capillary hemangioma (strawberry nevus) is commonly seen in neonates, appearing most often on the head. A hamartoma consisting of closely packed blood vessels, it may grow rapidly and ulcerate, suggestive of malignancy. Characteristically, the capillary hemangioma regresses during the first 5 years of life, fading from bright red to paler hues of pink and white. When polypoid, these are usually bright red to rich purple or blue. They are firm on palpation and blanch partially on diascopy. The cherry angioma is the capillary hemangioma of adulthood. Unlike hemangiomas of infancy, these do not regress. They are usually multiple 1- to 2-mm bright to dark red papules, with a predilection for the upper trunk. Thrombosis may supervene, simulating NM.

The glomus tumor (glomangioma) is a vascular hamartoma derived in most cases from the glomus cells (pericytes) of arteriovenous anastamoses. Often multiple, these may occur at any site but are usually located on the upper extremities, especially the hand. The tumor appears as a tender, solitary blue to red nodule of less than 1 cm in diameter. The glomus tumor will blanch at least partially on diascopy. At times, they are characterized by paroxysms of sharp pain, although when multiple, may be painless. A helpful differential point is that NM is neither painful nor tender and does not blanch. Glomus tumors have a subungual predilection, especially in females, and must be distinguished from subungual melanoma, which has a strong predilection for the thumb and great toe.

The capillary aneurysm begins as a deeply pigmented papule on previously uninvolved skin of the face and grows rapidly without ulceration. It closely mimics the growing nodule of NM.

Traumatic lesions

Traumatic lesions are frequently pigmented. The pigment may be endogenous (e.g., blood or melanin) or exogenous (e.g., an asphalt tattoo). Subungual hematoma, black heel, clavus vasculare, and traumatic tattoo may all simulate melanoma. Of these, the most common to be distinguished from melanoma is subungual hematoma. Although subungual hematoma is usually posttraumatic, a history of trauma does not clearly differentiate subungual hemorrhage from melanoma [272], as a history of antecedent trauma is common with subungual melanomas. Hutchinson's sign, the leaching of brown-black pigment onto the proximal and lateral nail fold, was first described in 1886 [88]. However, this periungual extension of pigmentation is seen in only a minority of subungual melanomas and may reflect benign disorders as well as Bowen's disease of the nail unit [89].

Subungual hematoma is usually sudden in onset, in contrast with the more gradual development of melanoma. Subungual hemorrhage will migrate distally as the nail grows; melanoma will not. Blood can be evacuated from a subungual hemorrhage by puncture of the nail, in contrast to melanoma. Nontraumatic causes of nail bed pigmentation are noteworthy. Melonychia may occur as a side effect of phototherapy, x-ray exposure, electron-beam therapy, and topical and systemic medications [260,273].

Black heel and clavus vasculare must be differentiated from acral melanoma. Black heel occurs on the lateral and posterior aspect of the heel and may be bilateral. The pigment is extravasated hemoglobin. It is seen in athletes, especially basketball players, and tends to resolve within 6 weeks after cessation of participation in the sport. It is painless, as is melanoma. Clavus vasculare, as its name implies, is a corn with a prominent vascular component. It usually results from ill-fitting shoes and occurs along the junction of plantar and dorsal surfaces and at the distal ends of the lateral toes. In contrast to black heel, which it resembles, clavus vasculare is painful, even when the foot is unshod. Melanoma, in contrast, is painless. Additionally, targetoid hemosiderotic nevus is a distinctive traumatized acquired melanocytic nevus that may simulate melanoma [274].

Exogenous dermal pigment (a tattoo) may simulate melanoma. Unintended tattoos may be induced by the introduction into the skin of asphalt in a cycling accident, a pencil stab wound introducing graphite, or gunpowder following an explosion. Unusual cases have been described. For example, finely particulate silver contaminating the finger of a jewelry maker produced an enlarging linear blue-black streak, highly suggestive of acral melanoma [275]. The traumatic introduction into the forearm of mercury from a broken thermometer produced, after 2 years, a bluish brown, friable nodule, simulating NM [276].

Prognosis

Primary cutaneous melanoma exhibits a broad spectrum of biologic behaviors in the course of its evolution. From microscopic beginnings in situ, it progressively expands in a circumferential fashion (radially) until the invasive vertical phase of growth supervenes. With penetration of the basement membrane, the tumor can reach lymphatic and blood vessels to facilitate nodal and visceral metastases. When locally invasive (stage I or II), the dominant prognostic variable is Breslow tumor thickness, a more powerful prognostic indicator than Clark levels of invasion [277–279]. Ulceration of the primary tumor is the second most important prognostic factor [277,280,281]. Once regional nodal metastases have occurred (stage III), the dominant variable is the extent of nodal involvement, especially the number of positive nodes [277,278,282]. Ulceration predicts adverse outcome in stage III disease as well [203]. Disseminated disease (stage IV; Fig. 11.16) carries an almost uniformly poor prognosis, with survival measured in months, although remarkable examples of tumor regression with significantly long remissions have been documented [203]. In a study of lymph node melanoma, the relatively favorable long-term survival noted in patients with melanoma of unknown primary suggested that these patients have a prognosis similar to, if not better than, many patients with stage III disease [199].

Clinical staging of melanoma

Accurate assessment begins with careful examination of the entire body surface, including scalp, mucosal surfaces (conjunctival, oral, anogenital areas), and subungual and volar surfaces. The tumor

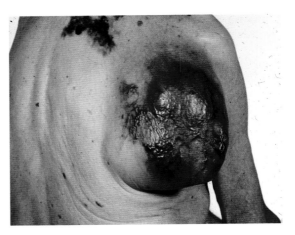

Fig. 11.16 Disseminated melanoma with a large tumor nodule on the back, in proximity to a superficial spreading melanoma.

should be inspected for dimension, color, nodularity, and ulceration. The skin and subcutaneous tissue must be examined for satellite lesions, in-transit metastases, and lymphadenopathy.

In the early 1960s, the TNM (tumor-node-metastasis) staging system of breast cancer was extended to melanoma and employed three stages (Table 11.12). Subsequently, a more complex TNM staging system was proposed by the American Joint Commission on Cancer (AJCC), extending the system for prognosticating breast cancer to melanoma [283]. The AJCC staging system was last modified

Table 11.12 Obsolete system for clinical staging of cutaneous melanoma (1960s)

Stage I: localized disease
    A. Primary lesion alone
    B. Primary lesion and satellites (i.e., within 5 cm of the primary)
    C. Local recurrence within 5 cm of a previously resected primary
    D. In-transit metastases: >5 cm from the primary, but within the primary lymphatic drainage area
Stage II: regional nodal disease
Stage III: disseminated disease (cutaneous, lymphatic, visceral)

Source: MacNeer & Das Gupta [318].

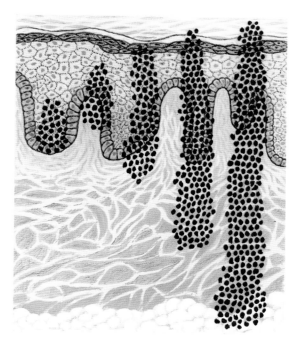

Fig. 11.17 Clark levels of invasion. The upward component is variable and does not contribute to the assignment of level.

in 2001, based on a data base of 17,600 melanoma patients from the United States, Europe, and Australia [277]. The new staging system for cutaneous melanoma identified as the most important prognostic factors Breslow tumor thickness, ulceration, satellite and distant metastasis, the number of involved lymph nodes, and lymph node metastatic mass as "clinically occult" (microscopic) or "clinically apparent" (macroscopic) metastases. Clark levels of invasion are considered only for staging T1 melanomas of tumor thickness less than or equal to 1.0 mm (Tables 11.13 and 11.14).

Depth of tumor invasion

The most widely recognized systems of measurement of depth of invasion are Clark levels of invasion [284] and Breslow tumor thickness [285]. Clark levels of invasion (Fig. 11.17) are defined as follows:

• Level I: All tumor cells are above the basement membrane (in situ)

• Level II: Tumor extends through the basement membrane into the loose papillary dermis but not filling the papillary dermis

• Level III: Tumor fills the papillary dermis and impinges upon but does not invade the reticular dermis

• Level IV: Tumor invades the collagen of the reticular dermis, infiltrating between the thick collagen bundles

• Level V: Tumor extends into the subcutaneous fat Breslow tumor thickness is obtained by the use of an ocular micrometer to measure maximum vertical dimension of the tumor from the top of the granular layer to the deepest point of invasion [286]. When ulcerated, it is measured from the base of the ulcer to the deepest point of invasion.

Although there is a direct correlation between Clark levels of invasion and Breslow tumor thickness, there are also notable incongruities, particularly the wide variation of thicknesses and survival rates for Clark levels III and IV [284,286,287]. Clark levels of invasion better predict thin (T1) melanomas than thicker ones [277]. The use of Clark levels is further hindered by the subjectivity of these determinations [286,288]. Tumor thickness, in contrast, is a continuous variable and relatively more reproducible than Clark levels of invasion. However, level of invasion may be more applicable to exophytic or pedunculated lesions, in which the upward growth component obscures the determination of tumor thickness [288].

Breslow [286] identified three distinct populations of melanoma patients: those whose tumors measured less than 0.76 mm, all of whom did well; those whose tumors measured 0.76 to 1.50 mm thick, whose survival was apparently unaffected by prophylactic lymph node dissection; and those with tumors greater than 1.50 mm in thickness, for whom lymph node dissection appeared to double survival. Subsequently, one group [289] found prognostic breakpoints at 0.85 mm, 1.70 mm, and 3.65 mm, whereas another proposed breakpoints at 1.0 mm, 1.5 mm, 2.75 mm, and 4.0 mm [290]. In 1988, the AJCC system employed 0.75 mm, 1.5 mm, and 4 mm as breakpoints distinguishing thin, intermediate, and thick melanomas. These were accepted widely. In 2001, the revised AJCC staging system defined tumor thickness (T) category

Table 11.13 The TNM classification of melanoma (revised 2001)

Primary Tumor (T)	Thickness	Ulceration
TX	Cannot be assessed (e.g., shave biopsy, regressed tumor)	
T0	No evidence of primary tumor	
Tis	Melanoma in situ	
T1	≤1.0 mm	a: without ulceration and level II/III b: with ulceration or level IV/V
T2	1.01–2.0 mm	a: without ulceration b: with ulceration
T3	2.01–4.0 mm	a: without ulceration b: with ulceration
T4	>4.0 mm	a: without ulceration b: with ulceration

Regional Nodes (N)	Number of Metastatic Nodes	Nodal Metastatic Mass
NX	Cannot be assessed	
N0	No nodal metastasis	
N1	1 node	a: micrometastasis b: macrometastasis
N2	2–3 nodes, or intralymphatic metastasis *without* nodes	a: micrometastasis b: macrometastasis c: satellite or in-transit *without* nodes
N3	≥4 nodes or matted metastatic nodes, or in-transit metastasis or satellite(s) *with* metastatic nodes	

Distant Metastases (M)	Site	Lactate Dehydrogenase
MX	Cannot be assessed	
M0	No distant metastasis	

M1	Distant metastasis
	  To skin, subcutaneous tissues, distant lymph nodes
	  To lung
	  To all other visceral sites
	  To any site
		a: normal
		
		b: normal
		c: normal
		c: elevated

Source: Balch et al. [278].

thresholds in whole integers (1.0 mm, 2.0 mm, and 4.0 mm). Accordingly, the new T classification differentiates among four different subgroups of tumor thickness ($\leq$1.0 mm, >1.0 to 2.0 mm, >2.0 to 4.0 mm, and >4.0 mm) [278] (Table 11.13).

Ulceration

Ulceration of melanoma is defined histopathologically and results when the tumor invades through the overlying epidermis rather than pushing it upward, yielding an absent epidermis overlying the major portion of the tumor [291,292]. Ulceration is easily distinguished from artifactual or traumatic disruption of the epidermis, which is associated with hemorrhage and an eosinophilic fibrin exudation at the site. The interpretation of melanoma ulceration is highly reproducible among pathologists [293,294].

The prognostic relevance of ulceration in primary cutaneous melanoma was first observed by Allen and Spitz [256] and was confirmed in following decades [278]. In 2001, histologic ulceration was introduced as a pivotal parameter in the AJCC staging system [278] (Tables 11.13 and 11.14). For melanomas thicker than 1.0 mm, ulceration strongly predicts survival outcome, whereas for melanomas less than or equal to 1.0 mm (T1), ulceration appears a weaker predictor than Clark level of invasion.

Under the revised staging system, all melanoma patients with stage I, II, or III disease are upstaged when the primary tumor is ulcerated (Table 11.14). It is estimated that 25% of patients are upstaged when ulceration is taken into consideration [295]. The prognostic significance of ulceration in thin (T1) melanomas, however, is controversial [277,280,296,297].

Regression

Depigmented areas deserve particular attention, as they may represent areas of regression. A Wood's lamp aids in their evelution. Because prognosis is most strongly correlated with the maximum depth of tumor invasion, one would suspect that regression may cause underestimation of its original maximum thickness. In "thin" melanomas, regression has been linked to increased risk of metastases [52,298,299]. In a study of 486 melanoma patients with clinical stage I ($\leq$1 mm in maximal thickness), a past history of regression without fibrotic scar formation had no significant effect on survival, but regression in the presence of fibrotic scar tissue adversely affected survival. The 10-year survival was 95% for patients without regression versus 79% for patients with a history of regression [300]. In contrast, some studies have found the prognosis of thin melanomas to be unaffected by regression [301–303], whereas others consider regression a favorable prognostic indicator [165]. In the new AJCC staging classification, regression is not considered a prognostic factor [277,278].

Anatomic site

Reports decades ago had found the BANS region (upper part of back, posterior aspects of arms, posterior and lateral aspects of neck, posterior aspect of scalp) to be of prognostic significance [304]. Subsequently, two multivariate analysis studies confirmed that location of melanoma in the so-called BANS distribution had no prognostic significance, either for intermediate thickness melanomas or for localized melanomas in general [305,306]. In a multivariate analysis of 13,581 patients with stage I or II disease, anatomic site had no prognostic value [277]. Similarly, a multivariate analysis of 1151 patients with stage III disease found anatomic site to have no prognostic value [277]. However, based on a multivariate analysis of 1158 patients with stage IV disease, 1-year survival was greater for metastasis to skin (59%) and lung (57%) than for all other visceral sites (41%) [277]. Thus, based on 1-year survival, the new AJCC staging classification stratified M1 into three groups by site of metastasis:
• M1a: Metastasis to skin, subcutaneous tissues, or *distant* lymph nodes
• M1b: Metastasis to lung
• M1c: Metastasis to all other visceral sites
In addition, elevated serum lactate dehydrogenase (LDH), found to be strongly predictive of poor outcome in metastatic melanoma [307–310], was included in the new AJCC staging. An elevated LDH upstages to M1c for any site of distant metastasis [277].

Table 11.14 AJCC staging groups for cutaneous invasive melanoma (revised 2001)[a]

Stage	Clinical Staging			Pathologic Staging			10-Year Survival, %[b]
	T	N	M	T	N	M	
0	Tis	N0	M0	Tis	N0	M0	–[c]
IA	T1a	N0	M0	T1a	N0	M0	88
IB	T1b	N0	M0	T1b	N0	M0	83
	T2a	N0	M0	T2a	N0	M0	79
IIA	T2b	N0	M0	T2b	N0	M0	64
	T3a	N0	M0	T3a	N0	M0	64
IIB	T3b	N0	M0	T3b	N0	M0	51
	T4a	N0	M0	T4a	N0	M0	54
IIC	T4b	N0	N0	T4b	N0	N0	32
III	any T	N1	M0				–[c]
	any T	N2	M0				–[c]
	any T	N3	M0				–[c]
IIIA				T1-T4a	N1a	M0	63
				T1-T4a	N2a	M0	57
IIIB				T1-T4b	N1a	M0	38
				T1-T4b	N2a	M0	36
				T1-T4a	N1b	M0	48
				T1-T4a	N2b	M0	39
				T1-4a/b	N2c	M0	–[c]
IIIC				T1-T4b	N1b	M0	24
				T1-T4b	N2b	M0	15
				any T	N3	M0	18
IV	any T	any N	M1	any T	any N	M1	6

[a] *Source:* Balch et al. [278].
[b] *Source:* Balch et al. [277].
[c] No data.
M, distant metastasis; N, regional nodal metastasis; T, primary tumor.

Prognosis of stage III disease

The major determinants of outcome for patho-logic stage III melanoma are (1) the number of metastatic lymph nodes; (2) whether the tumor burden is "clinically occult" (microscopic), having been detected by sentinel or elective lymphadenec-tomy, or "clinically apparent" (macroscopic), hav-ing been clinically detected and verified patholog-ically; (3) the presence or absence of ulceration of the primary melanoma; and (4) the presence or ab-sence of satellite or in-transit metastases. Survival rates for patients with microscopic and macroscopic lymph node metastases are significantly different [66,311].

The previous AJCC melanoma staging system relied on the maximum measured dimension of nodal metastases. In the revised AJCC staging sys-tem, the number of metastatic lymph nodes is the primary criterion for defining the N category, as this most strongly correlates with 10-year sur-vival [278]. According to the revised AJCC stag-ing system, regional lymph nodes are classified by the number of metastatic nodes and presence or absence of intralymphatic metastases (in-transit or satellite metastasis). Thus, patients with one metastatic node are categorized as N1, those with two to three metastatic nodes are N2, and those with four or more metastatic nodes are N3. A second

Table 11.15 Palpation of lymph nodes in assessing lymph node metastases: sensitivity and specificity

Reference	Sensitivity, %	Specificity, %
Karakousis et al. [319]	71	74
Cohen et al. [320]	79	91
Goldsmith et al. [321]	83	84
Gumport and Harris [322]	45	94
Fortner et al. [323]	61	93
Guiss & MacDonald [324]	82	93

Table 11.16 Correlation of the number of involved regional lymph nodes with 5-year survival

Reference	Positive Nodes, no. (% survival)		
Balch et al. [325]	1 (57)	2–4 (27)	>4 (10)
Karakousis et al. [319]	1 (41)	2 (30)	>2 (18)
Cohen et al. [320]	1–3 (55)	>3 (26)	
Guiss & MacDonald [324]	1 (40)	>1 (31)	
Milton et al. [76]	1 (47)	>1 (12)	
Fortner et al. [323]	1 (46)	>1 (9)	
Day et al. [326]	1–3 (48)	>3 (17)	
Karakousis et al. [327]	1 (46)	2–3 (32)	>3 (10)
Drepper et al. [328]	1 (47)	2–4 (31)	>4 (20)

determinant, not included in the previous AJCC staging system, is tumor burden, classified as "clinically occult" (microscopic) metastasis or "clinically apparent" (macroscopic) metastasis (Table 11.13).

- N1: Metastasis to 1 lymph node
  N1a: Clinically occult (microscopic) metastasis
  N1b: Clinically apparent (macroscopic) metastasis
- N2: Metastasis to two or three lymph nodes or intralymphatic metastasis *without* nodal metastasis
  N2a: Clinically occult (microscopic) metastasis
  N2b : Clinically apparent (macroscopic) metastasis
  N2c: Satellite or in-transit metastasis
- N3: Metastasis to 4+ nodes; or matted metastatic nodes; or satellite or in-transit metastasis *with* nodal metastasis

In the new classification, satellite metastasis, which formerly modified the T category, is part of the N category and is merged with in-transit metastasis (in categories N2c and N3).

Stage III disease may be clinically apparent or inapparent. Clinical findings may contradict histologic ones. For example, palpable regional lymph nodes (clinically positive) may be histologically negative (false positive). Table 11.15 illustrates the extent to which the clinical assessment of lymph node status may err. The assessment of nodal involvement is ultimately a tissue diagnosis. Dissection with histologic evaluation is the gold standard [312].

Once stage III disease is clinically apparent, risk for distant metastases increases and prognosis worsens (Table 11.14). Whereas tumor thickness is the best prognostic variable for the localized primary melanoma, the number of histologically positive regional lymph nodes is the dominant prognostic variable in stage III disease. Patients with the fewest positive nodes will have the greatest chance of surgical cure. Table 11.16 presents the relationship between the number of involved nodes and survival. The management of melanoma is the subject of Chapter 31.

Conclusion

An appropriately high index of suspicion must be maintained for the early recognition and treatment of melanoma. Even in the most skilled hands, clinical diagnostic accuracy may be a challenge [313] (Table 11.9).

The incidence of melanoma appears to be rising faster than that of any other malignancy, except lung cancer [13]. Most melanomas should be entirely preventable. Risk factors for melanoma are easily identified in children, and sunscreen and other appropriate preventive measures should be instituted early [47,143]. The dysplastic nevus syndrome, the subject of Chapter 10, may serve as a marker for those at greatest risk. Multiple solar lentigines on the upper back and shoulders of adults may be clinical markers of past severe sunburn which, in turn, may identify a population at higher risk for developing cutaneous melanoma [311]. Moreover, since first- and second-degree relatives of melanoma patients have been shown to be at increased risk for melanoma as well as other malignancies, suggesting heritable cancer syndromes, individuals with a family history of melanoma should strictly adhere to recommended screenings for all cancers. With earlier recognition, better public education, and changes in sun exposure habits, the incidence of melanoma should markedly diminish.

References

1 Urteaga O, Pack GT. On the antiquity of melanoma. Cancer 1966;19:607–10.

2 Carswell R. Pathological anatomy: part 9. Melanoma. London: Longman; 1838.

3 Becker SW. Pitfalls in the diagnosis and treatment of melanoma. AMA Arch Dermatol Syphilol 1954;69:11–30.

4 Driver JR, MacVicar DN. Cutaneous melanomas: a clinical study of sixty cases. JAMA 1943;131:413–20.

5 Graadt van Roggen JF, Mooi WJ, Hogendoorn PC. Clear cell sarcoma of tendons and aponeuroses (malignant melanoma of soft parts) and cutaneous melanoma: exploring the histogenetic relationship between these two clinicopathological entities. J Pathol 1998;186:3–7.

6 Safioleas M, Agapitos E, Kontzoglou K, et al. Primary melanoma of the gallbladder: does it exist? Report of a case and review of the literature. World J Gastroenterol 2006;12:4259–61.

7 Kundranda MN, Clark CT, Chaudhry AA, et al. Primary malignant melanoma of the lung: a case report and review of the literature. Clin Lung Cancer 2006;7:279–81.

8 Wong JA, Bell DG. Primary malignant melanoma of the prostate: case report and review of the literature. Can J Urol 2006;13:3053–6.

9 Dargent JL, Lespagnard L, Heenen M, et al. Malignant melanoma occurring in a case of oculocutaneous albinism. Histopathology 1992;21:74–6.

10 Harasymowycz P, Boucher MC, Corriveau C, et al. Choroidal amelanotic melanoma in a patient with oculocutaneous albinism. Can J Ophthalmol 2005; 40: 754–8.

11 Rees J. Melanoma rates remain high in Australia. Nature 2006;443:750.

12 Coory M, Baade P, Aitken J, et al. Trends for in situ and invasive melanoma in Queensland, Australia, 1982–2002. Cancer Causes Control 2006;17:21–7.

13 Jemal A, Siegel R, Ward E, et al. Cancer statistics, 2007. CA Cancer J Clin 2007;57:43–66.

14 Ries LAG, Hankey BF, Miller BA, et al. Cancer statistics review 1973–1988. Bethesda, MD: National Cancer Institute; 1991.

15 Cutler SJ, Scotto J, Devesa SS, et al. Third national cancer survey—an overview of available information. J Natl Cancer Inst 1974;53:1565–75.

16 Horm JW, Asire AJ, Young JLJ, et al. SEER Program. Cancer incidence and mortality in the United States 1973–1981. Bethesda, MD: National Cancer Institute; 1984.

17 Marks R. Epidemiology of melanoma. Clin Exp Dermatol 2000;25:459–63.

18 National Cancer Institute. Surveillance epidemiology and end results (SEER), cancer statistics review 1975–2003. Bethesda, MD: National Cancer Institute.

19 Hall HI, Miller DR, Rogers JD, et al. Update on the incidence and mortality from melanoma in the United States. J Am Acad Dermatol 1999;40:35–42.

20 Mansson-Brahme E, Johansson H, Larsson O, et al. Trends in incidence of cutaneous malignant melanoma in a Swedish population 1976–1994. Acta Oncol 2002;41:138–46.

21 Vinceti M, Bergomi M, Borciani N, et al. Rising melanoma incidence in an Italian community from 1986 to 1997. Melanoma Res 1999;9:97–103.

22 de Vries E, Bray FI, Coebergh JW, et al. Changing epidemiology of malignant cutaneous melanoma in Europe 1953–1997: rising trends in incidence and mortality but recent stabilizations in western Europe and decreases in Scandinavia. Int J Cancer 2003;107:119–26.

23 Australian Institute of Health and Welfare (AIHW) and Australian Associations of Cancer Registries (AACR). Cancer in Australia 1998. Canberra: Australian Institute of Health and Welfare; 1998. p. 42.

24 Jones WO, Harman CR, Ng AK, et al. Incidence of malignant melanoma in Auckland, New Zealand: highest rates in the world. World J Surg 1999;23:732–5.

25 Bliss JM, Ford D, Swerdlow AJ, et al. Risk of cutaneous melanoma associated with pigmentation characteristics and freckling: systematic overview of 10 case-control studies. The International Melanoma Analysis Group (IMAGE). Int J Cancer 1995;62:367–76.

26 Hakulinen T, Andersen A, Malker B, et al. Trends in cancer incidence in the Nordic countries. A collaborative study of the five Nordic Cancer Registries. Acta Pathol Microbiol Immunol Scand Suppl. 1986;288:1–151.

27 Hinds MW, Kolonel LN. Malignant melanoma of the skin in Hawaii, 1960–1977. Cancer 1980;45:811–7.

28 Holman CD, Armstrong BK. Pigmentary traits, ethnic origin, benign nevi, and family history as risk factors for cutaneous malignant melanoma. J Natl Cancer Inst 1984;72:257–66.

29 Dubin N, Moseson M, Pasternack BS. Epidemiology of malignant melanoma: pigmentary traits, ultraviolet radiation, and the identification of high-risk populations. Recent Results Cancer Res 1986;102:56–75.

30 Swerdlow AJ, English J, MacKie RM, et al. Benign melanocytic naevi as a risk factor for malignant melanoma. Br Med J (Clin Res Ed) 1986;292:1555–9.

31 Holly EA, Kelly JW, Shpall SN, et al. Number of melanocytic nevi as a major risk factor for malignant melanoma. J Am Acad Dermatol 1987;17:459–68.

32 Green A, Bain C, McLennan R, et al. Risk factors for cutaneous melanoma in Queensland. Recent Results Cancer Res 1986;102:76–97.

33 Naldi L, Lorenzo Imberti G, Parazzini F, et al. Pigmentary traits, modalities of sun reaction, history of sunburns, and melanocytic nevi as risk factors for cutaneous malignant melanoma in the Italian population: results of a collaborative case-control study. Cancer 2000;88:2703–10.

34 Garbe C, Buttner P, Weiss J, et al. Risk factors for developing cutaneous melanoma and criteria for identifying persons at risk: multicenter case-control study of the Central Malignant Melanoma Registry of the German Dermatological Society. J Invest Dermatol 1994;102:695–9.

35 Green A, MacLennan R, Siskind V. Common acquired naevi and the risk of malignant melanoma. Int J Cancer 1985;35:297–300.

36 Tucker MA, Fraser MC, Goldstein AM, et al. A natural history of melanomas and dysplastic nevi: an atlas of lesions in melanoma-prone families. Cancer 2002;94:3192–209.

37 Rampen FH, van der Meeren HL, Boezeman JB. Frequency of moles as a key to melanoma incidence? J Am Acad Dermatol 1986;15:1200–3.

38 Kopf AW, Gold RS, Rogers GS, et al. Relationship of lumbosacral nevocytic nevi to sun exposure in dysplastic nevus syndrome. Arch Dermatol 1986;122:1003–6.

39 Viola MV, Houghton A, Munster EW. Solar cycles and malignant melanoma. Med Hypotheses 1979;5:153–60.

40 Thompson JF, Scolyer RA, Kefford RF. Cutaneous melanoma. Lancet 2005;365:687–701.

41 Whiteman DC, Milligan A, Welch J, et al. Germline CDKN2A mutations in childhood melanoma. J Natl Cancer Inst 1997;89:1460.

42 Curtin JA, Fridlyand J, Kageshita T, et al. Distinct sets of genetic alterations in melanoma. N Engl J Med 2005;353:2135–47.

43 Elwood JM, Gallagher RP, Worth AJ, et al. Etiological differences between subtypes of cutaneous malignant melanoma: Western Canada Melanoma Study. J Natl Cancer Inst 1987;78:37–44.

44 Gilchrest BA, Eller MS, Geller AC, et al. The pathogenesis of melanoma induced by ultraviolet radiation. N Engl J Med 1999;340:1341–8.

45 Singh AD, Rennie IG, Seregard S, et al. Sunlight exposure and pathogenesis of uveal melanoma. Surv Ophthalmol 2004;49:419–28.

46 Scelo G, Boffetta P, Autier P, et al. Associations between ocular melanoma and other primary cancers: An international population-based study. Int J Cancer 2007;120:152–9.

47 Schwartz RA. Cutaneous malignant melanoma risk assessment. G Ital Dermatol Venereol 2005;140:315–6.

48 Cormier JN, Xing Y, Ding M, et al. Ethnic differences among patients with cutaneous melanoma. Arch Intern Med 2006;166:1907–14.

49 Elwood JM. Could melanoma be caused by fluorescent light? A review of relevant epidemiology. Recent Results Cancer Res 1986;102:127–36.

50 Walter SD, Marrett LD, Shannon HS, et al. The association of cutaneous malignant melanoma and fluorescent light exposure. Am J Epidemiol 1992;135:749–62.

51 Clark WH Jr, From L, Bernardino EA, et al. The histogenesis and biologic behavior of primary human malignant melanomas of the skin. Cancer Res 1969;29:705–27.

52 McGovern VJ. The classification of melanoma and its relationship with prognosis. Pathology 1970;2:85–98.

53 McGovern VJ, Cochran AJ, Van der Esch EP, et al. The classification of malignant melanoma, its histological reporting and registration: a revision of the 1972 Sydney classification. Pathology 1986;18:12–21.

54 Clark WH Jr, Elder DE, Van Horn M. The biologic forms of malignant melanoma. Hum Pathol 1986;17:443–50.

55 Puig S, Castro J, Ventura PJ, et al. Large deletions of chromosome 9p in cutaneous malignant melanoma identify patients with a high risk of developing metastases. Hospital Clinic Malignant Melanoma Group, University of Barcelona. Melanoma Res 2000;10:231–6.

56 Bani MR, Rak J, Adachi D, et al. Multiple features of advanced melanoma recapitulated in tumorigenic

variants of early stage (radial growth phase) human melanoma cell lines: evidence for a dominant phenotype. Cancer Res 1996;56:3075–86.

57 Chin L, Garraway LA, Fisher DE. Malignant melanoma: genetics and therapeutics in the genomic era. Genes Dev 2006;20:2149–82.

58 Gallagher WM, Bergin OE, Rafferty M, et al. Multiple markers for melanoma progression regulated by DNA methylation: insights from transcriptomic studies. Carcinogenesis 2005;26:1856–67.

59 Ackerman AB, David KM. A unifying concept of malignant melanoma: biologic aspects. Hum Pathol 1986;17:438–40.

60 Ishihara K, Saida T, Yamamoto A. Updated statistical data for malignant melanoma in Japan. Int J Clin Oncol 2001;6:109–16.

61 Krementz ET, Sutherland CM, Carter RD, et al. Malignant melanoma in the American Black. Ann Surg 1976;183:533–42.

62 Swetter SM, Boldrick JC, Jung SY, et al. Increasing incidence of lentigo maligna melanoma subtypes: northern California and national trends 1990–2000. J Invest Dermatol 2005;125:685–91.

63 Cox NH, Aitchison TC, MacKie RM. Extrafacial lentigo maligna melanoma: analysis of 71 cases and comparison with lentigo maligna melanoma of the head and neck. Br J Dermatol 1998;139:439–43.

64 Savin JA, Hardie RA. Proprietary depigmenting cream used wrongly for lentigo maligna. Br Med J (Clin Res Ed) 1981;282:1666–7.

65 McKenna JK, Florell SR, Goldman GD, et al. Lentigo maligna/lentigo maligna melanoma: current state of diagnosis and treatment. Dermatol Surg 2006;32:493–504.

66 Balch CM, Soong S, Ross MI, et al. Long-term results of a multi-institutional randomized trial comparing prognostic factors and surgical results for intermediate thickness melanomas (1.0 to 4.0 mm). Intergroup Melanoma Surgical Trial. Ann Surg Oncol 2000;7:87–97.

67 Phillips ME, Margolis RJ, Merot Y, et al. The spectrum of minimal deviation melanoma: a clinicopathologic study of 21 cases. Hum Pathol 1986;17:796–806.

68 Hayashi H, Kawashima T, Hosokawa K, et al. Epidermotropic metastatic malignant melanoma with a pedunculated appearance. Clin Exp Dermatol 2003;28:666–8.

69 Mihm MC Jr, Clark WH Jr, Reed RJ. The clinical diagnosis of malignant melanoma. Semin Oncol 1975;2:105–18.

70 Arrington JH 3rd, Reed RJ, Ichinose H, et al. Plantar lentiginous melanoma: a distinctive variant of human cutaneous malignant melanoma. Am J Surg Pathol 1977;1:131–43.

71 Seiji M, Mihm MC Jr, Sober AJ, et al. Malignant melanoma of the palmar-plantar-subungual-mucosal type: clinical and histopathological features. In: Klaus SN, editor. Pigment cell. Vol. 5. Basel: Karger; 1979. p. 95–104.

72 Phan A, Touzet S, Dalle S, et al. Acral lentiginous melanoma: a clinicoprognostic study of 126 cases. Br J Dermatol 2006;155:561–9.

73 Collins RJ. Melanoma in the Chinese of Hong Kong. Emphasis on volar and subungual sites. Cancer 1984;54:1482–8.

74 Feibleman CE, Stoll H, Maize JC. Melanomas of the palm, sole, and nailbed: a clinicopathologic study. Cancer 1980;46:2492–504.

75 Miura S, Jimbow K. Clinical characteristics of subungual melanomas in Japan: case report and a questionnaire survey of 108 cases. J Dermatol 1985;12:393–402.

76 Milton GW, Shaw HM, McCarthy WH. Occult primary malignant melanoma: factors influencing survival. Br J Surg 1977;64:805–8.

77 Jimbow K, Takahashi H, Miura S, et al. Biological behavior and natural course of acral malignant melanoma. Clinical and histologic features and prognosis of palmoplantar, subungual, and other acral malignant melanomas. Am J Dermatopathol 1984;6 Suppl:43–53.

78 Chang JW, Yeh KY, Wang CH, et al. Malignant melanoma in Taiwan: a prognostic study of 181 cases. Melanoma Res 2004;14:537–41.

79 Fleming ID, Barnawell JR, Burlison PE, et al. Skin cancer in black patients. Cancer 1975;35:600–5.

80 Seiji M, Takematsu H, Hosokawa M, et al. Acral melanoma in Japan. J Invest Dermatol 1983;80 Suppl:56s–60s.

81 Bellows CF, Belafsky P, Fortgang IS, et al. Melanoma in African-Americans: trends in biological behavior and clinical characteristics over two decades. J Surg Oncol 2001;78:10–6.

82 Milton GW, Shaw HM, McCarthy WH. Subungual malignant melanoma: a disease entity separate from other forms of cutaneous melanoma. Australas J Dermatol 1985;26:61–4.

83 Clarkson JH, McAllister RM, Cliff SH, et al. Subungual melanoma in situ: two independent streaks in one nail bed. Br J Plast Surg 2002;55:165–7.

84 de Giorgi V, Stante M, Carelli G, et al. Subungual melanoma: an insidious erythematous nodule on the nail bed. Arch Dermatol 2005;141:398–9.

85 Kato T, Tanita Y, Takematsu H, et al. Pigmented freckles on the sole of acral lentiginous melanoma in situ. J Dermatol 1985;12:263–6.

86 O'Leary JA, Berend KR, Johnson JL, et al. Subungual melanoma. A review of 93 cases with identification of prognostic variables. Clin Orthop Relat Res 2000:206–12.

87 Mikhail GR. Hutchinson's sign. J Dermatol Surg Oncol 1986;12:519–21.

88 Hutchinson J. Melanosis often not black: melanotic whitlow. Br Med J 1886;1:519–21.

89 Baran R, Kechijian P. Hutchinson's sign: a reappraisal. J Am Acad Dermatol 1996;34:87–90.

90 Stalkup JR, Orengo IF, Katta R. Controversies in acral lentiginous melanoma. Dermatol Surg 2002;28:1051–9; discussion 1059.

91 Colver GB, Millard PR, Dawber RP. Atypical malignant melanoma of the nail apparatus. Br J Dermatol 1986;114:389–92.

92 Chang AE, Karnell LH, Menck HR. The National Cancer Data Base report on cutaneous and noncutaneous melanoma: a summary of 84,836 cases from the past decade. The American College of Surgeons Commission on Cancer and the American Cancer Society. Cancer 1998;83:1664–78.

93 Singh AD, Topham A. Incidence of uveal melanoma in the United States: 1973–1997. Ophthalmology 2003;110:956–61.

94 Singh AD, Bergman L, Seregard S. Uveal melanoma: epidemiologic aspects. Ophthalmol Clin North Am 2005;18:75–84, viii.

95 Didolkar MS, Elias EG, Barber NA, et al. Biologic behavior of ocular malignant melanoma and comparison with melanoma of the head and neck. Am J Surg 1980;140:522–6.

96 Layton C, Glasson W. Clinical aspects of conjunctival melanoma. Clin Experiment Ophthalmol 2002;30:72–9.

97 Friedman RJ, Rodriguez-Sains R, Jakobiec F. Ophthalmologic oncology: conjunctival malignant melanoma in association with sporadic dysplastic nevus syndrome. J Dermatol Surg Oncol 1987;13:31–4.

98 Roper JP, Jones T, Common JD. Desmoplastic malignant melanoma masquerading as chalazion. Br J Ophthalmol 1986;70:907–10.

99 Folberg R, McLean IW. Primary acquired melanosis and melanoma of the conjunctiva: terminology, classification, and biologic behavior. Hum Pathol 1986;17:652–4.

100 Jeffrey IJ, Lucas DR, McEwan C, et al. Malignant melanoma of the conjunctiva. Histopathology 1986;10:363–78.

101 Demirci H, Shields CL, Shields JA, et al. Malignant melanoma arising from unusual conjunctival blue nevus. Arch Ophthalmol 2000;118:1581–4.

102 Shields JA, Shields CL, Eagle RC Jr, et al. Conjunctival metastasis as initial sign of disseminated cutaneous melanoma. Ophthalmology 2004;111:1933–4.

103 Wechter ME, Gruber SB, Haefner HK, et al. Vulvar melanoma: a report of 20 cases and review of the literature. J Am Acad Dermatol 2004;50:554–62.

104 Weinstock MA. Malignant melanoma of the vulva and vagina in the United States: patterns of incidence and population-based estimates of survival. Am J Obstet Gynecol 1994;171:1225–30.

105 Orlandini V, Kolb F, Spatz A, et al. [Melanoma of the penis: 6 cases]. Ann Dermatol Venereol 2004;131:541–4.

106 Sanchez-Ortiz R, Huang SF, Tamboli P, et al. Melanoma of the penis, scrotum and male urethra: a 40-year single institution experience. J Urol 2005;173:1958–65.

107 Jorda E, Verdeger JM, Moragon M, et al. Desmoplastic melanoma of the penis. J Am Acad Dermatol 1987;16:619–20.

108 Forrer JA, Sugrue DL. Malignant melanoma of prepuce: case report. Genitourin Med 1986;62:399–401.

109 Das G, Gupta S, Shukla PJ, et al. Anorectal melanoma: a large clinicopathologic study from India. Int Surg 2003;88:21–4.

110 Chute DJ, Cousar JB, Mills SE. Anorectal malignant melanoma: morphologic and immunohistochemical features. Am J Clin Pathol 2006;126:93–100.

111 Cagir B, Whiteford MH, Topham A, et al. Changing epidemiology of anorectal melanoma. Dis Colon Rectum 1999;42:1203–8.

112 Rhodes AR, Wood WC, Sober AJ, et al. Nonepidermal origin of malignant melanoma associated with a giant congenital nevocellular nevus. Plast Reconstr Surg 1981;67:782–90.

113 Cruz MA, Cho ES, Schwartz RA, et al. Congenital neurocutaneous melanosis. Cutis 1997;60:178–81.

114 Swetter SM, Ecker PM, Johnson DL, et al. Primary dermal melanoma: a distinct subtype of melanoma. Arch Dermatol 2004;140:99–103.

115 Ariyanayagam-Baksh SM, Baksh FK, Finkelstein SD, et al. Malignant blue nevus: a case report and molecular analysis. Am J Dermatopathol 2003;25:21–7.

116 Lambert WC, Brodkin RH. Nodal and subcutaneous cellular blue nevi. A pseudometastasizing pseudomelanoma. Arch Dermatol 1984;120:367–70.

117 Dorsey CS, Montgomery H. Blue nevus and its distinction from Mongolian spot and the nevus of Ota. J Invest Dermatol 1954;22:225–36.

118 Bisceglia M, Carosi I, Fania M, et al. [Nevus of Ota. Presentation of a case associated with a cellular blue nevus with suspected malignant degeneration and review of the literature]. Pathologica 1997;89:168–74.

119 Sinha S, Cohen PJ, Schwartz RA. Nevus of Ota. Cutis. In press.

120 Mones JM, Ackerman AB. "Atypical" blue nevus, "malignant" blue nevus, and "metastasizing" blue nevus: a critique in historical perspective of three concepts flawed fatally. Am J Dermatopathol 2004;26:407–30.

121 Magro CM, Crowson AN, Mihm MC. Unusual variants of malignant melanoma. Mod Pathol 2006;19 Suppl 2:S41–70.

122 Bauer J, Curtin JA, Pinkel D, et al. Congenital melanocytic nevi frequently harbor NRAS mutations but no BRAF mutations. J Invest Dermatol 2007;127:179–82.

123 Berg P, Lindelof B. Congenital melanocytic naevi and cutaneous melanoma. Melanoma Res 2003;13:441–5.

124 Krengel S, Hauschild A, Schafer T. Melanoma risk in congenital melanocytic naevi: a systematic review. Br J Dermatol 2006;155:1–8.

125 Makkar HS, Frieden IJ. Congenital melanocytic nevi: an update for the pediatrician. Curr Opin Pediatr 2002;14:397–403.

126 Illig L, Weidner F, Hundeiker M, et al. Congenital nevi less than or equal to 10 cm as precursors to melanoma. 52 cases, a review, and a new conception. Arch Dermatol 1985;121:1274–81.

127 Hale EK, Stein J, Ben-Porat L, et al. Association of melanoma and neurocutaneous melanocytosis with large congenital melanocytic naevi—results from the NYU-LCMN registry. Br J Dermatol 2005;152:512–7.

128 Wiltz H, Kollmer WL, Rauscher GE, et al. Excision of the large congenital melanocytic nevus facilitated by the use of the tissue expander. J Surg Oncol 1988;38:104–7.

129 Gibstein LA, Abramson DL, Bartlett RA, et al. Tissue expansion in children: a retrospective study of complications. Ann Plast Surg 1997;38:358–64.

130 Swerdlow AJ, English JS, Qiao Z. The risk of melanoma in patients with congenital nevi: a cohort study. J Am Acad Dermatol 1995;32:595–9.

131 Sahin S, Levin L, Kopf AW, et al. Risk of melanoma in medium-sized congenital melanocytic nevi: a follow-up study. J Am Acad Dermatol 1998;39:428–33.

132 Abecassis S, Spatz A, Cazeneuve C, et al. [Melanoma within naevus spilus: 5 cases]. Ann Dermatol Venereol 2006;133:323–8.

133 Kopf AW, Bart RS, Hennessey P. Congenital nevocytic nevi and malignant melanomas. J Am Acad Dermatol 1979;1:123–30.

134 Ingordo V, Gentile C, Iannazzone SS, et al. Congenital melanocytic nevus: an epidemiological study in Italy. Dermatology 2007;214:227–30.

135 Schwartz RA, Cohen-Addad N, Lambert MW, et al. Congenital melanocytosis with myelomeningocele and hydrocephalus. Cutis 1986;37:37–9.

136 Huynh PM, Grant-Kels JM, Grin CM. Childhood melanoma: update and treatment. Int J Dermatol 2005;44:715–23.

137 Richardson SK, Tannous ZS, Mihm MC Jr. Congenital and infantile melanoma: review of the literature and report of an uncommon variant, pigment-synthesizing melanoma. J Am Acad Dermatol 2002;47:77–90.

138 Makkar HS, Frieden IJ. Neurocutaneous melanosis. Semin Cutan Med Surg 2004;23:138–44.

139 Bett BJ. Large or multiple congenital melanocytic nevi: occurrence of neurocutaneous melanocytosis in 1008 persons. J Am Acad Dermatol 2006;54:767–77.

140 Marghoob AA, Dusza S, Oliveria S, et al. Number of satellite nevi as a correlate for neurocutaneous melanocytosis in patients with large congenital melanocytic nevi. Arch Dermatol 2004;140:171–5.

141 Yu HS, Tsaur KC, Chien CH, et al. Neurocutaneous melanosis: electron microscopic comparison of the pigmented melanocytic nevi of skin and meningeal melanosis. J Dermatol 1985;12:267–76.

142 Rahimi-Movaghar V, Karimi M. Meningeal melanocytoma of the brain and oculodermal melanocytosis (nevus of Ota): case report and literature review. Surg Neurol 2003;59:200–10.

143 Azfar RS, Schwartz RA, Berwick M. Primary melanoma prevention in children. G Ital Dermatol Venereol 2004;139:267–72.

144 Ceballos PI, Ruiz-Maldonado R, Mihm MC Jr. Melanoma in children. N Engl J Med 1995;332:656–62.

145 Lefkowitz A, Schwartz RA, Janniger CK. Melanoma precursors in children. Cutis 1999;63:321–4.

146 Jafarian F, Powell J, Kokta V, et al. Malignant melanoma in childhood and adolescence: report of 13 cases. J Am Acad Dermatol 2005;3:816–22.

147 Peters MS, Goellner JR. Spitz naevi and malignant melanomas of childhood and adolescence. Histopathology 1986;10:1289–302.

148 Helm KF, Schwartz RA, Janniger CK. Juvenile melanoma (Spitz nevus). Cutis 1996;58:35–9.

149 Top H, Aygit AC, Bas S, et al. Spitzoid melanoma in childhood. Eur J Dermatol 2006;16:276–80.

150 Papadopoulos AJ, Schwartz RA, Sarasin A, et al. The xeroderma pigmentosum variant in a Greek patient. Int J Dermatol 2001;40:442–5.

151 Lambert MW, Lambert WC, Schwartz RA, et al. Colonization of nonmelanocytic cutaneous lesions by dendritic melanocytic cells: a simulant of acral-lentiginous (palmar-plantar-subungual-mucosal) melanoma. J Surg Oncol 1985;28:12–8.

152 Cleaver JE. Cancer in xeroderma pigmentosum and related disorders of DNA repair. Nat Rev Cancer 2005;5:564–73.

153 Chaudru V, Laud K, Avril MF, et al. Melanocortin-1 receptor (MC1R) gene variants and dysplastic nevi modify penetrance of CDKN2A mutations in French melanoma-prone pedigrees. Cancer Epidemiol Biomarkers Prev 2005;14:2384–90.

154 Streutker CJ, McCready D, Jimbow K, et al. Malignant melanoma in a patient with oculocutaneous albinism. J Cutan Med Surg 2000;4:149–52.

155 Luande J, Henschke CI, Mohammed N. The Tanzanian human albino skin. Natural history. Cancer 1985;55:1823–8.

156 Novakovic B, Clark WH Jr, Fears TR, et al. Melanocytic nevi, dysplastic nevi, and malignant melanoma in children from melanoma-prone families. J Am Acad Dermatol 1995;33:631–6.

157 Larson AA, Leachman SA, Eliason MJ, et al. Population-based assessment of non-melanoma cancer risk in relatives of cutaneous melanoma probands. J Invest Dermatol 2007;127:183–8.

158 Puig S, Malvehy J, Badenas C, et al. Role of the CDKN2A locus in patients with multiple primary melanomas. J Clin Oncol 2005;23:3043–51.

159 Marian C, Scope A, Laud K, et al. Search for germline alterations in CDKN2A/ARF and CDK4 of 42 Jewish melanoma families with or without neural system tumours. Br J Cancer 2005;92:2278–85.

160 Goldstein AM, Chan M, Harland M, et al. High-risk melanoma susceptibility genes and pancreatic cancer, neural system tumors, and uveal melanoma across GenoMEL. Cancer Res 2006;66:9818–28.

161 Clark WHJ. A classification of malignant melanoma in man correlated with histogenesis and biologic behavior In: Montagna W, Hu F, editors. Advances in biology of skin. London: Pergamon Press; 1967. p. 621–47. (The pigment system; vol 8).

162 Kuehnl-Petzoldt C, Berger H, Wiebelt H. Verrucous-keratotic variations of malignant melanoma: a clinicopathological study. Am J Dermatopathol 1982;4:403–10.

163 Blessing K, Evans AT, al-Nafussi A. Verrucous naevoid and keratotic malignant melanoma: a clinico-pathological study of 20 cases. Histopathology 1993;23:453–8.

164 Kolm I, Di Stefani A, Hofmann-Wellenhof R, et al. Dermoscopy patterns of halo nevi. Arch Dermatol 2006;142:1627–32.

165 Bystryn JC, Rigel D, Friedman RJ, et al. Prognostic significance of hypopigmentation in malignant melanoma. Arch Dermatol 1987;123:1053–5.

166 Giuliano AE, Cochran AJ, Morton DL. Melanoma from unknown primary site and amelanotic melanoma. Semin Oncol 1982;9:442–7.

167 Pizzichetta MA, Canzonieri V, Massarut S, et al. Pigmented mammary Paget's disease mimicking melanoma. Melanoma Res 2004;14:S13–5.

168 Liu W, Dowling JP, Murray WK, et al. Rate of growth in melanomas: characteristics and associations of rapidly growing melanomas. Arch Dermatol 2006;142:1551–8.

169 Koch SE, Lange JR. Amelanotic melanoma: the great masquerader. J Am Acad Dermatol 2000;42:731–4.

170 Stringa O, Valdez R, Beguerie JR, et al. Primary amelanotic melanoma of the esophagus. Int J Dermatol 2006;45:1207–10.

171 Borkovic SP, Schwartz RA. Amelanotic lentigo maligna melanoma manifesting as a dermatitislike plaque. Arch Dermatol 1983;119:423–5.

172 Soucek P, Cihelkova I. Primary treatment of choroidal amelanotic melanoma with photodynamic therapy [comment]. Clin Experiment Ophthalmol 2006;34:721; author reply 722.

173 Bongiorno MR, Lodato G, Affronti A, et al. Amelanotic conjunctival melanoma. Cutis 2006;77:377–81.

174 Huvos AG, Shah JP, Goldsmith HS. A clinicopathologic study of amelanotic melanoma. Surg Gynecol Obstet 1972;135:917–20.

175 Krebs JA, Roenigk HH Jr, Deodhar SD, et al. Halo nevus: competent surveillance of potential melanoma? Cleve Clin Q 1976;43:11–5.

176 Ferrari A, Bono A, Baldi M, et al. Does melanoma behave differently in younger children than in adults? A retrospective study of 33 cases of childhood melanoma from a single institution. Pediatrics 2005;115:649–54.

177 Goldberg DJ. Amelanotic melanoma presenting as Bowen's disease. J Dermatol Surg Oncol 1983;9:902–4.

178 Allan SJ, Dicker AJ, Tidman MJ, et al. Amelanotic lentigo maligna and amelanotic lentigo maligna melanoma: a report of three cases mimicking intraepidermal squamous carcinoma. J Eur Acad Dermatol Venereol 1998;11:78–81.

179 Pechman KJ, Bailin P. Recurrent amelanotic lentigo maligna melanoma: a case report. Cleve Clin Q 1983;50:173–5.

180 Rosen T. Acral lentiginous melanoma misdiagnosed as verruca plantaris: a case report. Dermatol Online J 2006;12:3.

181 Chun JK, Singer E, Kong A, et al. Desmoplastic amelanotic melanoma in an irradiated burn scar. Dermatol Surg 2006;32:161–4.

182 Harrington P, O'Kelly A, Trail IA, et al. Amelanotic subungual melanoma mimicking pyogenic granuloma in the hand. J R Coll Surg Edinb 2002;47:638–40.

183 Lemont H, Brady J. Amelanotic melanoma masquerading as an ingrown toenail. J Am Podiatr Med Assoc 2002;92:306–7.

184 Aragona F, Maio G, Piazza R, et al. Primary malignant melanoma of the female urethra: a case report. Int Urol Nephrol 1995;27:107–11.

185 Amenssag L, el Idrissi F, Erchidi I, et al. [Primary malignant melanoma of the cervix]. Presse Med 2002;31:976–8.

186 Haddad F, Nadir S, Benkhaldoun L, et al. [Primary anorectal melanoma]. Presse Med 2005;34:85–8.

187 Dube P, Elias D, Bonvalot S, et al. [Primary anorectal melanoma. Apropos of 19 cases]. J Chir (Paris) 1997;134:3–8.

188 Johnson IJ, Warfield AT, Smallman LA, et al. Primary malignant melanoma of the pharynx. J Laryngol Otol 1994;108:275–7.

189 Dong XD, DeMatos P, Prieto VG, et al. Melanoma of the gallbladder: a review of cases seen at Duke University Medical Center. Cancer 1999;85:32–9.

190 DeMatos P, Tyler DS, Seigler HF. Malignant melanoma of the mucous membranes: a review of 119 cases. Ann Surg Oncol 1998;5:733–42.

191 Jahnke A, Makovitzky J, Briese V. Primary melanoma of the female genital system: a report of 10 cases and review of the literature. Anticancer Res 2005;25:1567–74.

192 Boscaino A, D'Antonio A, Orabona P, et al. Primary malignant melanoma of the ovary. Pathologica 1995;87:685–8.

193 Piris A, Rosai J. Pigmented lesions in unusual anatomic sites. Semin Diagn Pathol 2003;20:249–59.

194 Titus-Ernstoff L, Perry AE, Spencer SK, et al. Multiple primary melanoma: two-year results from a population-based study. Arch Dermatol 2006;142:433–8.

195 Doubrovsky A, Menzies SW. Enhanced survival in patients with multiple primary melanoma. Arch Dermatol 2003;139:1013–8.

196 Stratigos AJ, Yang G, Dimisianos R, et al. Germline CDKN2A mutations among Greek patients with early-onset and multiple primary cutaneous melanoma. J Invest Dermatol 2006;126:399–401.

197 Millikan RC, Hummer A, Begg C, et al. Polymorphisms in nucleotide excision repair genes and risk of multiple primary melanoma: the Genes Environment and Melanoma Study. Carcinogenesis 2006;27:610–8.

198 Katz KA, Jonasch E, Hodi FS, et al. Melanoma of unknown primary: experience at Massachusetts General Hospital and Dana-Farber Cancer Institute. Melanoma Res 2005;15:77–82.

199 Cormier JN, Xing Y, Feng L, et al. Metastatic melanoma to lymph nodes in patients with unknown primary sites. Cancer 2006;106:2012–20.

200 Schwartz RA, Kist JM, Thomas I, et al. Ocular melanoma metastatic to skin: the value of HMB-45 staining. Dermatol Surg 2004;30:942–4.

201 Baab GH, McBride CM. Malignant melanoma: the patient with an unknown site of primary origin. Arch Surg 1975;110:896–900.

202 Blessing K, McLaren KM. Histological regression in primary cutaneous melanoma: recognition, prevalence and significance. Histopathology 1992;20:315–22.

203 High WA, Stewart D, Wilbers CR, et al. Completely regressed primary cutaneous malignant melanoma with nodal and/or visceral metastases: a report of 5 cases and assessment of the literature and diagnostic criteria. J Am Acad Dermatol 2005;53:89–100.

204 Tsao H, Cosimi AB, Sober AJ. Ultra-late recurrence (15 years or longer) of cutaneous melanoma. Cancer 1997;79:2361–70.

205 Raderman D, Giler S, Rothem A, et al. Late metastases (beyond ten years) of cutaneous malignant melanoma. Literature review and case report. J Am Acad Dermatol 1986;15:374–8.

206 Schmid-Wendtner MH, Baumert J, Schmidt M, et al. Late metastases of cutaneous melanoma: an analysis of 31 patients. J Am Acad Dermatol 2000;43:605–9.

207 Bulkley GB, Cohen MH, Banks PM, et al. Long-term spontaneous regression of malignant melanoma with visceral metastases. Report of a case with immunologic profile. Cancer 1975;36:485–94.

208 Hayes AJ, Clark MA, Harries M, et al. Management of in-transit metastases from cutaneous malignant melanoma. Br J Surg 2004;91:673–82.

209 Kang JC, Wanek LA, Essner R, et al. Sentinel lymphadenectomy does not increase the incidence of in-transit metastases in primary melanoma. J Clin Oncol 2005;23:4764–70.

210 Bohm M, Schiller M, Nashan D, et al. Diffuse melanosis arising from metastatic melanoma: pathogenetic function of elevated melanocyte peptide growth factors. J Am Acad Dermatol 2001;44:747–54.

211 Alexander A, Harris RM, Grossman D, et al. Vulvar melanoma: diffuse melanosis and metastasis to the placenta. J Am Acad Dermatol 2004;50:293–8.

212 Saghari S, Bakshandeh H, Kerdel F. Sudden onset of melanuria in a patient with metastatic melanoma and toxic epidermal necrolysis. Int J Dermatol 2002;41:116–8.

213 Konrad K, Wolff K. Pathogenesis of diffuse melanosis secondary to malignant melanoma. Br J Dermatol 1974;91:635–55.

214 Eide J. Pathogenesis of generalized melanosis with melanuria and melanoptysis secondary to malignant melanoma. Histopathology 1981;5:285–94.

215 Fitzpatrick TB, Montgomery H, Lerner AB. Pathogenesis of generalized dermal pigmentation secondary to malignant melanoma and melanuria. J Invest Dermatol 1954;22:163–72.

216 Kittler H, Pehamberger H, Wolff K, et al. Diagnostic accuracy of dermoscopy. Lancet Oncol 2002;3:159–65.

217 Ascierto PA, Palmieri G, Celentano E, et al. Sensitivity and specificity of epiluminescence microscopy: evaluation on a sample of 2731 excised cutaneous pigmented lesions. The Melanoma Cooperative Study. Br J Dermatol 2000;142:893–8.

218 Nachbar F, Stolz W, Merkle T, et al. The ABCD rule of dermatoscopy. High prospective value in the diagnosis of doubtful melanocytic skin lesions. J Am Acad Dermatol 1994;30:551–9.

219 Menzies S, Crotty K, Ingvar C, et al. An atlas of surface microscopy of pigmented skin lesions. New York: McGraw-Hill; 1996.

220 Argenziano G, Fabbrocini G, Carli P, et al. Epiluminescence microscopy for the diagnosis of doubtful melanocytic skin lesions. Comparison of the ABCD rule of dermatoscopy and a new 7-point checklist based on pattern analysis. Arch Dermatol 1998;134:1563–70.

221 Blum A, Rassner G, Garbe C. Modified ABC-point list of dermoscopy: A simplified and highly accurate dermoscopic algorithm for the diagnosis of cutaneous melanocytic lesions. J Am Acad Dermatol 2003;48:672–8.

222 Henning JS, Dusza SW, Wang SQ, et al. The CASH (color, architecture, symmetry, and homogeneity) algorithm for dermoscopy. J Am Acad Dermatol 2007;56:45–52.

223 Weatherhead SC, Haniffa M, Lawrence CM. Melanomas arising from naevi and de novo melanomas—does origin matter? Br J Dermatol 2007;156:72–6.

224 Duray PH, Ernstoff MS. Dysplastic nevus in histologic contiguity with acquired nonfamilial melanoma. Clinicopathologic experience in a 100-bed hospital. Arch Dermatol 1987;123:80–4.

225 Tarlow MM, Nemlick AS, Rothenberg J, et al. Pseudoglandular melanoma: a rare melanoma variant. J Cutan Pathol. In press.

226 Breier F, Feldmann R, Fellenz C, et al. Primary invasive signet-ring cell melanoma. J Cutan Pathol 1999;26:533–6.

227 Penneys NS. Microinvasive lentigo maligna melanoma. J Am Acad Dermatol 1987;17:675–80.

228 Schwartz RA. Histopathologic aspects of cutaneous metastatic disease. J Am Acad Dermatol 1995;33:649–57.

229 Lambert WC, Lambert MW, Mesa ML, et al. Melanoacanthoma and related disorders. Simulants of acral-lentiginous (P-P-S-M) melanoma. Int J Dermatol 1987;26:508–10.

230 Mark GJ, Mihm MC, Liteplo MG, et al. Congenital melanocytic nevi of the small and garment type. Clinical, histologic, and ultrastructural studies. Hum Pathol 1973;4:395–418.

231 Ellis DL, Wheeland RG, Solomon H. Estrogen and progesterone receptors in melanocytic lesions. Occurrence in patients with dysplastic nevus syndrome. Arch Dermatol 1985;121:1282–5.

232 Podnos YD, Jimenez JC, Zainabadi K, et al. Minimal deviation melanoma. Cancer Treat Rev 2002;28:219–21.

233 Reed RJ. Minimal deviation melanoma. Borderline and intermediate melanocytic neoplasia. Clin Lab Med 2000;20:745–58.

234 Nychay SG, Thomas I, Schwartz RA, et al. Metastatic minimal deviation melanoma. J Cutan Pathol 1991;18:382.

235 Reed RJ, Leonard DD. Neurotropic melanoma. A variant of desmoplastic melanoma. Am J Surg Pathol 1979;3:301–11.

236 Posther KE, Selim MA, Mosca PJ, et al. Histopathologic characteristics, recurrence patterns, and survival of 129 patients with desmoplastic melanoma. Ann Surg Oncol 2006;13:728–39.

237 Kay PA, Pinheiro AD, Lohse CM, et al. Desmoplastic melanoma of the head and neck: histopathologic and immunohistochemical study of 28 cases. Int J Surg Pathol 2004;12:17–24.

238 Hui JI, Linden KG, Barr RJ. Desmoplastic malignant melanoma of the lip: a report of 6 cases and review of the literature. J Am Acad Dermatol 2002;47:863–8.

239 Quinn MJ, Crotty KA, Thompson JF, et al. Desmoplastic and desmoplastic neurotropic melanoma: experience with 280 patients. Cancer 1998;83:1128–35.

240 Kao GF, Helwig EB, Graham JH. Balloon cell malignant melanoma of the skin. A clinicopathologic study of 34 cases with histochemical, immunohistochemical, and ultrastructural observations. Cancer 1992;69:2942–52.

241 Kato T, Demitsu T, Tomita Y, et al. New primary malignant melanoma, epidermotropism and Indian-file arrangement of metastatic tumor cells in a case with intransit metastases of acral type of malignant melanoma. Dermatologica 1986;173:95–100.

242 Kornberg R, Ackerman AB. Pseudomelanoma: recurrent melanocytic nevus following partial surgical removal. Arch Dermatol 1975;111:1588–90.

243 Ronnen M, Sokol MS, Huszar M, et al. Pseudomelanoma following treatment with surgical excision and intralesional triamcinolone acetonide to prevent keloid formation. Int J Dermatol 1986;25:533–4.

244 Grunwald MH, Gat A, Amichai B. Pseudomelanoma after Solcoderm treatment. Melanoma Res 2006;16:459–60.

245 Dwyer CM, Kerr RE, Knight SL, et al. Pseudomelanoma after dermabrasion. J Am Acad Dermatol 1993;28:263–4.

246 Lee HW, Ahn SJ, Lee MW, et al. Pseudomelanoma following laser therapy. J Eur Acad Dermatol Venereol 2006;20:342–4.

247 Thomas I, Kihiczak NI, Rothenberg J, et al. Melanoma within the seborrheic keratosis. Dermatol Surg 2004;30:559–61.

248 MacKie RM, English J, Aitchison TC, et al. The number and distribution of benign pigmented moles (melanocytic naevi) in a healthy British population. Br J Dermatol 1985;113:167–74.

249 Coombs BD, Sharples KJ, Cooke KR, et al. Variation and covariates of the number of benign nevi in adolescents. Am J Epidemiol 1992;136:344–55.

250 Valiukeviciene S, Miseviciene I, Gollnick H. The prevalence of common acquired melanocytic nevi and the relationship with skin type characteristics and sun exposure among children in Lithuania. Arch Dermatol 2005;141:579–86.

251 Brodell RT, Helms SE. The changing mole. Additional warning signs of malignant melanoma. Postgrad Med 1998;104:145–8.

252 Friedman RJ, Rigel DS, Kopf AW. Early detection of malignant melanoma: the role of physician examination and self-examination of the skin. CA Cancer J Clin 1985;35:130–51.

253 Benelli C, Roscetti E, Dal Pozzo V. Reproducibility of the clinical criteria (ABCDE rule) and dermatoscopic features (7FFM) for the diagnosis of malignant melanoma. Eur J Dermatol 2001;11:234–9.

254 Strayer SM, Reynolds PL. Diagnosing skin malignancy: assessment of predictive clinical criteria and risk factors. J Fam Pract 2003;52:210–8.

255 Spitz S. Melanoma of childhood. Am J Pathol 1948;24:591–609.

256 Allen AC, Spitz S. Malignant melanoma; a clinicopathological analysis of the criteria for diagnosis and prognosis. Cancer 1953;6:1–45.

257 Okun MR. Melanoma resembling spindle and epithelioid cell nevus. Arch Dermatol 1979;115:1416–20.

258 Moretti S, Spallanzani A, Pinzi C, et al. Fibrosis in regressing melanoma versus nonfibrosis in halo nevus upon melanocyte disappearance: could it be related to a different cytokine microenvironment? J Cutan Pathol 2007;34:301–8.

259 Schwartz RA, Hill WE, Hansen RC, et al. Verrucous malignant melanoma. J Dermatol Surg Oncol 1980;6:719–24.

260 Fitzpatrick TB, Gilchrest BA. Dimple sign to differentiate benign from malignant pigmented cutaneous lesions. N Engl J Med 1977;296:1518.

261 Lambert WC, Wiener BD, Schwartz RA, et al. The giant apocrine hidrocystoma. J Surg Oncol 1984;27:146–51.

262 Bickley LK, Goldberg DJ, Imaeda S, et al. Treatment of multiple apocrine hidrocystomas with the carbon dioxide (CO_2) laser. J Dermatol Surg Oncol 1989;15:599–602.

263 Schwartz RA, Hansen RC, Maize JC. The blue-gray cystic basal cell epithelioma. J Am Acad Dermatol 1980;2:155–60.

264 Kihiczak GG, Centurion SA, Schwartz RA, et al. Giant cutaneous melanoacanthoma. Int J Dermatol 2004;43:936–7.

265 Goldman L, Gibson SH, Richfield DF. Thrombotic angiokeratoma circumscriptum simulating melanoma. Arch Dermatol 1981;117:138–9.

266 Schwartz RA. Kaposi's sarcoma: an update. J Surg Oncol 2004;87:146–51.

267 Lin RL, Janniger CK. Pyogenic granuloma. Cutis 2004;74:229–33.

268 Mooney MA, Janniger CK. Pyogenic granuloma. Cutis 1995;55:133–6.

269 McBurney EI, Herron CB. Melanoma mimicking plantar wart. J Am Acad Dermatol 1979;1:144–6.

270 Schwartz RA, Sidor MI, Micali G, Lin RI. Hemangiomas: a challenge in pediatric dermatology. J Eur Acad Dermatol Venereol. In press.

271 Lin RL, Schwartz RA. Hemangiomas of infancy—a clinical review. Acta Dermatovenerol Croat 2006; 14:109–16.

272 Patterson RH, Helwig EB. Subungual malignant melanoma: a clinical-pathologic study. Cancer 1980;46:2074–87.

273 Andre J, Lateur N. Pigmented nail disorders. Dermatol Clin 2006;24:329–39.

274 Tomasini C, Broganelli P, Pippione M. Targetoid hemosiderotic nevus. A trauma-induced simulator of malignant melanoma. Dermatology 2005;210:200–5.

275 McMahon JT, Bergfeld WF. Metallic cutaneous contaminant mimicking malignant melanoma. Cleve Clin Q 1983;50:177–81.

276 Kadykow M. [Mercury-induced granuloma simulating malignant melanoma]. Przeglad Dermatologiczny 1986;73:147–51.

277 Balch CM, Soong SJ, Gershenwald JE, et al. Prognostic factors analysis of 17,600 melanoma patients: validation of the American Joint Committee on Cancer melanoma staging system. J Clin Oncol 2001;19:3622–34.

278 Balch CM, Buzaid AC, Soong SJ, et al. Final version of the American Joint Committee on Cancer staging system for cutaneous melanoma. J Clin Oncol 2001;19:3635–48.

279 Owen SA, Sanders LL, Edwards LJ, et al. Identification of higher risk thin melanomas should be based on Breslow depth not Clark level IV. Cancer 2001;91:983–91.

280 Eigentler TK, Buettner PG, Leiter U, et al. Impact of ulceration in stages I to III cutaneous melanoma as staged by the American Joint Committee on Cancer Staging System: an analysis of the German Central Malignant Melanoma Registry. J Clin Oncol 2004;22:4376–83.

281 Buttner P, Garbe C, Bertz J, et al. Primary cutaneous melanoma. Optimized cutoff points of tumor thickness and importance of Clark's level for prognostic classification. Cancer 1995;75:2499–506.

282 Drepper H, Biess B, Hofherr B, et al. The prognosis of patients with stage III melanoma. Prospective long-term study of 286 patients of the Fachklinik Hornheide. Cancer 1993;71:1239–46.

283 Beahrs OH, Myers MH. Manual for staging of cancer. Philadephia: JB Lippincott; 1983.

284 Clark WH Jr, Ainsworth AM, Bernardino EA, et al. The developmental biology of primary human malignant melanomas. Semin Oncol 1975;2:83–103.

285 Breslow A. Thickness, cross-sectional areas and depth of invasion in the prognosis of cutaneous melanoma. Ann Surg 1970;172:902–8.

286 Breslow A. Tumor thickness, level of invasion and node dissection in stage I cutaneous melanoma. Ann Surg 1975;182:572–5.

287 Wanebo HJ, Woodruff J, Fortner JG. Malignant melanoma of the extremities: a clinicopathologic study using levels of invasion (microstage). Cancer 1975;35:666–76.

288 Prade M, Sancho-Garnier H, Cesarini JP, et al. Difficulties encountered in the application of Clark classification and the Breslow thickness measurement in cutaneous malignant melanoma. Int J Cancer 1980;26:159–63.

289 Day CL Jr, Lew RA, Mihm MC Jr, et al. The natural break points for primary-tumor thickness in clinical stage I melanoma. N Engl J Med 1981;305: 1155.

290 Kuehnl-Petzold C, Wiebelt H, Berger H, et al. A proposal for staging malignant melanoma. Arch Dermatol Res 1983;275:255–6.

291 Balch CM, Wilkerson JA, Murad TM, et al. The prognostic significance of ulceration of cutaneous melanoma. Cancer 1980;45:3012–7.

292 Balch CM, Mihm MC. Reply to the article "The AJCC staging proposal for cutaneous melanoma: comments by the EORTC Melanoma Group," by DJ Ruiter et al. (Ann Oncol 2001;12:9–11). American Joint Committee on Cancer. Ann Oncol 2002;13:175–6.

293 Lock-Andersen J, Hou-Jensen K, Hansen JP, et al. Observer variation in histological classification of

cutaneous malignant melanoma. Scand J Plast Reconstr Surg Hand Surg 1995;29:141–8.

294 Corona R, Mele A, Amini M, et al. Interobserver variability on the histopathologic diagnosis of cutaneous melanoma and other pigmented skin lesions. J Clin Oncol 1996;14:1218–23.

295 Spatz A, Cook MG, Elder DE, et al. Interobserver reproducibility of ulceration assessment in primary cutaneous melanomas. Eur J Cancer 2003;39:1861–5.

296 McKinnon JG, Yu XQ, McCarthy WH, et al. Prognosis for patients with thin cutaneous melanoma: long-term survival data from New South Wales Central Cancer Registry and the Sydney Melanoma Unit. Cancer 2003;98:1223–31.

297 McCarthy WH, Shaw HM, McCarthy SW, et al. Cutaneous melanomas that defy conventional prognostic indicators. Semin Oncol 1996;23:709–13.

298 Trau H, Rigel DS, Harris MN, et al. Metastases of thin melanomas. Cancer 1983;51:553–6.

299 Naruns PL, Nizze JA, Cochran AJ, et al. Recurrence potential of thin primary melanomas. Cancer 1986;57:545–8.

300 Sondergaard K, Hou-Jensen K. Partial regression in thin primary cutaneous malignant melanomas clinical stage I. A study of 486 cases. Virchows Arch A Pathol Anat Histopathol 1985;408:241–7.

301 Wanebo HJ, Cooper PH, Hagar RW. Thin (less than or equal to 1 mm) melanomas of the extremities are biologically favorable lesions not influenced by regression. Ann Surg 1985;201:499–504.

302 Kelly JW, Sagebiel RW, Blois MS. Regression in malignant melanoma. A histologic feature without independent prognostic significance. Cancer 1985;56:2287–91.

303 Leiter U, Buettner PG, Eigentler TK, et al. Prognostic factors of thin cutaneous melanoma: an analysis of the central malignant melanoma registry of the German Dermatological Society. J Clin Oncol 2004;22:3660–7.

304 Day CL Jr, Mihm MC Jr, Sober AJ, et al. Prognostic factors for melanoma patients with lesions 0.76–1.69 mm in thickness. An appraisal of "thin" level IV lesions. Ann Surg 1982;195:30–4.

305 Cascinelli N, Vaglini M, Bufalino R, et al. BANS. A cutaneous region with no prognostic significance in patients with melanoma. Cancer 1986;57:441–4.

306 Rogers GS, Kopf AW, Rigel DS, et al. Influence of anatomic location on prognosis of malignant melanoma: attempt to verify the BANS model. J Am Acad Dermatol 1986;15:231–7.

307 Franzke A, Probst-Kepper M, Buer J, et al. Elevated pretreatment serum levels of soluble vascular cell adhesion molecule 1 and lactate dehydrogenase as predictors of survival in cutaneous metastatic malignant melanoma. Br J Cancer 1998;78:40–5.

308 Sirott MN, Bajorin DF, Wong GY, et al. Prognostic factors in patients with metastatic malignant melanoma. A multivariate analysis. Cancer 1993;72:3091–8.

309 Deichmann M, Benner A, Bock M, et al. S100-Beta, melanoma-inhibiting activity, and lactate dehydrogenase discriminate progressive from nonprogressive American Joint Committee on Cancer stage IV melanoma. J Clin Oncol 1999;17:1891–6.

310 Eton O, Legha SS, Moon TE, et al. Prognostic factors for survival of patients treated systemically for disseminated melanoma. J Clin Oncol 1998;16:1103–11.

311 Derancourt C, Bourdon-Lanoy E, Grob JJ, et al. Multiple large solar lentigos on the upper back as clinical markers of past severe sunburn: a case-control study. Dermatology 2007;214:25–31.

312 Juttner FM, Smolle J, Popper H, et al. Pitfalls in the diagnosis of pulmonary metastases in malignant melanoma. Dermatologica 1986;172:113–5.

313 Koh HK, Sober AJ, Fitzpatrick TB. Late recurrence (beyond ten years) of cutaneous malignant melanoma. Report of two cases and a review of the literature. JAMA 1984;251:1859–62.

314 McMullan FH, Hubener L. Malignant melanoma: a statistical review of clinical and histological diagnosis. Arch Dermatol 1956;74:618–9.

315 Swerdlow M. Nevi; a problem of misdiagnosis. Am J Clin Pathol 1952;22:1054–60.

316 Kopf AW, Mintzis M, Bart RS. Diagnostic accuracy in malignant melanoma. Arch Dermatol 1975;111:1291–2.

317 Bono A, Tolomio E, Trincone S, et al. Micro-melanoma detection: a clinical study on 206 consecutive cases of pigmented skin lesions with a diameter < or = 3 mm. Br J Dermatol 2006;155:570–3.

318 MacNeer G, Das Gupta T. Prognosis in malignant melanoma. Surgery 1964;56:512–8.

319 Karakousis CP, Seddiq MK, Moore R. Prognostic value of lymph node dissection in malignant melanoma. Arch Surg 1980;115:719–22.

320 Cohen MH, Ketcham AS, Felix EL, et al. Prognostic factors in patients undergoing lymphadenectomy for malignant melanoma. Ann Surg 1977;186:635–42.

321 Goldsmith HS, Shah JP, Kim DH. Prognostic significance of lymph node dissection in the treatment of malignant melanoma. Cancer 1970;26:606–9.

322 Gumport SL, Harris MN. Results of regional lymph node dissection for melanoma. Ann Surg 1974;179:105–8.

323 Fortner JG, Dasgupta T, McNeer G. Primary malignant melanoma on the trunk: an analysis of 194 cases. Ann Surg 1965;161:161–9.

324 Guiss LW, MacDonald I. The role of radical regional lymphadenectomy in treatment of melanoma. Am J Surg 1962;104:135–42.

325 Balch CM, Soong SJ, Murad TM, et al. A multifactorial analysis of melanoma: III. prognostic factors in melanoma patients with lymph node metastases (stage II). Ann Surg 1981;193:377–88.

326 Day CL Jr, Sober AJ, Lew RA, et al. Malignant melanoma patients with positive nodes and relatively good prognoses: microstaging retains prognostic significance in clinical stage I melanoma patients with metastases to regional nodes. Cancer 1981;47:955–62.

327 Karakousis CP, Goumas W, Rao U, et al. Axillary node dissection in malignant melanoma. Am J Surg 1991;162:202–7.

328 Drepper H, Kohler CO, Bastian B, et al. Benefit of elective lymph node dissection in subgroups of melanoma patients. Results of a multicenter study of 3616 patients. Cancer 1993;72:741–9.

CHAPTER 12

Dermoscopy for skin cancer

Giuseppe Micali, Francesco Lacarrubba, Beatrice Nardone,
and Robert A. Schwartz

Dermoscopy, also known as dermatoscopy, epiluminescence microscopy, surface microscopy, and incident light microscopy, is an in vivo noninvasive technique for the evaluation of pigmented lesions of the skin and accessible mucosa. In the last decades, studies have shown dermoscopy to be a method for improving accuracy in the diagnosis of skin cancer, especially melanoma. If performed by an expert, it significantly improves sensitivity and specificity, compared with clinical observation without it, of virtually all pigmented lesions, sometimes avoiding the need for biopsy or excision [1–5].

History

In 1951, Leon Goldman [6], the "father of dermatologic laser surgery," was the first to employ skin surface microscopy as a diagnostic procedure to evaluate pigmented skin lesions. In 1971, MacKie [7] used surface microscopy in the differential diagnosis of benign and malignant lesions. In 1980, Fritsch [8] first described the "pigment network" of melanocytic lesions. Since the late 1980s, this technique has developed in Europe, mainly through the contributions of Austrian, German, and Italian study groups [2]. In 1987, Pehamberger [9] proposed the "pattern analysis" model for the diagnosis of pigmented cutaneous lesions, using the term *epiluminescence microscopy*. In 1989, a standardized terminology of dermoscopic features was established by the first Consensus Meeting held in Hamburg [10]. In 2000, a consensus meeting held via the Internet focused on the reproducibility and validity of dermoscopic diagnostic features and algorithms [11]. Today, dermoscopy is routinely used by many dermatologists worldwide and is gaining in popularity [2,5].

Technique

Dermoscopy uses optic magnification to visualize morphologic features that are not visible to the naked eye. Typically, the technique involves the coverage of the examined skin lesion with a transparent medium (mineral oil, alcohol, or water) and then the inspection with a magnifying lens system provided with a light source such as a dermatoscope, a stereomicroscope, or a videodermatoscope [12]. The liquid functions by eliminating surface light reflection of the stratum corneum, thus enabling in vivo visualization of pigmented structures within the epidermis and the superficial dermis [5]. In this regard, the term *epiluminescence microscopy* seems to be more correct, although today it is not often used. Alternatively, similar results may be obtained with new dermoscopy systems using polarized light, which renders the use of the fluid unnecessary [3,13].

A widely used instrument for dermoscopy is the handheld dermatoscope. Its advantages include ease of use, low cost, and a fixed 10- or 20-fold magnification, sufficient for routine assessment in daily clinical practice [3]. On the other hand, it requires a clinician to be in close proximity to the skin being examined.

The binocular stereomicroscope, which provides a high-quality three-dimensional view of a lesion, with magnification ranging from ×6 to ×80, may be equipped with a camera for image storage; the equipment, however, is cumbersome and expensive [3].

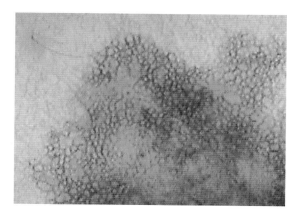

Fig. 12.1 Typical pigment network in a junctional nevus.

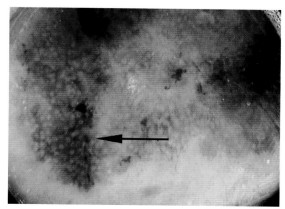

Fig. 12.2 Atypical pigment network (*arrow*) in a melanoma.

Videodermatoscopy, first introduced in the 1990s, consists of a digital system. The images are obtained by a high-resolution color video camera equipped with lenses that currently allow magnifications ranging from ×4 to ×1000. They are indirectly visualized on a high-definition monitor and may be digitalized and stored on a personal computer to allow recognition and comparison of changes over time, thus facilitating the follow-up of suspicious pigmented cutaneous lesions [3,14].

Dermoscopic semiology

Dermoscopy facilitates the identification of different morphologic structures located from the epidermis down to the upper dermis usually not seen by clinical observation [2,5,11,12,15,16]. Several studies have demonstrated a precise correlation between these structures, observed in a horizontal plane, and specific histopathologic findings, observed in the vertical plane [17]. Therefore, dermoscopy represents a link between clinical and histopathologic examination; however, dermatopathology remains the "gold standard" diagnostic procedure [1].

Common dermoscopic findings

The pigmented network probably represents the most important dermoscopic feature. It consists of a grid of brownish lines over a tan background and may be typical (regular, thin, narrow; Fig. 12.1) or atypical (irregular, thick, wide; Fig. 12.2) in benign

and malignant melanocytic lesions, respectively [9,18]. Histopathologically, the lines correspond to melanin pigment contained in keratinocytes or in melanocytes outlining the pattern of the epidermal rete ridges, whereas the holes correspond to the dermal papillae tips [1,2,11,17–19]. On palms and soles, the melanin pigment follows the furrows or the ridges of dermatoglyphics: in this case a typical parallel pattern (Fig. 12.3) is observed [11].

In diffuse pigmentation, localization of cutaneous melanin pigment determines the different colors seen. Melanin pigmentation within the epidermal stratum corneum appears black; in the lower epidermal layers, light to dark brown; and in the papillary

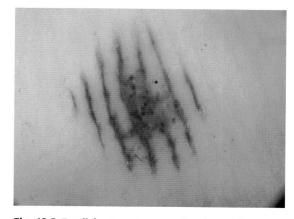

Fig. 12.3 Parallel pattern in an acral melanocytic nevus.

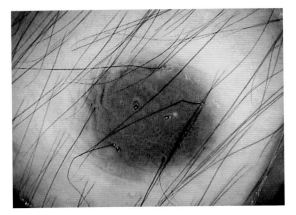

Fig. 12.4 Diffuse homogeneous blue pigmentation in a blue nevus.

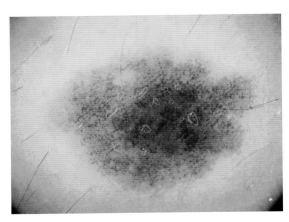

Fig. 12.6 Multiple brown globules in a compound nevus.

dermis, gray; whereas pigmentation of the reticular dermis is steel blue (Fig. 12.4) [18,19]. Even and uneven pigmentation is usually found in both benign and malignant lesions [19].

Hypopigmentation represents localized or diffuse areas of decreased pigmentation and is commonly observed in benign melanocytic lesions [2].

Black dots are small, round structures that may be regularly or irregularly distributed in benign and malignant melanocytic lesions (Fig. 12.5). They represent focal collections of melanin in the stratum corneum [2,9,17,19].

Brown globules are round to oval, variously sized structures that show a regular or irregular distribution in benign (Fig. 12.6) and malignant melanocytic lesions. They correspond to nests of melanin-containing melanocytes in the lower epidermis.

Streaks is a term comprising radial streaming and pseudopods, which radiate from the lesion border; the former are narrow, closely arranged, parallel lines; the latter appear as digitiform extensions (Fig. 12.7). Streaks may be regularly or irregularly distributed within both a pigmented Spitz nevus and a melanoma. Radial streaming and pseudopods show the same histopathology, namely peripheral, confluent, and heavily pigmented junctional nests of melanocytes.

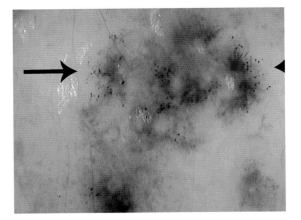

Fig. 12.5 Asymmetrical dots in a melanoma (*arrows*)

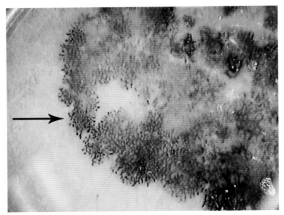

Fig. 12.7 Pseudopods (*arrow*) in a melanoma.

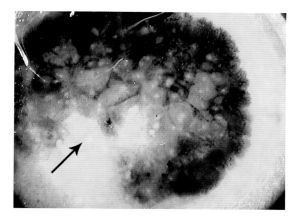

Fig. 12.8 White scar-like depigmentation (*arrow*) in a melanoma.

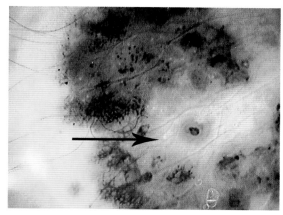

Fig. 12.10 Blue-white veil (*arrow*) in a melanoma.

Regression consists of an area of abnormal pigment distribution. It comprises white scar-like depigmentation, which corresponds to areas lighter than the normal skin (Fig. 12.8), and the so-called peppering, which consists of speckled multiple blue-gray granules within a hypopigmented area (Fig. 12.9). These two commonly associated aspects are the result of microscopic fibrosis and melanosis. Regression is frequently observed in melanoma.

Blue-white veil is an irregular, ill-defined gray-blue to whitish blue pigmentation dimming the underlying structures (Fig. 12.10). Histopathologically, it shows an acanthotic epidermis with focal hyper-granulosis above sheets of melanophages and/or heavily pigmented melanocytes in the superficial dermis. It is highly suggestive of melanoma.

Milia-like cysts, also called horny pseudocysts, are round luminescent whitish or yellowish structures (Fig. 12.11) that correspond to small intraepithelial cysts filled with keratinized material [2,9,11,17,19,20]. They are mainly observed in seborrheic keratoses.

Comedo-like openings are round or oval-shaped yellow to brown areas (Fig. 12.12) that correspond to keratin-filled epidermal invaginations. They are mainly observed in seborrheic keratoses,

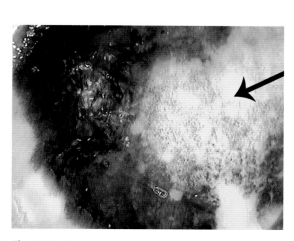

Fig. 12.9 "Peppering" (*arrow*) in a melanoma.

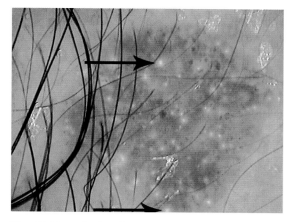

Fig. 12.11 Multiple milia-like cysts (*arrows*) in seborrheic keratosis.

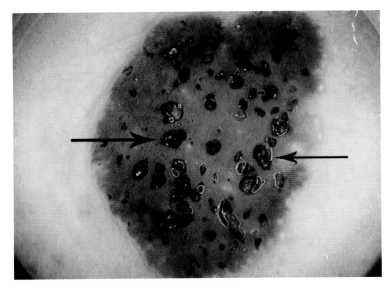

Fig. 12.12 Comedo-like openings (*arrows*) in seborrheic keratosis.

occasionally in papillomatous melanocytic nevi, rarely in melanoma.

A brain-like appearance is the result of the presence of irregular linear keratin-filled fissures (or sulci) alternating with yellowish to brownish ridges, or gyri (Fig. 12.13). This aspect is typical of seborrheic keratoses [2,11].

Exophytic papillary structures are dome-shaped formations that correspond to pronounced papillomatosis, observed in dermal nevi and in seborrheic keratoses [2,17].

Fingerprint-like structures consist of light brown delicate network-like configurations seen at the pe-

riphery of a lesion, producing a pattern that resembles fingerprints [11,20,21]. They are typical of flat seborrheic keratoses.

The moth-eaten border is a concave rim that has been compared to a moth-eaten garment (Fig. 12.14). It is typical of flat seborrheic keratoses [20,21].

Leaf-like areas consist of brown-gray or gray-blue regions located at the lesion periphery, forming a leaf-like pattern (Fig. 12.15). Histopathologically, a leaf-like area corresponds to clumps of pigmented basaloid cells and is typical of basal cell carcinoma [2,11,17].

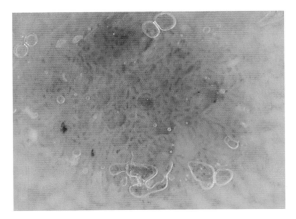

Fig. 12.13 Brain-like appearance in seborrheic keratosis.

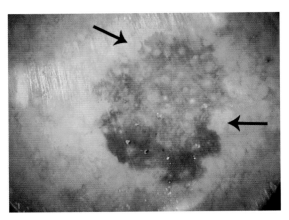

Fig. 12.14 Moth-eaten border (*arrows*) in flat seborrheic keratosis.

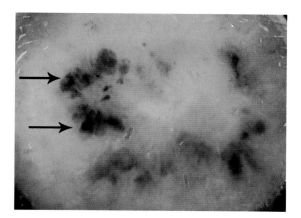

Fig. 12.15 Leaf-like areas (*arrows*) in pigmented basal cell carcinoma.

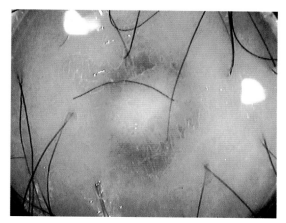

Fig. 12.17 Central white patch surrounded by delicate pigment network in a dermatofibroma.

Spoke-wheel areas are well-circumscribed gray, blue, or brown radial projections meeting at a darker central axis. They are highly suggestive of basal cell carcinoma [2,11].

Blue-gray globules and large blue-gray ovoid nests are well-circumscribed round to oval structures, of different size, not intimately connected to a pigmented tumor body (Fig. 12.16) [2,11]. Both features histopathologically consist of pigmented basaloid cells and are suggestive of basal cell carcinoma.

The central white patch is a relatively sharply circumscribed, round to oval, sometimes irregularly outlined whitish area within the center of a pigmented lesion (Fig. 12.17). It is the result of epidermal hyperplasia overlying a variable amount of dermal fibrosis and is specific for a dermatofibroma [2,17,22].

Red-blue areas, also identified as red lacunae or red lagoons, are roundish or oval structures with a reddish or red-bluish coloration (Fig. 12.18) that histopathologically correspond to widened vascular lacunae located in the superficial dermis [2,11,17]. They are typical of angiomas and may acquire a deep blue to black color after thrombosis.

Vascular structures include the following: "Comma-like" vessels are short, strongly curved blood vessels predominantly seen in dermal nevi [2,20,23]. "Hairpin-like" vessels are long capillary

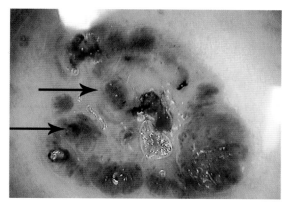

Fig. 12.16 Large blue-gray ovoid nests (*arrows*) in pigmented basal cell carcinoma.

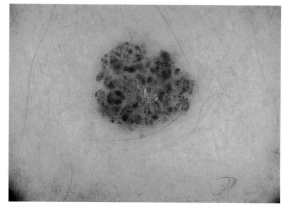

Fig. 12.18 Red-blue areas in a senile angioma.

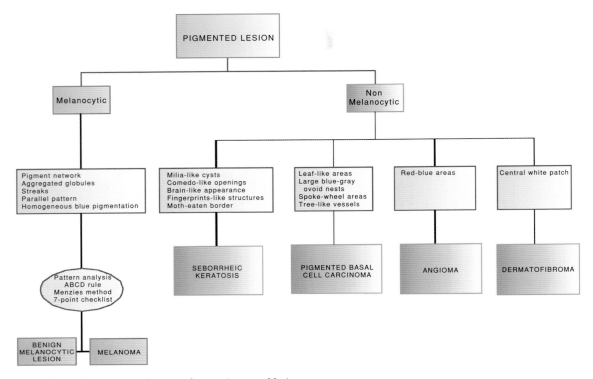

Flow Chart 12.1 Suggested approach to a pigmented lesion.

loops, usually present at the periphery of thicker tumors, which are mainly seen in melanomas and in seborrheic keratoses. "Dotted" vessels are small pinpoint vessels corresponding to short capillary loops, which are commonly seen in all types of melanocytic tumors, including melanoma. "Tree-like" vessels are thick and arborized structures commonly observed in basal cell carcinoma. "Linear-irregular" vessels are predominantly seen in melanoma.

Dermoscopy in the differential diagnosis of pigmented lesions

In the case of a pigmented lesion approached by dermoscopy, the observer should first distinguish melanocytic lesions from nonmelanocytic ones (Flow Chart 12.1). This is the first of a two-step procedure; the second step differentiates benign melanocytic lesions from malignant ones [2,11,16,18].

Melanocytic lesions

A lesion is considered to be melanocytic if dermoscopy reveals the presence of at least one of the following features: pigment network, aggregated globules, streaks, parallel pattern, or blue pigmentation (Flow Chart 12.1). In the latter case, the lesion is diagnosed as a blue nevus. If the lesion does not demonstrate any of the specific structures of nonmelanocytic lesions (Flow Chart 12.1), it should be considered melanocytic and consequently excised, to rule out a structureless melanoma [18].

Diagnostic methods

If a lesion is classified as melanocytic, several diagnostic methods may be used to identify it (Flow Chart 12.1).

Pattern analysis, as proposed by Pehamberger and associates [9] in 1987, was the first method used. It was based on subjective, qualitative, critical, simultaneous evaluation of several dermoscopic criteria. The authors characterized the general appearance of the pigmented skin lesion (uniform or

Table 12.1 Diagnostic methods: modified pattern analysis [11,16]

Global features
Reticular pattern
Globular pattern
Cobblestone pattern
Homogeneous pattern
Starburst pattern
Parallel pattern
Multicomponent pattern
Nonspecific pattern

Local features
Pigment network: typical/atypical
Dots/globules: regular/irregular
Streaks: regular/irregular
Blue-whitish veil
Regression structures
Hypopigmentation
Blotches symmetric/asymmetric
Vascular structures

Site-related features
Face: typical pseudo-network, annular–granular structures, gray pseudo-network, rhomboidal structures, asymmetric pigmented follicles
Palms/soles: parallel-furrow pattern, lattice-like pattern, fibrillar pattern, parallel-ridge pattern

heterogeneous), pattern of pigmentation (type and distribution of color, presence of depigmentation, pigment network, brown globules and black dots), and lesion margins (regular or irregular for the presence of pseudopods and/or radial streaming) as the most important dermoscopic criteria [2,5]. In 2000, a modified pattern analysis was proposed [11,16]. Compared with the original description, the authors introduced the "global pattern," simplified some criteria, and added the evaluation of vascular features (Table 12.1). Pattern analysis evaluation requires special knowledge of the criteria and specifically trained observers for it to be used with confidence [5,24].

To make dermoscopy more functional, new diagnostic algorithms have been introduced. They consist of dermoscopic score systems that can be used by less experienced observers, providing a high rate of diagnostic accuracy [2,5,18,25]. Of these, three simplified algorithms were validated in the Internet Consensus Meeting: the ABCD rule, the Men-

zies method, and the seven-point checklist [26,27]. Other algorithms, including the CASH (color, architecture, symmetry, and homogeneity) method and three-point checklist, are under evaluation [26,28].

The ABCD rule of dermatoscopy [29], developed in 1993, is a semiquantitative score system approach. It evaluates four criteria: asymmetry (A), borders (B), colors (C), and different structural components (D). The score descriptions are listed in Table 12.2. By the addition of each subscore (multiplied by a weight factor), a total dermoscopic score (TDS), ranging from 1.0 to 8.9, is ultimately obtained. A lesion with a TDS of 4.75 or less is considered benign, between 4.75 and 5.45 is suggestive of malignancy and should be excised or followed closely, and greater than 5.45 is highly suspicious for melanoma [2,27].

The Menzies method [30], proposed in 1996, evaluates two negative and nine positive features (Table 12.3). To make the diagnosis of melanoma, at least one positive feature and none of the negative features must be present. [2,27]

The seven-point checklist [31], developed in 1998, is based on the identification of three major criteria and four minor criteria (Table 12.4). Each major criterion receives two points, whereas each minor criterion receives one point. A score of 3 or greater is highly suspicious for melanoma [2,27].

A comparative study conducted by highly expert dermoscopists concluded that pattern analysis has the highest diagnostic accuracy [11]. On the other hand, a similar effort by relatively nonexpert practitioners favored the Menzies method for the highest diagnostic accuracy in melanoma diagnosis [32]. In conclusion, according to most authors, pattern analysis, although complex, is the most rapid and complete approach. When the observer achieves good dermoscopic experience, this modality's application becomes intuitive and automatic; this is of great utility, especially in patients with multiple lesions [5,26].

Dermoscopy of melanocytic neoplasms
Junctional melanocytic nevus is characterized by the presence of a regular, delicate pigment network that gradually fades at its periphery. In its central portion, multiple black dots or a uniform dark pigmentation may be present [9,19,33].

Table 12.2 Diagnostic methods: the ABCD rule of dermatoscopy [11,29]

		Points	Weight Factor	Subscore Range
Asymmetry	In 0, 1, or 2 perpendicular axes; assess contour, colors, and structures	0–2	1.3	0–2.6
Border	Abrupt ending of pigment pattern at the periphery in 0–8 segments	0–8	0.1	0–0.8
Color	1 point for each color: white, red, light brown, dark brown, blue-gray, black	1–6	0.5	0.5–3.0
Different structures	1 point for every structure: pigment network, structureless areas, dots, globules, streaks	1–5	0.5	0.5–2.5
Total score range:				1.0–8.9

Table 12.3 Diagnostic methods: the Menzies method [11,30]

Negative Features
Symmetry of pattern
Presence of a single color

Positive Features
Blue-white veil
Multiple brown dots
Pseudopods
Radial streaming
Scar-like depigmentation
Peripheral black dots–globules
Multiple colors (5 or 6)
Multiple blue/gray dots
Broadened network

Table 12.4 Diagnostic methods: the 7-point checklist according to Argenziano and colleagues [11,31]

Criteria	Score
Major	
Atypical pigment network	2
Blue-white veil	2
Atypical vascular pattern	2
Minor	
Irregular streaks	1
Irregular blotches	1
Irregular dots/globules	1
Regression structures	1

Compound melanocytic nevus typically shows the presence of a pigment network with stronger background brown pigmentation; it also exhibits brown globules regularly distributed throughout (Fig. 12.19) [9,16,19,33].

Dermal melanocytic nevus is characterized by the absence of pigment network and presence of brown globules varying in size and color; sometimes, they may be arranged to create a "cobblestone" effect (Fig. 12.20). Comma-like vessels are commonly observed.

Pigmented Spitz nevus frequently shows a characteristic starburst pattern formed by a prominent gray-blue to black diffuse pigmentation and by pseudopods radially and regularly located along the periphery (Fig. 12.21) [34]. In its center, a reticular black-whitish to blue-whitish veil, called reticular depigmentation, may be present [33]. The starburst pattern rarely may also be seen in melanoma; thus, in adult patients, a biopsy should be performed when such spitzoid features are detected by dermoscopy [35].

The typical feature of blue nevus consists of a homogeneous blue pigmentation with complete absence of other findings (Fig. 12.4). Multiple areas of hypopigmentation corresponding to fibrosis may be observed (Fig. 12.22) [33,36].

Melanoma usually shows a multicomponent pattern, with a combination of three or more dermoscopic structures (Figs. 12.23 to 12.26) [33].

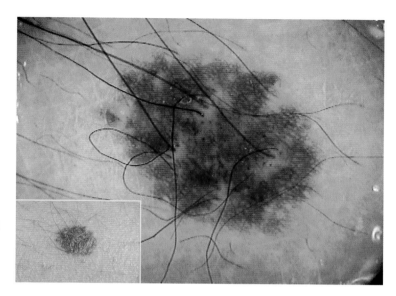

Fig. 12.19 Compound nevus: typical pigment network at the periphery and diffuse brown pigmentation and regular globules in the central portion of the lesion. *Inset*, clinical presentation.

Melanoma in situ and early invasive melanomas (Breslow index <0.76 mm) are characterized by a diffuse pigmentation irregular in color and/or distribution, atypical pigment network with wide and irregular meshes and thick lines ending abruptly at the periphery, dots or globules variously sized and haphazardly distributed, irregularly dispersed pseudopods, and/or radial streaming [9,11,19,33].

In intermediate and thick melanomas (Breslow index ≥0.76 mm), the previous findings are associated with a blue-whitish veil and, frequently, with dotted, linear irregular, and/or hairpin vessels. Regression may also be present and, if extensive, should always be biopsied, despite the presence of other dermoscopic criteria, to avoid missing a melanoma [35]. Finally, desmoplastic melanoma

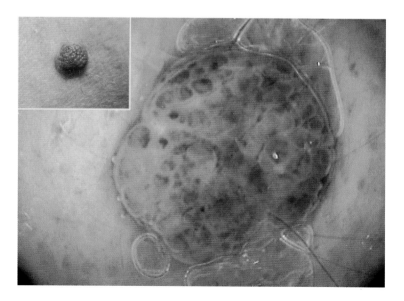

Fig. 12.20 Dermal nevus: "cobblestone" aspect. *Inset*, clinical presentation.

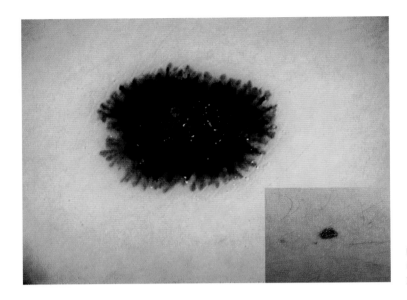

Fig. 12.21 Pigmented Spitz nevus: starburst pattern. *Inset,* clinical presentation.

may mimic a nonpigmented, benign inflammatory lesion, with dermoscopic examination showing a nonspecific pigment pattern atypical enough to biopsy.

Nonmelanocytic lesions

If a nonmelanocytic lesion is recognized in the first step, no further evaluation through algorithm methods is needed, as the diagnosis is readily made [2,11,16] (Flow Chart 12.1).

Dermoscopy of nonmelanocytic lesions

Pigmented basal cell carcinoma is usually characterized by leaf-like areas, spoke-wheel areas, blue-gray globules, and/or large blue-gray ovoid nests, with absence of pigment network (Fig. 12.27). The

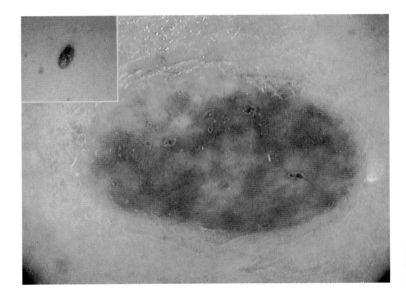

Fig. 12.22 Sclerotic blue nevus: blue pigmentation alternated with multiple areas of hypopigmentation. *Inset,* clinical presentation.

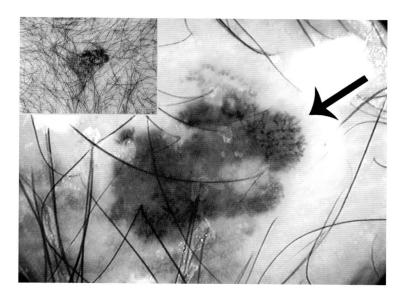

Fig. 12.23 Melanoma (Breslow thickness 0.45 mm): irregular pigmentation and irregular streaks (*arrow*). *Inset*, clinical presentation.

presence of tree-like vessels and/or ulcerations is also typical [33,37]. Dermoscopy may be particularly useful in the basal cell nevus syndrome, in which tumors less than 3 mm in diameter can be detected in early stages by the presence of blue-gray globules [38,39].

The hallmarks of superficial basal cell carcinoma are a shiny white to red appearance and the presence of irregularly dispersed, short, fine telangiectasias. In addition, about 70% have homogeneous red to brown to black structureless areas, corresponding to multiple small surface ulcerations [38].

The peculiar findings of seborrheic keratoses are milia-like cysts and comedo-like openings (Fig. 12.28). Background may considerably vary from opaque light brown to dark brown or black. A

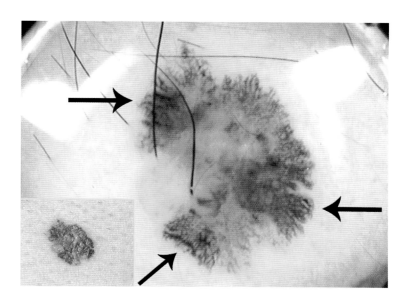

Fig. 12.24 Melanoma (Breslow thickness 0.48 mm): irregular pigmentation and irregular streaks (*arrows*). *Inset*, clinical presentation.

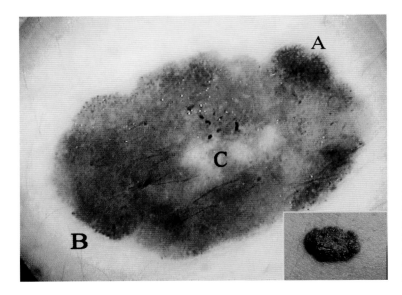

Fig. 12.25 Melanoma (Breslow thickness 0.93 mm): irregular pigmentation, atypical pigment network (*A*), irregular streaks (*B*), and a central white scar-like depigmentation (*C*). *Inset*, clinical presentation.

pronounced black pigmentation camouflaging the pathognomonic features may be seen in a melano-acanthoma [33]. Hairpin and dotted vessels may be present, mainly at the periphery of the lesions [20]. Other morphologic findings that sometimes may be observed include a brain-like appearance (Fig. 12.13) and exophytic papillary structures. Some flat seborrheic keratoses (also known as solar lentigines) may show either a fingerprint-like pattern or a moth-eaten border [2]. The presence of a brown-gray and blue-gray granular pattern is typical of lichen planus–like keratosis or benign lichenoid keratosis, which may be an inflammatory stage of regressing skin tumors, mainly solar lentigines and seborrheic keratoses [40].

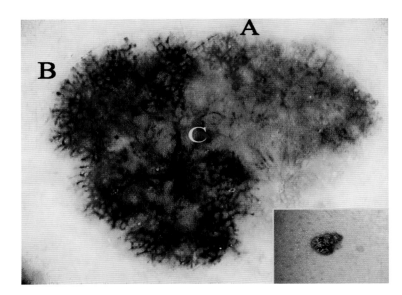

Fig. 12.26 Melanoma (Breslow thickness 1.33 mm): irregular pigmentation, atypical pigment network (*A*), irregular streaks (*B*), and a blue-white veil (*C*). *Inset*, clinical presentation.

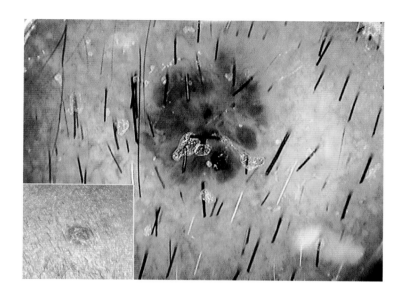

Fig. 12.27 Pigmented basal cell carcinoma: multiple confluent large blue-gray ovoid nests. *Inset*, clinical presentation.

Dermatofibroma shows a central white patch surrounded by a delicate, regular, usually light brown pigment network (Fig. 12.17). Sometimes within the central patch, several small round to oval globules of light brown coloration may be found [33].

With regard to vascular lesions, senile angiomas are characterized by the presence of several red-blue areas. Darker red-blue or red-black colors are signs of thrombi within the vascular spaces (Fig. 12.29). In angiokeratomas, whitish keratotic areas or a blue-whitish veil may be observed [41]. Hemorrhagic lesions, such as subcorneal hematomas, show a homogeneous dark-brown pattern or dark-red globules.

Dermoscopy at particular sites

Face

The conventional pigment network is rarely found on facial lesions because of the special architecture

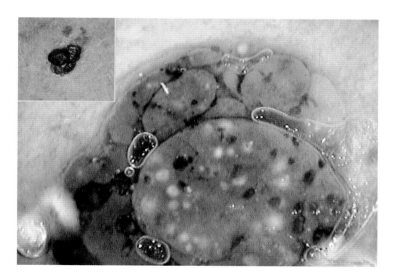

Fig. 12.28 Seborrheic keratosis: comedo-like openings and milia-like cysts. *Inset*, clinical presentation.

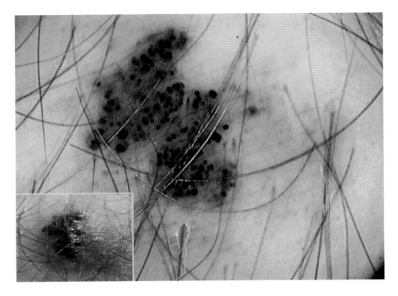

Fig. 12.29 Thrombosed angioma: multiple red-black areas. *Inset*, clinical presentation.

of the dermal–epidermal junction at this site, in which the rete ridges are flat to absent. Instead, a "pseudopigment network" with a broad mesh and holes, as the result of the numerous follicular and sweat gland openings, may be seen [15,42]. This finding may be seen in both melanocytic and nonmelanocytic lesions, so other criteria are necessary to distinguish the lesion type. Common pigmented lesions of the face include lentigo maligna,

flat seborrheic keratoses (or lentigo solaris), and pigmented actinic keratoses. A dermoscopic progression model has been identified for lentigo maligna [41]. In the first stage, hyperpigmented asymmetric follicular openings may be detected, with successively fine streaks, dots, and globules developing around the follicles and creating the so-called annular–granular pattern along with the formation of rhomboidal structures (Fig. 12.30). In its later

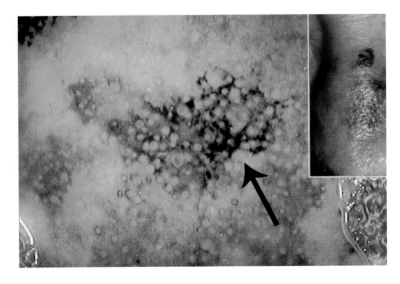

Fig. 12.30 Lentigo maligna: rhomboidal structures (*arrow*). *Inset*, clinical presentation.

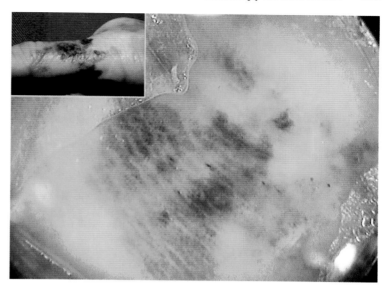

Fig. 12.31 In situ acral melanoma: parallel ridge pattern. *Inset*, clinical presentation.

stages, hyperpigmentation becomes homogeneous enough to obliterate follicular openings [5,42]. Flat seborrheic keratoses are usually characterized by milia-like cysts, yellow opaque areas, fingerprint-like structures, and a moth-eaten border. Specific dermoscopic criteria for pigmented actinic keratoses are lacking; a superficial, prominent, broken-up pseudonetwork is the most frequent finding, but the presence of rhomboidal structures, annular–granular structures, and a moth-eaten border may be evident [43].

Palms and soles

In the palms and soles, the pigment gives rise to parallel lines that follow the skin grooves [19,44]. Acral melanocytic nevi may show three different types of dermoscopic patterns: the "parallel-furrow pattern," the "lattice-like pattern," and the "fibrillar pattern" [45]. The parallel-furrow pattern, the most frequent, shows linear pigmentation along the sulci of the skin markings (Fig. 12.3) and two linear lines along both sides of each sulcus; single or double dotted lines along the sulci may be present as variants. In the lattice-like pattern, there is a linear pigmentation that follows and crosses the surface sulci. In the fibrillar pattern, fine fibrillar pigmentation runs in a slanting direction to the skin markings. In situ acral melanoma shows the so-called parallel ridge pattern, a diffuse and fine reticular,

irregularly shaped pigmentation that follows the papillary tips (Fig. 12.31). It is not seen in benign lesions, and thus exhibits a high specificity and sensitivity [5,44,45].

Advanced dermoscopy diagnosis

The use of dermoscopy has been recently extended to the differential diagnosis of some non-pigmented skin lesions, both melanocytic and non-melanocytic, by the evaluation of vascular patterns [23,46,47].

Amelanotic melanoma is characterized by the presence of polymorphous vessels, which may be dotted, hairpin, and/or linear irregular. Moreover, milky red globules or milky red areas that appear as localized or diffuse areas of reddish white color may be seen; these findings are thought to represent highly vascularized amelanotic tumor cell complexes [23,45,47]. The atypical vascular pattern and milky red areas are considered melanoma-specific criteria [47].

Bowen's disease is characterized by the presence of a scaly surface and "glomerular" vessels in a multicomponent global pattern. These distinctive, prominent "glomuleroid" dotted vessels are usually larger in size than "classic" dotted vessels. Pigmented Bowen's disease may have the additional presence of irregular diffuse gray to

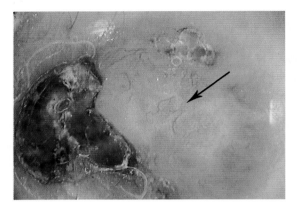

Fig. 12.32 Nonpigmented basal cell carcinoma: tree-like vessels (*arrow*) and ulcerations.

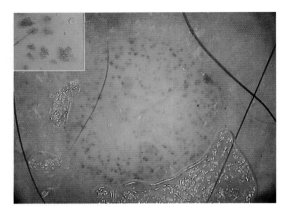

Fig. 12.33 Clear-cell acanthoma: symmetrical dotted vessels arranged in a netlike pattern. *Inset*: bush-like aspect at higher magnification (×200).

brown homogeneous pigmentation or irregularly distributed dots and globules [48].

Nonpigmented basal cell carcinoma is characterized by the presence of tree-like vessels and multiple ulcerations (Fig. 12.32) [23].

Nonpigmented facial actinic keratosis is characterized by the presence of a peculiar "strawberry" appearance, produced by four dermoscopic features: a pink-to-red "pseudo-network," a white-to-yellow surface scale, fine linear-wavy vessels, and hair follicle openings filled with yellowish keratotic plugs and/or surrounded by a white halo [49].

Clear-cell acanthoma is characterized by the presence, at low magnification, of symmetric dotted vessels arranged in a netlike pattern throughout the entire lesion; at higher magnification (×200), the vessels show a bush-like aspect (Fig. 12.33) [50].

Conclusions

The introduction of dermoscopy, particularly digital systems, has had a great impact on the management of pigmented skin lesions. Dermoscopy has been shown to significantly improve the early detection of skin cancer, increasing diagnostic accuracy between 5% and 30% over clinical visual inspection, depending on lesion type and physician experience [1,2,4,51,52]. However, dermoscopy requires sufficient familiarity and cannot be recommended for novice users. A study has shown that for untrained

observers, the diagnostic accuracy may be lower than that of the simple clinical examination [24].

Dermoscopic examination may confirm clinical suspicion. Correct use of dermoscopy results in a substantial decrease in unnecessary biopsies and excisions of benign but clinically equivocal pigmented skin lesions, such as thrombosed angiomas and seborrheic keratoses. On the other hand, dermoscopy may help increase the index of suspicion in the context of melanomas clinically mimicking benign lesions [43].

Dermoscopy may identify suspicious lesions not found with the naked eye. As many lesions as possible should be evaluated. However, special attention should be paid to the following types: lesions with a history of change (in color, size, shape, symptoms, etc.) or one lesion clinically different from the other pigmented lesions of the patient (the "ugly duckling" sign), and those that look clinically like a melanoma [25]. Although so far there are no digital dermoscopic criteria that can clearly distinguish dysplastic nevi from in situ melanomas [53], further advances may facilitate this distinction.

Adaptations are constantly being made. For example, photography illustrating the visualized alterations may be challenging with a regular dermoscope. However, a handheld digital camera can be used to capture dermoscopic images. The technique of Rushing and associates [54] uses a 5-megapixel

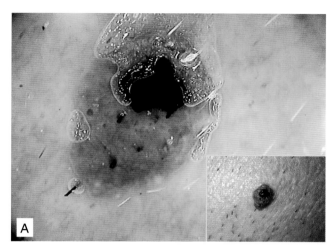

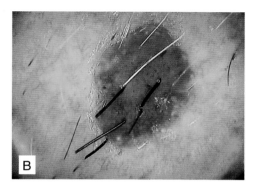

Fig. 12.34 *A*, Dermoscopy of a clinically suspicious lesion showing some milia-like cysts and comedo-like openings and a homogeneous black area (*inset*, clinical presentation). *B*, An image at 7 days' follow-up shows the disappearance of the black area. A diagnosis of traumatized seborrheic keratosis was made.

camera with a 3× optical zoom and 1.8-inch high-resolution LCD screen. The digital camera is placed above the dermoscope with the camera lens positioned directly against the posterior aspect of the dermoscope lens. With the digital camera's flash disabled and light provided by the dermoscope's halogen illumination, the camera's automatic focus is activated and applied to the image projected by the dermoscope. When the focused image appears on the LCD screen, the photograph is taken and immediately reviewed for accuracy.

Digital systems (videodermatoscopy), which allow for easy storage and retrieval of dermoscopic images, provide several advantages. One is the possibility to perform a dermoscopic follow-up of pigmented skin lesions to detect minimal changes for the early diagnosis of melanoma; the monitoring may reduce the number of biopsies, being a helpful tool to decide which neoplasms should be removed [13,55]. Long-term follow-up allows comparison of atypical nevi over 6 to 12 months in patients with multiple lesions (e.g., patients with atypical mole syndrome). Short-term follow-up (generally at 1 to 3 months) is performed on single suspicious lesions (i.e., anamnesis of changes) that lack features of melanoma (Fig. 12.34) [13]. Complete excision should be considered in a neoplasm that

shows significant dermoscopic changes on follow-up.

Further prospective studies are needed to determine the real impact of dermoscopic follow-up on the clinical management of patients with pigmented skin lesions. Moreover, digital dermoscopy facilitates research concerning the natural evolution of pigmented skin lesions, the influence of ultraviolet light, and the progression of atypical melanocytic nevi. Another advantage is the possibility of computer-assisted diagnosis, based on computerized analysis of digital images [2,56]. Automated diagnostic systems require no input by the clinician but rather report a likely diagnosis based on computer algorithms [13]. Many software programs are available that are approved for medical use; however, further evaluation of the reliability of these methods is recommended before their routine application. There are no formal clinical trials evaluating trained dermatologists' ability versus automated instruments [13,57]. Finally, it is possible to electronically transmit dermoscopic images via the Internet for teleconsultation [58]. Teledermoscopy may be used between physicians to exchange difficult or unusual images. An example of this potentiality was shown in the Internet Consensus Meeting held in 2000 [11].

References

1 Menzies SW, Zalaudek I. Why perform dermoscopy? The evidence for its role in the routine management of pigmented skin lesions. Arch Dermatol 2006;142:1211–2.

2 Braun RP, Rabinovitz HS, Oliviero M, et al. Dermoscopy of pigmented skin lesions. J Am Acad Dermatol 2005;52:109–21.

3 Ruocco V, Argenziano G, Soyer HP. Commentary: dermoscopy. Clin Dermatol 2002;20:199.

4 Bafounta ML, Beauchet A, Aegerter P, et al. Is dermoscopy (epiluminescence microscopy) useful for the diagnosis of melanoma? Results of a meta-analysis using techniques adapted to the evaluation of diagnostic tests. Arch Dermatol 2001;137:1343–50.

5 Carli P, De Giorgi V, Soyer HP, et al. Dermatoscopy in the diagnosis of pigmented skin lesions: a new semiology for the dermatologist. J Eur Acad Dermatol Venereol 2000;14:353–69.

6 Goldman L. Some investigative studies of pigmented nevi with cutaneous microscopy. J Invest Dermatol 1951;16:407–26.

7 MacKie RM. An aid to the preoperative assessment of pigmented lesions of the skin. Br J Dermatol 1971;85:232–8.

8 Fritsch P, Pechlaner R. The pigmented network: a new tool for the clinical diagnosis of pigmented lesions. J Invest Dermatol 1980;74:458.

9 Pehamberger H, Steiner A, Wolff K. In vivo epiluminescence microscopy of pigmented skin lesions. I. Pattern analysis of pigmented skin lesions. J Am Acad Dermatol 1987;17:571–83.

10 Bahmer FA, Fritsch P, Kreusch J, et al. Terminology in surface microscopy. Consensus meeting of the Committee on Analytical Morphology of the Arbeitsgemeinschaft Dermatologische Forschung, Hamburg, Federal Republic of Germany, Nov. 17, 1989. J Am Acad Dermatol 1990;23:1159–62.

11 Argenziano G, Soyer HP, Chimenti S, et al. Dermoscopy of pigmented skin lesions: results of a consensus meeting via the Internet. J Am Acad Dermatol 2003;48:679–93.

12 Soyer HP, Argenziano G, Chimenti S, et al. Dermoscopy of pigmented skin lesions. Eur J Dermatol 2001;11:270–6; quiz 277.

13 Menzies SW. Cutaneous melanoma: making a clinical diagnosis, present and future. Dermatol Ther 2006;19:32–9.

14 Micali G, Lacarrubba F. Possible applications of videodermatoscopy beyond pigmented lesions. Int J Dermatol 2003;42:430–3.

15 Argenziano G, Soyer HP, De Giorgi V. Interactive atlas of dermoscopy. Milan: Edra Medica Publishing and New Media; 2000.

16 Soyer HP, Argenziano G, Chimenti S. Dermoscopy of pigmented skin lesions. An atlas based on the Consensus Net Meeting on Dermoscopy 2000. Milan: Edra Medica Publishing and New Media; 2001.

17 Ferrara G, Argenziano G, Soyer HP, et al. Dermoscopic-pathologic correlation: an atlas of 15 cases. Clin Dermatol 2002;20:228–35.

18 Scope A, Benvenuto-Andrade C, Agero AL, et al. Non-melanocytic lesions defying the two-step dermoscopy algorithm. Dermatol Surg 2006;32:1398–406.

19 Dal Pozzo V, Benelli C. Atlas of dermoscopy. Milan: Edra Medica Publishing and New Media; 1997.

20 Braun RP, Rabinovitz H, Oliviero M, et al. Dermoscopic diagnosis of seborrheic keratosis. Clin Dermatol 2002;20:270–2.

21 Schiffner R, Schiffner-Rohe J, Vogt T, et al. Improvement of early recognition of lentigo maligna using dermatoscopy. J Am Acad Dermatol 2000;42:25–32.

22 Puig S, Romero D, Zaballos P, et al. Dermoscopy of dermatofibroma. Arch Dermatol 2005;141:122.

23 Kreusch JF. Vascular patterns in skin tumors. Clin Dermatol 2002;20:248–54.

24 Binder M, Schwarz M, Winkler A, et al. Epiluminescence microscopy. A useful tool for the diagnosis of pigmented skin lesions for formally trained dermatologists. Arch Dermatol 1995;131:286–91.

25 Bowling J, Argenziano G, Azenha A, et al. Dermoscopy key points: recommendations from the international dermoscopy society. Dermatology 2007;214:3–5.

26 Henning JS, Dusza SW, Wang SQ, et al. The CASH (color, architecture, symmetry, and homogeneity) algorithm for dermoscopy. J Am Acad Dermatol 2007;56:45–52.

27 Johr RH. Dermoscopy: alternative melanocytic algorithms-the ABCD rule of dermatoscopy, Menzies scoring method, and 7-point checklist. Clin Dermatol 2002;20:240–7.

28 Zalaudek I, Argenziano G, Soyer HP, et al. Three-point checklist of dermoscopy: an open internet study. Br J Dermatol 2006;154:431–7.

29 Nachbar F, Stolz W, Merkle T, et al. The ABCD rule of dermatoscopy. High prospective value in the diagnosis of doubtful melanocytic skin lesions. J Am Acad Dermatol 1994;30:551–9.

30 Menzies SW, Ingvar C, McCarthy WH. A sensitivity and specificity analysis of the surface microscopy features of invasive melanoma. Melanoma Res 1996;6:55–62.

31 Argenziano G, Fabbrocini G, Carli P, et al. Epiluminescence microscopy for the diagnosis of doubtful melanocytic skin lesions. Comparison of the ABCD rule of dermatoscopy and a new 7-point checklist based on pattern analysis. Arch Dermatol 1998;134: 1563–70.

32 Dolianitis C, Kelly J, Wolfe R, et al. Comparative performance of 4 dermoscopic algorithms by nonexperts for the diagnosis of melanocytic lesions. Arch Dermatol 2005;141:1008–14.

33 Soyer HP, Argenziano G, Ruocco V, et al. Dermoscopy of pigmented skin lesions (part II). Eur J Dermatol 2001;11:483–98.

34 Peris K, Ferrari A, Argenziano G, et al. Dermoscopic classification of Spitz/Reed nevi. Clin Dermatol 2002;20:259–62.

35 Argenziano G, Zalaudek I, Ferrara G, et al. Dermoscopy features of melanoma incognito: indications for biopsy. J Am Acad Dermatol 2007;56:508–13.

36 Grichnik JM. Dermoscopy of melanocytic neoplasms: sclerotic blue nevi. Arch Dermatol 2003;139: 1522.

37 Menzies SW. Dermoscopy of pigmented basal cell carcinoma. Clin Dermatol 2002;20:268–9.

38 Giacomel J, Zalaudek I. Dermoscopy of superficial basal cell carcinoma. Dermatol Surg 2005;31:1710–3.

39 Kolm I, Puig S, Iranzo P, et al. Dermoscopy in Gorlin-Goltz syndrome. Dermatol Surg 2006;32:847–51.

40 Zaballos P, Marti E, Cuellar F, et al. Dermoscopy of lichenoid regressing seborrheic keratosis. Arch Dermatol 2006;142:410.

41 Wolf IH. Dermoscopic diagnosis of vascular lesions. Clin Dermatol 2002;20:273–5.

42 Stolz W, Schiffner R, Burgdorf WH. Dermatoscopy for facial pigmented skin lesions. Clin Dermatol 2002;20:276–8.

43 Zalaudek I, Ferrara G, Leinweber B, et al. Pitfalls in the clinical and dermoscopic diagnosis of pigmented actinic keratosis. J Am Acad Dermatol 2005;53:1071–4.

44 Tanaka M. Dermoscopy. J Dermatol 2006;33:513–7.

45 Saida T, Oguchi S, Miyazaki A. Dermoscopy for acral pigmented skin lesions. Clin Dermatol 2002;20:279–85.

46 Zalaudek I. Dermoscopy subpatterns of nonpigmented skin tumors. Arch Dermatol 2005;141:532.

47 Johr R, Stolz W. Lessons on dermoscopy. Dermatol Surg 2002;28:299–300.

48 Zalaudek I, Di Stefani A, Argenziano G. The specific dermoscopic criteria of Bowen's disease. J Eur Acad Dermatol Venereol 2006;20:361–2.

49 Zalaudek I, Giacomel J, Argenziano G, et al. Dermoscopy of facial nonpigmented actinic keratosis. Br J Dermatol 2006;155:951–6.

50 Lacarrubba F, de Pasquale R, Micali G. Videodermatoscopy improves the clinical diagnostic accuracy of multiple clear cell acanthoma. Eur J Dermatol 2003;13:596–8.

51 Steiner A, Pehamberger H, Wolff K. In vivo epiluminescence microscopy of pigmented skin lesions. II. Diagnosis of small pigmented skin lesions and early detection of malignant melanoma. J Am Acad Dermatol 1987;17:584–91.

52 Kittler H, Pehamberger H, Wolff K, et al. Diagnostic accuracy of dermoscopy. Lancet Oncol 2002;3:159–65.

53 Burroni M, Sbano P, Cevenini G, et al. Dysplastic naevus vs. in situ melanoma: digital dermoscopy analysis. Br J Dermatol 2005;152:679–84.

54 Rushing ME, Hurst E, Sheehan D. Clinical pearl: the use of the handheld digital camera to capture dermoscopic and microscopic images. J Am Acad Dermatol 2006;55:314–5.

55 Rubegni P, Burroni M, Andreassi A, et al. The role of dermoscopy and digital dermoscopy analysis in the diagnosis of pigmented skin lesions. Arch Dermatol 2005;141:1444–6.

56 Malvehy J, Puig S. Follow-up of melanocytic skin lesions with digital total-body photography and digital dermoscopy: a two-step method. Clin Dermatol 2002;20:297–304.

57 Blum A, Hofmann-Wellenhof R, Luedtke H, et al. Value of the clinical history for different users of dermoscopy compared with results of digital image analysis. J Eur Acad Dermatol Venereol 2004;18:665–9.

58 Piccolo D, Peris K, Chimenti S, et al. Jumping into the future using teledermoscopy. Skinmed 2002;1:20–4.

CHAPTER 13
Merkel cell carcinoma

Mary S. Brady

Merkel cell carcinoma (MCC) is an uncommon but deadly dermal malignancy that was originally called "trabecular carcinoma" when first described by Toker [1] in 1972. Merkel cells are neural crest–derived cells that were documented by Friedrich Merkel in 1875 [2]. They are found in the basal layer of the epidermis and may play a role in proprioception and hair movement. MCC typically occurs in older white individuals, with a median age at presentation of 69 years [3]. The cause of the disease is unknown, although its propensity to be located on the head, neck, and extremities suggests that sun exposure, in addition to increased age, is a risk factor. MCC may also occur in association with immunosuppression related to hematologic malignancy, AIDS, or organ transplantation [4–6]. The disease appears to have tripled in incidence in North America from 0.15 cases per 100,000 in 1986 to 0.44 cases per 100,000 in 2001 [7]. This may represent a real increase in incidence or be a result of improved recognition, particularly in the examination of biopsy specimens [8].

In several important ways, MCC behaves like cutaneous melanoma. It is a deadly dermal malignancy that can metastasize widely. Distant disease is usually preceded by the development of regional nodal failure, suggesting an orderly progression of disease from primary site to regional nodes to distant sites [9]. Whereas cure is uncommon in melanoma patients with distant metastases, those with systemic MCC *cannot* be cured and have a median survival of 9 months [3].

Pathologic diagnosis

Immunohistochemical staining is critical to confirming the diagnosis of MCC. The tumor consists of sheets of small round blue cells, an appearance similar to that of melanoma and metastatic small cell carcinoma. MCC has immunohistochemical features of both neuroendocrine and epithelial cells. It is usually positive for cytokeratins, particularly CK20 (unlike melanoma and metastatic squamous cell carcinoma). MCC is usually negative for S-100 and thyroid transcription factor 1, a newly described nuclear protein that appears to be specific for small cell tumors of lung origin [10].

Clinical presentation

Merkel cell carcinoma typically appears as a pink/purplish dermal nodule, resembling an insect bite or low-grade squamous or basal cell carcinoma of the skin (Fig 13.1). It should be included in the differential diagnosis of a solitary nonspecific dermal nodule in a patient over the age of 40. Some MCCs may have a subtly translucent clinical appearance, resembling a basal cell carcinoma [8]. As a large firm reddish nodule on the eyelid, it may mimic an angioma [11]. Less commonly, it may appear as bright red to purple confluent nodules and plaques on the scalp, similar to malignant angioendothelioma [12]. Recurrent MCC is often evident as dermal and subcutaneous nodules (Figs. 13.2 and 13.3). MCC may develop synchronously with multiple actinic keratoses, squamous cell carcinomas, and basal cell carcinomas [13–15].

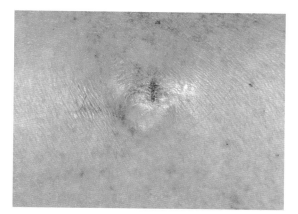

Fig. 13.1 Primary 3-cm MCC on the dorsal left forearm of a 55-year-old woman.

Staging and prognosis

Survival of patients with Merkel cell carcinoma is dependent on the stage of the disease at presentation, although overall survival at 5 years for all patients is approximately 65% (Table 13.1). Although no American Joint Committee on Cancer staging system for MCC exists, data from the Memorial Sloan-Kettering Cancer Center (MSKCC) supports one based on tumor size, nodal status, and distant metastasis [3], as illustrated in Table 13.2. Patients who present with clinically localized disease are

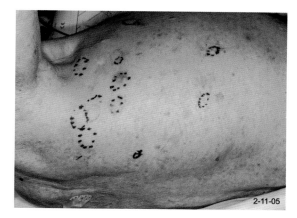

Fig. 13.2 Regionally recurrent subcutaneous MCC (*dotted circles*) on the back of an 88-year-old man following excision of a primary MCC.

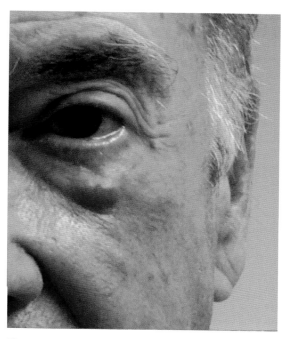

Fig. 13.3 Recurrent MCC in a 77-year-old man after empiric wide excision of the left cheek primary site, with 1 cm radial margins. Despite no pathologic evidence of residual tumor in a wide-excision specimen, the patient developed locally recurrent disease 3 months later.

stage I if the tumor is less than 2 cm and stage II if it is 2 cm or greater. Those with pathologically confirmed nodal metastasis are stage III. Patients with distant metastasis are stage IV.

Table 13.1 Five-year survival of patients with Merkel cell carcinoma

Author	Center	Patients, no.	Survival, %
Bielamowicz et al. [36]	UCLA	34	64
Smith et al. [37]	UCLA (Kaiser)	35	62[a]
Meeuwissen et al. [28]	Royal Brisbane	80	68[b]
Allen et al. [3]	MSKCC	251	64

[a]Projected.
[b]Thirty-six months survival.

Table 13.2 Memorial Sloan-Kettering staging system for patients with Merkel cell carcinoma

Tumor (T)	Nodes (N)	Metastases (M)	Stage
1 (< 2 cm)	0	0	I
2 (≥2 cm)	0	0	II
Any	1	0	III
Any	Any	1	IV

Source: Allen et al. [3].

Patients with a locally advanced primary lesion (stage II), regional nodal disease (stage III), or evidence of distant metastasis (stage IV) should undergo an extent of disease evaluation consisting of cross-sectional imaging of the head, chest, abdomen, and pelvis. Alternatively, or in addition, whole-body positron emission tomography scanning may be used [16]. Like melanoma, MCC has a propensity to metastasize to many sites, particularly regional nodes, lung, liver, brain, and bone.

In a large single-institution experience of patients with stage I and II disease, factors associated with improved survival in univariate analysis were primary tumor less than 2 cm, negative surgical margins, and head and neck site. The only independent predictor of outcome was presentation with early-stage disease. The disease-free survival for all patients with a median follow-up of 35 months was 76% [3]. Optimal local and regional control makes long-term survival or cure possible in more than half of patients with initially localized disease [9].

Management of the primary lesion

Wide local excision of the primary MCC is an essential component of management in patients with localized disease (Table 13.3). Optimal surgical margins are at least 2 cm [9]. Excision margins of less than 3 cm were associated with a trend toward increased local recurrence in a large retrospective analysis of a single-institution experience. The excision should include the skin and subcutaneous tissue, as well as the underlying fascia when the tumor is close to it. In anatomic areas where optimal surgical margins cannot be obtained, adjuvant radiation therapy to the primary site after optimal surgical excision should be used, when feasible. Dermal lymphatic spread is a common route of dissemination. Procedures that are performed with the goal of obtaining "negative" surgical margins are meaningless. Wide empiric margins should be obtained.

Table 13.3 Local and regional management of Merkel cell carcinoma

Primary Site	Management
Trunk, proximal extremity	Excision, with 2–3 cm margins
Head and neck, distal extremity	Excision, with 1–2 cm margins; adjuvant RT[a]
Locally recurrent disease	Re-excision; consider adjuvant RT[a]
Any site, positive or close margin	Adjuvant RT[a] following optimal excision
Regional Nodes	
Trunk, extremity, SLN (+)	Completion lymphadenectomy
Trunk, extremity, clinically node (+)	Therapeutic lymphadenectomy; consider adjuvant RT
Head and neck, SLN (+) or clinically node (+)	Completion lymphadenectomy; consider adjuvant RT[a]
Head and neck, SLN (−)	Consider adjuvant RT to primary and regional basin
Recurrent Disease	
Local	Excision and RT[a] if not already given
Regional	Excision and RT[a] if not already given

[a]5500 to 6000 cGy over 4 to 6 weeks.

(+), positive; (−), negative; RT, radiation therapy; SLN, sentinel lymph node.

Although positive margins are clearly concerning, negative margins do not mean that adequate local therapy has been performed.

It is often difficult to excise MCC of the head/neck or distal extremity with a wide margin. Adjuvant radiotherapy (5500 to 6000 cGy over 6 weeks) should be strongly considered in this setting. Patients who develop a local recurrence following primary excision, regardless of site, should undergo re-excision, if possible. Adjuvant radiotherapy should be considered.

Mohs micrographic surgery has been proposed as a reasonable therapeutic option in patients with MCC. O'Connor and colleagues [17] retrospectively evaluated 12 patients treated with Mohs surgery alone for their primary tumor compared with eight patients treated with Mohs surgery and adjuvant radiation therapy (RT). Of the patients treated with Mohs surgery alone, one had a local recurrence and four developed regional metastasis. Of patients treated with Mohs surgery and adjuvant RT, none developed a local or regional recurrence. This observation was confirmed by Boyer and colleagues [18], who noted four locoregional recurrences in 25 patients treated with Mohs surgery alone and none in 20 treated with Mohs and adjuvant RT to the primary site (8/20) or primary site and regional nodes (12/20). The capacity for MCC to disseminate in a noncontiguous fashion via the dermal lymphatics may eliminate the advantage of Mohs surgery alone in the management of primary MCC. Obtaining wide empiric margins of grossly normal tissue and judicious use of adjuvant RT is, in my opinion, a more rational strategy.

Regional lymph nodes

Controversy regarding the management of clinically negative regional lymph nodes has been eliminated with the use of sentinel lymph node (SLN) mapping for patients with MCC [19–21] (Table 13.3). Approximately 25% of patients with MCC will be found to have metastatic disease in the SLN [22,23]. When the SLN is found to contain metastatic MCC, a completion lymphadenectomy should be performed. Early removal of microscopic disease in regional nodes detected by SLN biopsy may afford the patient a greater opportunity for cure than expectant management of the regional nodal basin, although this remains unproven [24]. In our experience, patients with clinically node-negative MCC who undergo pathologic nodal staging with either an elective lymph node dissection or SLN biopsy have a 5-year disease-specific survival of 97% (n = 55) [3].

Unfortunately, more than half of patients who undergo regional lymphadenectomy for clinically positive nodes (palpable disease) will die of distant disease, [3,9,25] an experience similar to that of patients with metastatic melanoma [26].

Adjuvant chemotherapy and radiation therapy

Merkel cell carcinoma is a highly malignant tumor. The treating physician should enlist the assistance of radiation and medical oncology colleagues for individuals at high risk for recurrence due to suboptimal surgical margins, advanced tumor size, or stage III disease, or poor prognostic features of the primary MCC, such as lymphatic tumor emboli.

Merkel cell carcinoma is a radiosensitive tumor. Adjuvant RT has been advocated for local as well as regional disease control [27,28]. In a recent review, Lewis and colleagues [29] reported significant reductions in local (hazard ratio [HR], 0.27) and regional (HR, 0.34) recurrence when adjuvant radiation was given to the primary or regional nodal bed, respectively. Allen and associates [3] found that local recurrence after surgical resection of primary MCC was uncommon, occurring in only 8% of patients. It was not more common in those who did not receive adjuvant radiotherapy after resection of the primary cancer. Others have observed a much higher risk of local recurrence for surgical resection alone, although these reports are difficult to interpret because of the heterogeneous nature of the patients described [28]. The use of RT as a primary, adjuvant, or therapeutic modality in the patient with MCC must be individualized and requires considerable judgment on the part of the treating physician.

Radiation therapy is important when wide radial margins cannot be obtained or in those found to have pathologically close or involved margins after optimal excision of the primary tumor. Adjuvant radiation to the nodal bed following complete lymphadenectomy in patients with microscopically positive lymph nodes is rarely required for regional control, as nodal basin recurrence in this setting is uncommon [3,24]. As in patients with advanced regional melanoma, adjuvant radiation to a nodal basin following removal of clinically apparent regional disease should be strongly considered. It is always important to consider, however, that management of patients with local or regional recurrence of MCC may be particularly difficult in the setting of previous RT.

Patients with large primary tumors or palpable disease in regional nodes are at significant risk for systemic failure. Adjuvant chemotherapy in an otherwise fit patient should be strongly considered. Although the rarity of the tumor precludes randomized trials to assess the value of adjuvant chemotherapy, recurrent MCC in lymph nodes or distant sites is almost invariably fatal. In this setting, it is certainly reasonable to consider adjuvant chemotherapy in an attempt to decrease this risk. Patients with systemic metastasis are commonly treated with chemotherapy similar to that used for patients with small cell carcinoma, with response rates reported in 50% to 60% of patients. For this reason, these same agents are rational choices in the adjuvant setting. As in patients with small cell carcinoma, concurrent chemotherapy and RT is a common approach.

Poulsen and colleagues [30] reported no survival advantage in a prospective cohort of 40 patients with high-risk MCC treated with concurrent chemotherapy (carboplatin and etoposide) and radiotherapy (50 Gy in 25 fractions over 5 weeks) to the primary site and regional nodal basin as part of a phase II trial when compared with 62 historical controls who met the eligibility criteria. It is difficult to generalize from this study because the patients were quite heterogeneous. A significant proportion who were treated had residual disease; therefore, the therapy was not "adjuvant." In addition, the ability of the study to detect an advantage to chemoradiation was limited.

The toxicity of concurrent chemoradiation is considerable. Poulsen and colleagues [31] reported that the most significant finding was neutropenia,

although 35 of 40 patients were able to complete the planned four cycles. The median age of patients in the trial was 67 years. There were no treatment-related deaths.

Adjuvant chemotherapy should be considered in the high-risk patient who is otherwise well. High-risk patients include those with advanced primary tumors, locally recurrent disease, and regional nodal metastasis. Appropriate regimens include cisplatin, carboplatin, or etoposide. Concurrent RT may be given in patients who are otherwise fit, although evidence for a survival advantage with this approach is lacking. The dosage of RT administered is generally 4500 to 5000 cGy in 180 to 200 cGy fractions [32].

Chemotherapy for metastatic disease

Several investigators observed favorable response rates in patients with metastatic MCC using a variety of agents [33,34]. Complete responses were noted in 33% of patients (median duration, 6 months) and partial responses in 23%. Chemotherapy using a small cell regime with platinum-based chemotherapy was used [35] and is currently recommended in the National Comprehensive Cancer Network guidelines for MCC [32]. Treatment is considered palliative, as cure of patients with distant metastatic disease has not been documented.

Follow-up of patients with clinically localized disease

The median time to recurrence for patients with clinically localized MCC that will recur after treatment is short, approximately 8 months [17,30]. The vast majority (>90%) who develop local or regional disease that recurs will have the recurrence within the first 2 years [3]. Consequently, close clinical surveillance during this interval is important, although there is no evidence that early detection of recurrence will affect outcome.

Conclusions

The opportunity to cure patients with MCC occurs at presentation with clinically localized disease.

Wide radial margins of excision, regional nodal staging, and selective use of adjuvant RT form the cornerstone of treatment for patients in this setting [3,24,30,33]. SLN mapping should be strongly considered in patients with clinically negative regional nodes because it provides important prognostic information and allows selection of patients for additional regional nodal therapy as well as consideration of adjuvant chemotherapy. Adjuvant RT and chemotherapy, often given simultaneously, may be recommended in patients found to have clinically positive regional lymph nodes, although convincing evidence for a benefit is lacking. Treatment of patients with distant metastasis is palliative, but clinical responses may be obtained in approximately half of them.

References

1 Toker C. Trabecular carcinoma of the skin. Arch Dermatol 1972;105:107–10.

2 Halata Z, Grim M, Bauman KI. Friedrich Sigmund Merkel and his "Merkel cell," morphology, development, and physiology: review and new results. Anat Rec A Discov Mol Cell Evol Biol 2003;271:225–39.

3 Allen PJ, Bowne WB, Jaques DP, et al. Merkel cell carcinoma: prognosis and treatment of patients from a single institution. J Clin Oncol 2005;23:2300–9.

4 An KP, Ratner D. Merkel cell carcinoma in the setting of HIV infection. J Am Acad Dermatol 2001;45:309–12.

5 Boyle F, Pendlebury S, Bell D. Further insights into the natural history and management of primary cutaneous neuroendocrine (Merkel cell) carcinoma. Int J Radiat Oncol Biol Phys 1995;31:315–23.

6 Catlett JP, Todd WM, Carr ME Jr. Merkel cell tumor in an HIV-positive patient. Va Med Q 1992;119:256–8.

7 Hodgson NC. Merkel cell carcinoma: changing incidence trends. J Surg Oncol 2005;89:1–4.

8 Schwartz RA, Lambert WC. The Merkel cell carcinoma: a 50-year retrospect. J Surg Oncol 2005;89:5.

9 Yiengpruksawan A, Coit DG, Thaler HT, et al. Merkel cell carcinoma. Prognosis and management. Arch Surg 1991;126:1514–9.

10 Leech SN, Kolar AJ, Barrett PD, et al. Merkel cell carcinoma can be distinguished from metastatic small cell carcinoma using antibodies to cytokeratin 20 and thyroid transcription factor 1. J Clin Pathol 2001;54:727–9.

11 Kase S, Yoshida K, Osaki M, et al. Expression of erythropoietin receptor in human Merkel cell carcinoma of the eyelid. Anticancer Res 2006;26:4535–7.

12 Tyring SK, Lee PC, Omura EF, et al. Recurrent and metastatic cutaneous neuroendocrine (Merkel cell) carcinoma mimicking angiosarcoma. Arch Dermatol 1987;123:1368–70.

13 Aydin A, Kocer NE, Bekerecioglu M, et al. Cutaneous undifferentiated small (Merkel) cell carcinoma, that developed synchronously with multiple actinic keratoses, squamous cell carcinomas and basal cell carcinoma. J Dermatol 2003;30:241–4.

14 Boutilier R, Desormeau L, Cragg F, et al. Merkel cell carcinoma: squamous and atypical fibroxanthoma-like differentiation in successive local tumor recurrences. Am J Dermatopathol 2001;23:46–9.

15 Cottoni F, Montesu MA, Lissia A, et al. Merkel cell carcinoma, Kaposi's sarcoma, basal cell carcinoma and keratoacanthoma: multiple association in a patient with chronic lymphatic leukaemia. Br J Dermatol 2002;147:1029–31.

16 Belhocine T, Pierard GE, Fruhling J, et al. Clinical added-value of 18FDG PET in neuroendocrine-Merkel cell carcinoma. Oncol Rep 2006;16:347–52.

17 O'Connor WJ, Roenigk RK, Brodland DG. Merkel cell carcinoma. Comparison of Mohs micrographic surgery and wide excision in eighty-six patients. Dermatol Surg 1997;23:929–33.

18 Boyer JD, Zitelli JA, Brodland DG, et al. Local control of primary Merkel cell carcinoma: review of 45 cases treated with Mohs micrographic surgery with and without adjuvant radiation. J Am Acad Dermatol 2002;47:885–92.

19 Pfeifer T, Weinberg H, Brady MS. Lymphatic mapping for Merkel cell carcinoma. J Am Acad Dermatol 1997;37:650–1.

20 Ames SE, Krag DN, Brady MS. Radiolocalization of the sentinel lymph node in Merkel cell carcinoma: a clinical analysis of seven cases. J Surg Oncol 1998;67:251–4.

21 Hill AD, Brady MS, Coit DG. Intraoperative lymphatic mapping and sentinel lymph node biopsy for Merkel cell carcinoma. Br J Surg 1999;86:518–21.

22 Allen PJ, Zhang ZF, Coit DG. Surgical management of Merkel cell carcinoma. Ann Surg 1999;229:97–105.

23 Messina JL, Reintgen DS, Cruse CW, et al. Selective lymphadenectomy in patients with Merkel cell (cutaneous neuroendocrine) carcinoma. Ann Surg Oncol 1997;4:389–95.

24 Mehrany K, Otley CC, Weenig RH, et al. A meta-analysis of the prognostic significance of sentinel

lymph node status in Merkel cell carcinoma. Dermatol Surg 2002;28:113–7; discussion 117.

25 Shaw JH, Rumball E. Merkel cell tumour: clinical behaviour and treatment. Br J Surg 1991;78:138–42.

26 Balch CM, Buzaid AC, Soong SJ, et al. Final version of the American Joint Committee on Cancer staging system for cutaneous melanoma. J Clin Oncol 2001;19: 3635–48.

27 Suntharalingam M, Rudoltz MS, Mendenhall WM, et al. Radiotherapy for Merkel cell carcinoma of the skin of the head and neck. Head Neck 1995;17:96–101.

28 Meeuwissen JA, Bourne RG, Kearsley JH. The importance of postoperative radiation therapy in the treatment of Merkel cell carcinoma. Int J Radiat Oncol Biol Phys 1995;31:325–31.

29 Lewis KG, Weinstock MA, Weaver AL, et al. Adjuvant local irradiation for Merkel cell carcinoma. Arch Dermatol 2006;142:693–700.

30 Poulsen MG, Rischin D, Porter I, et al. Does chemotherapy improve survival in high-risk stage I and II Merkel cell carcinoma of the skin? Int J Radiat Oncol Biol Phys 2006;64:114–9.

31 Poulsen M, Rischin D, Walpole E, et al. Analysis of toxicity of Merkel cell carcinoma of the skin treated with synchronous carboplatin/etoposide and radiation: a Trans-Tasman Radiation Oncology Group study. Int J Radiat Oncol Biol Phys 2001;51:156–63.

32 Miller SJ, Alam M, Andersen J, et al. Merkel cell carcinoma. J Natl Compr Canc Netw 2006;4:704–12.

33 Voog E, Biron P, Martin JP, et al. Chemotherapy for patients with locally advanced or metastatic Merkel cell carcinoma. Cancer 1999;85:2589–95.

34 Tai PT, Yu E, Winquist E, et al. Chemotherapy in neuroendocrine/Merkel cell carcinoma of the skin: case series and review of 204 cases. J Clin Oncol 2000;18:2493–9.

35 Feun LG, Savaraj N, Legha SS, et al. Chemotherapy for metastatic Merkel cell carcinoma. Review of the M.D. Anderson Hospital's experience. Cancer 1988;62:683–5.

36 Bielamowicz S, Smith D, Abemayor E. Merkel cell carcinoma: an aggressive skin neoplasm. Laryngoscope. 1994;104:528–32.

37 Smith DE, Bielamowicz S, Kagan AR, Anderson PJ, Peddada AV. Cutaneous neuroendocrine (Merkel cell) carcinoma. A report of 35 cases. Am J Clin Oncol 1995;18:199–203.

CHAPTER 14
Dermatitic precursors of mycosis fungoides

W. Clark Lambert and Robert A. Schwartz

It has long been recognized in dermatology that certain apparent longstanding, recalcitrant dermatoses have the potential to develop into an overt cutaneous lymphoma or lymphoma-like condition, particularly mycosis fungoides, [1–3] as discussed in Chapter 15 on cutaneous lymphomas. Some of these apparent longstanding dermatoses were considered to be definable as one or another of a cluster of diseases known as the parapsoriasis group; the remainder, despite resemblance in some cases to diseases such as atopic or seborrheic dermatitis early in their course, were considered to have been lymphoma/mycosis fungoides all along but not to have manifested themselves clearly as such until quite late in their course. This led, in turn, to a theory that certain disorders in the parapsoriasis group are also, in fact, early stages of mycosis fungoides.

The concepts of development of mycosis fungoides and related conditions in skin that are currently evolving are quite different from the above. Epidemiologic studies show that certain cohorts of cases of industrial contact dermatitis develop mycosis fungoides in a high proportion of cases [4]. Some mycosis fungoides patients have an occupational etiology, but only a small fraction of exposed workers are apparently susceptible, because the disease is so rare [5]. Most cases of mycosis fungoides develop following dermatitic conditions other than the parapsoriases [6,7]; it now appears that a large number of, and perhaps any, longstanding dermatitic conditions may give rise to lymphoma/mycosis fungoides and that they do so in a small minority of cases [1]. This is analogous to development of cancer in other organs following a chronic non-neoplastic condi-

tion; examples are development of bladder cancer following schistosomiasis and development of liver cancer following certain types of cirrhosis [8]. Classical experiments performed by Dr. Michael Potter and others of the National Cancer Institute in animals [9] and equally classical observations of Dr. Elliot Osserman and his colleagues at Columbia on human tissue [10] have established that a similar development of cancer following longstanding pathologic stimulation occurs in the immune system (reviewed in Lambert [1]). Such "premycotic eruptions" (i.e., pre–mycosis fungoides eruptions) thus consist of at least several longstanding, usually severe, recalcitrant inflammatory dermatoses [1].

Clinical recognition of dermatitic precursors of mycosis fungoides

Dermatitis

It has been clearly documented that longstanding contact dermatitis may eventuate in malignancy [4]. In our experience, a number of cases of atopic dermatitis and a few with seborrheic dermatitis in which involvement was severe and widespread have developed this complication. Epidemiologic studies have given inconsistent results regarding whether or not frequent inflammatory dermatoses or industrial exposure progress to mycosis fungoides [3,5,7,11,12]. The small frequency of this complication as well as the heterogeneity of some of the population studied would appear to account for this discrepancy.

Among dermatitides other than the parapsoriasis group, there is no clear information regarding which type of dermatitis is likely to give rise to a malignancy. Rather, there are certain common features of these dermatoses that are clues that mycosis fungoides may be developing. There are (1) pruritus in a lesion that has been only slightly pruritic or nonpruritic in the past; (2) induration, especially in an irregular "blotchy" distribution; and (3) progressive lymphadenopathy correlating with affected regions. A fourth sign, which is completely absent in some cases but quite striking in others, is poikiloderma. *Poikiloderma* is a contraction of the full term, *poikiloderma vasculare atrophicans*, meaning mottled hypo- and hyperpigmentation (*poikilo-*) with vascular involvement (*vasculare*) and, most of all, progressive atrophy (*atrophicans*; note the Latin ablative case [ending in -*ans* rather than -*us*], indicating "toward"—hence progressive atrophy of the skin [*derma*]). All these changes must be evident for poikiloderma to be said to be present. In current usage, the full term, *poikiloderma vasculare atrophicans*, is reserved to denote individuals who show a generalized poikiloderma, as opposed to those who show only a more localized distribution of it [13]. In addition to cutaneous lymphoma, poikiloderma may be a precursor of squamous cell carcinoma [14,15].

Poikiloderma may occur as a part of, particularly a late stage of, a number of disorders, including lichen planus and chronic exposure to cold. It may occur in a case of frank mycosis fungoides as well, but this should not cause one to regard all examples of poikiloderma as mycosis fungoides; it is just further evidence that this is a cutaneous syndrome that may be seen in a large number of quite different conditions. The term *poikiloderma vasculare atrophicans* has also been misused as a synonym for large plaque parapsoriasis, discussed below. Although large plaque parapsoriasis may indeed present as poikiloderma, and even as an example of generalized poikiloderma, it is inappropriate to use the term *poikiloderma vasculare atrophicans* as a synonym for it. There are clear examples of generalized poikiloderma that are neither a parapsoriasis nor mycosis fungoides. Perhaps the most unique example of which the authors are aware is of an erotic dancer who consumed large quantities of phenolphthalein to cause her skin to glow under the weak long-wavelength ultravio-

let (UV) light used in her place of work [16]. She subsequently developed generalized poikiloderma.

Parapsoriasis

Although they are grouped under a single heading, there is considerable doubt regarding the extent to which the diseases in this group are actually related. The term *parapsoriasis* was coined by Brocq [17] in 1902 as part of a now long-forgotten grand scheme to link together in an organized way all the inflammatory dermatoses. It is thus not clear whether anyone ever intended this to be an organized group designation. The nomenclature of this group has been badly confused. The diseases and their synonyms are listed in Table 14.1. We now examine each of these in turn, beginning with large plaque parapsoriasis, which has a 10% to 20% chance (with some authors claiming up to 50%; see Chapter 15) of giving rise to a cutaneous lymphoma and which is thus particularly relevant to our discussion. A brief summary of the major features of these disorders is provided in Table 14.2.

Large plaque parapsoriasis

Large plaque parapsoriasis (Figs. 14.1 and 14.2) is an uncommon but not rare disorder that occurs in middle life [2]. It has an extremely slow onset and tends to persist for years to decades, with little tendency toward clearing. One sees large, very poorly defined plaques, which are usually atrophic and may be poikilodermatous. The lesions are usually nonindurated or only very slightly indurated. Lesions tend to occur on the buttocks, thighs, and axillae, and in women, on and under the breasts. Retiform parapsoriasis (Fig. 14.3) is a variant in which the lesions are extremely atrophic, tend to be generalized, and show a netlike or retiform pattern that is probably related to the underlying vasculature, although this has not been proven.

In large plaque parapsoriasis, as in other potentially premycotic dermatoses, one must be concerned that mycosis fungoides may be developing if the lesions become increasingly pruritic; if the lesions become indurated, especially in a blotchy or irregular pattern; and if lymphadenopathy develops or increases. Perhaps the most significant predisposing sign is progressive poikiloderma,

Table 14.1 Nomenclature of the parapsoriases

Disease Entity	Synonyms
Large plaque parapsoriasis[a,b]	Large plaque (atrophic) parapsoriasis[c] LPAP[c] Atrophic parapsoriasis[c] Poikilodermatous parapsoriasis[c] Parapsoriasis en plaques,[c] large plaque type Parapsoriasis en plaques,[d] atrophic type Parapsoriasis en grandes plaques simples Parapsoriasis en grandes plaques poikilodermiques Lichenoid stage of mycosis fungoides Poikilodermic mycosis fungoides Prereticulotic dermatitis Prereticulotic poikiloderma Parapsoriasis en plaques[b,d,e] Poikiloderma vasculare atrophicans[e,f] Parapsoriasis lichenoides[e,g]
Variant: retiform parapsoriasis[h]	Parapsoriasis variegata[c,g] Parakeratosis variegata[c] Lichen variegatus Parapsoriasis lichenoides[e,g]
Small plaque parapsoriasis[a,b]	Parapsoriasis en plaque,[d] small plaque type Parapsoriasis en plaques,[d] simple discrete type Parapsoriasis en plaques,[d] benign type Leopard-spot parapsoriasis Chronic superficial dermatitis[e] Parapsoriasis en plaques[b,d,e]
Variant: digitate dermatosis[i] perstans[i,j,k]	Fingerprint parapsoriasis[i]
Pityriasis lichenoides[l] Acute[l]	Parapsoriasis guttata[c,g,e] Pityriasis lichenoides et varioliformis acuta[c] PLEVA[c] PLVA[c] Mucha-Habermann disease[c] Parapsoriasis lichenoides et varioliformis acuta Parapsoriasis varioliformis Parapsoriasis acuta[g] Acute guttate parapsoriasis Acute pityriasis lichenoides
Chronic[l]	Pityriasis lichenoides chronica[c,g] Parapsoriasis lichenoides chronica[g] Chronic guttate parapsoriasis

especially progressive atrophy, in affected areas. The more common form of large plaque parapsoriasis, with poorly demarcated, atrophic plaques on the buttocks, thighs, axillae, and, in women, breasts, gives rise to mycosis fungoides in about 10% to 20% of cases. Retiform parapsoriasis, perhaps because of its more widespread distribution and more severe atrophy, appears to progress toward a malignancy in a high proportion of cases–certainly more than half. Retiform parapsoriasis is extremely rare, however, so much so that there are simply not enough cases reported to give an accurate probability that this will happen in any one case. It is an extremely striking lesion in most cases, so it is easily recognized despite its rarity. It was the first of the parapsoriases to be reported in the literature [18].

---

[a]Some authorities consider large plaque and small plaque parapsoriasis to be a single entity, usually termed *parapsoriasis en plaques*.
[b]The term *Brocq's disease* is sometimes used to denote small and large plaque parapsoriasis together as a single entity; less commonly, it is used to denote one or more of the other parapsoriases.
[c]Preferred synonyms, based on frequent usage.
[d]*Parapsoriasis en plaques* is pronounced with the final *s* silent, misleading some English-speaking authors to misspell it *parapsoriasis en plaque*.
[e]These terms are frequently used by different authors to denote completely different diseases. For this reason, their use is not recommended.
[f]Poikiloderma vasculare atrophicans is sometimes labeled *poikiloderma atrophicans vasculare*. Either term is acceptable.
[g]When equivalent terms in different languages are in common use, only the Latin name is given (e.g., parapsoriasis guttata [guttate parapsoriasis, parapsoriasis en gouttes, or en gotas]; parapsoriasis lichenoides [lichenoid parapsoriasis, parapsoriasis lichenoides]; parapsoriasis variegata [variegate parapsoriasis]).
[h]Some authorities regard retiform parapsoriasis as a separate entity.
[i]Some authors regard digitate dermatosis, of which fingerprint parapsoriasis is a synonym and xanthoerythrodermia perstans a variant, as a separate entity.
[j]Xanthoerythrodermia perstans is a variant of digitate dermatosis in which the lesions are yellow in color on clinical examination. It is sometimes incorrectly applied to other forms of parapsoriasis with yellow lesions.
[k]*Xanthoerythrodermia perstans* is an unnecessary term that should be avoided.
[l]Some authors consider acute and chronic pityriasis lichenoides to be separate entities.
Source: Adapted from Lambert WC, Everett MA. The nosology of parapsoriasis. J Am Acad Dermatol 1981;5:373–395.

Table 14.2 Major characteristics of the parapsoriases (including pityriasis lichenoides)

Type	Clinical Features	Histopathology	Prognosis
Large plaque parapsoriasis	Slightly indurated, reddish blue, scaly plaques with indiscrete, irregular borders that occur mainly on the buttocks, proximal extremities, and in women, the breasts; most are <10 cm in diameter; atrophy is often present	Early, not diagnostic; later atypical large lymphocytes may be seen, notably in epidermis	Persists for years to decades; about 10% progress to lymphoma cutis
Variant: retiform parapsoriasis	Generalized netlike distribution of red to brown, shiny, flat-topped scaling papules; atrophy is usually prominent	Similar to large plaque parapsoriasis with atrophic changes most prominent	Same as above
Small plaque parapsoriasis	Nonindurated reddish blue to yellowish scaling plaques with distinct, regular borders that occur mainly on the trunk; most are <5 cm in diameter; lesions on the proximal extremities may be larger	Not diagnostic, but some features may be useful in differential diagnosis	Persists for years to decades with no malignancy potential
Variant: digitate dermatosis	Same as above, but lesions are in a palisaded pattern following dermatomes	Same as above	Same as above
Pityriasis lichenoides Acute	Generalized red to brown, often necrotic, vesicular or hemorrhagic scaling papules at different stages of evolution; the lesions may recur in acute exacerbations	Broad regions of parakeratosis, focal epidermal necrosis, dilatation and hemorrhage of small blood vessels in the papillary dermis; wedge-shaped lymphohistiocytic inflammatory infiltrate; atypical lymphocytes may be present	Lesions clear spontaneously after weeks to months, leaving scars
Chronic	Lesions as described above but less severe, less variable, sometimes more scaly	Similar to but milder than above and with no necrosis or atypical cells in most patients	Individual lesions may persist for weeks, process for years

Small plaque parapsoriasis

Small plaque parapsoriasis has no potential to give rise to a cutaneous lymphoma; it is mentioned here solely because of the possibility of confusing it with large plaque parapsoriasis, a completely different disease. In the older literature, the two were lumped together as a single entity [8]. Small plaque parapsoriasis, like large plaque parapsoriasis, occurs primarily in adulthood, in middle life, and shows plaques on the trunk, but there the clinical similarity ends. In small plaque parapsoriasis, erythematous, slightly scaly lesions occur over the entire torso and extend out to involve the proximal aspects of the extremities. Lesions are well demarcated, nonatrophic, and small, averaging less than 5 cm in diameter, although a few larger or confluent areas may

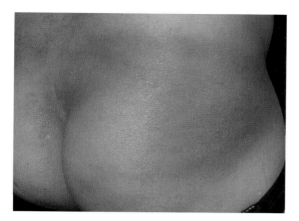

Fig. 14.1 Parapsoriasis, large plaque, early, without atrophy (courtesy of Professor Wiesław Gliński, Chairman, Dermatology, Medical University of Warsaw).

be seen on the proximal aspects of the extremities (Fig. 14.4).

Digitate dermatosis is a disorder that is quite similar to small plaque parapsoriasis in most respects and may represent a variation of it [8,19–22]. The two entities have indistinguishable histopathologies and differ clinically only by the shape and distribution of plaques, which in digitate dermatosis are elongated and tend to occur on the trunk with the long axis along dermatomes. *Xanthoerythrodermia perstans* is an older term that denotes cases of digitate dermatosis in which the lesions have a yellow color.

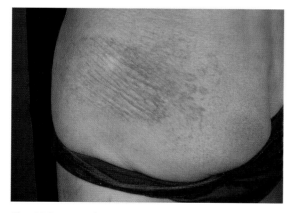

Fig. 14.2 Large plaque parapsoriasis, showing large atrophic plaque.

The origin of the yellow color is not clear, but it does not appear to be the result of lipid accumulation. Lesions of this color are also sometimes seen in the ordinary form of small plaque parapsoriasis.

Like large plaque parapsoriasis, small plaque parapsoriasis is uncommon but by no means rare. We are not aware of any reports of small plaque parapsoriasis eventuating in malignancy. One recent study suggested that "digitiform parapsoriasis" could be an early stage of mycosis fungoides [23].

Pityriasis lichenoides and lymphomatoid papulosis

Pityriasis lichenoides is a completely different disorder, both clinically and histologically, from either large plaque parapsoriasis or small plaque parapsoriasis [24–28]. It includes pityriasis lichenoides et varioliformis acuta (PLEVA), febrile ulceronecrotic Mucha-Habermann disease (a subtype of PLEVA), and pityriasis lichenoides chronica. It occurs in a slightly younger age group, mostly teenage to middle life, although there is broad overlap between the age distributions. Clinically, one sees numerous papules, distributed over the entire trunk, each of which shows a progression from a simple erythematous lesion to a scaly process that may show ulceration, hemorrhage, and even necrosis (Fig. 14.5). Each individual lesion tends to last for several weeks; the entire process lasts from weeks to years. The lesions are asymptomatic and tend to resolve, each leaving a small scar. The single most diagnostic feature of the disease is that each lesion progresses through its course completely independently of the others, so a lesion at the beginning of its course may be alongside an advanced or resolving lesion. The lesions may, however, occur in acute exacerbations, or "crops." In the acute form, the above changes are observed and the course of the disease is weeks to months; in chronic pityriasis lichenoides, the lesions are less severe and less variable, with less tendency to ulcerate, but may be more scaly, and the disease lasts for months to years. Despite earlier convictions that pityriasis lichenoides is a benign inflammatory dermatosis, some consider both acute and chronic pityriasis lichenoides to be a form of indolent cutaneous T-cell dyscrasia with limited

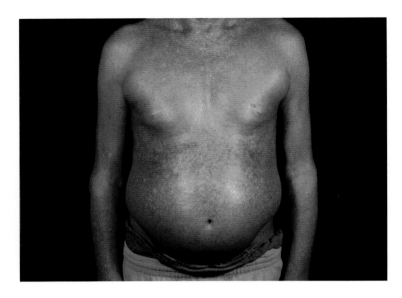

Fig. 14.3 Retiform parapsoriasis with netlike distribution of atrophic lesions and associated erythroderma.

propensity for progression into mycosis fungoides [28].

In *lymphomatoid papulosis* [29–32], lesions appear clinically quite similar to those of pityriasis lichenoides but histologically show large numbers of atypical lymphoid cells in the dermis. Although some authors feel that lesions of lymphomatoid papulosis tend to be larger, more indurated, and more plaque-like than those of pityriasis lichenoides [1], in our experience there is such extensive clinical overlap that they are for all useful purposes indistinguishable. A follicular variant of lymphomatoid papulosis has also been reported [32]. A distribution along hair follicles, or follicular lymphomatoid

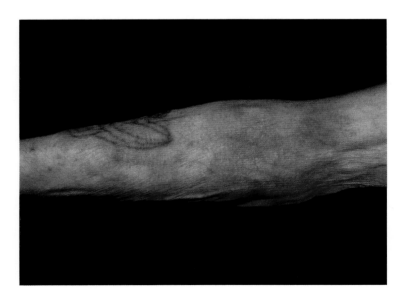

Fig. 14.4 Small plaque parapsoriasis.

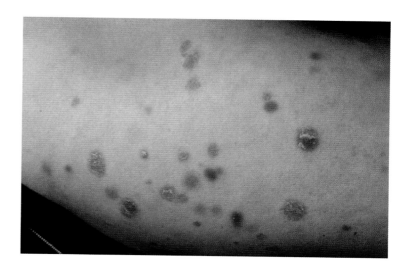

Fig. 14.5 Lymphomatoid papulosis.

papulosis, was observed in five biopsy specimens of 85 cases examined in one series.

Lymphomatoid papulosis is a lymphoproliferative disorder of CD30+ T cells that may be associated with other lymphoid malignancies, particularly Hodgkin's disease, mycosis fungoides, and anaplastic T-cell lymphomas [32–35]. Some cases of lymphomatoid papulosis may show, histologically, varying numbers of large atypical cells with hypertetraploid karyotype (Willemze type A), whereas others show predominantly small, medium-sized, and large cerebriform mononuclear cells (Willemze type B). Other cases may show both cell types (Willemze type C). In one series of 85 patients, 78 had only one histopathologic subtype of lymphomatoid papulosis (64 had type A, 3 had type B, and 11 had type C) [32]. Type A lesions are said to be related to Hodgkin's disease and type B to mycosis fungoides. This separation of lesion types is by no means universally accepted or established.

Whereas pityriasis lichenoides does not give rise to malignancy, approximately 10% of cases of lymphomatoid papulosis eventuate in either mycosis fungoides or another lymphoma, particularly Hodgkin's disease [1]. It is thus essential to obtain at least three biopsies of all patients suspected of having either pityriasis lichenoides or lymphomatoid papulosis. Three biopsies are recommended to

rule out sampling error (see below). In very rare instances, lesions clinically, and to some extent histologically, resembling pityriasis lichenoides may be seen within lesions of otherwise typical large plaque parapsoriasis. This is the only known relationship between the two disorders.

Histopathological features

Both large plaque parapsoriasis and small plaque parapsoriasis show relatively nonspecific histopathology that may be indistinguishable from many inflammatory disorders. This consists of slight hyperkeratosis and acanthosis with a mild to moderate, diffuse perivascular lymphocytic infiltrate in the superficial dermis. In both large plaque parapsoriasis and chronic dermatitis of any type, when progression toward malignancy occurs, either of two patterns may be observed. In the first, the epidermis is not appreciably atrophic and is often acanthotic. Changes characteristic of the primary dermatosis may persist, or they may be difficult to recognize. For example, in cases of chronic widespread seborrheic dermatitis progressing toward a malignancy, one may see mounds of scale crust in the stratum corneum near sebaceous/pilosebaceous ostia. The dermis shows variable edema and a very variable lymphohistiocytic infiltrate, from barely perceptible to very marked, composed entirely of non-atypical cells. In the epidermis, however, one sees markedly atypical lymphocytes with convoluted, hyperchromatic nuclei occurring singly at all levels. These tend to be surrounded by a clear space, giving a "lump of coal on a pillow" appearance. A collection of these markedly atypical cells occurring together in the epidermis constitutes a Pautrier microabscess, which represents a later step in the process and is diagnostic of fully developed mycosis fungoides. Alternatively, one may see five or more such cells lined up just above the epidermal basement membrane; this is also diagnostic of mycosis fungoides. It is important to remember that non-atypical lymphocytes may occur singly or in nests in the epidermis in a number of conditions, including several different types of dermatitis and large and small plaque parapsoriasis. It is critical to not mistake these cells for the frankly atypical cells of the above processes.

In the second pattern showing development of mycosis fungoides in chronic dermatitis or large plaque parapsoriasis, the entire epidermis is markedly atrophic, with a thin, mainly orthokeratotic hyperkeratotic stratum corneum, basal vacuolar degeneration, and loss of distinctness of the basement membrane, with a variable lymphocytic infiltrate [36]. Atypical lymphocytes in the epidermis may become evident only relatively late in the process.

If either of these patterns is observed, incipient mycosis fungoides should be assumed and appropriate management measures taken. It is our belief that one should not wait until frank mycosis fungoides is present to initiate treatment of these patients, as discussed below. The histologic end point for development of mycosis fungoides from a precursor is very difficult to ascertain, and much disagreement exists among dermatopathologists. However, because the process is gradual, the diagnosis is not urgent, and one may wait for more definitive changes in subsequent biopsies.

In pityriasis lichenoides, a characteristic and often distinctive histologic presentation is observed. One sees broad and relatively uniform parakeratotic hyperkeratosis overlying the entire lesion. Neutrophils in the stratum corneum may also be seen. The epidermis shows inconsistent edema,

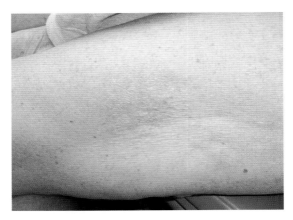

Fig. 14.6 Pagetoid reticulosis, evident as slightly scaly erythematous patch.

exocytosis of lymphocytes and neutrophils, and sometimes ulceration. In the dermis, a perivascular and partially bandlike junctional lymphocytic infiltrate is observed that extends into the dermis in a wedge-like manner, so as to resemble an inverted triangle with the apex deep and the base at the dermal–epidermal interface. Up to 10% of these lymphocytes may show mild to moderate atypia.

In lymphomatoid papulosis, one sees a process much like the above except that the lymphocytic infiltrate is denser and contains numerous markedly atypical cells. These are found in the dermis in contrast to early lesions of mycosis fungoides arising in a dermatitis or large plaque parapsoriasis. These atypical cells may resemble lymphocytes, histiocytes, or both, as noted above.

Sampling error is an important aspect of diagnosis and management of all of these conditions. Taking several biopsies at intervals of 6 months to 1 year is highly recommended.

Pagetoid reticulosis (Woringer-Kolopp disease)

Pagetoid reticulosis manifests clinically as slightly scaly or nonscaly erythematous patches that may occur anywhere on the skin (Fig. 14.6) [37–39]. Histologically, one sees a striking intraepidermal infiltration of mononuclear cells in a diffuse, scattered distribution more or less resembling that of a melanoma or Paget's disease. An underlying lymphohistiocytic inflammatory infiltrate is also seen. Several dozen cases of this rare disorder have been reported, predominately in middle-aged patients, about half appearing as localized patches and half as generalized disease clinically resembling mycosis fungoides, the so-called Ketron Goodman variant.

Ultrastructural and cell marker studies have shown that the epidermotropic infiltrate of this disease contains both T lymphocytes and cells of the macrophage series. Whether pagetoid reticulosis is best considered a precursor or a variant of mycosis fungoides is a matter of current debate, with the numbers of cases followed and reported at present too few to provide sufficient data to provide a clear answer. Individual cases of pagetoid reticulosis have been described in association with both large plaque parapsoriasis and mycosis fungoides [40,41]. Because of unequivocal similarities between pagetoid reticulosis and mycosis fungoides histologically, it is our opinion that pagetoid reticulosis is best considered a variant of mycosis fungoides.

Management

When faced with a dermatosis of whatever type that appears to be progressing toward a cutaneous lymphoma, it is the practice in some centers to offer no therapy, reserving treatment for the day that frank mycosis fungoides has manifested itself. There is some merit to this, because the patient is spared long and sometimes costly treatment until it is really needed, and because treatments that may be given for only a limited length of time or in limited dosages, such as electron-beam therapy, or to which the patient may become sensitized, such as topical nitrogen mustard, are saved for later when the disease is more advanced. If the disease is localized, photodynamic therapy [42] or direct laser therapy [37] may be considered.

The authors' approach, however, is quite different. We believe that a patient whose dermatosis is beginning to give rise to mycosis fungoides should be treated. It is possible to withhold certain therapies, such as those mentioned above, while giving frequent and comprehensive treatment with modalities such as fluorinated steroids or imiquimod [43],

usually given with an emollient; midrange UV-B light, with or without tar; or PUVA (psoralen plus long-wavelength UV-A light). Etretinate may also be useful and may reduce the amount of other modalities needed. One of us (WCL) used etretinate in patients from overseas before its release in the United States, with uniformly good results. These treatments may be used in any combination that keeps the dermatosis under good control, as near to clear as possible. The rule to follow is "very aggressive treatment with nonaggressive modalities." We have recommended this approach to a number of patients who have been referred to us precisely because their dermatosis was converting to a lymphoma. To date, none of those who have followed this type of regimen has developed mycosis fungoides to our knowledge. Further studies are needed, of course, to confirm and extend these findings or to modify them.

References

1 Lambert WC. Premycotic eruptions. Dermatol Clin 1985;3:629–45.

2 Vakeva L, Sarna S, Vaalasti A, et al. A retrospective study of the probability of the evolution of parapsoriasis en plaques into mycosis fungoides. Acta Derm Venereol 2005;85:318–23.

3 Morales-Suarez-Varela MM, Olsen J, Johansen P, et al. Occupational sun exposure and mycosis fungoides: a European multicenter case-control study. J Occup Environ Med 2006;48:390–3.

4 Cohen SR, Stenn KS, Braverman IM, et al. Clinicopathologic relationships, survival, and therapy in 59 patients with observations on occupation as a new prognostic factor. Cancer 1980;46:2654–66.

5 Morales-Suarez-Varela MM, Olsen J, Johansen P, et al. Occupational exposures and mycosis fungoides. A European multicentre case-control study (Europe). Cancer Causes Control 2005;16:1253–9.

6 Lambert WC, Cohen PJ, Schwartz RA. Surgical management of mycosis fungoides. J Med 1997;28:211–22.

7 Greene MH, Dalager NA, Lamberg SI, et al. Mycosis fungoides: epidemiologic observations. Cancer Treat Rep 1979;63:597–606.

8 Lambert WC, Everett MA. The nosology of parapsoriasis. J Am Acad Dermatol 1981;5:373–95.

9 Potter M, Pumphrey JG, Bailey DW. Genetics of susceptibility to plasmacytoma induction. I. BALB/cAnN

(C), C57BL/6N (B6), C57BL/Ka (BK), (C times B6)F1, (C times BK)F1, and C times B recombinant-inbred strains. J Natl Cancer Inst 1975;54:1413–7.

10 Isobe T, Osserman EF. Pathologic conditions associated with plasma cell dyscrasias: a study of 806 cases. Ann N Y Acad Sci 1971;190:507–18.

11 Whittemore AS, Holly EA, Lee IM, et al. Mycosis fungoides in relation to environmental exposures and immune response: a case-control study. J Natl Cancer Inst 1989;81:1560–7.

12 Teixeira F, Ortiz-Plata A, Cortes-Franco R, et al. Do environmental factors play any role in the pathogenesis of mycosis fungoides and Sezary syndrome? Int J Dermatol 1994;33:770–2.

13 Wain EM, Orchard GE, Whittaker SJ, et al. Outcome in 34 patients with juvenile-onset mycosis fungoides: a clinical, immunophenotypic, and molecular study. Cancer 2003;98:2282–90.

14 Colver G, Mortimer P, Dawber R. Premycotic poikiloderma, mycosis fungoides and cutaneous squamous cell carcinoma. Two cases and a discussion of their relevance. Int J Dermatol 1986;25:376–8.

15 Kreuter A, Hoffmamm K, Altmeyer P. A case of poikiloderma vasculare atrophicans, a rare variant of cutaneous T-cell lymphoma, responding to extracorporeal photopheresis. J Am Acad Dermatol 2005;52:706–8.

16 Zimmerman MC. Poikiloderma? Arch Dermatol 1971;104:450–1.

17 Brocq L. Les parapsoriasis. Ann Dermatol Syphilig (Paris) 1902;3:433–68.

18 Unna PG, Santi S, Pollitzer S. Ueber die Parakeratosen in Allegemeinen und eine neue Form derselben (Parakeratosis variegata). Monatschr Praktische Dermatol 1890;10:404–12.

19 Malhomme de la Roche HJ, Bunker CB. Digitate dermatosis responding to bicalutamide therapy. Clin Exp Dermatol 2006;31:590.

20 Hu CH, Winkelmann RK. Digitate dermatosis. A new look at symmetrical, small plaque parapsoriasis. Arch Dermatol 1973;107:65–9.

21 Radcliffe-Crocker H. Xanthoerythrodermia perstans. Br J Dermatol Syph 1905;17:119–34.

22 Alagheband M, Cairns ML, Chuang TY. Xanthoerythrodermia perstans and alopecia mucinosa in a patient with CD-30 cutaneous T-cell lymphoma. Cutis 1997;60:41–2.

23 Bernier C, Nguyen JM, Quereux G, et al. CD13 and TCR clone: markers of early mycosis fungoides. Acta Derm Venereol 2007;87:155–9.

24 Patel DG, Kihiczak G, Schwartz RA, et al. Pityriasis lichenoides. Cutis 2000;65:17–20, 23.

25 Ersoy-Evans S, Greco MF, Mancini AJ, et al. Pityriasis lichenoides in childhood: a retrospective review of 124 patients. J Am Acad Dermatol 2007;56:205–10.

26 Bowers S, Warshaw EM. Pityriasis lichenoides and its subtypes. J Am Acad Dermatol 2006;55:557–72; quiz 573–6.

27 Tsuji T, Kasamatsu M, Yokota M, et al. Mucha-Habermann disease and its febrile ulceronecrotic variant. Cutis 1996;58:123–31.

28 Magro CM, Crowson AN, Morrison C, et al. Pityriasis lichenoides chronica: stratification by molecular and phenotypic profile. Hum Pathol 2007;38:479–90.

29 Nijsten T, Curiel-Lewandrowski C, Kadin ME. Lymphomatoid papulosis in children: a retrospective cohort study of 35 cases. Arch Dermatol 2004;140:306–12.

30 Macaulay WL. Lymphomatoid papulosis. A continuing self-healing eruption, clinically benign–histologically malignant. Arch Dermatol 1968;97:23–30.

31 Macaulay WL. Lymphomatoid papulosis update. A historical perspective. Arch Dermatol 1989;125:1387–9.

32 El Shabrawi-Caelen L, Kerl H, Cerroni L. Lymphomatoid papulosis: reappraisal of clinicopathologic presentation and classification into subtypes A, B, and C. Arch Dermatol 2004;140:441–7.

33 Ribeiro-Silva A, Chang D, Arruda D, et al. Lymphomatoid papulosis in a patient with Waldenstrom's macroglobulinemia. J Dermatol 2005;32:132–6.

34 Gallardo F, Costa C, Bellosillo B, et al. Lymphomatoid papulosis associated with mycosis fungoides: clinicopathological and molecular studies of 12 cases. Acta Derm Venereol 2004;84:463–8.

35 Amir AR, Sheikh SS. Hodgkin's lymphoma with concurrent systemic amyloidosis, presenting as acute renal failure, following lymphomatoid papulosis. J Nephrol 2006;19:361–5.

36 Everett MA. Early diagnosis of mycosis fungoides: vacuolar interface dermatitis. J Cutan Pathol 1985;12:271–8.

37 Goldberg DJ, Stampien TM, Schwartz RA. Mycosis fungoides palmaris et plantaris: successful treatment with the carbon dioxide laser. Br J Dermatol 1997;136:617–9.

38 Cribier B. History: Frederic Woringer (1903–1964) and Woringer-Kolopp disease. Am J Dermatopathol 2005;27:534–45.

39 Steffen C. Ketron-Goodman disease, Woringer-Kolopp disease, and pagetoid reticulosis. Am J Dermatopathol 2005;27:68–85.

40 Pagnanelli G, Bianchi L, Cantonetti M, et al. Disseminated pagetoid reticulosis presenting as cytotoxic CD4/CD8 double negative cutaneous T-cell lymphoma. Acta Derm Venereol 2002;82:314–6.

41 Lu D, Patel KA, Duvic M, et al. Clinical and pathological spectrum of CD8-positive cutaneous T-cell lymphomas. J Cutan Pathol 2002;29:465–72.

42 Berroeta L, Lewis-Jones MS, Evans AT, et al. Woringer-Kolopp (localized pagetoid reticulosis) treated with topical photodynamic therapy (PDT). Clin Exp Dermatol 2005;30:446–7.

43 Hughes PS. Treatment of lymphomatoid papulosis with imiquimod 5% cream. J Am Acad Dermatol 2006;54:546–7.

CHAPTER 15

Cutaneous lymphoma, leukemia, and related disorders

Günter Burg, Werner Kempf, and Reinhard Dummer

Almost 200 years ago Alibert [1] described a group of diseases, which he referred to as *pian fungoide* or *frambosia mycoides*. Bontius, an Italian physician, already in the 16th century had described similar skin changes in a book that was edited by Gulielmo Piso in 1658 [2]. When it became clear that most of these disorders were proliferations of T lymphocytes, specifically of helper T lymphocytes [3], or of B lymphocytes [4,5], the terms *cutaneous T-cell lymphoma* (CTCL) and *cutaneous B-cell lymphoma* (CBCL), respectively, were created [6]. Cutaneous lymphomas (CLs) are "illegitimate" lymphoproliferative skin infiltrates of either T, B, or undefined lymphocyte lineage that primarily occur in and remain confined to the skin without detectable extracutaneous manifestation for at least 6 months. Because the skin provides a unique structural and humoral microenvironment to which T and B cells can migrate, it is reasonable that CLs are different from nodal lymphomas in terms of biologic behavior, spreading pattern, prognosis, and treatment strategies. Nevertheless, classification of CLs has to be in accordance with the classification of nodal lymphomas without neglecting the distinct peculiarities of the skin as a special homing organ.

Epidemiology of cutaneous lymphomas

The overall frequency of CLs is approximately 0.3 per 100,000 population per year [7]. Sixty-five percent of CLs are T-cell types, 25% are B-cell types, and the rest comprise unclassified, undefined, or suspicious types of lymphoproliferative skin infiltrates. There is, however, substantial geographic variation. CBCLs seem to be more frequent in Europe than in other parts of the world. Excessive CTCL or mycosis fungoides mortality rates were found in areas where petroleum, rubber, primary and fabricated metal, machinery, and printing industries were located [8,9]. However, other studies have failed to confirm a relationship between disease frequency and professional activities [10,11].

The difficulties in discriminating between early patch stage mycosis fungoides and what has been referred to in the past as parapsoriasis en plaques [12] have led to the tendency to lump everything together under the label *mycosis fungoides*, disregarding their completely different biological behaviors and prognoses. This misconception is reflected in an apparent increase in disease frequency beyond that of lymphoma in general between 1980 and 1985 and a prolongation of survival time in these "mycosis fungoides" patients [13]. Similarity does not mean identity; including orangutans—our evolutionary ancestors—within a population census would constitute an analogous misconception.

Diagnostic approach to cutaneous lymphomas

Clinical staging

Besides physical examination and blood analysis, skin biopsies should be taken at multiple sites. Additional investigations include chest radiography, computed tomography (CT) scan, or ultrasound of the abdomen and of enlarged peripheral lymph nodes. A bone marrow biopsy in advanced stages of progressive malignant CTCL is optional but should be performed in all cases of CBCL. Biopsy of enlarged lymph nodes is mandatory in CTCL and CBCL. 18F-fluorodeoxyglucose (FDG)–positron emission tomography (PET) has been advocated as having higher diagnostic value than CT in the detection of tumor spread [14,15].

The classical Alibert Bazin system [1,16] divided mycosis fungoides into three stages:

I Premycotic eczematous stage, clinically and histologically suspicious but not unambiguously diagnosable

II Plaque or infiltrate stage, unambiguous clinical and histologic diagnostic criteria

III Tumor stage, unambiguous clinical and histologic diagnostic criteria

These stages usually develop sequentially, although they may be seen simultaneously. The current TNM (tumor, nodes, metastases) staging system for CTCL takes into account the body surface area involved: less (T1) or more (T2) than 10%; the quality of skin manifestation, that is, patches/plaques or tumors (T3) or erythroderma (T4); in conjunction with the presence or absence of lymph node (N0–N3) or visceral organ involvement (M0–M1) [17].

The International Society for Cutaneous Lymphomas (ISCL) and the Cutaneous Lymphoma Task Force of the European Organization of Research and Treatment of Cancer (EORTC) recently proposed revisions to the staging classification of mycosis fungoides and Sézary syndrome [18,19]. Future staging systems for CTCL must be designed to reflect prognostically relevant categories of tumor burden by taking into account the types, numbers, and severity of skin lesions, weighing the quality (patch, plaque, tumor) and quantity (absent or present, more or less than 30%) of neoplastic infiltrates (tumor burden index [TBI]) [20,21].

Diagnostic tools

In addition to clinical features, which are most characteristic in CTCL, histo- and cytomorphology both provide helpful methods for the diagnosis of CL. Immunophenotyping and genotyping by either Southern blot or polymerase chain reaction (PCR) are important diagnostic tools to confirm the final diagnosis, which must be based on a constellation of criteria, including clinical, histopathologic, immunophenotypic, and molecular findings. Translocation of the bcl-2 gene (t14;18) [22] or of the anaplastic lymphoma kinase (ALK) gene (t2;5) [23], although regularly seen in follicle center cell lymphomas and in anaplastic large cell lymphomas of the lymph node, respectively, is usually negative in CL and thus cannot be regarded as a helpful diagnostic tool in these cases. Analysis of single cells using microdissection techniques to more precisely identify the tumor cell(s) and its clonal and subclonal expansion is an interesting concept [24] but is not likely to become a routine diagnostic procedure. Genetic defects in CL are heterogeneous [25]. Accordingly, the detection of chromosomal abnormalities has limited diagnostic or prognostic value in CTCL and CBCL.

Analysis and profiling of tissue-specific gene expression by microarray technology are promising and may be a future basis for new lymphoma classifications [26,27].

Classification of cutaneous lymphomas

Various nosologic entities of malignant lymphoma deserve different strategies for treatment and follow-up. These diversities should be reflected in an appropriate classification that discriminates between entities with varying biologic behavior. It should be based on simple, reproducible clinical, histologic, and cytologic markers that may be supplemented by additional phenotypic or genotypic information.

There is no logical reason for classifying cutaneous or other extranodal lymphomas differently from nodal lymphomas. A more global rather than provincial approach for classification, as reflected in the new World Health Organization (WHO)/EORTC classification of CLs, is mandatory to speak a common language with oncologists, pathologists, and hematologists. However, because of some organ-specific peculiarities, there probably never will be one single classification system that adequately encompasses all specific nosologic features of both nodal and extranodal lymphomas.

Table 15.1 WHO/EORTC classification of cutaneous lymphomas[a]

MATURE T-CELL AND NK-CELL NEOPLASMS
Mycosis fungoides
   Variants
   -Pagetoid reticulosis (localized disease)
   -Follicular, syringotropic, granulomatous variants
   Subtype
   -Granulomatous slack skin
Sézary syndrome
CD30[+] T-cell lymphoproliferative disorders of the skin
Lymphomatoid papulosis
Primary cutaneous anaplastic large cell lymphoma
Subcutaneous panniculitis-like T-cell lymphoma[b]
Primary cutaneous peripheral T-cell lymphoma (PTL), unspecified
   Subtypes of PTL
   -Primary cutaneous aggressive epidermotropic
   -CD8[+] T-cell lymphoma (provisional)
   -Cutaneous γ/δ-positive T-cell lymphoma
   -Primary cutaneous CD4[+] small/medium-sized
    pleomorphic T-cell lymphoma (provisional)
Extranodal NK/T-cell lymphoma, nasal type
Hydroa vacciniformia-like lymphoma (variant)
Adult T-cell leukemia/lymphoma
Angioimmunoblastic T-cell lymphoma

MATURE B-CELL NEOPLASMS
**Cutaneous marginal zone B-cell lymphoma
(MALT-type)**
   Variants
   -Immunocytoma
Primary cutaneous follicle center lymphoma
   Variants (according to growth pattern)
   -follicular
   -follicular and diffuse
   -diffuse
Cutaneous diffuse large B-cell lymphoma
   Variants
   -leg type
   -others
Intravascular large B-cell lymphoma
Lymphomatoid granulomatosis
Chronic lymphocytic leukemia
Mantle cell lymphoma
Burkitt lymphoma

Table 15.1 (*Continued*)

IMMATURE HEMATOPOIETIC MALIGNANCIES
Blastic NK-cell lymphoma[c]
CD4[+]/CD56[+] hematodermic neoplasm
**Precursor lymphoblastic leukemia/
lymphoma**
T-lymphoblastic lymphoma
B-lymphoblastic lymphoma

**MYELOID AND MONOCYTIC
LEUKEMIAS**

HODGKIN'S LYMPHOMA

[a] This table also contains entities of extracutaneous lymphomas frequently involving the skin as a secondary site (printed in *italics*).
[b] Definition is restricted to lymphomas of α/β T-cell origin.
[c] Recent evidence suggests an origin from a dendritic cell precursor. In recognition of uncertain histogenesis, the term *CD4[+]/CD56[+] hematodermic neoplasm* is preferred.
Sources: Burg et al. [28,29], Willemze et al. [31], and LeBoit et al. [32].

In the past, CLs also have been classified in the context of nodal lymphoma classification systems [28]. The new WHO/EORTC classification for CL [29–31], which in its original version was published in volume X of the WHO book series on skin tumors [32], fits into the conceptual framework of the current WHO classifications for nodal lymphomas. The main categories are (a) mature T-cell and natural killer (NK)-cell neoplasms, (b) mature B-cell neoplasms, and (c) immature hematopoietic malignancies (Table 15.1). Among the almost 30 entities, only seven represent the most important types of CL (Table 15.2). They are discussed in more detail later in this chapter as clinicopathologic entities.

Moreover, with respect to their clinical and biological behavior, a categorization of CL is recommended: (a) "Semi-malignant" (abortive) lymphomas have a chronic, incurable clinical course. They remain confined to the skin, do not spread systemically, and are not life-threatening. Prelymphomatous parapsoriasis, lymphomatoid papulosis, and rare circumscribed variants of mycosis fungoides, such as syringolymphoid hyperplasia and

Woringer-Kolopp–type pagetoid reticulosis, belong to this category. Transformation of such cases into progressive lymphoma is the exception rather than the rule. (b) Indolent progressive malignant lymphomas, such as mycosis fungoides and Sézary syndrome, are "definite" lymphomas in the context of the Revised European American Lymphoma (REAL)/WHO classification, showing a progressive course with a tendency to spread systemically in advanced stages. They exhibit a chronic but ultimately fatal course. There is a risk of transformation into the aggressive lymphoma category. Survival time is 5 to 10 years. (c) Aggressive progressive malignant lymphomas include disseminated large B- or T-cell, NK-cell, and hematodermic (CD4$^+$, CD56$^+$) lymphomas. Survival time is less than 5 years. (d) Pseudolymphomas in this context are reactive lymphoproliferative disorders, which regress either spontaneously or by nonaggressive therapy, such as antibiotics, within 6 months and do not recur.

Clinicopathologic entities of cutaneous lymphomas

Table 15.2 gives an overview of the relative frequency, synonyms in other classifications, clinical and histologic features, immunophenotype, molecular genetics, and prognostic category in mycosis fungoides, Sézary syndrome, subcutaneous panniculitis-like T-cell lymphoma (SPTCL), CD30$^+$ T-cell lymphoma, marginal zone lymphoma (MZL), follicle center lymphoma (FCL), and diffuse large B-cell lymphoma (DLBCL), which together comprise more than 90% of primary CLs [33].

Cutaneous T-cell lymphomas
Mycosis fungoides

WHO/EORTC classification (2005): mycosis fungoides
WHO classification (2001): mycosis fungoides
REAL classification (1997): mycosis fungoides
EORTC classification (1997): mycosis fungoides
Biological category: indolent progressive CL
Characteristics
- Incidence (% of CL): 44%
- Prognosis (5-year survival rate): greater than 88%
- Clinical features: male-to-female ratio (M:F) = 2:1; patches-plaques-tumors
- Histologic features: lichenoid, epidermotropic infiltrate; lining-up, cerebriform nuclei; cytoplasmic halo; edema; fibrosis; eosinophils; plasma cells; postcapillary venules
- Immunophenotype: CD2$^+$, CD3$^+$, CD5$^+$, CD4$^+$, CD8$^-$, CD7$^-$, CD30$^-$, CD45RO$^+$, bF1$^+$
- Genotype: clonal *TCRβ* gene rearrangement

Mycosis fungoides is the prototype of the peripheral non-Hodgkin's T-cell lymphomas initially presenting in the skin. Clinically, mycosis fungoides is characterized by the sequential appearance of patches, which usually are diagnostically nonspecific [34,35], developing into plaques and finally tumors (Fig. 15.1). In the early initial stages, the histologic diagnosis of mycosis fungoides usually is difficult to establish, as the disease may closely resemble dermatitis [34,36]. Intraepidermal Pautrier microabscesses are the most specific findings, which are seen in only 10% to 20% of lesions (Fig. 15.2). Typical but not specific features are the presence of medium to large hyper-convoluted cerebriform cells in the epidermis larger than dermal lymphocytes showing a clear perinuclear halo (haloed lymphocytes), lymphocytes in clusters in the dermis, and lymphocytes aligned within the basal layer [37–39] (Fig. 15.2A). In early mycosis fungoides, the presence of lymphocytes with strikingly irregular nuclear contours and/or variable nuclear and cytoplasmic features is of diagnostic value, with a sensitivity of 53.3% and a specificity of 88.9% [40].

In the plaque stage, the histologic findings usually are fully diagnostic. There is a dense infiltrate with lymphocytes lining up in the basal layer, especially at the tips of the rete ridges with prominent epidermotropism of single cells. The majority of cells are small, differentiated lymphocytes with round or only slightly cerebriform nuclei. The infiltrate may contain eosinophils, plasma cells, macrophages, and dermal dendritic cells. There may be prominent subepidermal edema (Fig. 15.2C) and proliferation of postcapillary venules (Fig. 15.2D). The dermal infiltrates become more diffuse when progression from plaque stage to tumor stage occurs, and epidermotropism may disappear.

Table 15.2 The seven most important types of cutaneous lymphoma, which together comprise more than 90% of primary cutaneous lymphomas

	MF	SS	SPTCL	CD30⁺	MZL	FCL	DLBCL
Rel. Frequ.	45%	2%	<1%	24%	10%	12%	6%
Synonyms[a]	WHO, REAL, EORTC: mycosis fungoides	WHO, REAL, EORTC: Sézary syndrome	WHO, REAL, EORTC: subcutaneous panniculitis-like T-cell lymphoma	WHO, REAL, EORTC: ALCL, CD30⁺	WHO, REAL: extran. MZL; EORTC: pc immunocytoma/marginal zone B-cell lymphoma	WHO, REAL, EORTC: follicle center lymphoma	WHO, REAL: DLBCL; EORTC: large B-cell lymphoma of the lower leg
Clinical features	M:F 2:1; patches, plaques, tumors; dissemination; pruritus **(Fig. 15.1)**	Erythroderma, palmoplantar hyperkeratosis, alopecia, marked lymphadenopathy, edema, pruritus, leukemic blood picture	Panniculitis-like plaques or nodules, predominantly on lower extremities **(Fig. 15.4)**	Solitary or grouped rapidly growing ulcerated nodule(s) **(Fig. 15.4)**	Solitary or multiple nodules or tumors	Solitary or grouped nodules or plaques **(Fig. 15.9)**	Solitary or grouped violaceous nodules, ulceration, elderly women > men, lower leg **(Fig. 15.10)**
Histologic features	Lichenoid, epidermotropic infiltrate; lining-up, cerebriform nuclei; cytoplasmic Halo; edema; fibrosis; eosinophils; plasma cells; postcapillary venules **(Figs. 15.2 and 15.3)**	Lichenoid bandlike, epidermotropic and perivascular infiltrate; lining-up, cerebriform nuclei of lymphocytes; edema; fibrosis; eosinophils; plasma cells; postcapillary venules	Predominantly lobular lymphoid infiltrate with karyorrhexis and rimming of tumor cells around fat lobules **(Fig. 15.5)**	Cohesive sheets of anaplastic tumor cells; sparse reactive inflammatory infiltrate **(Fig. 15.6)**	Nodular or diffuse infiltrates, inverse pattern; small lymphoid cells with indented nuclei and abundant pale cytoplasm; numerous plasma cells **(Fig. 15.7)**	Nodular or diffuse infiltrates; Grenz zone, follicular pattern; centroblasts/centrocytes	Dense diffuse infiltrates: dermis and subcutis; centroblasts/immunoblasts; high mitotic activity
I'phenotype	CD2⁺, CD3⁺, CD5⁺, CD4⁺, CD8⁻, CD7⁻, CD30⁻, CD45RO⁺, bF1⁺	CD2⁺, CD3⁺, CD4⁺ > CD8⁺, CD5⁺, CD45RO⁺, CD30⁻	TCR α/β (βF1⁺), CD2⁺, CD3⁺, CD5⁺, CD4⁻, CD8⁺, CD43⁺, and cytotoxic proteins such as TIA-1, granzyme B, and perforin	CD2⁺, CD3⁺, CD4⁺, CD8⁻, CD5⁺, CD30⁺ **(Fig. 15.6)**, ALK⁻	CD20⁺, CD43⁺, CD79a⁺, CD5⁻, CD10⁻, bcl-2⁺ **(Fig. 15.8)**, bcl-6⁻, KiM1p⁺, reactive follicles	CD20⁺/⁻, CD43⁺, CD79a⁺, CD10⁺/⁻ bcl-6⁺; bcl-2⁻; clonal κ/λ, irregular networks of CD21⁺ FDC, T cells	CD20⁺, CD79a⁺, bcl-2⁺, bcl-6⁺ MUM1⁺, CD10⁻/⁺; clonal κ/λ.
Mol.Gen.	Clonal TCRβ gene rearrangement	Clonal TCR gene rearrangement	Clonal TCRβ gene rearrangement in the majority of cases	Clonal TCR gene rearrangement	Clonal IgH gene rearrangement	Clonal IgH gene rearrangement	Clonal IgH gene rearrangement
5-year SRV	>88%	24%	>80%	>95%	99%	95%	55%
Progn. Categ.	Good	Poor	Usually indolent (α/β phenotype)	Good	Good	Good	Intermediate

[a] In various classification systems.

ALCL, anaplastic large cell lymphoma; CD30⁺, CD30⁺ T-cell lymphoma; DLBCL, diffuse large B-cell lymphoma; FCL, follicle center lymphoma; IgH, immunoglobulin H; I'phenotype, immunophenotype; MF, mycosis fungoides; M:F, male-to-female ratio; Mol.Gen., molecular genetics; MZL, marginal zone lymphoma; Progn.Categ., prognostic category; Rel.Frequ., relative frequency; SPTCL, subcutaneous panniculitis-like T-cell lymphoma; SRV, survival; SS, Sézary syndrome; TCR, T-cell receptor.

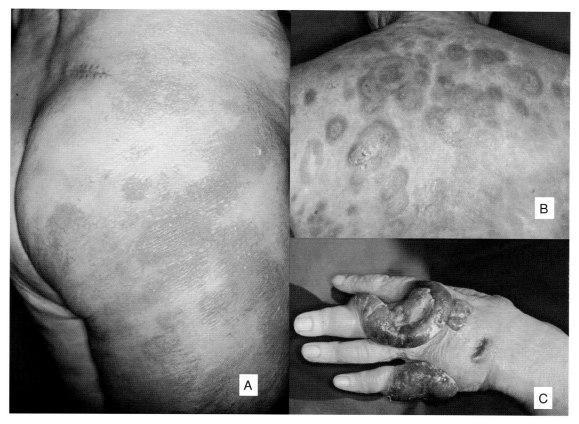

Fig. 15.1 Mycosis fungoides in (*A*) patch, (*B*) plaque, and (*C*) tumor stage. © 2008, Dr. Günter Burg, Universität Zürich, Switzerland.

Immunophenotypically, mycosis fungoides is a disease of T helper 2 (Th2) lymphocytes expressing T-cell–associated antigens (CD2+, CD3+, CD5+, CD4+, CD8−, CD7−, CD30−, CD45RO+, bF1+) and clonally rearranged T-cell receptor (TCR) genes. The cytokines produced by the tumor cells (interleukin [IL]-4, IL-5, IL-10) account for the many systemic changes associated with mycosis fungoides, such as eosinophilia, increased immunoglobulin E (IgE) or IgA, and impaired delayed-type reactivity [41,42].

Cases of mycosis fungoides showing similar histologic and phenotypic features like the prototype are referred to as *variants*.

Pagetoid reticulosis
Biological category: semimalignant (abortive) CL

Pagetoid reticulosis, in its localized form also referred to as Woringer-Kolopp's disease [43], clinically presents as a solitary, slowly growing psoriasiform crusty or hyperkeratotic patch or plaque, typically on a distal limb. The histologic hallmark is the pagetoid pattern due to the sponge-like disaggregation of the epidermis by lymphoid cells. The immunophenotype of the neoplastic cells corresponds to the findings in mycosis fungoides [5]. Rare CD8+ and γ/δ positive variants have been reported [44].

Syringotropic cutaneous T-cell lymphoma
Syringotropic CTCL is a rare variant of mycosis fungoides exclusively reported in men. The lesions are usually red-brown patches, slightly infiltrated scaling plaques, or small red or skin-colored papules. There may be anhidrosis, with hair loss in the

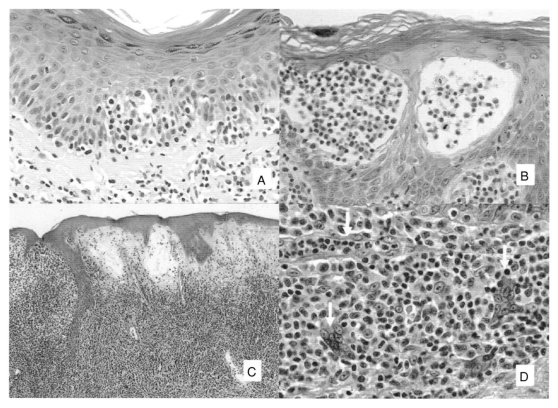

Fig. 15.2 Mycosis fungoides, histologic features. *A*, Patch stage showing epidermotropism of lymphocytes. *B*, Formation of intraepidermal (Pautrier's) abscesses. *C*, Dense dermal infiltrate with strong subepidermal edema. *D*, Postcapillary venules surrounded by neoplastic cells. (Hematoxylin-eosin [H&E] stain.) © 2008, Dr. Günter Burg, Universität Zürich, Switzerland.

affected area. A specific histopathologic pattern with predominant involvement of eccrine sweat glands by small cerebriform lymphocytes is seen [45]. The neoplastic cells express a T helper cell phenotype (CD3+, CD4+, CD8−) and clonal rearrangement of TCR genes in most cases.

Mycosis fungoides with follicular mucinosis
This variant of mycosis fungoides has specific histologic features [46,47]. It is more refractory to treatment, and has a worse prognosis than the classic type of mycosis fungoides [48] (Fig. 15.3).

Other variants of mycosis fungoides
Other variants of mycosis fungoides include bullous, follicular, granulomatous, pustular, hyperkeratotic, hyperpigmented or hypopigmented, adnexotropic, and purpuric forms [49].

Granulomatous slack skin
WHO/EORTC classification (2005): granulomatous slack skin (subtype of mycosis fungoides)
WHO classification (2001): not listed
REAL classification (1997): not listed
EORTC classification (1997): granulomatous slack skin
The clinical and histologic features of this subtype of mycosis fungoides show clear differences from classical mycosis fungoides. The clinical hallmark is hanging, bulky folds of lax skin in flexural areas. This rare condition also occurs in children [50] and originally was reported in a 15-year-old youngster [51]. The histopathology shows a lymphocytic infiltrate with almost complete loss of both papillary and reticular dermal elastic tissue, which may be found as small fragments in the cytoplasm of huge giant

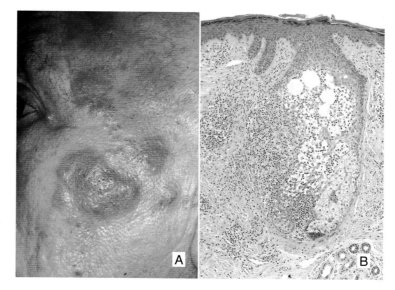

Fig. 15.3 Symptomatic follicular mucinosis, a variant of mycosis fungoides. *A*, Plaque-like lesions on the face. *B*, Mucinous degeneration in adnexal structures with lymphoid infiltrate. (H&E stain.) © 2008, Dr. Günter Burg, Universität Zürich, Switzerland.

cells [52]. Immunophenotyping and genotyping reveal lymphocytes with a mature helper T-cell phenotype showing clonal rearrangement of TCR genes [53].

Sézary syndrome

WHO/EORTC classification (2005): Sézary syndrome

WHO classification (2001): Sézary syndrome

REAL classification (1997): Sézary syndrome

EORTC classification (1997): Sézary syndrome

Biological category: progressive CL, more frequently aggressive than indolent.

Characteristics

- Incidence (% of CL): 3%
- Prognosis (5-year survival rate): greater than 24%
- Clinical features: erythroderma, palmoplantar hyperkeratosis, alopecia, marked lymphadenopathy, edema, pruritus, leukemic blood picture
- Histologic features: lichenoid band–like, epidermotropic, and perivascular infiltrate; lining-up; cerebriform nuclei of lymphocytes; edema; fibrosis, eosinophils; plasma cells; postcapillary venules
- Immunophenotype: $CD2^+$, $CD3^+$, $CD4^+$ > $CD8^+$, $CD5^+$, $CD7^-$, $CD45RO^+$, $CD30^-$
- Genotype: clonal *TCRβ* gene rearrangement

The typical features, described by von Zumbusch [54], later by Sézary [55] and Baccaredda [56], have been reviewed [57]. An international working group [58,59] has elaborated the criteria, consisting of erythroderma (Fig.15.4A) and circulating atypical lymphoid cells expressing the Th2 phenotype at a concentration of more than 1000/mL blood [60,61]. Additional symptoms are edematous swelling of the skin, pruritus, adenopathy of peripheral lymph nodes, hair loss, dystrophy of nails, and hyperkeratosis of the palms and soles.

Histologically, there is edema in the upper dermis and a subepidermal bandlike infiltrate composed of predominantly small atypical lymphocytes, which is nonspecific in one third of the cases; Pautrier's microabscesses are seen in only half the cases [62]. There is little difference compared to the features of mycosis fungoides in the plaque stage [63].

Immunophenotypically, tumor cells in Sézary syndrome express a T helper phenotype ($CD2^+$, $CD3^+$, $CD4^+$ > $CD8^+$, $CD5^+$, $CD7^-$, $CD45RO^+$, $CD30^-$) and CL antigen (CLA). Loss of T-cell antigens, mostly CD2, is seen in two thirds of the cases [64]. The lack of T(reg) cells (FOXP3) in Sézary syndrome may account for the more aggressive nature of this lymphoma compared with other CTCLs [65].

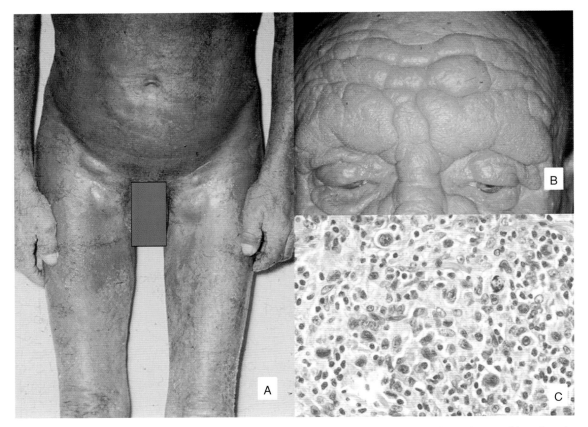

Fig. 15.4 Sézary syndrome (*A*) showing typical (melano-)erythroderma, scaling, and swelling of inguinal lymph nodes. (*B*) Transformation into high-grade malignant ALCL, showing thick plaques and nodules with (*C*) large atypical anaplastic cells. (H&E stain.) © 2008, Dr. Günter Burg, Universität Zürich, Switzerland.

Molecular biology: Clonal T-cell gene rearrangement can be detected by Southern blot or PCR in the skin or peripheral blood in up to 90% of cases. Cytogenetic studies have not shown any distinct diagnostic profile [66]. In advanced stages of the disease, transformation into large cell anaplastic lymphoma may be seen, which is indicative of a worsening prognosis (Fig. 15.4B,C).

CD30+ T-cell lymphoproliferative disorders of the skin

Lymphomatoid papulosis (LYP), primary cutaneous anaplastic large-cell lymphoma (ALCL) and so-called borderline cases [67] are clinically and morphologically distinct entities in the spectrum of

CD30+ lymphoproliferative disorders of the skin [68].

Lymphomatoid papulosis

WHO/EORTC classification (2005): CD30 lymphoproliferative disorders of the skin—lymphomatoid papulosis

WHO classification (2001): CD30 lymphoproliferative disorders of the skin—lymphomatoid papulosis

REAL classification (1997): not listed

EORTC classification (1997): lymphomatoid papulosis

Biological category: semimalignant (abortive) CL

Characteristics

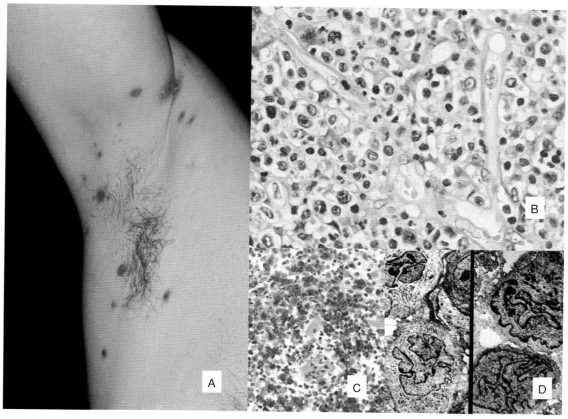

Fig. 15.5 Lymphomatoid papulosis. (*A*) Multiple papules in various stages of regression in the axillary region. (*B*) Histology, besides postcapillary venules, shows an infiltrate of atypical lymphoid cells, which express CD30 (*C*) and show highly convoluted nuclear contours on electron microscopy (*D*). © 2008, Dr. Günter Burg, Universität Zürich, Switzerland.

• Incidence (% of CL): 10%
• Prognosis (5-year survival rate): greater than 95%
• Clinical features: chronic recurrent self-healing papular, papulonecrotic, and/or nodular skin lesions at different stages of development; scars
• Histologic features: variable, depending on the age of the lesion biopsied; large atypical cells may be suggestive of high-grade malignant lymphoma. There may be a very few of these cells, up to sheets of them.
• Immunophenotype: CD2$^+$, CD3$^+$, CD4$^+$, CD8$^-$, CD56$^+$ (10%), CD45RO$^+$, CD30$^+$
• Genotype: clonal *TCRβ* gene rearrangement in most cases

Lymphomatoid papulosis (Fig. 15.5) described by Macaulay [69] is a chronic recurrent self-healing "rhythmic paradoxical" papulonodular skin eruption with an indolent course and histologic features of a malignant lymphoma. Transformation into aggressive malignant lymphoma, usually with features of ALCL, occurs in about 10% of cases [70].

Clinically (Fig. 15.5A), LYP is characterized by a few to hundreds of disseminated papules or nodules, which evolve and regress over a few weeks, sometimes leaving behind scars. Although no definite predilection site has been identified, LYP tends to arise on the trunk, especially the buttocks, and on extremities.

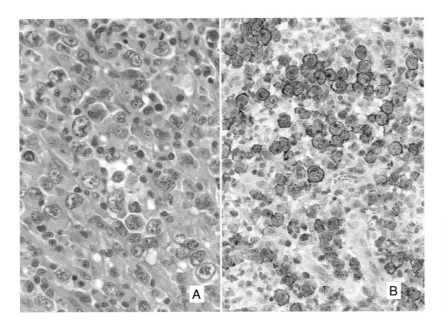

Fig. 15.6 Anaplastic large cell lymphoma showing sheets of large atypical cells in the H&E stain (*A*) that express CD30 (*B*). © 2008, Dr. Günter Burg, Universität Zürich, Switzerland.

The phenotypic hallmark is pleomorphic cells (Fig. 15.5B) expressing CD30 (Fig. 15.5C) [71,72] and showing highly atypical nuclear contours (Fig. 15.5D). These features indicate the cytogenetic relationship between the tumor cells in LYP, mycosis fungoides, Hodgkin's disease [73], and ALCL [74].

Anaplastic large T-cell lymphoma

WHO/EORTC classification (2005): primary cutaneous anaplastic large cell lymphoma

WHO classification (2001): primary cutaneous anaplastic large cell lymphoma

REAL classification (1997): anaplastic large cell lymphoma, CD30+

EORTC classification (1997): primary cutaneous large cell T-cell lymphoma, CD30+

Biological category: indolent (solitary) or intermediate (disseminated) progressive CD30+

CL with favorable prognosis.

Characteristics
- Incidence (% of CL): 12%
- Prognosis (5-year survival rate): greater than 95%
- Clinical features: solitary or grouped, rapidly growing ulcerated nodule(s)

- Histologic features: cohesive sheets of anaplastic tumor cells, sparse reactive inflammatory infiltrate
- Immunophenotype: CD2+, CD3+, CD4+, CD8−, CD5+, CD 30+ (>75% of cells), ALK−
- Genotype: clonal *TCRβ* gene rearrangement

The CD30+ ALCL is closely related to Hodgkin's disease and LYP [73]. Primary cutaneous and primary nodal CD30+ ALCL are distinct clinical entities that have identical morphologic features, but differ in age of onset, immunophenotype, and prognosis [75]. Clinically, the skin tumors usually are solitary or multiple, confined to an extremity or a circumscribed area of the body. As in LYP, spontaneous regression may be observed, usually following ulceration. Histologically (Fig. 15.6A), dense sheets of large bizarre cells with abundant, clear, or eosinophilic cytoplasm and large round, irregularly shaped nuclei extend through all levels of the dermis.

Immunophenotyping shows positivity of the large anaplastic cells for CD30 (Fig. 15.6B). Primary cutaneous CD30+ ALCL usually lacks expression of the ALK fusion protein resulting from t(2;5) translocation [76].

Subcutaneous panniculitis-like T-cell lymphoma

WHO/EORTC classification (2005): subcutaneous panniculitis-like T-cell lymphoma

WHO classification (2001): subcutaneous panniculitis-like T-cell lymphoma

REAL classification (1997): subcutaneous panniculitis-like T-cell lymphoma

EORTC classification (1997): subcutaneous panniculitis-like T-cell lymphoma

Biological category: usually indolent (α/β phenotype) progressive

Characteristics

- Incidence (% of CL): less than 1%
- Prognosis (5-year survival rate): greater than 80%
- Clinical features: panniculitis-like plaques or nodules, predominantly on lower extremities
- Histologic features: predominantly lobular lymphoid infiltrate with karyorrhexis and rimming of tumor cells around fat lobules
- Immunophenotype: TCR α/β ($\beta F1^+$), $CD2^+$, $CD3^+$, $CD5^+$, $CD4^-$, $CD8^+$, $CD43^+$, and cytotoxic proteins such as TIA-1, granzyme B, and perforin
- Genotype: clonal $TCR\beta$ gene rearrangement in the majority of cases

Only SPTCLs expressing an α/β phenotype are referred to as SPTCL sui generis in the WHO/EORTC classification, whereas cases with a γ/δ phenotype are included in the group of peripheral T-cell lymphomas, cytotoxic type [77]. The histopathologic hallmark of this type of CTCL is predominant involvement of subcutaneous fat lobules, simulating lobular panniculitis [78–81]. Therefore deep biopsies are required to establish the diagnosis. There also may be karyorrhexis and fat necrosis. Rimming of adipocytes by tumor, even though frequently present in SPTCL, cannot be considered specific of subcutaneous panniculitis-like T-cell lymphoma [82]. Panniculitis and lupus profundus have to be differentiated; repeat biopsies are important [83].

Cutaneous peripheral T-cell lymphomas, unspecified

This category constitutes a heterogeneous group of diseases, representing less than 10% of all CTCLs [84]. By definition, it includes all T-cell neoplasms that do not fit into any of the other categories of T-cell lymphoma/leukemia. Their biologic behavior is aggressively progressive in most cases.

The following disorders have been included in the group of peripheral T-cell lymphomas:

1 Cutaneous γ/δ T-cell lymphoma

2 Primary cutaneous aggressive epidermotropic CD8+ cytotoxic T-cell lymphoma

3 Primary cutaneous $CD4^{-+}$ small/medium-sized pleomorphic T-cell lymphoma

4 T-zone lymphoma

Extranodal NK/T-cell lymphoma

WHO/EORTC classification (2005): extranodal NK/T-cell lymphoma, nasal type

WHO classification (2001): extranodal NK/T-cell lymphoma, nasal type

REAL classification (1997): extranodal NK/T-cell lymphoma, nasal type

EORTC classification (1997): not listed

There is a considerable heterogeneity—clinical as well as histologic and immunophenotypic—among extranodal NK/T-cell lymphoma [85]. The classic nasal extranodal NK/T-cell lymphoma occurs more frequently in Asia and Latin America and is associated with Epstein-Barr virus (EBV). Tumor cells express CD56 and cytotoxic proteins such as TIA-1, granzyme B, and perforin. Large ulcerations in the area of the nose are the hallmark of the disease and led to the old term *lethal midline granuloma*. Hydroa-like lymphoma shows many features of this group of diseases and is best categorized here [86,87].

Adult T-cell leukemia/lymphoma

WHO/EORTC classification (2005): adult T-cell leukemia/lymphoma

WHO classification (2001): adult T-cell leukemia/lymphoma

REAL classification (1997): adult T-cell leukemia/lymphoma

EORTC classification (1997): not included

This peripheral T-cell lymphoma is etiologically associated with human T-cell leukemia virus I (HTLV-1) and is endemic in southwestern Japan and the Caribbean but also occurs outside these areas [88]. There is a considerable spectrum of clinical manifestations and histologic features. Skin involvement occurs in about 50% of the cases during the course of the disease and presents as purpuric plaques, papules, nodules, tumors, or erythroderma, simulating mycosis fungoides in nonendemic areas [89].

Cutaneous B-cell lymphomas

B-cell lymphomas are much more common in lymph nodes than in skin. Because CBCLs have a benign overall prognosis, proper recognition is vital to avoid overtreatment. The subclassification and the extent of cutaneous involvement are the two most relevant prognostic factors in primary CBCL [90].

Cutaneous marginal zone B-cell lymphoma (mucosa-associated lymphoid tissue [MALT] type)

Marginal zone B-cell lymphoma arises from the marginal zone cells of the lymph follicle.

WHO/EORTC classification (2005): cutaneous marginal zone B-cell lymphoma

WHO classification (2001): extranodal marginal zone lymphoma of MALT type

REAL classification (1997): extranodal marginal zone B-cell lymphoma

EORTC classification (1997): primary cutaneous marginal zone B-cell lymphoma

Biological category: indolent progressive CL

Characteristics

- Incidence (% of CL): 7%
- Prognosis (5-year survival rate): greater than 95%
- Clinical features: solitary or multiple nodules or tumors
- Histologic features: nodular or diffuse infiltrates, inverse pattern. Small lymphoid cells with indented nuclei and abundant pale cytoplasm, numerous plasma cells
- Immunophenotype: CD20$^+$, CD43$^+$, CD79a$^+$; CD5$^-$, CD10$^-$, bcl-2$^+$, bcl-6$^-$, KiM1p$^+$, reactive follicles
- Genotype: clonal IgH gene rearrangement

Extranodal low-grade B-cell lymphoma of the MALT type and FCL are the most frequent types of peripheral B-cell neoplasms seen primarily in the skin [91–93]. Extranodal MZLs are thought to develop from reactive infiltrates that represent immune responses to external or autoantigens [33]. An etiopathologic relationship to *Borrelia burgdorferi* has been suggested in some cases [94,95]; however, direct evidence in tissue biopsies is lacking [96].

Clinically, MZL presents with solitary or clustered reddish dome-shaped papules, nodules, or erythematous plaques, frequently located in the head and neck area (Fig. 15.7A). Histologically, there is a nodular or diffuse infiltrate. Tumor cells are small to medium-sized with indented nuclei and an abundant pale cytoplasm (monocytoid B-cells, marginal zone cells) [97]. Pale-staining cells surround a zone of darker chromatin-dense cells, which display a characteristic "inverse pattern."

Primary cutaneous MZLs with high numbers of monotypic plasma cells and lymphoplasmacytoid cells showing intranuclear periodic acid-Schiff–positive globular inclusions (Dutcher bodies) have been previously referred to as *cutaneous immunocytoma* [94,98].

The tumor cells express the following immunophenotype: CD19$^+$, CD20$^+$, CD22$^+$, CD43$^+$, CD79a$^+$, CD5$^-$, CD10$^-$, CD23$^-$, bcl-6$^-$, bcl-2$^+$, KiM1p$^+$ (monocytoid B-cell related antibody). The cells also show monotypic expression of immunoglobulin light chain κ more frequently than λ. Plasmacytoid cells may be present in confluent aggregates. There are a variable number of reactive CD3$^+$ T cells, usually in the periphery of the neoplastic infiltrates, and of reactive follicles, colonized by tumor cells. Molecular analysis has shown that IgH genes are clonally rearranged in almost 80% of cases [99]. Translation of t(11;18) involving the *API2/MLT* genes, which usually is found in gastric MZL, is not found in primary cutaneous MZL.

Follicle center lymphoma

Follicle center lymphoma is a neoplasm with differentiation of follicle center cells (centrocytes and centroblasts).

WHO/EORTC classification (2005): primary cutaneous follicle center lymphoma

WHO classification (2001): cutaneous follicle center lymphoma

REAL classification (1997): follicle center lymphoma, follicular

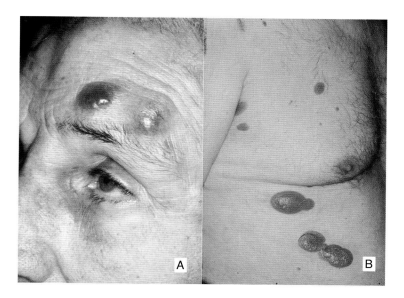

Fig. 15.7 Nodules and tumors in CBCL. Marginal zone lymphoma (*A*) and follicle center lymphoma (*B*). © 2008, Dr. Günter Burg, Universität Zürich, Switzerland.

EORTC classification (1997): primary cutaneous follicle center cell lymphoma
Biological category: indolent progressive CL
Characteristics
 • Incidence (% of CL): 12%
 • Prognosis (5-year survival rate): greater than 95%
 • Clinical features: solitary or grouped nodules or plaques
 • Histologic features: nodular or diffuse infiltrates; Grenz zone; follicular pattern; centroblasts/centrocytes
 • Immunophenotype: CD20$^+$, CD43$^+$, CD79a$^+$, CD10$^{+/-}$, bcl-6$^+$, bcl-2$^-$, clonal κ/λ, irregular networks of CD21$^+$ follicular dendritic cells, admixture of many reactive T cells
 • Genotype: clonal IgH gene rearrangement
Clinically (Figs. 15.7B and 15.8A), nodules and tumors of firm consistency without ulceration most frequently are located in the head and neck area but also in other locations of the body [100,101]. Histologically (Fig. 15.8B,C), three growth patterns can be differentiated: follicular, nodular, and diffuse. A subepidermal Grenz zone is present in most cases (Fig. 15.8B). There are many CD21$^+$ dermal dendritic cells (Fig. 15.8C) accompanying in an irregular pattern the neoplastic centrocytes and centroblasts (Fig. 15.8D). Mitoses, tin-

gible body macrophages, and starry sky features, which are typical for reactive lymphoid hyperplasia (pseudolymphoma) [102], are rare or absent in FCL.

Immunophenotypically, the cells in FCL express CD19$^+$, CD20$^+$, CD22$^+$, CD43$^+$, CD79a$^+$, CD5$^-$, CD23$^{+/-}$, CD43, bcl-6$^+$, bcl-2$^-$, and CD10$^+$ in cases with follicular growth pattern. Follicular dendritic cells (CD21$^+$) are arranged in an irregular ring-like pattern (Fig 15.8C). The MUM/IRF4 antigen, which is positive in DLBCL, is not expressed in FCL. Molecular analysis shows clonal rearrangement of immunoglobulin genes. Chromosomal translocation of t(14;18) and *BCL-2* gene rearrangement are absent in most cases [22,99,103,104]; if present in cutaneous sites, it indicates secondary skin involvement. Gene expression studies have shown distinct profiles in various types of cutaneous B-cell lymphoma [26,27]. Reticulohistiocytoma of the back or Crosti's lymphoma is a variant of cutaneous FCL [105].

Diffuse large B-cell lymphoma

WHO/EORTC classification (2005): cutaneous diffuse large B-cell lymphoma
 DLBCL, leg type
 DLBCL, other

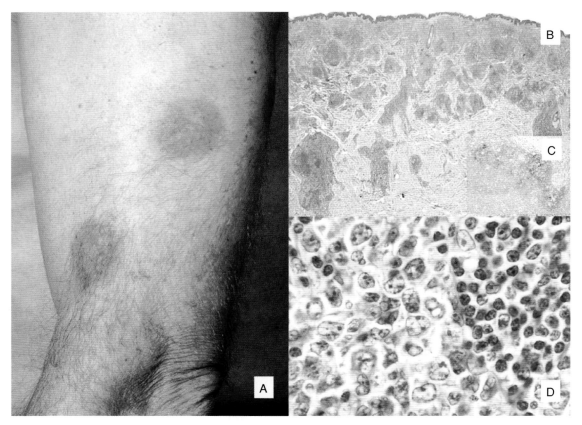

Fig. 15.8 (*A*) Follicle center lymphoma showing plaque-like lesions. Histology reveals a nodular infiltrate displaying a typical B-cell pattern (*B*) with an irregular network of CD21⁺ dendritic cells (*C*). (*D*) Large and small follicular center cells. (H&E stain.) © 2008, Dr. Günter Burg, Universität Zürich, Switzerland.

WHO classification (2001): diffuse large B-cell lymphoma

REAL classification (1997): diffuse large B-cell lymphoma

EORTC classification (1997): primary cutaneous large B-cell lymphoma of the leg

Biological category: aggressive progressive CL

Characteristics
- Incidence (% of CL): 4%
- Prognosis (5-year survival rate): 55%
- Clinical features: solitary or grouped violaceous nodules, ulceration, elderly women more affected than men, lower leg
- Histologic features: dense diffuse infiltrates: dermis and subcutis; centroblasts/immunoblasts; high mitotic activity

- Immunophenotype: CD19⁺, CD20⁺, CD22⁺, CD5⁻, CD10⁻, CD79a⁺, bcl-2⁺, bcl-6⁺, MUM1⁺, CD138⁻, cyclin D1⁻, clonal κ/λ
- Genotype: clonal IgH gene rearrangement

Clinically, these lymphomas usually present as solitary or multiple tumors restricted to one anatomic area. In contrast to other CBCL types, they show a poorer prognosis and tend to have extracutaneous involvement. In the WHO/EORTC classification, two forms are distinguished. The most common variant, DLBCL, leg type (Fig. 15.9A), usually occurs on the leg and less frequently at other sites. Other variants are referred to as DLBCL and comprise T-cell/histiocyte-rich DLBCL, plasmablastic lymphoma, and others that do not fulfill the criteria for a DLBCL, leg type.

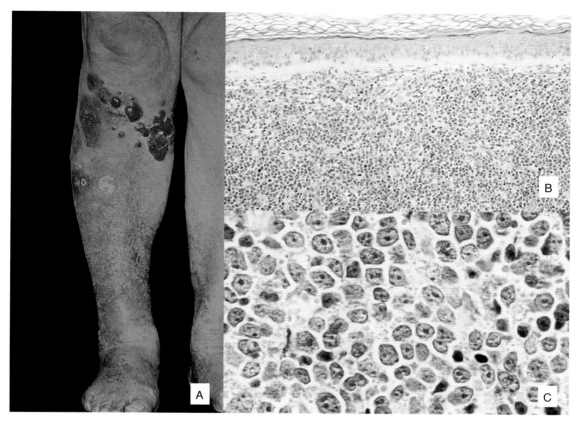

Fig. 15.9 (*A*) Diffuse large B-cell lymphoma, leg type. Histology shows a dense infiltrate in the dermis, sparing a subepidermal Grenz zone (*B*) composed of large atypical lymphoid cells (*C*). (H&E stain.) © 2008, Dr. Günter Burg, Universität Zürich, Switzerland.

Histology reveals a diffuse growth pattern of monomorphous cells involving the entire dermis, destroying adnexal structures and extending into the subcutaneous tissue. There is a subepidermal Grenz zone (Fig. 15.9B). The cytomorphologic hallmark of DLBCL is large B cells (Fig. 15.9C): centroblasts and immunoblasts [106]. Centrocytes, which are typically seen in FCL, are missing in DLBCL.

The neoplastic cells express the following immunophenotype: CD19$^+$, CD20$^+$, CD22$^+$, CD5$^-$, CD10$^-$, CD79a$^+$, bcl-2$^+$, bcl-6$^+$, MUM1$^+$, CD138$^-$, cyclin D1$^-$. The strong positivity for Bcl-2 protein and MUM-1/IRF-4 [107] allows differentiation from FCL with diffuse growth pattern. Studies using tissue microarrays have shown that expression of bcl-6 and MUM1 correlates with survival [108].

Molecular analysis reveals clonal rearrangement of immunoglobulin genes. The t(14; 18) and the bcl-2/JH translocation cannot be detected in primary cutaneous DLBCL [109]. Studies on gene expression profiles have revealed some differences between primary and secondary cutaneous large B-cell lymphomas as well as between DLBCL and FCL with diffuse growth pattern [26,27,110].

Diffuse large B-cell lymphoma, leg type
This type of DLBCL is located on the leg, mostly of elderly women.

The pathologic, immunophenotypic, and molecular features are similar to those seen at other sites.

Therefore, it is justified to refer to all together as DLBCL, leg type, in analogy to similar terms in the classification of lymphomas such as "nasal type."

Diffuse large B-cell lymphoma, other
This term refers to other lymphomatous proliferations of large transformed B cells showing the same phenotypic and genotypic profile as those of the leg type but differing in their localization at other sites of the body. They also include large B-cell lymphomas with distinct growth pattern, such as T-cell–rich/histiocytic DLBCL [111,112] and intravascular large B-cell lymphoma [113–115].

B-cell lymphomas with common secondary cutaneous involvement
Lymphomatoid granulomatosis
Lymphomatoid granulomatosis was originally described by Liebow and colleagues [116]. It is a rare multisystemic angiocentric and angiodestructive lymphoproliferative disease that involves extranodal sites, especially the lungs, skin, and nervous system. It is EBV positive in most cases and may progress to DLBCL.

Burkitt lymphoma
Burkitt lymphoma is an aggressive B-cell lymphoma associated with EBV infection in most cases and featuring translocation of the *c-myc* gene. This lymphoma occurs endemically in children in the so-called lymphoma belt of Central Africa [117]. Sporadic cases are less closely associated with EBV and may also be seen in association with HIV-induced immunodeficiency [118].

Mantle cell lymphoma
Mantle cell lymphoma is a B-cell lymphoma involving the mantle cells in the mantle zone of the lymphoid follicle. Skin involvement is rare and usually secondary [119].

Waldenström macroglobulinemia
Waldenström macroglobulinemia (WM) is a hematologic malignancy characterized by a clonal expansion of lymphocytes with plasmacytoid features that produce a monoclonal IgM protein and infiltrate bone marrow, lymph nodes, and spleen [120]. Non-specific cutaneous changes of WM include urticarial and purpuric eruptions, ulcers, bulla, and vasculitides. The specific cellular infiltration presents as asymptomatic infiltrative papules, plaques, or nodules [121,122].

Hyperkeratotic spicules are typically found on the face of patients with monoclonal gammopathy due to multiple myeloma (Fig. 15.10A) [123].

Immature hematopoietic malignancies
Blastic "hematodermic NK-cell lymphoma" (CD4$^+$/CD56$^+$)
WHO/EORTC classification (2005): CD4$^+$/CD56$^+$ hematodermic neoplasm; blastic NK-cell lymphoma
WHO classification (2001): blastic NK-cell lymphoma
REAL classification (1997): not listed
EORTC classification (1997): not listed
In future classifications, this precursor hematologic neoplasm that frequently first presents in the skin [124] will probably no longer be categorized as T- or NK-cell lymphoma because cytogenetically the neoplastic cells are related to myeloid and to lymphoid precursor cells (type 2 dendritic cells).
Biological category: highly aggressive progressive cutaneous neoplasm
Characteristics
- Incidence (% of CL): less than 1%
- Prognosis: extremely poor
- Clinical features: multiple nodules or plaques, contusiform (bruising) aspect; mucosal involvement; lymphadenopathy
- Histologic features: monomorphous infiltrate, no epidermotropism; pleomorphic medium-sized cells; erythrocyte extravasation
- Immunophenotype: CD4$^+$, CD56$^+$, CD43$^+$, CD45$^+$, CD123$^+$; other T- and B-cell markers: negative; CD68$^+$; CD14, MPO, lysozyme negative
- Genotype: no clonal TCR gene rearrangement
Clinically (Fig 15.10B), in almost 90% of the cases, contusiform, brownish infiltrated plaques or nodules of the skin manifest early during the course of the disease [124–129]. Involvement of the oral mucosa is a typical feature. Generalization of the disease with involvement of lymph nodes and other extracutaneous sites develops early and rapidly.

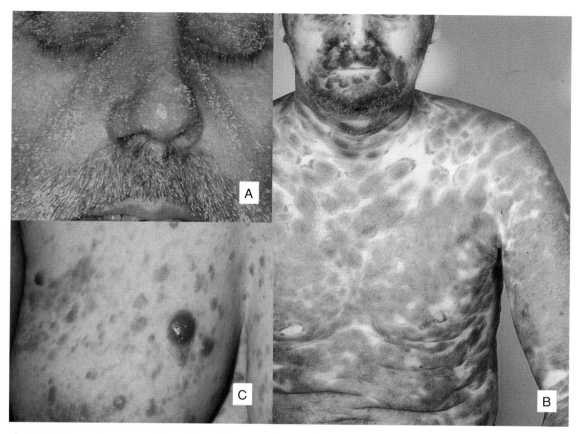

Fig. 15.10 Rare cutaneous manifestations of hematopoietic neoplasia. *A,* Hyperkeratotic spicules (Nazzarro syndome) in a patient with multiple myeloma and monoclonal gammopathy. *B,* Hematodermic (CD4$^+$, CD56$^+$) lymphoma showing hemorrhagic plaques involving almost 100% of the skin. *C,* Violet plaques and tumors in a patient with myelomonocytic leukemia. © 2008, Dr. Günter Burg, Universität Zürich, Switzerland.

Histologically, there is a nonepidermotropic infiltrate consisting of medium- to large-sized tumor cells. Erythrocyte extravasation is responsible for the bruise-like appearance. The immunophenotypic profile (CD4$^+$, CD56$^+$, CD123$^+$) of the neoplastic cell indicates its cytogenetic relationship to activated type 2 dendritic cells (plasmacytoid monocyte) [130]. Other markers for T, B, NK, or myeloid cells are negative.

Precursor lymphoblastic leukemia/lymphoma

Neoplasms of B lymphoblasts or T lymphoblasts involve bone marrow, peripheral blood, nodal and extranodal sites. Eighty-five percent to 90% of lymphoblastic lymphomas are precursor T lymphoblasts. Unlike T lymphoblasts, which commonly affect lymph nodes and the mediastinum, B lymphoblasts usually encompass extranodal sites [131].

Hodgkin's disease

Cutaneous manifestations associated with Hodgkin's disease have been described in a few case reports and literature reviews. Studies have shown either paraneoplastic cutaneous manifestations associated with Hodgkin's disease in about 4% of the patients or specific cutaneous Hodgkin's disease in about 0.3% of a large series of more than 1000 patients with Hodgkin's disease [132,133]. Pruritus is the most commonly recognized presenting symptom. Mycosis fungoides, observed in 1% of the patients with Hodgkin's disease, was 290 times more common in patients with Hodgkin's disease than in the general population. Primary cutaneous Hodgkin's disease is an extremely rare event [134]; most experts doubt the existence of extranodal primary Hodgkin's disease.

Cutaneous pseudolymphomas

Cutaneous pseudolymphomas are defined as reactive benign lymphoproliferative processes composed predominantly of B or T cells that heal spontaneously and do not recur after elimination of the causative agent (e.g., drugs, bacteria, viruses) or following nonaggressive therapy for which one would not expect serious side effects after long-term use, such as antibiotics. There is no evidence for systemic involvement in pseudolymphomas during a period of at least 6 months.

In 1923, Biberstein [135] coined the term *lymphocytoma cutis*. Subsequently, Bafverstedt [136] in 1943 introduced the term *lymphadenosis benigna cutis*. The term *pseudolymphoma* is not well accepted by pathologists, who prefer *cutaneous lymphoid hyperplasia* [137]. Pseudolymphomas are divided into B-cell pseudolymphomas, which are more frequent, and T-cell pseudolymphomas, depending on the predominant cell type. Pseudolymphomas are of great clinical relevance because they may be difficult to distinguish from CL. For some pseudolymphomas, both clinical manifestations and etiology are clearly defined, for example, *Borrelia*-associated lymphadenosis cutis benigna. In most cases, however, the etiology of pseudolymphomas cannot be identified.

Clinically, pseudolymphomas are variable and usually present as solitary nodules, sometimes nodules grouped in a circumscribed area, or rarely disseminated nodules or infiltrated plaques. Histologically, in T-cell pseudolymphomas a sleeve-like pattern around blood vessels and adnexal structures is seen, whereas a follicular pattern is common in B-cell pseudolymphomas, also known as follicular lymphoid hyperplasia. In addition to routine

microscopy, immunohistochemistry and molecular studies may be helpful in the distinction from CL. Detection of monoclonal T or B cells argues for the presence of a lymphoma, although exceptions exist. The final diagnosis should always be based on a clinicopathologic correlation and should never be based on one single criterion.

Parapsoriasis: a debatable issue

The term *parapsoriasis*, which was created by Brocq (1856–1928) [138,139] 100 years ago, is confusing and requires explanation. It encompasses a number of different pathologic states clinically manifested by chronic recalcitrant erythematous scaling lesions. The common features of these subgroups are (i) long duration of the disease, (ii) good general health, (iii) absence of itching, (iv) erythema and pityriasiform scaling, (v) control of disease without cure by topical treatment, and (vi) round cell infiltrate in the papillary dermis. Brocq differentiated three conditions: (i) "parapsoriasis en gouttes" (guttate parapsoriasis), (ii) "parapsoriasis lichenoide," and (iii) "parapsoriasis en plaques." The third condition, later referred to as Brocq's disease, is important in the context of cutaneous lymphomas and prelymphomatous conditions [140].

Today, two groups of parapsoriasis are differentiated: the benign form ("parapsoriasis en plaques" [Brocq's disease in a strict sense]) and large plaque forms with or without poikiloderma. The small plaque form never evolves into mycosis fungoides or CTCL, whereas in up to 50% of the cases, the large plaque forms may evolve into mycosis fungoides or other CTCLs after several decades. The most useful criteria for distinguishing between benign and premalignant forms of parapsoriasis en plaques are summarized in Table 15.3.

Skin involvement in leukemias

Histologically specific cutaneous infiltrates are much less common than nonspecific ones, which may be first evident as eczema, pruritic papules, or purpuric patches. In addition, the immunocompromised state of patients with leukemia is often associated with an enhanced susceptibility to bacterial, fungal, and viral infections. Although the majority of histologically specific infiltrates occur in the

Table 15.3 Most useful criteria for distinguishing between benign and premalignant forms of parapsoriasis en plaques

	Benign Form (Small Patch Type)	Premalignant Form (Large Patch Type) with or without Poikiloderma
Age distribution	Adults	All ages
Sex incidence (M:F)	5:1	2:1
Clinical features	Small (2–6 cm in diameter); mostly oval or finger-like patches; slightly erythematous (pseudo-atrophy) and wrinkled surface uniformly pinkish or yellowish, with pityriasiform scaling	Few large patches; pityriasiform scaling with or without telangiectases and netlike pigmentation
Preferential locations	Trunk and upper extremities	Breast and buttocks
Histologic features	Patchy parakeratosis; slight perivascular patchy infiltrate; no edema; no epidermotropism	Slight epidermal atrophy with loss of rete ridges; significant bandlike dermal lymphocytic infiltrate sparing the subepidermal zone; no epidermotropism; no edema; telangiectases, either prominent (poikilodermatous variant) or absent
Prognosis	Life expectancy normal; no progress to mycosis fungoides	Life expectancy normal in most cases; progress to mycosis fungoides may occur

Source: Burg et al. [140].

setting of established hematologic malignancy, they may be the initial clue to the diagnosis of an unrecognized systemic leukemia [141].

The diagnosis of specific skin infiltrates is based on the recognition of the preponderant cell type and pattern of infiltration in the skin and on correlation with clinical and hematologic findings in lymph nodes, peripheral blood, and bone marrow. In the large majority of cases, an objective diagnosis of specific cutaneous infiltrate in patients with leukemia can be made based on distinctive clinicopathologic features, which may be supplemented by immunohistochemical and molecular studies.

Chronic lymphocytic leukemia

B-cell chronic lymphocytic leukemia (CLL) is the most common leukemia of elderly people in the western world. Histologically, specific skin lesions occur in approximately 8% of patients. They usually present as red or violaceous macules, papules, or nodules typically located on the face, particularly the ears, but may also frequently be seen on the scalp, trunk, and extremities. Histologically, the infiltrate is typically nodular, well circumscribed, and separated from the epidermis by a narrow Grenz zone. It tends to be monomorphous and consists of small to medium-sized lymphocytes with a round nucleus, dense nuclear chromatin, small nucleoli, and scant cytoplasm. In contrast to B-cell pseudolymphomas, eosinophils, neutrophils, and plasma cells usually are lacking.

Immunophenotypically, besides the classical B-cell markers, the neoplastic cells aberrantly express the T-cell marker CD5. The detection of a monoclonal restriction to either κ or λ is an important feature of B-cell CLL cells.

T-cell CLL is less frequent than B-cell CLL. However, T cells have a stronger tendency to home to the skin than do B cells. Clinically, the most commonly reported skin lesions are a diffuse maculopapular eruption, nodules, and erythroderma, which may simulate Sézary syndrome.

Specific infiltrates show a monomorphous collection of small to medium-sized lymphocytes, variably admixed with eosinophils and neutrophils. These cells immunophenotypically express CD4+, CD8−, or less frequently, CD4+, CD8+.

Myeloid and monocytic leukemia

Histologically specific skin lesions (Fig. 15.10C) present as multiple disseminated or even generalized erythematous papules, plaques, or nodules that show a magenta or violet color and may become purpuric and ulcerated. Acute febrile neutrophilic dermatosis (Sweet's syndrome) frequently is associated with myeloid and monocytic leukemia. Histology in specific skin infiltrates of myeloid and monocytic leukemia is very typical, showing an interstitial Indian file– or netlike spread of tumor cells. The infiltrate is pleomorphic and dominated by mature and immature cells of the granulocytic series, including atypical myelocytes, metamyelocytes, eosinophils, and neutrophils. The myeloid and monocytic leukemia cells stain for CD43, CD45, CD68, myeloperoxidase, lysozyme, and naphthol AS-D chloracetate esterase (NASDCE).

Etiology and pathogenesis of cutaneous lymphomas

The development of CL is a multifactorial and multistep process due to the impact of various etiologic aspects on a susceptible "genotraumatic" clone of lymphoid cells over a long period of time [142]. The disease mostly starts as a reactive, inflammatory process. Genetic, environmental, infectious, and immunologic factors may be important in initiating the pathogenetic process. Deficits in cell proliferation, regulation and defective oncogene and/or suppressor gene expression promote transition from pre-neoplastic conditions to neoplasia.

Cytokines that play an important role in this process are IL-15, IL-7 and IL-2 [143–145]. Programmed cell death (apoptosis) is blocked by increased bcl-2 protein expression [146]. Moreover, the enzyme telomerase, by which cells overcome the natural "aging" process, shows a significant increase of activity in CTCL [147]. Finally, a highly abnormal cell clone evolves that grows independently from external stimuli as the result of autocrine stimulation by IL-15, IL-7, or other cytokines produced by the tumor cells themselves [145,148]. This

hypothesis, that carcinogenesis is a multifactorial, stepwise evolutionary process arising from the accumulation of gene mutations [149], provides a reasonable explanation for the broad spectrum of CTCLs observed.

Therapy of cutaneous lymphomas

Almost completely lacking are large randomized therapeutic trials in the heterogeneous group of CLs that have sufficient stratification of subgroups while producing data that is statistically significant [150]. Standard and experimental treatment modalities recently have been reviewed [151]. The EORTC consensus recommendations for the treatment of mycosis fungoides/Sézary syndrome have been elaborated. They indicate that skin-directed therapies are the most appropriate option for early-stage mycosis fungoides and Sézary syndrome, whereas patients with advanced disease should be encouraged to participate in clinical trials [152].

Treatment strategies may be topical or systemic, nonaggressive or aggressive (i.e., severe side effects to be expected), or combinations. In CTCL, long-term disease-free survival is not improved by an early aggressive treatment [153]; therefore, a stage-adapted therapy is recommended. Current treatment modalities are depicted in Table 15.4. Besides the type of lymphoma, the choice of treatment modality depends on the extent and morphology of skin lesions and the aggressiveness of the lymphoma, the age and physical condition of the patient, the presence of concurrent diseases, the availability of treatment techniques, and the patient's compliance.

Lymphomas expressing the IL-2 receptor can be targeted by fusion proteins containing diphtheria toxin fragments, which split off and kill the "labeled" cells [154,155]. Gemcitabine is an effective monotherapy in patients with advanced, heavily pretreated CTCL [156]. Future experimental treatment modalities include topical immune-response modifiers and monoclonal antibodies. Imiquimod binds to Toll-like receptor 7 [157]. Bexarotene is a retinoid derivate binding to the retinoid X receptor [158,159]. Rituximab acts as a recombinant chimeric monoclonal antibody

Table 15.4 Treatment strategies[a]

	Topical	Systemic
Nonaggressive	Glucosteroids PUVA UV-B narrow band Topical retinoids	Interferon-α Retinoids Photopheresis
Aggressive	HN2 Carmustine X-rays TSEB	Chemotherapy • Single agent • Combination

[a] Treatment may be topical or systemic; nonaggressive or aggressive, i.e., with severe side effects to be expected; or a combination of these.

HN2, mechlorethamine; PUVA, psoralen–ultraviolet A; TSEB, total-skin electron-beam radiation; UV-B, ultraviolet B.

directed against the CD20 antigen expressed by B lymphocytes [160,161]. The humanized monoclonal antibody alemtuzumab (Campath-1H, Genzyme) binds to the CD52 antigen, a glycoprotein that is widely expressed on normal and malignant B and T lymphocytes [162,163]. Another human monoclonal anti-CD4 antibody that has been used successfully for the treatment of CD4+ refractory peripheral T-cell lymphoma is zanolimumab (HuMax-CD4, Genmab) [164].

The application of IL-12 may restore the reduced T helper-1 activity in CTCL [165]. Overall response rate was reported to be approximately 50% in 32 patients [166]. Histone deacetylase inhibitors such as suberoylanilide hydroxamic acid can restore the expression of the tumor-suppressor and/or cell-cycle regulatory genes in cancer cells and block the cellular proliferation of these cells without major toxic side effects. There are several ongoing trials investigating this new group of drugs [156]. Recombinant measles virus induces cytolysis of CTCL. In a phase I clinical trial, measles virus vaccine induced tumor regression in CTCL patients [167]. Progress in molecular biology and immunology has to be translated into biology-based treatment approaches [151]. Nevertheless, controlling rather than curing the disease is the best approach for treatment in most cases, because complete healing of the disease—that is, clearing of skin lesions without recurrence over a follow-up time of at least 1 year—usually is not possible.

Prognostic parameters in cutaneous lymphomas

The course and prognosis of CLs differ significantly from those of their nodal counterparts. There also is a wide range of biologic behavior among the various types of CL [30]. In CTCL the clinical stage at the time of diagnosis represents the most relevant prognostic factor. In addition to clinical stage, there are many other parameters, including histologic features, immunophenotype of tumor cells, presence of tumor cells in the peripheral blood, and serologic findings. In CBCL, there still is no widely used system for classifying stage. In contrast to CTCL, type and spread of the tumor do not correlate well with prognosis. Various prognostic parameters include clinical features, histomorphologic pattern, cytomorphologic and immunocytologic characteristics, and genetic profile of the neoplastic cells.

References

1 Alibert JLM. Tableau du pian fongoide. Description des maladies de la peau, observées à l'Hôpital Saint-Louis et exposition des meilleurs méthodes suivies pour leur traitement. Paris: Barrois L'Ainé & Fils; 1806.

2 Bontius J. De medicina indorum libri IV. Piso; 1642.

3 Brouet JC, Flandrin G, Seligmann M. Indications of the thymus-derived nature of the proliferating cells in six patients with Sezary's syndrome. N Engl J Med 1973;289:341–4.

4 Burg G, Braun-Falco O. Classification and differentiation of cutaneous lymphomas. Enzyme-cytochemical and immunocytological studies. Br J Dermatol 1975;93:597–9.

5 Burg G, Braun-Falco O. Morphological and functional differentiation and classification of cutaneous lymphomas. Bull Cancer 1977;64:225–40.

6 Kerl H, Cerroni L. Primary cutaneous B-cell lymphomas: then and now. J Cutan Pathol 2006;33 Suppl 1:1–5.

7 Weinstock MA, Gardstein B. Twenty-year trends in the reported incidence of mycosis fungoides and associated mortality. Am J Public Health 1999;89:1240–4.

8 Greene MH, Dalager NA, Lamberg SI, et al. Mycosis fungoides: epidemiologic observations. Cancer Treat Rep 1979;63:597–606.

9 Cohen SR, Stenn KS, Braverman IM, et al. Clinicopathologic relationships, survival, and therapy in 59 patients with observations on occupation as a new prognostic factor. Cancer 1980;46:2654–66.

10 Whittemore AS, Holly EA, Lee IM, et al. Mycosis fungoides in relation to environmental exposures and immune response: a case-control study. J Natl Cancer Inst 1989;81:1560–7.

11 Teixeira F, Ortiz PA, Cortes FR, et al. Do environmental factors play any role in the pathogenesis of mycosis fungoides and Sezary syndrome? Int J Dermatol 1994;33:770–2.

12 Samman PD. The natural history of parapsoriasis en plaques (chronic superficial dermatitis) and prereticulotic poikiloderma. Br J Dermatol 1972;87:405–11.

13 Weinstock MA. Epidemiology of mycosis fungoides. Semin Dermatol 1994;13:154–9.

14 Kumar R, Xiu Y, Zhuang HM, et al. 18F-fluorodeoxyglucose-positron emission tomography in evaluation of primary cutaneous lymphoma. Br J Dermatol 2006;155:357–63.

15 Tsai EY, Taur A, Espinosa L, et al. Staging accuracy in mycosis fungoides and Sezary syndrome using integrated positron emission tomography and computed tomography. Arch Dermatol 2006;142:577–84.

16 Bazin P. Leçons sur le traitement des maladies chroniques en général, affections de la peau en particulier, par l'emploi comparé des eaux minérales, de l'hydrothérapie et des moyens pharmaceutiques. Paris: Delahaye; 1870.

17 Bunn PA Jr, Lamberg SI. Report of the Committee on Staging and Classification of Cutaneous T-Cell Lymphomas. Cancer Treat Rep 1979;63:725–8.

18 Olsen E, Vonderheid E, Pimpinelli E, et al. Revisions to the staging and classification of mycosis fungoides and Sézary syndrome: a proposal of the International Society for Cutaneous Lymphomas (ISCL) and the Cutaneous Lymphoma Task Force of the European Organization of Research and Treatment of Cancer (EORTC) [published online ahead of print on May 31, 2007]. Blood.

19 Kim YH, Willemze R, Pimpinelli N, et al. TNM classification system for primary cutaneous lymphomas other than mycosis fungoides and Sezary syndrome: a proposal of the International Society for Cutaneous Lymphomas (ISCL) and the Cutaneous Lymphoma Task Force of the European Organization of Research and Treatment of Cancer (EORTC). Blood 2007; 110:479–84.

20 Schmid MH, Bird P, Dummer R, et al. Tumor burden index as a prognostic tool for cutaneous T-cell lymphoma: a new concept. Arch Dermatol 1999;135:1204–8.

21 Stevens SR, Ke MS, Parry EJ, et al. Quantifying skin disease burden in mycosis fungoides-type cutaneous T-cell lymphomas: the severity-weighted assessment tool (SWAT). Arch Dermatol 2002;138:42–8.

22 Cerroni L, Volkenandt M, Rieger E, et al. bcl-2 protein expression and correlation with the interchromosomal 14;18 translocation in cutaneous lymphomas and pseudolymphomas. J Invest Dermatol 1994;102: 231–5.

23 Beylot-Barry M, Lamant L, Vergier B, et al. Detection of t(2;5)(p23;q35) translocation by reverse transcriptase polymerase chain reaction and in situ hybridization in CD30-positive primary cutaneous lymphoma and lymphomatoid papulosis. Am J Pathol 1996;149:483–92.

24 Cerroni L, Minkus G, Putz B, et al. Laser beam microdissection in the diagnosis of cutaneous B-cell lymphoma. Br J Dermatol 1997;136:743–6.

25 Kempf W, Cozzio A, Kazakov DV, et al. Cytogenetic studies in cutaneous lymphomas. In: Burg G, Kempf W, editors. Cutaneous lymphomas. Boca Raton: Francis & Taylor Group; 2005. p. 69–72.

26 Storz MN, van de Rijn M, Kim YH, et al. Gene expression profiles of cutaneous B cell lymphoma. J Invest Dermatol 2003;120:865–70.

27 Hoefnagel JJ, Dijkman R, Basso K, et al. Distinct types of primary cutaneous large B-cell lymphoma identified by gene expression profiling. Blood 2005;105:3671–8.

28 Burg G, Dummer R, Kerl H. Classification of cutaneous lymphomas. Dermatol Clin 1994;12: 213–7.

29 Burg G, Jaffe ES, Kempf W, et al. WHO/EORTC classification of cutaneous lymphomas. In: LeBoit P, Burg G, Weedon D, et al., editors. WHO Books: Tumors of the skin, vol. X. Lyon: WHO IARC; 2006. p. 166–8.

30 Burg G, Kempf W, Hess Schmid M. Prognostic parameters in cutaneous lymphomas. In: Burg G, Kempf W, editors. Cutaneous lymphomas. Boca Raton: Francis & Taylor Group; 2005. p. 529–42.

31 Willemze R, Jaffe ES, Burg G, et al. WHO-EORTC classification for cutaneous lymphomas. Blood 2005;105:3768–85.

32 LeBoit P, Burg G, Weedon D, et al., editors. Tumors of the skin, vol. X. Lyon: WHO IARC; 2006.

33 Bahler DW, Kim BK, Gao A, et al. Analysis of immunoglobulin V genes suggests cutaneous marginal zone B-cell lymphomas recognise similar antigens. Br J Haematol 2006;132:571–5.

34 Santucci M, Burg G, Feller AC. Interrater and intrarater reliability of histologic criteria in early cutaneous T-cell lymphoma: an EORTC Cutaneous Lymphoma Project Group study. Dermatol Clin 1994; 12:323–7.

35 Smoller BR, Detwiler SP, Kohler S, et al. Role of histology in providing prognostic information in mycosis fungoides. J Cutan Pathol 1998;25:311–5.

36 Smoller BR, Bishop K, Glusac E, et al. Reassessment of histologic parameters in the diagnosis of mycosis fungoides. Am J Surg Pathol 1995;19:1423–30.

37 Massone C, Kodama K, Kerl H, et al. Histopathologic features of early (patch) lesions of mycosis fungoides: a morphologic study on 745 biopsy specimens from 427 patients. Am J Surg Pathol 2005;29: 550–60.

38 Santucci M, Biggeri A, Feller AC, et al. Efficacy of histologic criteria for diagnosing early mycosis fungoides: an EORTC Cutaneous Lymphoma Study Group investigation. European Organization for Research and Treatment of Cancer. Am J Surg Pathol 2000;24:40–50.

39 Guitart J, Kennedy J, Ronan S, et al. Histologic criteria for the diagnosis of mycosis fungoides: proposal for a grading system to standardize pathology reporting. J Cutan Pathol 2001;28:174–83.

40 Pimpinelli N, Olsen EA, Santucci M, et al. Defining early mycosis fungoides. J Am Acad Dermatol 2005;53:1053–63.

41 Dummer R, Kohl O, Gillessen J, et al. Peripheral blood mononuclear cells in patients with nonleukemic cutaneous T-cell lymphoma. Reduced proliferation and preferential secretion of a T helper-2-like cytokine pattern on stimulation. Arch Dermatol 1993;129:433–6.

42 Vowels BR, Lessin SR, Cassin M, et al. Th2 cytokine mRNA expression in skin in cutaneous T-cell lymphoma. J Invest Dermatol 1994;103:669–73.

43 Woringer F, Kolopp P. Lesion erythemato-squameuse polycyclique de l'avant-bras evoluant depuis 6 ans chez un garconnet de 13 ans. Ann Dermatol Syphilol 1939;10:945–58.

44 Fujiwara Y, Abe Y, Kuyama M, et al. CD8+ cutaneous T-cell lymphoma with pagetoid epidermotropism and angiocentric and angiodestructive infiltration. Arch Dermatol 1990;126:801–4.

45 Burg G, Schmockel C. Syringolymphoid hyperplasia with alopecia—a syringotropic cutaneous T-cell lymphoma? Dermatology 1992;184:306–7.

46 Cerroni L, Kerl H. Primary follicular mucinosis and association with mycosis fungoides and other cutaneous T-cell lymphomas. J Am Acad Dermatol 2004;51:146–7; author reply 7–8.

47 Cerroni L, Fink-Puches R, Back B, et al. Follicular mucinosis: a critical reappraisal of clinicopathologic features and association with mycosis fungoides and Sezary syndrome. Arch Dermatol 2002;138: 182–9.

48 van Doorn R, Scheffer E, Willemze R. Follicular mycosis fungoides, a distinct disease entity with or without associated follicular mucinosis: a clinicopathologic and follow-up study of 51 patients. Arch Dermatol 2002;138:191–8.

49 Kazakov DV, Burg G, Kempf W. Clinicopathological spectrum of mycosis fungoides. J Eur Acad Dermatol Venereol 2004;18:397–415.

50 Camacho FM, Burg G, Moreno JC, et al. Granulomatous slack skin in childhood. Pediatr Dermatol 1997;14:204–8.

51 Convit J, Kerdel F, Goihman M, et al. Progressive, atrophying, chronic granulomatous dermohypodermitis. Autoimmune disease? Arch Dermatol 1973;107:271–4.

52 LeBoit PE. Granulomatous slack skin. Dermatol Clin 1994;12:375–89.

53 LeBoit PE, Beckstead JH, Bond B, et al. Granulomatous slack skin: clonal rearrangement of the T-cell receptor beta gene is evidence for the lymphoproliferative nature of a cutaneous elastolytic disorder. J Invest Dermatol 1987;89:183–6.

54 von Zumbusch L. Fallbericht. Arch Dermatol Syphilol 1915;51:119.

55 Sézary A, Bouvrain Y. Erythrodermie avec presence de cellules monstueuses dansle dermeetlesang circulant. Bull Soc Fr Dermatol Syphiligr 1938;45: 254–60.

56 Baccaredda A. Reticulohistiocytosis cutanea hyperplastica benigna cum melanodermia. Arch Dermatol Syphilol 1939;179:209–56.

57 Kerl H, Aubock L, Bayer U. [Formation and treatment of pathologic scars—clinical and micromorphologic investigations (author's transl)]. Z Hautkr 1981;56:282–300.

58 Vonderheid EC, Bernengo MG, Burg G, et al. Update on erythrodermic cutaneous T-cell lymphoma: report of the International Society for Cutaneous Lymphomas. J Am Acad Dermatol 2002;46:95–106.

59 Vonderheid EC, Pena J, Nowell P. Sezary cell counts in erythrodermic cutaneous T-cell lymphoma: implications for prognosis and staging. Leuk Lymphoma 2006;47:1841–56.

60 Dummer R, Posseckert G, Nestle F, et al. Soluble interleukin-2 receptors inhibit interleukin 2-dependent proliferation and cytotoxicity: explanation for diminished natural killer cell activity in cutaneous T-cell lymphomas in vivo? J Invest Dermatol 1992;98:50–4.

61 Vowels BR, Cassin M, Vonderheid EC, et al. Aberrant cytokine production by Sezary syndrome patients: cytokine secretion pattern resembles murine Th2 cells. J Invest Dermatol 1992;99:90–4.

62 Trotter MJ, Whittaker SJ, Orchard GE, et al. Cutaneous histopathology of Sezary syndrome: a study of 41 cases with a proven circulating T-cell clone. J Cutan Pathol 1997;24:286–91.

63 Kamarashev J, Burg G, Kempf W, et al. Comparative analysis of histological and immunohistological features in mycosis fungoides and Sezary syndrome. J Cutan Pathol 1998;25:407–12.

64 Harmon CB, Witzig TE, Katzmann JA, et al. Detection of circulating T cells with CD4+CD7- immunophenotype in patients with benign and malignant lymphoproliferative dermatoses. J Am Acad Dermatol 1996;35:404–10.

65 Klemke CD, Fritzsching B, Franz B, et al. Paucity of FOXP3+ cells in skin and peripheral blood distinguishes Sezary syndrome from other cutaneous T-cell lymphomas. Leukemia 2006;20:1123–9.

66 Scarisbrick JJ, Woolford AJ, Russell-Jones R, et al. Allelotyping in mycosis fungoides and Sezary syndrome: common regions of allelic loss identified on 9p, 10q, and 17p. J Invest Dermatol 2001;117:663–70.

67 Paulli M, Berti E, Rosso R, et al. CD30/Ki-1-positive lymphoproliferative disorders of the skin—clinicopathologic correlation and statistical analysis of 86 cases: a multicentric study from the European Organization for Research and Treatment of Cancer Cutaneous Lymphoma Project Group. J Clin Oncol 1995;13:1343–54.

68 Bekkenk MW, Geelen FA, van Voorst Vader PC, et al. Primary and secondary cutaneous CD30(+) lymphoproliferative disorders: a report from the Dutch Cutaneous Lymphoma Group on the long-term follow-up data of 219 patients and guidelines for diagnosis and treatment. Blood 2000;95:3653–61.

69 Macaulay WL. Lymphomatoid papulosis. A continuing self-healing eruption, clinically benign—histologically malignant. Arch Dermatol 1968;97:23–30.

70 Gruber R, Sepp NT, Fritsch PO, et al. Prognosis of lymphomatoid papulosis. Oncologist 2006;11:955–7; author reply 7.

71 Kadin M, Nasu K, Sako D, et al. Lymphomatoid papulosis. A cutaneous proliferation of activated helper T cells expressing Hodgkin's disease-associated antigens. Am J Pathol 1985;119:315–25.

72 Kaudewitz P, Burg G, Stein H, et al. Monoclonal antibody patterns in lymphomatoid papulosis. Dermatol Clin 1985;3:749–57.

73 Davis TH, Morton CC, Miller-Cassman R, et al. Hodgkin's disease, lymphomatoid papulosis, and cutaneous T-cell lymphoma derived from a common T-cell clone. N Engl J Med 1992;326:1115–22.

74 Amagai M, Kawakubo Y, Tsuyuki A, et al. Lymphomatoid papulosis followed by Ki-1 positive anaplastic large cell lymphoma: proliferation of a common T-cell clone. J Dermatol 1995;22:743–6.

75 Stein H, Foss HD, Durkop H, et al. CD30(+) anaplastic large cell lymphoma: a review of its histopathologic, genetic, and clinical features. Blood 2000;96:3681–95.

76 Herbst H, Sander C, Tronnier M, et al. Absence of anaplastic lymphoma kinase (ALK) and Epstein-Barr virus gene products in primary cutaneous anaplastic large cell lymphoma and lymphomatoid papulosis. Br J Dermatol 1997;137:680–6.

77 Burg G, Dummer R, Wilhelm M, et al. A subcutaneous delta-positive T-cell lymphoma that produces interferon gamma. N Engl J Med 1991;325:1078–81.

78 Mehregan DA, Su WP, Kurtin PJ. Subcutaneous T-cell lymphoma: a clinical, histopathologic, and immunohistochemical study of six cases. J Cutan Pathol 1994;21:110–7.

79 Salhany KE, Macon WR, Choi JK et al. Subcutaneous panniculitis-like T-cell lymphoma: clinico-pathologic, immunophenotypic, and genotypic analysis of alpha/beta and gamma/delta subtypes. Am J Surg Pathol 1998;22:881–93.

80 Gonzalez CL, Medeiros LJ, Braziel RM, et al. T-cell lymphoma involving subcutaneous tissue. A clinicopathologic entity commonly associated with hemophagocytic syndrome. Am J Surg Pathol 1991;15:17–27.

81 Perniciaro C, Zalla MJ, White JW Jr, et al. Subcutaneous T-cell lymphoma. Report of two additional

cases and further observations. Arch Dermatol 1993;129:1171–6.

82 Lozzi GP, Massone C, Citarella L, et al. Rimming of adipocytes by neoplastic lymphocytes: a histopathologic feature not restricted to subcutaneous T-cell lymphoma. Am J Dermatopathol 2006;28:9–12.

83 Weenig RH, Ng CS, Perniciaro C. Subcutaneous panniculitis-like T-cell lymphoma: an elusive case presenting as lipomembranous panniculitis and a review of 72 cases in the literature. Am J Dermatopathol 2001;23:206–15.

84 Bekkenk MW, Vermeer MH, Jansen PM, et al. Peripheral T-cell lymphomas unspecified presenting in the skin: analysis of prognostic factors in a group of 82 patients. Blood 2003;102:2213–9.

85 Santucci M, Pimpinelli N, Massi D, et al. Cytotoxic/natural killer cell cutaneous lymphomas. Report of EORTC Cutaneous Lymphoma Task Force Workshop. Cancer 2003;97:610–27.

86 Iwatsuki K, Ohtsuka M, Harada H, et al. Clinicopathologic manifestations of Epstein-Barr virus-associated cutaneous lymphoproliferative disorders. Arch Dermatol 1997;133:1081–6.

87 Barrionuevo C, Anderson VM, Zevallos-Giampietri E, et al. Hydroa-like cutaneous T-cell lymphoma: a clinicopathologic and molecular genetic study of 16 pediatric cases from Peru. Appl Immunohistochem Mol Morphol 2002;10:7–14.

88 Levine PH, Jaffe ES, Manns A, et al. Human T-cell lymphotropic virus type I and adult T-cell leukemia/lymphoma outside Japan and the Caribbean Basin. Yale J Biol Med 1988;61:215–22.

89 D'Incan M, Antoniotti O, Gasmi M, et al. HTLV-I-associated lymphoma presenting as mycosis fungoides in an HTLV-I non-endemic area: a viromolecular study. Br J Dermatol 1995;132:983–8.

90 Zinzani PL, Quaglino P, Pimpinelli N, et al. Prognostic factors in primary cutaneous B-cell lymphoma: the Italian Study Group for Cutaneous Lymphomas. J Clin Oncol 2006;24:1376–82.

91 Cerroni L, Signoretti S, Hofler G, et al. Primary cutaneous marginal zone B-cell lymphoma: a recently described entity of low-grade malignant cutaneous B-cell lymphoma. Am J Surg Pathol 1997;21:1307–15.

92 Bailey EM, Ferry JA, Harris NL, et al. Marginal zone lymphoma (low-grade B-cell lymphoma of mucosa-associated lymphoid tissue type) of skin and subcutaneous tissue: a study of 15 patients. Am J Surg Pathol 1996;20:1011–23.

93 Pimpinelli N, Santucci M. The skin-associated lymphoid tissue-related B-cell lymphomas. Semin Cutan Med Surg 2000;19:124–9.

94 Braun-Falco O, Guggenberger K, Burg G, et al. [Immunocytoma simulating chronic acrodermatitis atrophicans]. Hautarzt 1978;29:644–7.

95 Garbe C, Stein H, Gollnick H, et al. [Cutaneous B cell lymphoma in chronic Borrelia burgdorferi infection. Report of 2 cases and a review of the literature]. Hautarzt 1988;39:717–26.

96 LeBoit PE, McNutt NS, Reed JA, et al. Primary cutaneous immunocytoma. A B-cell lymphoma that can easily be mistaken for cutaneous lymphoid hyperplasia. Am J Surg Pathol 1994;18:969–78.

97 Tomaszewski MM, Abbondanzo SL, Lupton GP. Extranodal marginal zone B-cell lymphoma of the skin: a morphologic and immunophenotypic study of 11 cases. Am J Dermatopathol 2000;22:205–11.

98 Rijlaarsdam JU, van der Putte SC, Berti E, et al. Cutaneous immunocytomas: a clinicopathologic study of 26 cases. Histopathology 1993;23:117–25.

99 Child FJ, Woolford AJ, Calonje E, et al. Molecular analysis of the immunoglobulin heavy chain gene in the diagnosis of primary cutaneous B cell lymphoma. J Invest Dermatol 2001;117:984–9.

100 Pimpinelli N, Santucci M, Bosi A, et al. Primary cutaneous follicular centre-cell lymphoma—a lymphoproliferative disease with favourable prognosis. Clin Exp Dermatol 1989;14:12–9.

101 Rijlaarsdam JU, Meijer CJ, Willemze R. Differentiation between lymphadenosis benigna cutis and primary cutaneous follicular center cell lymphomas. A comparative clinicopathologic study of 57 patients. Cancer 1990;65:2301–6.

102 Cerroni L, Arzberger E, Putz B, et al. Primary cutaneous follicle center cell lymphoma with follicular growth pattern. Blood 2000;95:3922–8.

103 Bergman R, Kurtin PJ, Gibson LE, et al. Clinicopathologic, immunophenotypic, and molecular characterization of primary cutaneous follicular B-cell lymphoma. Arch Dermatol 2001;137:432–9.

104 Mirza I, Macpherson N, Paproski S, et al. Primary cutaneous follicular lymphoma: an assessment of clinical, histopathologic, immunophenotypic, and molecular features. J Clin Oncol 2002;20:647–55.

105 Berti E, Alessi E, Caputo R, et al. Reticulohistiocytoma of the dorsum. J Am Acad Dermatol 1988;19:259–72.

106 Kodama K, Massone C, Chott A, et al. Primary cutaneous large B-cell lymphomas: clinicopathologic features, classification, and prognostic factors in a large series of patients. Blood 2005;106:2491–7.

107 Paulli M, Viglio A, Vivenza D, et al. Primary cutaneous large B-cell lymphoma of the leg: histogenetic analysis of a controversial clinicopathologic entity. Hum Pathol 2002;33:937–43.

108 Sundram U, Kim Y, Mraz-Gernhard S, et al. Expression of the bcl-6 and MUM1/IRF4 proteins correlate with overall and disease-specific survival in patients with primary cutaneous large B-cell lymphoma: a tissue microarray study. J Cutan Pathol 2005;32:227–34.

109 Gronbaek K, Moller PH, Nedergaard T, et al. Primary cutaneous B-cell lymphoma: a clinical, histological, phenotypic and genotypic study of 21 cases. Br J Dermatol 2000;142:913–23.

110 Dijkman R, Tensen CP, Buettner M, et al. Primary cutaneous follicle center lymphoma and primary cutaneous large B-cell lymphoma, leg type, are both targeted by aberrant somatic hypermutation but demonstrate differential expression of AID. Blood 2006;107:4926–9.

111 Ramsay AD, Smith WJ, Isaacson PG. T-cell-rich B-cell lymphoma. Am J Surg Pathol 1988;12:433–43.

112 Dommann SN, Dommann-Scherrer CC, Zimmerman D, et al. Primary cutaneous T-cell-rich B-cell lymphoma. A case report with a 13-year follow-up. Am J Dermatopathol 1995;17:618–24.

113 Pfleger L, Tappeiner J. [On the recognition of systematized endotheliomatosis of the cutaneous blood vessels (reticuloendotheliosis?)]. Hautarzt 1959;10:359–63.

114 Perniciaro C, Winkelmann RK, Daoud MS, et al. Malignant angioendotheliomatosis is an angiotropic intravascular lymphoma. Immunohistochemical, ultrastructural, and molecular genetics studies. Am J Dermatopathol 1995;17:242–8.

115 Ferreri AJ, Campo E, Seymour JF, et al. Intravascular lymphoma: clinical presentation, natural history, management and prognostic factors in a series of 38 cases, with special emphasis on the 'cutaneous variant'. Br J Haematol 2004;127:173–83.

116 Liebow AA, Carrington CR, Friedman PJ. Lymphomatoid granulomatosis. Hum Pathol 1972;3:457–558.

117 Burkitt D. A sarcoma involving the jaws in African children. Br J Surg 1958;46:218–23.

118 Jacobson MA, Hutcheson AC, Hurray DH, et al. Cutaneous involvement by Burkitt lymphoma. J Am Acad Dermatol 2006;54:1111–3.

119 Motegi S, Okada E, Nagai Y, et al. Skin manifestation of mantle cell lymphoma. Eur J Dermatol 2006;16:435–8.

120 Waldenstroem J. Incipient myelomatosis or essential hyperglobulinemia with fibrinogenopenia—new syndrome? Acta Medica Scand 1944;117:216–47.

121 Mascaro JM, Montserrat E, Estrach T, et al. Specific cutaneous manifestations of Waldenstrom's macroglobulinaemia. A report of two cases. Br J Dermatol 1982;106:217–22.

122 Libow LF, Mawhinney JP, Bessinger GT. Cutaneous Waldenstrom's macroglobulinemia: report of a case and overview of the spectrum of cutaneous disease. J Am Acad Dermatol 2001;45:S202–6.

123 Requena L, Sarasa JL, Ortiz Masllorens F, et al. Follicular spicules of the nose: a peculiar cutaneous manifestation of multiple myeloma with cryoglobulinemia. J Am Acad Dermatol 1995;32:834–9.

124 Martin JM, Nicolau MJ, Galan A, et al. CD4+/CD56+ haematodermic neoplasm: a precursor haematological neoplasm that frequently first presents in the skin. J Eur Acad Dermatol Venereol 2006;20:1129–32.

125 Dummer R, Potoczna N, Haffner AC, et al. A primary cutaneous non-T, non-B CD4+, CD56+ lymphoma. Arch Dermatol 1996;132:550–3.

126 Kato N, Yasukawa K, Kimura K, et al. CD2– CD4+ CD56+ hematodermic/hematolymphoid malignancy. J Am Acad Dermatol 2001;44:231–8.

127 Ng AP, Lade S, Rutherford T, et al. Primary cutaneous CD4+/CD56+ hematodermic neoplasm (blastic NK-cell lymphoma): a report of five cases. Haematologica 2006;91:143–4.

128 Assaf C, Gellrich S, Whittaker S, et al. CD56 lymphoproliferative disorders of the skin: A multicenter study of the Cutaneous Lymphoma Project Group of the European Organization for Research and Treatment of Cancer (EORTC) [published online ahead of print on October 3, 2006]. J Clin Pathol.

129 Petrella T, Bagot M, Willemze R, et al. Blastic NK-cell lymphomas (agranular CD4+CD56+ hematodermic neoplasms): a review. Am J Clin Pathol 2005;123:662–75.

130 Petrella T, Comeau MR, Maynadie M, et al. "Agranular CD4+ CD56+ hematodermic neoplasm" (blastic NK-cell lymphoma) originates from a population of CD56+ precursor cells related to plasmacytoid monocytes. Am J Surg Pathol 2002;26:852–62.

131 Lin P, Jones D, Dorfman DM, et al. Precursor B-cell lymphoblastic lymphoma: a predominantly extranodal tumor with low propensity for leukemic involvement. Am J Surg Pathol 2000;24:1480–90.

132 Perifanis V, Sfikas G, Tziomalos K, et al. Skin involvement in Hodgkin's disease. Cancer Invest 2006;24:401–3.

133 Rubenstein M, Duvic M. Cutaneous manifestations of Hodgkin's disease. Int J Dermatol 2006;45:251–6.

134 Jurisic V, Bogunovic M, Colovic N, et al. Indolent course of the cutaneous Hodgkin's disease. J Cutan Pathol 2005;32:176–8.

135 Biberstein H. Lymphozytome. Zentralbl Hautkr 1923;6:70–1.

136 Bafverstedt B. Can benign lymphadenosis (lymphomatosis) of the orbit occasionally be a paraneoplasia? Acta Ophthalmol (Copenh) 1974;52:367–72.

137 Caro WA, Helwig HB. Cutaneous lymphoid hyperplasia. Cancer 1969;24:487–502.

138 Brocq L. Les érythrodermies pityriasiques en plaques disséminées. Rev Gen Clin J Pract 1897;11:577–90.

139 Brocq L. Les parapsoriasis. Ann Dermatol Syphilol 1902;3:433–68.

140 Burg G, Kempf W, Dummer R, et al. Parapsoriasis. In: Burg G, Kempf W, editors. Cutaneous lymphomas. Boca Raton: Francis & Taylor Group; 2005. p. 351–4.

141 Buechner SA, Su DWP. Skin involvement in leukemias. In: Burg G, Kempf W, editors. Cutaneous lymphomas. Boca Raton: Francis & Taylor Group; 2005. p. 373–405.

142 Thestrup-Pedersen K, Kaltoft K. Genotraumatic T cells and cutaneous T-cell lymphoma. A causal relationship? Arch Dermatol Res 1994;287:97–101.

143 Blauvelt A, Asada H, Klaus-Kovtun V, et al. Interleukin-15 mRNA is expressed by human keratinocytes Langerhans cells, and blood-derived dendritic cells and is downregulated by ultraviolet B radiation. J Invest Dermatol 1996;106:1047–52.

144 Grabstein KH, Eisenman J, Shanebeck K, et al. Cloning of a T cell growth factor that interacts with the beta chain of the interleukin-2 receptor. Science 1994;264:965–8.

145 Dobbeling U, Dummer R, Laine E, et al. Interleukin-15 is an autocrine/paracrine viability factor for cutaneous T-cell lymphoma cells. Blood 1998;92:252–8.

146 Dummer R, Michie SA, Kell D, et al. Expression of bcl-2 protein and Ki-67 nuclear proliferation antigen in benign and malignant cutaneous T-cell infiltrates. J Cutan Pathol 1995;22:11–7.

147 Taylor RS, Ramirez RD, Ogoshi M, et al. Detection of telomerase activity in malignant and nonmalignant skin conditions. J Invest Dermatol 1996;106:759–65.

148 Yamanaka K, Clark R, Dowgiert R, et al. Expression of interleukin-18 and caspase-1 in cutaneous T-cell lymphoma. Clin Cancer Res 2006;12:376–82.

149 Fearon ER, Vogelstein B. A genetic model for colorectal tumorigenesis. Cell 1990;61:759–67.

150 Vonderheid EC, Micaily B. Treatment of cutaneous T-cell lymphoma. Dermatol Clin 1985;3:673–87.

151 Dummer R, Cozzio A, Urosevic M. Pathogenesis and therapy of cutaneous lymphomas—progress or impasse? Exp Dermatol 2006;15:392–400.

152 Trautinger F, Knobler R, Willemze R, et al. EORTC consensus recommendations for the treatment of mycosis fungoides/Sezary syndrome. Eur J Cancer 2006;42:1014–30.

153 Kaye FJ, Bunn PA Jr, Steinberg SM, et al. A randomized trial comparing combination electron-beam radiation and chemotherapy with topical therapy in the initial treatment of mycosis fungoides. N Engl J Med 1989;321:1784–90.

154 Foss FM. Interleukin-2 fusion toxin: targeted therapy for cutaneous T cell lymphoma. Ann N Y Acad Sci 2001;941:166–76.

155 Foss F. Clinical experience with denileukin diftitox (ONTAK). Semin Oncol 2006;33:S11–6.

156 Duvic M, Talpur R, Ni X, et al. Phase II Trial of Oral Vorinostat (Suberoylanilide Hydroxamic Acid, SAHA) for Refractory Cutaneous T-cell Lymphoma (CTCL). Blood 2006;109:31–9.

157 Coors EA, Schuler G, Von Den Driesch P. Topical imiquimod as treatment for different kinds of cutaneous lymphoma. Eur J Dermatol 2006;16:391–3.

158 Foss F, Demierre MF, DiVenuti G. A phase-1 trial of bexarotene and denileukin diftitox in patients with relapsed or refractory cutaneous T-cell lymphoma. Blood 2005;106:454–7.

159 Stadler R, Kremer A. Therapeutic advances in cutaneous T-cell lymphoma (CTCL): from retinoids to rexinoids. Semin Oncol 2006;33:S7–10.

160 Shan D, Ledbetter JA, Press OW. Apoptosis of malignant human B cells by ligation of CD20 with monoclonal antibodies. Blood 1998;91:1644–52.

161 Heinzerling L, Dummer R, Kempf W, et al. Intralesional therapy with anti-CD20 monoclonal antibody rituximab in primary cutaneous B-cell lymphoma. Arch Dermatol 2000;136:374–8.

162 Kennedy GA, Seymour JF, Wolf M, et al. Treatment of patients with advanced mycosis fungoides and Sezary syndrome with alemtuzumab. Eur J Haematol 2003;71:250–6.

163 Dearden C. The role of alemtuzumab in the management of T-cell malignancies. Semin Oncol 2006;33:S44–52.

164 Hagberg H, Pettersson M, Bjerner T, et al. Treatment of a patient with a nodal peripheral T-cell lymphoma (angioimmunoblastic T-Cell lymphoma) with a human monoclonal antibody against the CD4 antigen (HuMax-CD4). Med Oncol 2005;22:191–4.

165 Rook AH, Kubin M, Cassin M, et al. IL-12 reverses cytokine and immune abnormalities in Sezary syndrome. J Immunol 1995;154:1491–8.

166 Rook AH, Kuzel TM, Olsen EA. Cytokine therapy of cutaneous T-cell lymphoma: interferons, interleukin-12, and interleukin-2. Hematol Oncol Clin North Am 2003;17:1435–48, ix.

167 Kunzi V, Oberholzer PA, Heinzerling L, et al. Recombinant measles virus induces cytolysis of cutaneous T-cell lymphoma in vitro and in vivo. J Invest Dermatol 2006;126:2525–32.

CHAPTER 16
Cutaneous metastatic disease

Robert A. Schwartz

Cutaneous metastatic disease is not unusual, although it may be overlooked [1,2]. Cutaneous metastases may represent the first evidence of a visceral malignancy. In addition, because cutaneous metastases may be the first sign of extranodal disease, alterations in therapy may be mandated by detection of cutaneous metastases. After treatment, skin metastases may be important as the first indication of recurrence. For patients in whom the tumor is considered resectable, especially when radical surgery is contemplated, the entire mucocutaneous surface should be thoroughly examined for possible metastases first. Demonstration of a small metastasis from lung, breast, or kidney cancer or melanoma has at times dramatically altered therapeutic plans. After correlating gross and microscopic features of the primary tumor with the metastatic one, there may be reasons to suspect a second primary tumor. Cutaneous metastatic disease may rarely be evident years after the primary has been treated. For example, analysis of data of 6298 patients with cutaneous melanoma seen at the Ludwig-Maximilians University of Munich identified 31 patients who first experienced metastatic disease 10 or more years after surgical treatment of the primary melanoma [3].

Cutaneous metastases occur in up to 9% of all patients with cancer, data that include melanoma, sarcoma, and cancer originating in bone marrow and lymph nodes [4]. In a series of patients with skin metastases as the first evidence of malignancy, the underlying cancer had been undiagnosed in 60% of patients with lung cancer, 53% with renal cancer, and 40% with ovarian cancer [5–7]. Of women with cutaneous metastatic disease, the metastases were the presenting sign in 6%. The figure was even higher in men.

Cutaneous involvement by cancer may occur either by direct extension from the primary tumor or by metastases, which may be either local or distant. Metastases may be defined as "a neoplastic lesion arising from another neoplasm with which it is no longer in continuity" or as "a neoplastic lesion arising from another neoplasm that is no longer in continuity or in close proximity within the same tissue." Thus, Paget's disease of breast may be viewed as a direct extension [8] but also as a local metastasis [1].

The frequency of metastatic skin disease correlates roughly with the types of primary cancer in each sex [9]. Women with skin metastases had the following distribution of primary cancers: breast, 69%; colon, 9%; melanoma, 5%; lung, 4%; ovary, 4%; sarcoma, 2%; uterine cervix, 2%; pancreas, 2%; squamous cell carcinoma (SCC) of the oral cavity, 1%; and bladder, 1%. In men, the distribution was as follows: lung, 24%; colon, 19%; melanoma, 13%; SCC of the oral cavity, 12%; kidney, 6%; stomach, 6%; esophagus, 3%; sarcoma, 3%; pancreas, 2%; urinary bladder, 2%; salivary glands, 2%; breast, 2%; and 1% each for prostate, thyroid, liver, and SCC of the skin (Figs. 16.1 to 16.7). The above data do not include the lymphoma and leukemia group, common malignancies found to spread to skin in 6.6% of patients in an autopsy series [4]. Nonhematopoietic tumors most likely to metastasize to the skin in children are rhabdomyosarcoma and neuroblastoma [10].

Breast cancer

Breast carcinoma, the most frequent fatal cancer in women, shows nine distinct clinicopathologic types of cutaneous metastases:

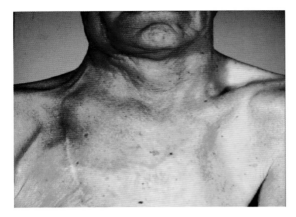

Fig. 16.1 Inflammatory metastatic carcinoma in a man with parotid adenocarcinoma rather than the usually associated breast cancer.

1 Inflammatory breast carcinoma is characterized by an erythematous patch or plaque with an active spreading border simulating erysipelas, usually involving the breast and nearby skin (Fig. 16.1). The clinical appearance of inflammation is the result of capillary congestion, sometimes suggesting a cellulitis or an allergic contact dermatitis. Histologically, there is no inflammatory infiltrate (Fig. 16.2). Rarely, metastases from carcinoma of pancreas, parotid, stomach, esophagus, rectum, melanoma, cervix and other pelvic organs, larynx, and lung may produce this clinical pattern [11–16]. General toxic symptoms resembling erysipelas may appear.

2 Carcinoma en cuirasse, characterized by a diffuse morphea-like induration of the skin, is usually the result of breast cancer but may rarely result from lung, lymphoma, gastrointestinal, and other metastasizing malignancies [17–21]. This description was chosen because of the resemblance of this type of metastatic cancer to the metal breastplate of a cuirassier [1]. Carcinoma en cuirasse usually occurs on the trunk but may be evident elsewhere, including on the scrotum (Fig. 16.3). Unusual keloid-like nodules or scars on the chest should be evaluated for this diagnosis.

3 Telangiectatic metastatic carcinoma shows violaceous papulovesicles resembling lymphangioma circumscriptum [17,22]. It is overwhelmingly of breast origin but may rarely be from other organs, such as the prostate [23]. Its violaceous color is the result of blood in dilated vascular channels. It may be pruritic. A rare variant of this type presenting as a purpuric plaque may mimic cutaneous vasculitis [24].

4 The nodular type of metastatic carcinoma is evident as multiple firm papules or nodules, sometimes

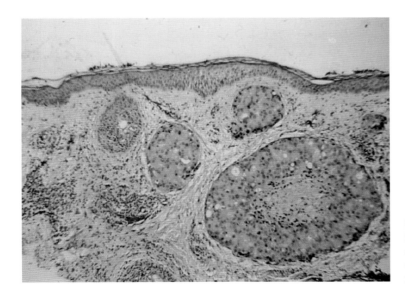

Fig. 16.2 Histology of metastatic inflammatory carcinoma shows nests of adenocarcinoma cells high in the dermis. Note the absence of inflammatory infiltrate.

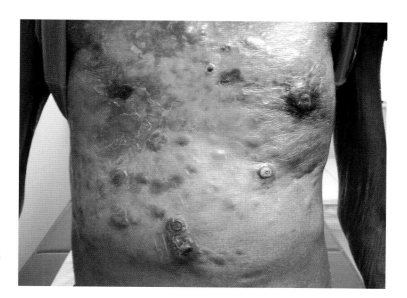

Fig. 16.3 Carcinoma en cuirasse form of metastatic breast cancer with localized nodulation.

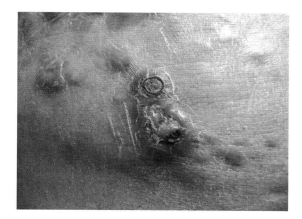

Fig. 16.4 Close-up view of these metastatic breast cancer cutaneous nodules, some of which appear hyperkeratotic.

in a zosteriform pattern [25–28]. This pattern is not restricted to breast cancer and may be seen with lymphomas and other cancers (Fig. 16.4), including melanoma [29,30].

5 Alopecia neoplastica, unlike the previous four types, is probably the result of hematogenous rather than lymphatic spread. It is evident as a circular plaque of scalp alopecia resembling alopecia areata. Because this may be the first clinical sign of metastatic breast cancer, a breast examination and a punch biopsy of atypical alopecia areata in adult women should be considered [31].

6 Paget's disease of the breast represents a distinct pattern of cutaneous metastases from breast cancer with a specific histology. It is a sharply demarcated area of erythema and scaling occurring on the nipple or areola and is regularly associated with an underlying breast cancer. Sir James Paget made this association in 1874 based on 15 cases of women between 40 and 60 years of age with clinically "long-persistent eczema" starting on the nipple and areola [32] (Fig. 16.5). It also occurs in men [33] and may develop from ectopic breast tissue in men and women [34]. An increased number of melanocytes may rarely be observed, producing pigmented Paget's disease. The prognosis is much better if there is no palpable tumor and no adenopathy [35]. Paget's disease is usually but not always associated with an underlying cancer [36].

7 Breast cancer of the inframammary crease produces a cutaneous exophytic nodule clinically suggestive of a primary cutaneous SCC, a basal cell carcinoma, or an epidermal inclusion cyst [37]. Diagnostic confusion may delay diagnosis.

8 Metastatic mammary cancer in the eyelid with histiocytoid microscopic features represents another distinct pattern [38].

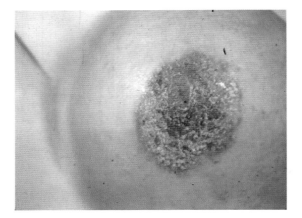

Fig. 16.5 Paget's disease of the breast.

9 Noninflammatory skin involvement in breast cancer, histologically confirmed, may be identified, sometimes when there is only nipple retraction or breast skin dimpling clinically apparent [39]. It is believed to be the result of infiltration of breast cancer cells inducing retraction of Cooper suspensory ligaments. This clinicopathologic entity is not a significant prognostic factor and should not result in a patient being misclassified as having T4 breast cancer, as it does not represent locally advanced breast cancer.

Extramammary Paget's disease

An eruption morphologically and histologically similar to Paget's disease of the breast, known as extramammary Paget's disease, may also occur in the axilla, external ear canal, eyelids, and anogenital region (Figs. 16.6 and 16.7)[40]. At times, it may appear rather verrucous. The eponym is well chosen. Paget's original description, "On Disease of the Mammary Areola Preceding Cancer of the Mammary Gland," had noted that "a similar sequence of events may occur in other parts," as on the penis [32]. There are three types of extramammary Paget's disease: one unassociated with an underlying cancer, one linked with an adjacent apocrine or eccrine gland carcinoma, and one as a result of gastrointestinal or genitourinary tract cancer [41].

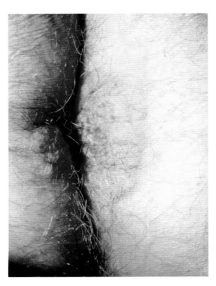

Fig. 16.6 Extramammary Paget's disease, perianal, in an elderly man with no indefinable associated or underlying cancer.

Neuroblastoma

Although most skin metastases do not have any specific or suggestive clinical appearance, a few are morphologically distinctive. Neuroblastoma, for example, is the most common cancer found at birth; 32% of such patients have subcutaneous metastases [42,43]. Neuroblastomas may appear as a generalized, seemingly randomly scattered eruption of firm, nontender, mobile, bluish, subcutaneous nodules. Infants with it have been described by the term "blueberry muffin baby" [44]. When rubbed, these nodules blanch for about 30 to 60 minutes, followed by a 1- to 2-hour refractory period. Periorbital ecchymoses ("raccoon eyes") and heterochromia iridis may be evident as well. Neonatal neuroblastoma with spread to liver, skin, and bone marrow usually regresses or matures; thus, these metastases do not portend certain death but rather the likely transformation into a benign ganglioneuroma (Table 16.1).

Scar metastases

Metastases may sometimes occur within other cutaneous eruptions or at radiation or surgical sites. Skin

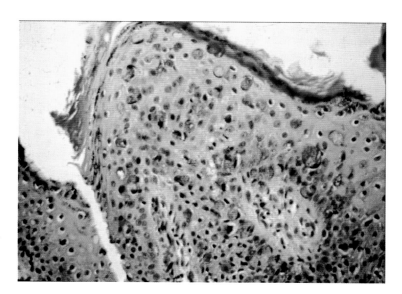

Fig. 16.7 Histology of extramammary Paget's disease, with clear Paget cells "shotgunned" throughout the epidermis.

Table 16.1 Cutaneous neuroblastoma metastases

Blueberry muffin baby: skin tumors in 70% of neonates at the time of diagnosis

Nodules blanch after rubbing, lasting 30–60 minutes, with a 2-hour refractory period

"Raccoon eyes" (periorbital ecchymoses) and heterochromia iridis

Stage IV-S usually remits or becomes benign

metastases may result from implantation following a surgical procedure such as a needle biopsy. Sometimes induced iatrogenically ("iatrogenic metastases"), local metastases in preexistent surgical scars are worthy of note [45–47]. They may be seen in or near the excision or procedure scar of a primary tumor, usually appearing within a year of surgery [48]. However, they may also be present in unrelated surgical or traumatic scar sites. They may be the first sign of breast, ovarian, colorectal, liver, oral, laryngeal, lung, renal, and endometrial cancers. Thus, new nodules in old scars should be examined histologically, as should nodules in new scars. This phenomenon may occur as cutaneous implantation metastasis of cholangiocarcinoma after percutaneous transhepatic biliary drainage [45]. Such metastases are often mistaken for a foreign body reaction, hypertrophic scar, granulation tissue,

traumatic neuroma, SCC developing within a scar, or calcification within a scar [48]. A patient may have a metastatic adenocarcinoma with heterotopic bone formation. Rarely, a cutaneous metastasis may be seen alongside a primary skin cancer [49].

Lymphoma cutis, leukemia cutis (see Chapter 15)

Cutaneous infiltration is relatively common in lymphoma and leukemia patients, sometimes as the first sign [1]. Aleukemic leukemia cutis is characterized by infiltration of leukemic cells into the skin before they appear in the peripheral blood. In addition, skin metastases may be the first sign of extranodal disease. It may be difficult to determine whether a cutaneous lymphoma is metastatic or primary in the skin, a distinction of importance. Lymphoma metastatic to skin may be more common than melanoma, as was the case in a series that found skin metastases in 61 of 674 patients (9%) with non-Hodgkin's lymphoma and 6 of 205 patients (3%) with Hodgkin's disease [4].

Histologically specific cutaneous lesions of both Hodgkin's and non-Hodgkin's lymphomas tend to appear as firm, raised, smooth, slightly violaceous to erythematous nodules or plaques varying in size from a few millimeters to a few centimeters.

Larger plaques and nodules may break down into deep ulcers with sharp, sometimes serpiginous borders. They may resemble a gumma of syphilis, be an indurated plaque meriting the designation "lymphoma en cuirasse," [21] or appear as subcutaneous nodules resembling erythema nodosum [50]. In addition, cutaneous infiltrations may be seen overlying involved lymph nodes, as a local extension rather than as distant spread of lymphoma. Although usually a late finding, occasionally cutaneous nodules may represent an early lymphoma from retrograde spread from a nearby node.

Leukemia cutis may be evident as macules, papules, plaques, nodules, ecchymoses, palpable purpura, or ulcers. As leukemia cutis often precedes or occurs concomitantly with the diagnosis of systemic leukemia, a skin biopsy specimen may be useful in detecting the leukemia and facilitating its evaluation. Specific cutaneous infiltrates are seen in about a quarter of infants with congenital leukemia, usually evident as widespread firm blue, red, or violaceous nodules (blueberry muffin baby—a description also employed for congenital neuroblastoma) and often preceding other manifestations of the leukemia by months [51,52]. Myeloid sarcoma is rare, characterized by the occurrence of one or more tumor masses of immature myeloid cells first evident at an extramedullary site, such as skin. It may develop de novo or concurrently with acute myeloid leukemia (AML), myeloproliferative disorder, or myelodysplastic syndrome, and may be the first evidence of AML or may precede it by months or years. The commonest site of presentation was the skin (28.2%) in a recent analysis of 92 adult patients [53]. These cutaneous tumors are also known as myeloblastomas or granulocytic sarcomas, which, when green in color from the elevated myeloperoxidase levels in the leukemic cells, are termed chloromas. Pernio-like plaques of leukemia cutis on the distal nose and fingers may be the first evidence of myelomonocytic leukemia [54]. Mucocutaneous involvement is particularly common in patients with monocytic leukemia, varying from papules and plum-colored nodules that may ulcerate or become bullous [55] to gingival infiltrations [56].

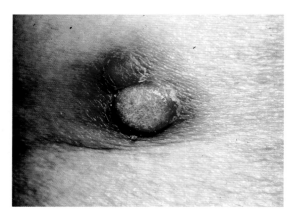

Fig. 16.8 Squamous cell carcinoma metastasis from hypopharyngeal primary.

General growth patterns of cutaneous metastases

Most cutaneous metastases appear as nonspecific painless dermal or subcutaneous nodules with intact, overlying epidermis. They may be flesh-colored, pink, violaceous, or brownish black and are often stone hard when palpated (Figs. 16.8 and 16.9). They may appear as multiple small papules sometimes numbering in the hundreds, as large tumors, as sclerotic plaques, or as hemangioma-like nodules. They may also become necrotic and ulcerated or be cystic. Scalp metastases resembling

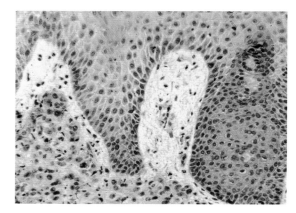

Fig. 16.9 Histology of SCC metastasis from hypopharyngeal primary, with tumor cells abutting the epidermis.

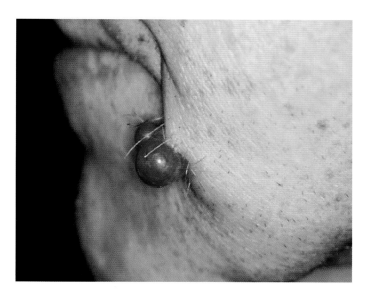

Fig. 16.10 Botryoid (grape-like cluster) metastases to the face from colon adenocarcinoma.

cylindromas or pilar cysts most commonly represent prostatic carcinoma. Metastases may be so hyperkeratotic as to suggest a cutaneous horn or a keratoacanthoma [57]. Rarely, metastases may be unilateral ("zosteriform") or grow like a cluster of grapes (botryoid) [25,58] (Fig. 16.10). Sometimes cutaneous metastases may become large (Fig. 16.11) or erupt with showers of nodules or tumors (Figs. 16.12 and 16.13). I have seen this eruptive metastatic disease phenomenon mostly with melanoma. One should recall that extracutaneous melanoma may be metastatic to skin [59]. A number of primary cutaneous disorders may be mimicked by cutaneous metastases (Table 16.2). Renal cell carcinoma metastases may resemble Kaposi's sarcoma or pyogenic granuloma or be so hyperkeratotic and proliferative as to suggest a keratoacanthoma [6,57]. Lymphoma cutis or a transitional cell carcinoma may resemble a penile chancre.

The growth pattern of skin metastases is unpredictable and may not reflect that of the primary tumor. They may grow rapidly and appear in showers, or they may be slow growing and solitary. The diagnosis of metastatic neoplasms should be considered in the differential diagnosis of any skin nodule or tumor that appears dermatologically atypical.

The localization of metastatic skin disease probably does not occur in a completely random fashion.

Tumors that tend to invade veins, such as kidney and lung cancer, often appear as distinct cutaneous metastases. Dissemination through the valveless vertebral venous system, which bypasses the lungs, may account for seemingly unexpected patterns of metastatic spread, such as prostate, cervix, and breast cancer in the scalp [60,61] (Table 16.3). It may occur early; on the other hand, cancers that invade the overlying skin by direct extension may appear late in the course of the malignant disease [5,9].

When both sexes are considered, colon and rectal carcinoma is the most common visceral cancer.

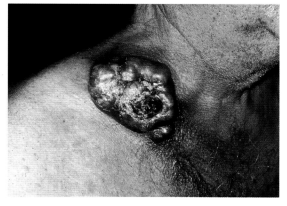

Fig. 16.11 Huge metastatic melanoma in a patient with disseminated metastatic melanoma.

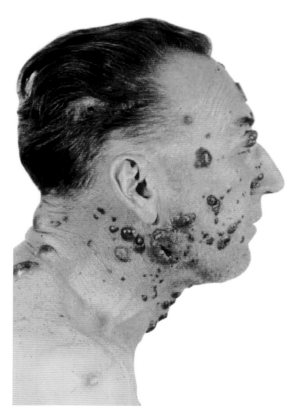

Fig. 16.12 Multiple pigmented tumors in a patient with disseminated metastatic melanoma.

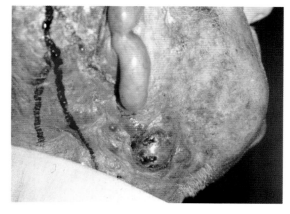

Fig. 16.13 Multiple tumors in a patient with disseminated Merkel cell carcinoma.

Table 16.2 Cutaneous metastases simulating other cutaneous diseases

May Clinically Resemble	Primary Site of Metastasis
"Blueberry muffin baby" (viral)	Neuroblastoma
Multiple cylindromas	Prostate
Large sebaceous cysts	Prostate
Pyogenic granuloma	Renal
Kaposi's sarcoma	Renal
Alopecia areata	Breast
Lymphangiomas	Breast, rarely lung, other
Morphea	Breast, rarely stomach, lung, mixed tumor lacrimal gland
Erysipelas	Breast (inflammatory type), rarely other sites
First-degree skin cancer, inframammary fold	Breast chancre lymphoma, nasopharyngeal transitional cell
Gumma	Lymphoma
Primary skin tumors of head, neck	Paranasal sinus tumors

Table 16.3 Vertebral venous system explains some metastatic sites

A set of valveless veins under low pressure

Includes epidural veins, periverbral veins, and veins of the head and neck

Parallels portal, pulmonary and caval system, connecting with and bypassing them

Bateson's experiments: injecting dye into the dorsal vein of the penis produces facial lesions

Its metastases are most often located in abdominal or perineal areas and tend to appear after the primary cancer has been identified [9]. The abdominal wall appears to be the most common site for tumors first evident as metastatic disease, with lung cancer most frequently seen. Of the metastatic tumors in the abdominal wall, about 10% affect the umbilicus [62], where a metastatic nodule has been called the "Sister Mary Joseph sign." This eponym honors the hospital administrator and frequent assistant who pointed out the sign to the famed Dr. William

Table 16.4 Cutaneous metastases from hypernephroma

Clinically resembles Kaposi's sarcoma, pyogenic
  granuloma, or cutaneous horn
May be histologically specific
Skin lesions may be presenting sign
Polymastia may be associated

Mayo [63]. Surprisingly, one large series of umbilical tumors revealed that 57% were benign and only 43% were either primary or metastatic cancer. Melanocytic nevi, acrochordons, and epithelial inclusion cysts accounted for the majority of the benign tumors; metastatic disease arising from the gastrointestinal tract accounted for most of the malignant ones [62]. Such cutaneous metastases originate predominately in the stomach, colon, ovary, and pancreas [64–67]. Most patients with cancer die within months of this ominous sign, which may occur by lymphatic, vascular, or direct contiguous extension from the underlying peritoneal surface, although there are rare exceptions [68,69]. Umbilical nodules must be differentiated from endometriosis, teratoma, primary skin cancers, dermatofibroma, condyloma acuminatum, foreign body and infectious granulomas, and other benign neoplasms. Endometriosis, a benign metastasizing disease, is a common umbilical tumor.

Suggestive histologic patterns

Cutaneous metastatic diseases may be clinically nonspecific yet reveal histologic characteristics identifying the primary tumor, sometimes by special studies [2]. Histologically recognizable tumors include choriocarcinoma [70], hepatoma [47,71], testicular seminoma [72], testicular Leydig cell tumor [73], hypernephroma [5,6,74–78] (Table 16.4), and malignant carcinoids and other neuroendocrine tumors [79,80]. A metastatic hypernephroma may mimic a clear cell hidradenoma [81]. Carcinoids from bronchus, pancreas, and stomach may show a trabecular histologic pattern, whereas carcinoids originating in the small intestine, proximal colon, or ovary may display nodular solid nests of tumor cells, and carcinoids of the distal colon and rectum may have a mixture of these features [76,79,82,83]. In

liver cancer, cutaneous metastases may show recognizable hepatocytes arranged in irregular columns, bile canniculi, and bile; acinar patterns with documentation of bile in lumina are also noted at times [84,85]. Highly suggestive findings may be seen with skin metastases of mesotheliomas [69,86,87], ameloblastomas [88,89], chondrosarcomas of bone (although their specific histologic pattern is shared by primary benign cutaneous cartilaginous tumors and rarely by sarcomatoid breast carcinoma) [90–92], malignant fibrous histiocytoma [93], papillary carcinoma of the thyroid [94–96], follicular carcinoma of the thyroid [95,97], and cardiac atrial myxoma [98].

Cutaneous metastases may display diagnostic clues. Carcinomas of the gastrointestinal tract may have mucinous metastases that suggest their origin, although they may be confused with primary mucinous carcinoma of the skin or with breast or lung cancer metastases [99]. The presence of psammoma bodies may suggest ovarian carcinoma or a meningoma [5,100]. Cutaneous metastases from chordomas and neuroblastomas may reflect their respective type of primary tumor [101,102]. Skin metastases of lung cancer often appear adenomatous, sometimes with well-formed mucin-secreting glandular structures [5]. Small cell carcinoma of the lung may show characteristic dense-core granules in cutaneous metastases [49,103]. Thyroid carcinoma metastases may test positive for antithyroglobulin antibodies or demonstrate thyroglobulin or triiodothyronine (T_3) in tumor cells [96,97,104]. Cutaneous metastases from medullary carcinoma of thyroid may stain for calcitonin and chromogranin A [105]. Likewise, the ability to demonstrate keratin by immunoperoxidase staining may confirm a squamous cell origin of metastatic disease [106] (Fig. 16.3).

Signet-ring cells may suggest adenocarcinoma of stomach or intestinal origin [107], but small numbers of signet-ring cells may also be present in carcinoma of lung or breast [48] and have been described with metastatic bladder carcinoma, sweat gland carcinoma, and melanoma [108–110]. Carcinoma cutis may be suggested by signet-ring–like cells and myxoid change as unusual findings within a cutaneous endometrioma [27]. Histologically, metastatic tumors from the prostate, breast, colon, larynx, penis, or vagina may have pronounced epidermotropism, producing pagetoid changes resembling either a primary melanoma or an in situ one, or both [31,111]. Pigmented epidermotropic metastasis of a breast carcinoma may mimic a melanoma [112]. HMB-45 may be of value in the detection of ocular melanoma metastatic to skin [113]. Anaplastic Paget's disease may resemble Bowen's disease more closely than the usual histologic pattern of Paget's disease [114]. Special stains may be used in distinguishing Paget's disease and extramammary Paget's disease from Bowen's disease and melanoma (Fig. 16.7). What appears to be a primary mucinous carcinoma may be a secondary mucinous carcinoma of the skin, representing metastatic breast cancer [99]. Adenoid cystic carcinoma may be a rare primary eccrine skin tumor or more commonly a metastasis from colon, salivary gland, bronchus, or breast cancer [115]. Cutaneous metastases of metaplastic breast cancer may contain elements of mesenchymal differentiation including osteogenic sarcoma and chondrosarcoma; they may require distinction from a primary malignant cutaneous mixed tumor [90]. Rarely, histologic sections show carcinoma cutis within a melanocytic nevus, underlying a basal cell carcinoma, or within a burn [116,117]. Immunohistochemical stains for estrogen and progesterone receptors and *CDX-2* (an intestinal homeobox gene) can distinguish metastatic inflammatory carcinoma of breast from that of esophageal origin [16]. Occasionally what appears to be an SCC metastasis may on careful scrutiny show transitional cells, suggesting a primary cancer of the urinary tract or nasopharyngeal origin [118,119]. However, poorly differentiated squamous and transitional cell carcinomas, in the absence of keratinization, cannot be distinguished. Immunohistochemical and ultrastructural analysis may be necessary to distinguish metastatic small cell carcinoma of the lung, primary or metastatic cutaneous Merkel cell carcinoma, lymphoma cutis, melanoma, neuroblastoma, primitive neuroectodermal tumor, rhabdomyosarcoma, and metastatic Ewing's sarcoma [2,120–122]. However, clinical information and morphologic evaluation are usually more reliable than the use of these ancillary techniques [123].

Lung cancer can usually only be classified as an adenocarcinoma, an SCC, or an undifferentiated carcinoma. In men, the most common cancer presenting with each of these three nondiagnostic patterns is lung cancer. A man with an unrecognized primary who presents with cutaneous metastases that show one of these three nondiagnostic patterns on biopsy should be evaluated for lung cancer [5]. Women smokers should be similarly considered.

Therapeutic approaches

Although metastatic skin cancer rarely requires more than symptomatic therapy and tends to respond to systemic anticancer treatment [124,125], surgical excision and/or radiotherapy may at times be beneficial [126–128]. Many cutaneous metastases are radiosensitive [129]. Photodynamic therapy is another choice [130]. Local chemotherapy or immunotherapy may also be useful, as pioneered by Klein in the 1960s [131–134]. I usually recommend intralesional or topical 5-fluorouracil as an excellent option. Imiquimod 5% cream has become a popular choice too; it has been described as eradicating skin metastases of melanoma [135–137]. A new option is 4,4'-dihydroxybenzophenone-2,4-dinitrophenylhydrazone (A-007), a topical treatment for cutaneous metastases from malignant cancers [138]. Intravenous pegylated liposomal doxorubicin in combination with hyperthermia has been successfully employed for skin metastases of breast carcinoma [139]. Paclitaxel may be beneficial by intralesional delivery into skin breast cancer metastases [140]. Cutaneous metastatic melanoma, breast cancer, and SCC have responded to topical miltefosine [141–143]. Efficient palliation of hemorrhaging melanoma skin metastases has been accomplished by electrochemotherapy [144].

Although the development of a skin metastasis is usually associated with a poor prognosis signifying final conquest of the patient by a cancer [145], there are exceptions [146,147]. Cutaneous metastasis may present the aware physician with an opportunity for a diagnosis, and dramatically alter therapeutic plans even if the primary cancer was already known. Some salient features of cutaneous metastases are summarized in Table 16.5. A timely diagnosis may signify cure or a much-prolonged life

Table 16.5 Salient features of cutaneous metastases

Lung, renal, and ovarian cancer: metastases often present before primary

Most frequent primaries for women: breast, colon, and melanoma

Most frequent primaries for men: lung, colon, and melanoma

Sister Mary Joseph sign: an umbilical nodule; the abdominal wall is the most common area for tumors that *present* as metastases; 10% of abdominal metastatic tumors are periumbilical, i.e., Sister Mary Joseph sign

Histology: few cutaneous metastases have specific histology; most are squamous, adenoid, or anaplastic

Histology occasionally specific or highly suggestive for:
Fetal testicular choriocarcinoma (curable even with metastases)
Hepatoma
Testicular seminoma
Follicular thyroid carcinoma
Malignant carcinoid
Chondrosarcoma of bone

expectancy. With our many new techniques, such as immunohistochemical and electron microscopic analyses, diagnosis of the primary from the metastasis can be greatly facilitated.

References

1 Schwartz RA. Cutaneous metastatic disease. J Am Acad Dermatol 1995;33:161–82; quiz 183–6.

2 Schwartz RA. Histopathologic aspects of cutaneous metastatic disease. J Am Acad Dermatol 1995;33: 649–57.

3 Schmid-Wendtner MH, Baumert J, Schmidt M, et al. Late metastases of cutaneous melanoma: an analysis of 31 patients. J Am Acad Dermatol 2000;43:605–9.

4 Spencer PS, Helm TN. Skin metastases in cancer patients. Cutis 1987;39:119–21.

5 Brownstein MH, Helwig EB. Metastatic tumors of the skin. Cancer 1972;29:1298–307.

6 Szepietowski J, Wasik F, Szybejko-Machaj J, et al. [Cutaneus metastases as the first diagnostic sign of renal carcinoma]. Przegl Dermatol 1995;82:293–7.

7 Molina Garrido MJ, Mora Rufete A, Guillen Ponce C, et al. Skin metastases as first manifestation of lung cancer. Clin Transl Oncol 2006;8:616–7.

8 Lookingbill DP, Spangler N, Sexton FM. Skin involvement as the presenting sign of internal carcinoma. A retrospective study of 7316 cancer patients. J Am Acad Dermatol 1990;22:19–26.

9 Brownstein MH, Helwig EB. Patterns of cutaneous metastasis. Arch Dermatol 1972;105:862–8.

10 Wesche WA, Khare VK, Chesney TM, et al. Non-hematopoietic cutaneous metastases in children and adolescents: thirty years experience at St. Jude Children's Research Hospital. J Cutan Pathol 2000;27: 485–92.

11 Schwartz RA, Rubenstein DJ, Raventos A. et al. Inflammatory metastatic carcinoma of the parotid. Arch Dermatol 1984;120:796–7.

12 Bottoni U, Innocenzi D, Mannooranparampil TJ, et al. Inflammatory cutaneous metastasis from laryngeal carcinoma. Eur J Dermatol 2001;11:124–6.

13 Schonmann R, Altaras M, Biron T, et al. Inflammatory skin metastases from ovarian carcinoma—a case report and review of the literature. Gynecol Oncol 2003;90:670–2.

14 Yang HI, Lee MC, Kuo TT, et al. Cellulitis-like cutaneous metastasis of uterine cervical carcinoma. J Am Acad Dermatol 2007;56:S26–8.

15 Ahn SJ, Oh SH, Chang SE, et al. Cutaneous metastasis of gastric signet ring cell carcinoma masquerading as allergic contact dermatitis. J Eur Acad Dermatol Venereol 2007;21:123–4.

16 Nebesio CL, Goulet RJ Jr, Helft PR, et al. Metastatic esophageal carcinoma masquerading as inflammatory breast carcinoma. Int J Dermatol 2007;46:303–5.

17 Lin JH, Lee JY, Chao SC, et al. Telangiectatic metastatic breast carcinoma preceded by en cuirasse metastatic breast carcinoma. Br J Dermatol 2004;151: 523–4.

18 Mullinax K, Cohen JB. Carcinoma en cuirasse presenting as keloids of the chest. Dermatol Surg 2004;30:226–8.

19 Ferguson MA, White BA, Johnson DE, et al. Carcinoma en cuirasse of the scrotum: an unusual presentation of lung carcinoma metastatic to the scrotum. J Urol 1998;160:2154–5.

20 Lopez-Tarruella Cobo S, Moreno Anton F, Sastre J, et al. Cuirasse skin metastases secondary to gastric adenocarcinoma. Clin Transl Oncol 2005;7:213–5.

21 Park KD, Kim YK, Chun SI. Lymphoma en cuirasse. J Am Acad Dermatol 1995;32:519–20.

22 Brasanac D, Boricic I, Todorovic V. Epidermotropic metastases from breast carcinoma showing different clinical and histopathological features on the trunk and on the scalp in a single patient. J Cutan Pathol 2003;30:641–6.

23 Reddy S, Bang RH, Contreras ME. Telangiectatic cutaneous metastasis from carcinoma of the prostate. Br J Dermatol 2007;156:598–600.

24 Pickard C, Callen JP, Blumenreich M. Metastatic carcinoma of the breast. An unusual presentation mimicking cutaneous vasculitis. Cancer 1987;59:1184–6.

25 Bassioukas K, Nakuci M, Dimou S, et al. Zosteriform cutaneous metastases from breast adenocarcinoma. J Eur Acad Dermatol Venereol 2005;19:593–6.

26 Damin DC, Lazzaron AR, Tarta C, et al. Massive zosteriform cutaneous metastasis from rectal carcinoma. Tech Coloproctol 2003;7:105–7.

27 Nogales FF, Martin F, Linares J, et al. Myxoid change in decidualized scar endometriosis mimicking malignancy. J Cutan Pathol 1993;20:87–91.

28 Torchia D, Palleschi GM, Terranova M, et al. Ulcerative carcinoma of the breast with zosteriform skin metastases. Breast J 2006;12:385.

29 Kondras K, Zalewska A, Janowski P, et al. Cutaneous multifocal melanoma metastases clinically resembling herpes zoster. J Eur Acad Dermatol Venereol 2006;20:470–2.

30 Garcia-Morales I, Herrera-Saval A, Rios JJ, et al. Zosteriform cutaneous metastases from Hodgkin's lymphoma in a patient with scrofuloderma and nodal tuberculosis. Br J Dermatol 2004;151:722–4.

31 Haas N, Hauptmann S. Alopecia neoplastica due to metastatic breast carcinoma vs. extramammary Paget's disease: mimicry in epidermotropic carcinoma. J Eur Acad Dermatol Venereol 2004;18:708–10.

32 Paget J. On disease of the mammary areola preceeding cancer of the mammary gland. St Bartholomews Hosp Rep 1874;10:87–9.

33 Menet E, Vabres P, Brecheteau P, et al. [Pigmented Paget's disease of the male nipple]. Ann Dermatol Venereol 2001;128:649–52.

34 Kao GF, Graham JH, Helwig EB. Paget's disease of the ectopic breast with an underlying intraductal carcinoma: report of a case. J Cutan Pathol 1986;13:59–66.

35 Helm KF, Billingsley EY, Zangwill BC, et al. Localized limb cutaneous metastases. J Surg Oncol 1998;67:261–4.

36 Jones RE Jr. Mammary Paget's disease without underlying carcinoma. Am J Dermatopathol 1985;7:361–5.

37 Sanki A, Spillane A. Diagnostic and treatment challenges of inframammary crease breast carcinomas. ANZ J Surg 2006;76:230–3.

38 Hood CI, Font RL, Zimmerman LE. Metastatic mammary carcinoma in the eyelid with histiocytoid appearance. Cancer 1973;31:793–800.

39 Gueth U, Wight E, Schoetzau A, et al. Non-inflammatory skin involvement in breast cancer, histologically proven but without the clinical and histological T4 category features. J Surg Oncol 2007; 95:291–7.

40 Ohira S, Itoh K, Osada K, et al. Vulvar Paget's disease with underlying adenocarcinoma simulating breast carcinoma: case report and review of the literature. Int J Gynecol Cancer 2004;14:1012–7.

41 Brenden LD, Schwartz RA. Extramammary Paget's disease. Am Fam Physician 1983;28:159–61.

42 Yanai T, Okazaki T, Yamataka A, et al. A rare case of bilateral stage IV adrenal neuroblastoma with multiple skin metastases in a neonate: diagnosis, management, and outcome. J Pediatr Surg 2004;39:1782–3.

43 Gunes T, Akcakus M. Congenital neuroblastoma with cutaneous metastases. Indian Pediatr 2002;39:308.

44 Holland KE, Galbraith SS, Drolet BA. Neonatal violaceous skin lesions: expanding the differential of the "blueberry muffin baby." Adv Dermatol 2005;21:153–92.

45 Balzani A, Clerico R, Schwartz RA, et al. Cutaneous implantation metastasis of cholangiocarcinoma after percutaneous transhepatic biliary drainage. Acta Dermatovenerol Croat 2005;13:118–21.

46 Zalaudek I, Leinweber B, Richtig E, et al. Cutaneous zosteriform melanoma metastases arising after herpes zoster infection: a case report and review of the literature. Melanoma Res 2003;13:635–9.

47 Nakamuta M, Tanabe Y, Ohashi M, et al. Transabdominal seeding of hepatocellular carcinoma after fine-needle aspiration biopsy. J Clin Ultrasound 1993;21:551–6.

48 Brownstein MH, Helwig EB. Spread of tumors to the skin. Arch Dermatol 1973;107:80–6.

49 Chikkamuniyappa S. Coexisting basal cell carcinoma and metastatic small cell carcinoma of lung. Dermatol Online J 2004;10:18.

50 Risulo M, Rubegni P, Sbano P, et al. Subcutaneous panniculitis lymphoma: erythema nodosum-like. Clin Lymphoma Myeloma 2006;7:239–41.

51 Torrelo A, Madero L, Mediero IG, et al. Aleukemic congenital leukemia cutis. Pediatr Dermatol 2004;21: 458–61.

52 Zhang IH, Zane LT, Braun BS, et al. Congenital leukemia cutis with subsequent development of leukemia. J Am Acad Dermatol 2006;54:S22–7.

53 Pileri SA, Ascani S, Cox MC, et al. Myeloid sarcoma: clinico-pathologic, phenotypic and cytogenetic analysis of 92 adult patients. Leukemia 2007;21:340–50.

54 Affleck AG, Ravenscroft JC, Leach IH. Chilblain-like leukemia cutis. Pediatr Dermatol 2007;24:38–41.

55 Chen L, Rodgers TR, Chaffins ML, et al. Acute monocytic leukemia with cutaneous manifestation. Arch Pathol Lab Med 2005;129:425–6.

56 Abdullah BH, Yahya HI, Kummoona RK, et al. Gingival fine needle aspiration cytology in acute leukemia. J Oral Pathol Med 2002;31:55–8.

57 Reich A, Kobierzycka M, Wozniak Z, et al. Keratoacanthoma-like cutaneous metastasis of lung cancer: a learning point. Acta Derm Venereol 2006;86:459–60.

58 Kamisawa T, Takahashi M, Nakajima H, et al. Gastrointestinal: zosteriform metastases to the skin. J Gastroenterol Hepatol 2006;21:620.

59 Yanagi T, Akiyama M, Kasai M, et al. Multiple skin metastases of amelanotic melanoma originating from the sinonasal mucosa. Acta Derm Venereol 2005;85:554–5.

60 Schwarz RA, Fleishman JS. Skin metastases from malignant neoplasms. Arch Dermatol 1982;118:289–90.

61 Maheshwari GK, Baboo HA, Ashwathkumar R, et al. Scalp metastasis from squamous cell carcinoma of the cervix. Int J Gynecol Cancer 2001;11:244–6.

62 Steck WD, Helwig EB. Tumors of the umbilicus. Cancer 1965;18:907–15.

63 Kundranda MN, Daw AH. Sister Mary Joseph nodule: an important sign of an ominous diagnosis. Intern Med J 2006;36:617.

64 Maeda S, Hara H, Morishima T. Zosteriform cutaneous metastases arising from adenocarcinoma of the colon: diagnostic smear cytology from cutaneous lesions. Acta Derm Venereol 1999;79:90–1.

65 Hopton BP, Wyatt JI, Ambrose NS. A case of Sister Mary Joseph nodule associated with primary gastric lymphoma. Ann R Coll Surg Engl 2005;87:W6–7.

66 Gabriele R, Conte M, Egidi F, et al. Umbilical metastases: current viewpoint. World J Surg Oncol 2005;3:13.

67 Jun DW, Lee OY, Park CK, et al. Cutaneous metastases of pancreatic carcinoma as a first clinical manifestation. Korean J Intern Med 2005;20:260–3.

68 Okamoto N, Yamafuji K, Asami A, et al. [A long-term survival case after resection for umbilical metastasis from gastric cancer treated with weekly paclitaxel]. Gan To Kagaku Ryoho 2006;33:1155–7.

69 Chen KT. Malignant mesothelioma presenting as Sister Joseph's nodule. Am J Dermatopathol 1991;13:300–3.

70 Ameur A, el Haouri M, Lezrek M, et al. [Cutaneous metastasis revealing a testicular choriocarcinoma]. Prog Urol 2002;12:690–1.

71 Kahn JA, Sinhamohapatra SB, Schneider AF. Hepatoma presenting as a skin metastasis. Arch Dermatol 1971;104:299–300.

72 Schiff BL. Tumors of testis with cutaneous metastases to scalp. AMA Arch Dermatol 1955;71:465–7.

73 Ahsan Z, Maloney DJ, English PJ. Metastasis to skin from Leydig cell tumour. Br J Urol 1993;72:510–1.

74 Barbagelata Lopez A, Ruibal Moldes M, Blanco Diez A, et al. [Cutaneous metastasis of a renal carcinoma: case report and review]. Arch Esp Urol 2005;58:247–50.

75 Rekhi B, Saxena S. Gastric outlet obstruction and cutaneous metastasis in adenocarcinoid tumor of stomach – unusual presentations with cytologic and ultra structural findings. Indian J Cancer 2005;42:99–101.

76 Haroske G, Dimmer V, Herrmann WR, et al. Metastasizing APUD cell tumours of the human gastrointestinal tract. Light microscopic and karyometric studies. Pathol Res Pract 1984;178:363–8.

77 Preetha R, Kavishwar VS, Butle P. Cutaneous metastasis from silent renal cell carcinoma. J Postgrad Med 2004;50:287–8.

78 Opper B, Elsner P, Ziemer M. Cutaneous metastasis of renal cell carcinoma. Am J Clin Dermatol 2006;7:271–2.

79 Hatta R, Nambu Y, Suzuki S, et al. [A case of atypical pulmonary carcinoid accompanying skin metastasis]. Nihon Kokyuki Gakkai Zasshi 2004;42:357–61.

80 Rodriguez G, Villamizar R. Carcinoid tumor with skin metastasis. Am J Dermatopathol 1992;14:263–9.

81 Volmar KE, Cummings TJ, Wang WH, et al. Clear cell hidradenoma: a mimic of metastatic clear cell tumors. Arch Pathol Lab Med 2005;129:e113–6.

82 Archer CB, Wells RS, MacDonald DM. Metastatic cutaneous carcinoid. J Am Acad Dermatol 1985;13:363–6.

83 Schmidt U, Metz KA, Schrader M, et al. Well-differentiated (oncocytoid) neuroendocrine carcinoma of the larynx with multiple skin metastases: a brief report. J Laryngol Otol 1994;108:272–4.

84 Bennett AJ, Kalra JK, Cortes EP. Hepatocellular carcinoma. Arch Dermatol 1982;118:69–70.

85 Ackerman D, Barr RJ, Elias AN. Cutaneous metastases from hepatocellular carcinoma. Int J Dermatol 2001;40:782–4.

86 Gaudy-Marqueste C, Dales JP, Collet-Villette AM, et al. [Cutaneous metastasis of pleural mesothelioma: two cases]. Ann Dermatol Venereol 2003;130:455–9.

87 Maiorana A, Giusti F, Cesinaro AM, et al. Cutaneous metastases as the first manifestation of pleural malignant mesothelioma. J Am Acad Dermatol 2006;54:363–5.

88 Abada RL, Kadiri F, Tawfik N, et al. [Multiple metastases of a mandibular ameloblastoma]. Rev Stomatol Chir Maxillofac 2005;106:177–80.

89 Charfi L, Mrad K, Abbes I, et al. [An unusual cutaneous metastasis]. Ann Pathol 2005;25:145–6.

90 Sexton CW, White WL. Chondrosarcomatous cutaneous metastasis. A unique manifestation of sarcomatoid (metaplastic) breast carcinoma. Am J Dermatopathol 1996;18:538–42.

91 Arce FP, Pinto J, Portero I, et al. Cutaneous metastases as initial manifestation of dedifferentiated chondrosarcoma of bone. An autopsy case with review of the literature. J Cutan Pathol 2000;27:262–7.

92 Ozcanli H, Oruc F, Aydin AT. Bilateral multiple cutaneous hand metastases of chondrosarcoma. J Eur Acad Dermatol Venereol 2006;20:893–4.

93 Lew W, Lim HS, Kim YC. Cutaneous metastatic malignant fibrous histiocytoma. J Am Acad Dermatol 2003;48:S39–40.

94 Junik R, Klubo-Gwiezdzinska J, Zuchora Z, et al. Papillary thyroid cancer with metastasis to the skin. Clin Nucl Med 2006;31:435–6.

95 Alwaheeb S, Ghazarian D, Boerner SL, et al. Cutaneous manifestations of thyroid cancer: a report of four cases and review of the literature. J Clin Pathol 2004;57:435–8.

96 Lissak B, Vannetzel JM, Gallouedec N, et al. Solitary skin metastasis as the presenting feature of differentiated thyroid microcarcinoma: report of two cases. J Endocrinol Invest 1995;18:813–6.

97 Ghfir I, Ccedil Aoui M, Ben Rais N. [Follicular thyroid carcinoma: metastasis to unusual skin locations]. Presse Med 2005;34:1145–6.

98 Okada N, Yamamura T, Kitano Y, et al. Metastasizing atrial myxoma: a case with multiple subcutaneous tumours. Br J Dermatol 1986;115:239–42.

99 Schwartz RA, Wiederkehr M, Lambert WC. Secondary mucinous carcinoma of the skin: metastatic breast cancer. Dermatol Surg 2004;30:234–5.

100 Chamberlain MC, Glantz MJ. Cerebrospinal fluid-disseminated meningioma. Cancer 2005;103:1427–30.

101 Ruiz HA, Goldberg LH, Humphreys TR, et al. Cutaneous metastasis of chordoma. Dermatol Surg 2000;26:259–62.

102 Rubin AI, Bagel J, Niedt G. Chordoma cutis. J Am Acad Dermatol 2005;52:S105–8.

103 D'Aniello C, Brandi C, Grimaldi L. Cutaneous metastasis from small cell lung carcinoma. Case report. Scand J Plast Reconstr Surg Hand Surg 2001;35:103–5.

104 Capezzone M, Giannasio P, De Sanctis D, et al. Skin metastases from anaplastic thyroid carcinoma. Thyroid 2006;16:513–4.

105 Jee MS, Chung YI, Lee MW, et al. Cutaneous metastasis from medullary carcinoma of thyroid gland. Clin Exp Dermatol 2003;28:670–1.

106 Schultz BM, Schwartz RA. Hypopharyngeal squamous cell carcinoma metastatic to skin. J Am Acad Dermatol 1985;12:169–72.

107 Kim BJ, Jeon EK, Seo YJ, et al. A case of signet-ring cell gastric carcinoma of which the first symptom was skin lesions. Korean J Dermatol 2006;44:1426–9.

108 Bellman B, Gregory NA, Silvers D, et al. Sweat gland carcinoma with metastases to the skin: response to 5-fluorouracil chemotherapy. Cutis 1995;55:221–4.

109 Lifshitz OH, Berlin JM, Taylor JS, et al. Metastatic gastric adenocarcinoma presenting as an enlarging plaque on the scalp. Cutis 2005;76:194–6.

110 Jaworsky C, Bergfeld WF. Metastatic transitional cell carcinoma mimicking zoster sine herpete. Arch Dermatol 1986;122:1357–8.

111 Segal R, Penneys NS, Nahass G. Metastatic prostatic carcinoma histologically mimicking malignant melanoma. J Cutan Pathol 1994;21:280–2.

112 Bourlond A. Pigmented epidermotropic metastasis of a breast carcinoma. Dermatology 1994;189 Suppl 2:46–9.

113 Schwartz RA, Kist JM, Thomas I, et al. Ocular melanoma metastatic to skin: the value of HMB-45 staining. Dermatol Surg 2004;30:942–4.

114 Rayne SC, Santa Cruz DJ. Anaplastic Paget's disease. Am J Surg Pathol 1992;16:1085–91.

115 Chang CH, Liao YL, Hong HS. Cutaneous metastasis from adenoid cystic carcinoma of the parotid gland. Dermatol Surg 2003;29:775–9.

116 Betke M, Suss R, Hohenleutner U, et al. Gastric carcinoma metastatic to the site of a congenital melanocytic nevus. J Am Acad Dermatol 1993;28:866–9.

117 Schwartz RA, Burgess GH, Milgrom H. Breast carcinoma and basal cell epithelioma after x-ray therapy for hirsutism. Cancer 1979;44:1601–5.

118 Schwartz RA, Fleishman JS. Transitional cell carcinoma of the urinary tract presenting with a cutaneous metastasis. Arch Dermatol 1981;117:513–5.

119 Caloglu M, Uygun K, Altaner S, et al. Nasopharyngeal carcinoma with extensive nodular skin metastases: a case report. Tumori 2006;92:181–4.

120 Biswas G, Khadwal A, Kulkarni P, et al. Ewing's sarcoma with cutaneous metastasis—a rare entity: report of three cases. Indian J Dermatol Venereol Leprol 2005;71:423–5.

121 Fernandez-Figueras MT, Puig L, Gilaberte M, et al. Merkel cell (primary neuroendocrine) carcinoma of the skin with nodal metastasis showing rhabdomyosarcomatous differentiation. J Cutan Pathol 2002;29:619–22.

122 Izquierdo MJ, Pastor MA, Carrasco L, et al. Cutaneous metastases from Ewing's sarcoma: report of two cases. Clin Exp Dermatol 2002;27:123–8.

123 Azoulay S, Adem C, Pelletier FL, et al. Skin metastases from unknown origin: role of immunohistochemistry in the evaluation of cutaneous metastases of carcinoma of unknown origin. J Cutan Pathol 2005;32:561–6.

124 Lejeune FJ, Monnier Y, Ruegg C. Complete and long-lasting regression of disseminated multiple skin melanoma metastases under treatment with cyclooxygenase-2 inhibitor. Melanoma Res 2006;16:263–5.

125 Rosati G, Rossi A, Germano D, et al. Responsiveness of skin metastases to CMF in a patient with urothelial carcinoma of the bladder: a case report. Tumori 2003;89:85–7.

126 Fruh M, Ruhstaller T, Neuweiler J, et al. Resection of skin metastases from gastric carcinoma with long-term follow-up: an unusual clinical presentation. Onkologie 2005;28:38–40.

127 Kouloulias VE, Plataniotis GA, Kouvaris JR, et al. Re-irradiation in conjunction with liposomal doxorubicin for the treatment of skin metastases of recurrent breast cancer: a radiobiological approach and 2 years of follow-up. Cancer Lett 2003;193:33–40.

128 Zuetenhorst JM, van Velthuysen ML, Rutgers EJ, et al. Pathogenesis and treatment of pain caused by skin metastases in neuroendocrine tumours. Neth J Med 2002;60:207–11.

129 Fritz P, Hensley FW, Berns C, et al. Long-term results of pulsed irradiation of skin metastases from breast cancer. Effectiveness and sequelae. Strahlenther Onkol 2000;176:368–76.

130 Sheleg SV, Zhavrid EA, Khodina TV, et al. Photodynamic therapy with chlorin e(6) for skin metastases of melanoma. Photodermatol Photoimmunol Photomed 2004;20:21–6.

131 Klein E. Tumors of skin. 8. Local chemotherapy of metastatic neoplasms. N Y State J Med 1968;68:877–85.

132 Klein E. Immunotherapeutic approaches to skin cancer. Hosp Pract 1976;11:107–16.

133 Klein E, Schwartz RA, Case RW, et al. Accessible tumors. In: LoBuglio AF, editor. Clinical immunotherapy. New York: Marcel Dekker; 1980. p. 31–71.

134 Trefzer U, Sterry W. Topical immunotherapy with diphenylcyclopropenone in combination with DTIC and radiation for cutaneous metastases of melanoma. Dermatology 2005;211:370–1.

135 Wolf IH, Richtig E, Kopera D, et al. Locoregional cutaneous metastases of malignant melanoma and their management. Dermatol Surg 2004;30:244–7.

136 Ugurel S, Wagner A, Pfohler C, et al. Topical imiquimod eradicates skin metastases of malignant melanoma but fails to prevent rapid lymphogenous metastatic spread. Br J Dermatol 2002;147:621–4.

137 Bong AB, Bonnekoh B, Franke I, et al. Imiquimod, a topical immune response modifier, in the treatment of cutaneous metastases of malignant melanoma. Dermatology 2002;205:135–8.

138 Eilender D, LoRusso P, Thomas L, et al. 4,4′-Dihydroxybenzophenone-2, 4-dinitrophenylhydrazone (A-007): a topical treatment for cutaneous metastases from malignant cancers. Cancer Chemother Pharmacol 2006;57:719–26.

139 Dvorak J, Zoul Z, Melichar B, et al. Pegylated liposomal doxorubicin in combination with hyperthermia for treatment of skin metastases of breast carcinoma: a case report. Onkologie 2001;24:166–8.

140 Rohr UD, Oberhoff C, Markmann S, et al. The safety of synthetic paclitaxel by intralesional delivery with OncoGeltrade mark into skin breast cancer metastases: method and results of a clinical pilot trial [published online ahead of print on November 29, 2005]. Arch Gynecol Obstet.

141 Ragnarsson-Olding B, Djureen-Martensson E, Mansson-Brahme E, et al. Loco-regional control of cutaneous metastases of malignant melanoma by treatment with miltefosine (Miltex). Acta Oncol 2005;44:773–7.

142 Mahieu-Renard L, Richard MA, Dales JP, et al. [Treatment of cutaneous metastases of a squamous cell carcinoma of the leg with topical miltefosine]. Ann Dermatol Venereol 2005;132:346–8.

143 Leonard R, Hardy J, van Tienhoven G, et al. Randomized, double-blind, placebo-controlled, multicenter trial of 6% miltefosine solution, a topical

chemotherapy in cutaneous metastases from breast cancer. J Clin Oncol 2001;19:4150–9.

144 Gehl J, Geertsen PF. Efficient palliation of haemorrhaging malignant melanoma skin metastases by electrochemotherapy. Melanoma Res 2000;10:585–9.

145 Dequanter D, Mboti FB, Lothaire P, et al. Skin metastases from a head and neck carcinoma: a prognostic factor? B-Ent 2005;1:113–5.

146 Segura Huerta A, Perez-Fidalgo JA, Lopez-Tendero P, et al. [Thirteen years' survival in a patient with isolated skin metastases of a gastric carcinoma. What kind of disease is that?]. An Med Interna 2003;20:251–3.

147 Ambrogi V, Nofroni I, Tonini G, et al. Skin metastases in lung cancer: analysis of a 10-year experience. Oncol Rep 2001;8:57–61.

CHAPTER 17
Cutaneous markers of internal malignancy

Robert A. Schwartz

The skin may display a number of reaction patterns and lesions that are important to recognize because they may reflect an internal cancer. Some skin processes or diseases linked to internal cancers, such as bullous pemphigoid, may either be unassociated when age-matched controls are used or are only coupled fortuitously.

Cutaneous disorders traditionally associated with internal cancers include the following cutaneous disorders: generalized pruritus, flushing, tylosis, nail clubbing with or without pachydermoperiostosis, erythroderma, Paget's disease, extramammary Paget's disease, caput medusae, Cushing's syndrome, arsenical keratoses, hepatic estrogenic effects, herpes simplex and zoster, candidiasis, erythema gyratum repens, acanthosis nigricans, Leser-Trélat sign, dermatomyositis, and acquired ichthyosis. A diffuse slate-gray hue may suggest hereditary hemochromatosis (occasionally associated with hepatoma) or the rare generalized melanosis of melanoma. Other associations with underlying cancer include psoriasiform acrokeratosis of Bazex and the yellow nail syndrome.

Emphasized disorders include the following: glucagonoma syndrome, porphyria cutanea tarda associated with hepatoma, acquired multiple mucosal neuromas with pheochromocytoma and medullary carcinoma of the thyroid, Werner's syndrome, acquired hypertrichosis, bullous pyoderma gangrenosum and leukemia, multicentric reticulohistiocytosis, paraneoplastic pemphigus, and pemphigus foliaceus with thymoma. Of considerable importance is the association of chronic cutaneous radiation damage on or near the thyroid or breast with the eventual development of cancer at these sites. Other linkages with malignancy discussed elsewhere in this book include those of the basal cell nevus syndrome, arsenicism, cutaneous metastases, and the cutaneous lymphoma-leukemia-myeloma manifestations (both specific and nonspecific, including the maculopapular rash of immunoblastic sarcoma).

There are a number of syndromes associating cutaneous changes and internal malignancies. In this chapter, we discuss a number of syndromes of special interest. Because some are autosomal dominant, with one diagnosis one may have identified many family members. A number of acquired syndromes are also discussed. Because we live in an age of carcinogenic hazards, arsenic exposure and radiation exposure are included as well.

Peutz-Jeghers syndrome

In 1921, Peutz in Holland described a case of familial polyposis of the intestinal tract with distinctive pigmented macules of the skin and oral mucosa. Jeghers in 1944 described two similar patients, and in 1949, Jeghers and associates reviewed eight additional patients with "generalized intestinal polyposis and melanin spots of the oral mucosa, lips and digits—a syndrome of diagnostic significance" [1]. Peutz-Jeghers syndrome (PJS) is a rare multiorgan familial cancer syndrome. The pigmentation appears as round, oval, and irregular patches of brown to black pigment, occasionally bluish if the melanin pigment is deep. These flat spots (macules) tend not to coalesce and appear as solid dots or as finely stippled aggregations. They may seem to be freckles clinically, but their location on the lips and around the skin adjacent to oral or nasal mucosa is distinctive. Although these have been called "ephelides inversae," reflecting this facial distribution as well as their occurrence on the fingers and toes, they are actually better classified clinically and histologically as simple lentigines. They may appear in unusual sites, such as in psoriatic plaques.

However, these multiple macules, which first appear at birth or in childhood, tend to fade after the age of 25 years, so the persistent mucosal pigmentation is the sine qua non of the syndrome. The gastrointestinal complications of this autosomal dominant, highly penetrant condition are usually manifest before the age of 30 years. Acute abdominal pain, usually from transient but often recurrent intussusceptions, is the most common complication of small bowel polyposis [2]. The most common complications of the gastric, colonic, and rectal polyps are bleeding and anemia.

Polyposis as well as gastrointestinal and non-gastrointestinal invasive malignancies may be evident [3]. Polyps tend to incorporate muscle in the polyp stroma, creating the impression of malignancy. Polyps in the duodenum may be at increased susceptibility for malignant change, but the stomach and large and small intestines may also house cancer in this syndrome. In one analysis of 52 PJS patients, the incidence of gastric polyps was 64.4%, colorectal polyps 76%, and small bowel polyps 95% [4]. A conservative surgical approach has been suggested. However, endoscopic resection of polyps seems appropriate and has revealed foci of adenocarcinoma in them [2]. Laparoscopically assisted endoscopic polypectomy is a good idea [5].

There are other associations with this syndrome, both benign and malignant [6]. Benign changes include polyps of the ureters, bladder, renal pelvis, bronchus, gall bladder, and nasal mucosa [7]. In women, ovarian neoplasms, cancerous and otherwise, may be seen, especially granulosa cell tumors, sex cord tumors with annular tubules, and sex cord stromal tumors with sexual precocity [8–12]. In the uterus, well-differentiated mucinous adenocarcinomas of the endocervix (adenoma malignum) may be evident. In women with PJS, the risk of breast

Table 17.1 Peutz-Jeghers syndrome: essential features

Autosomal dominant; mutated serine kinase gene *STK11*
Pigmented macules of skin, oral mucosa beginning at birth or childhood
Small bowel polyps with recurrent intussusceptions
Gastric, colonic, and rectal polyps with bleeding, anemia
Gastrointestinal condition before age 30
Malignant change in stomach, duodenal, colonic polyps
Chance of intestinal cancer: 2%–3%; breast and cervical cancer
Ovarian and testicular neoplasms (sex cord tumors)
Polyps of bladder, ureters, bronchi, gall bladder, nasal mucosa

cancer was substantially increased, being 8% and 31% at ages 40 and 60 years, respectively [13]. Females with PJS may also be at increased risk of bilateral breast cancer [14]. Men with this syndrome may be at risk of developing testicular tumors of apparent Sertoli cell nature [15]. The case of a 41-year-old woman with this syndrome who was diagnosed with an ovarian sex cord tumor with annular tubules diagnosed together with a minimal deviation adenocarcinoma of the uterine cervix, mucinous metaplasia of both the fallopian tubal mucosa and the endometrium, and a history of breast cancer emphasizes the diversity of neoplasms that may be seen [9].

The fact that this syndrome usually appears in complete form with cutaneous and mucosal pigmentation and gastrointestinal polyposis suggests a single pleiotropic gene. A number of germ line mutations in the *STK11* gene, encoding a serine threonine kinase, have been described in these patients. However, *STK11* mutations do not explain all PJS cases [16].

New endoscopic technologies may improve management of intestinal polyposis, exclude pregnancy, and document small bowel obstruction. The cutaneous stigmata may be treated with laser surgery [17]. Essentials of PJS are summarized in Table 17.1.

Muir-Torre syndrome

In 1967, Torre [18] presented to the New York Dermatologic Society a 57-year-old man with more

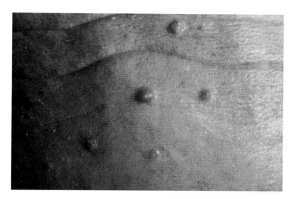

Fig. 17.1 Muir-Torre syndrome, with multiple sebaceous epitheliomas and sebaceous adenoma on the face, gut cancer, and polyps. (Reprinted with permission from Schwartz et al. [20].)

than 100 skin tumors scattered on his face, trunk, and scalp. Representative biopsy specimens showed sebaceous adenomas, sebaceous carcinomas, and basal cell epitheliomas with sebaceous differentiation. This patient had a history of primary carcinomas of the ampulla of Vater and colon and removal of one intestinal polyp with colonic cancer. In the same year, Muir and associates [19] described a Maltese man with multiple primary cancers of the colon, duodenum, and larynx associated with multiple facial keratoacanthomas and a sebaceous adenoma. No keratoacanthomas were noted in Torre's patient, although keratoacanthomas have been shown to occur in enough of these patients to be considered part of this syndrome [20,21].

This association of multiple sebaceous neoplasms and keratoacanthomas with multiple low-grade internal malignancies has been well described [21] (Fig. 17.1). The sebaceous adenoma is usually evident as a yellow papule or nodule. Sebaceous epitheliomas usually resemble a typical basal cell carcinoma, other than often having a more yellow coloration, and may appear hyperkeratotic enough to suggest a keratoacanthoma clinically. It should be noted that sebaceous adenomas, sebaceous carcinomas, and sebaceous epitheliomas are rare, whereas unassociated sebaceous hyperplasia is quite common. Rarely, sebaceous adenomas have been described as resembling sebaceous hyperplasia clinically [22]. The syndrome occurs in both sexes

and tends to manifest during the fifth and sixth decades of life. The skin lesions (sebaceous neoplasms or keratoacanthomas) may be noted before or after the visceral cancer(s). Of 139 patients with Muir-Torre syndrome, 31 (22%) had at least one keratoacanthoma. Despite multiple visceral malignancies, many of the patients had no metastatic disease evident and experienced prolonged survival after resection of the primary tumor. One patient was reported alive and well 14 years after a pulmonary metastasis was excised [23]. The number of sebaceous adenomas or other cutaneous tumors varies greatly from patient to patient. The cutaneous nodules may proliferate if a patient is immunosuppressed. Use of maintenance oral retinoids may stabilize the cutaneous neoplasms and possibly even prevent or discourage cutaneous and visceral neoplasms.

Of cancers that developed in 139 reported patients, over 80% are gastrointestinal in origin, mainly colon and rectal; 51% of all cancers were colorectal [21]. Unlike the latter in the general population, but like that of the cancer family syndrome, the majority (58%) had colorectal cancer proximal to or at the splenic flexure [24]. Urogenital tumors also occur, including those of vagina, ovary, and endometrium. In these 139 patients, multiple primary cancers have been the rule for a total of 282 primary visceral cancers. Thirty-seven percent had two or more visceral cancers, with 10% having four to nine of them. In addition, an association of colonic polyposis with Muir-Torre syndrome has been established. In 139 patients with this syndrome, one or more polyps were evidenced in 38 (27%).

This syndrome is inherited in an autosomal dominant fashion. It is the result of mutations in mismatch repair genes, *MLH-1*, *MSH-2*, or *MSH-6* [25], with a recent breakdown of 36 mutation carrier patients showing 32 (86%) *MSH-2*, 4 (11%) *MLH-1*, and 1 (3%) *MSH-6* [26]. Keratoacanthomas and sebaceous neoplasms may be analyzed for microsatellite instability (MSI) and by immunohistochemistry for concomitant *MSH-2* or *MLH-1* immunostaining. In addition, testing for MSI and mutations of these genes in sebaceous neoplasms and keratoacanthomas may be used as screening for the identification of families at risk [27]. After all, they are

Table 17.2 Muir-Torre syndrome: essential features

Autosomal dominant
Mutation in a mismatch repair gene
Multiple sebaceous neoplasms (adenomas, epitheliomas, carcinomas)
Keratoacanthomas may be present
Colonic polyps
Multiple primary low-grade visceral cancers, mainly of gut and genitourinary tract

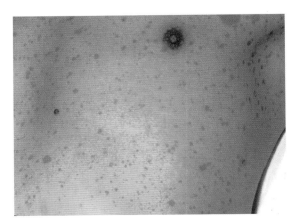

Fig. 17.2 Café-au-lait spot and smaller ones labeled "axillary freckles."

at increased risk for multiple primary malignancies and may have family members also at risk. It may also be useful to screen patients with gastrointestinal polyposis for this syndrome and to evaluate patients with keratoacanthoma for sebaceous neoplasms. When I do a consultation on our oncology service for possible Muir-Torre syndrome, the patient is cheerfully informed that the cancer associated with it has a good prognosis and that I hope to be able to make the diagnosis. A renal transplant recipient with Muir-Torre syndrome and a *MSH-2* mutation on a tacrolimus-based regimen switched to sirolimus with arrest of the disease [28]. Perhaps sirolimus may have a role in retarding and preventing both cutaneous and visceral neoplasms in this syndrome [29]. The essential features of Muir-Torre syndrome are summarized in Table 17.2. However, there is great clinical variability in this syndrome with the incomplete manifestations observed [30]. Nevertheless, a surveillance program should be offered to family members with pathogenic DNA mismatch repair (MMR) gene mutations or high clinical suspicion of them. They should undergo annual colonoscopy beginning at age 20 years, or 10 years earlier than the youngest age of colon cancer diagnosis in the family, and other appropriate evaluations for internal malignancy.

Neurofibromatosis

Von Recklinghausen's disease or neurofibromatosis type 1 (NF-1) is an autosomal dominant multisystem disorder with an incidence of one in 2500 live births [31–34]. The association of oval patches of pigmentation with a color prompting their description as café-au-lait spots may occur as the pretumorous stage of neurofibromatosis. Although neurofibromatosis may produce tremendous disfigurement both from skin tumors and skeletal alterations, grotesque examples of neurofibromatosis are fortunately rare. More commonly, the diagnosis of neurofibromatosis is subtle. Important clues include café-au-lait spots, axillary or inguinal "freckling," cutaneous neurofibromas (Fig. 17.2), neurofibromas of the areolae in postpubertal women, sphenoid wing dysplasia or congenital bowing or thinning of the long bone cortex, Lisch nodules in the iris, or a family history of neurofibromatosis.

Half of neurofibromatosis patients lack a family history of the disease, as they represent new mutations. The gene responsible for neurofibromatosis, the NF-1 gene, located on chromosome 17, encodes for neurofibromin, which may account for tumor formation in these patients [35]. Pathological mutations range from single nucleotide substitutions to large-scale genomic deletions dispersed throughout the gene [36]. A DNA chip microarray-based technology, combinational sequence-based hybridization, has been introduced to expedite mutation detection.

Crowe and Schull's [37] careful study of neurofibromatosis patients revealed that some 75% of them with proven neurofibromatosis possess six or more café-au-lait spots of 1.5 cm or more in diameter. In children, five or more café-au-lait spots 0.5 cm or more in size is probably diagnostic, because less than 1% of unaffected children have so many café-au-lait macules [38]. Careful observation often shows the café-au-lait spots to be present in the first few weeks of life; by the age of 5 years, they are fully developed. The original study by Crowe and Schull [37] noted that more than six café-au-lait spots over 1.5 cm in broadest diameter make a presumptive diagnosis, even in the absence of a positive family history, because neurofibromatosis appears to be a common mutation. If a person has fewer than six café-au-lait spots and no family history, the more numerous the spots, the greater the probability of the syndrome. If fewer than six café-au-lait spots are present, but there is a family history of neurofibromatosis, then the probability of involvement is a function of the pigmentary pattern similarity between this person and affected family members. Furthermore, Crowe and Schull observed that 10% of 6853 institutionalized patients had one to five café-au-lait spots over 1.5 cm in diameter, a figure comparable to the 8.6% found in a group of 1331 college males. Of 98 neurofibromatosis patients, 89.6% had one or more café-au-lait spots. Marked central nervous system (CNS), intrathoracic, or intra-abdominal involvement; segmental distribution; and late age of onset were more frequent in neurofibromatosis patients with three or fewer café-au-lait spots over 1.5 cm in broadest diameter. Segmental neurofibromatosis is a special form of neurofibromatosis with neurofibromas and café-au-lait macules limited to a circumscribed body segment [39].

The shape of the café-au-lait spots in neurofibromatosis is smooth, like the California coast, as opposed to those (usually less numerous) café-au-lait spots in Albright's syndrome, with borders that tend to be irregular and jagged, like the Maine coast. However, a review of 27 patients with Albright's syndrome and 19 with NF-1 showed that the configuration and coloration of both were of no help in differential diagnosis [40]. This study also observed that the histologic pattern was identical, although NF-1 is more likely to have giant pigment granules in the epidermal keratinocytes or melanocytes. A significant increase in melanocyte density was observed in NF-1 café-au-lait spots compared with the isolated ones in control individuals [41]. Others feel that quantitation of melanin macromelanosomes

may be useful [42]. Nevertheless, there is no consensus as to the value of biopsying these café-au-lait spots to assist in clarifying a diagnosis of NF-1. Small pigmented spots, of which the size is of no importance, have been described by Crowe [43]—Crowe's sign—as occurring in the axillae and occasionally in the perineal areas of people with NF-1. They tend to occur only when there is other pigmentary evidence of neurofibromatosis and as such represent an important diagnostic aid, because axillary freckling is very rare in people without NF-1. Clinically and histologically, these "freckles" are pigmented spots like café-au-lait ones and do not darken on exposure to ultraviolet light (as do freckles).

Iris nodules described by Lisch, or "Lisch nodules," are considered pathognomonic of neurofibromatosis [44]. They are small nonpigmented to highly pigmented iris hamartomas scattered randomly and usually bilaterally. On slit lamp examination, they appear as smooth, well-defined gelatinous masses protruding from the iris surface. Lisch nodules may be large enough to be seen with the naked eye. Histologically, these are melanocytic hamartomas. They tend to be seen with increasing age in patients with NF-1.

Cutaneous neurofibromas may be scattered anywhere on the cutaneous surface, tending to appear in late childhood or adolescence, often accompanied by the symptom of pruritus. Clinically, they are skin colored with a soft consistency and may be indented easily (Fig. 17.3). Neurofibromas of the areolae in postpubertal females occur with striking regularity [45] (Fig. 17.4). They may be small or large and may also be seen in males. Pendulous flabby masses called plexiform neurofibromas may be observed. Overlying hyperpigmentation and sometimes hypertrichosis or hypopigmentation may be seen. Subcutaneous neurofibromas may also be evident, sometimes overlain with blue-red macules and pseudo-atrophic macules. Among children, the presence of facial plexiform neurofibromas and pruritus was significantly associated with mortality [46].

Malignant degeneration of neurofibromas occurs most commonly in patients between 20 and 50 years of age [47]. Plexiform neurofibromas are more likely than others to have this malignant

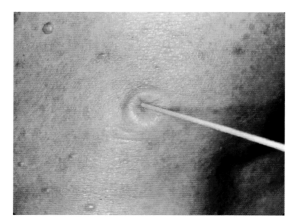

Fig. 17.3 Soft, compressible neurofibromas in an NF-1 patient.

alternation. Neurofibrosarcoma presumably arises from small cutaneous nerves, is locally aggressive, and may metastasize. The most common site is in the lower extremity, where it becomes evident as rapid growth of a preexistent mass, usually in the deep soft tissue. Clearly, neurofibrosarcoma occurs with excessive frequency among patients with NF-1, with an incidence of 3.5% [48]. In two other series, 3.1% and 16.4% of neurofibromatosis patients developed malignant degeneration. Because these are highly malignant tumors, all neurofibromatosis patients should be warned to watch for any rapid soft tissue growth or any sudden change in

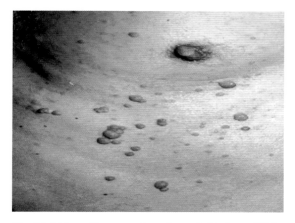

Fig. 17.4 Neurofibromas of areolae and skin in an NF-1 patient.

a preexistent lesion. 18-fluorodeoxyglucose (FDG) positron emission tomography (PET) is useful in determining malignant changes in plexiform neurofibromas in NF-1 [49]. Although the clinical and radiologic diagnosis of sarcomatous change remains difficult, FDG-PET can assess increased glucose metabolism in malignant tissue such as sarcomas and accurately distinguish malignant from benign neurofibromas [50]. The technique may be useful as a noninvasive screening tool for malignant transformation of neurofibromas. Neurofibrosarcomas (malignant schwannomas) may also develop in the retroperitoneum or elsewhere. PET has demonstrated that a sophisticated imaging technique also has a role in diagnosing malignant peripheral nerve sheath tumors [51]. One of the most clinically aggressive cancers associated with NF-1 is the malignant peripheral nerve sheath tumor, first evident as pain associated with a mass [52]. Thirty-four individuals (2%) were identified of 1475 NF-1 patients in one careful survey. Tumor standardized uptake values for the malignant peripheral nerve sheath tumor obtained by FDG-PET were a significant parameter for prediction of survival in NF-1 patients, whereas histopathologic tumor grading did not predict outcome [53].

Other neoplasms that develop in neurofibromatosis patients include gliomas of the optic nerve, astrocytomas, and intramedullary gliomas of the spinal cord. It is important to recognize that optic gliomas are an integral part of neurofibromatosis, with most occurring before the age of 12 years [54]. Because they may arise in children younger than 6 years of age, all NF-1 children should undergo annual ophthalmologic examination [55]. Failing vision and exophthalmos should prompt consideration of a computed tomography (CT) scan or magnetic resonance imaging scan to diagnose optic gliomas. There is an earlier and more severe clinical presentation of optic pathway gliomas in children with sporadic optic gliomas versus those associated with NF-1. Women with NF-1 have a five-fold risk of breast cancer after 50 years of age and should be considered for mammography from 40 years of age [56].

Children and young adults with NF-1 have a higher risk for non-neurogenic sarcomas than does the general population. Nephroblastoma (Wilms' tumor) accounts for 20% of all childhood solid tumors; between 80% and 90% of early cases are now curable. A series of 342 nephroblastoma patients found three cases of coexistent neurofibromatosis, making for a 29-fold higher incidence of neurofibromatosis in Wilms' tumor patients than what would be expected by chance [57]. Neural induction of nephrogenesis may link these two entities in utero. Rhabdomyosarcomas and childhood nonlymphocytic leukemia may also be more common than expected in neurofibromatosis patients [58]. Why chronic myelogenous leukemia and acute myelomonocytic leukemia should be increased in neurofibromatosis patients is unclear [59]. Bader and Miller [60], in reporting 12 new cases of childhood leukemia in neurofibromatosis patients and reviewing 17 earlier ones, also observed that three patients with "transient leukemia" and a second leukemia variant, "xantholeukemia" (nonlymphocytic leukemia with multiple skin xanthomas and normal cholesterol levels), may also be associated with neurofibromatosis patients. Pheochromocytomas and duodenal carcinoids also seem to develop in neurofibromatosis patients with a higher than normal frequency [61,62]. A subsequent malignant peripheral nerve sheath tumor may occur as a second malignant neoplasm [63]. Long-term follow-up of neurofibromatosis patients has shown that malignant neoplasms or benign CNS tumors occurred in 45% of 212 patients [64]. The essential features of neurofibromatosis are summarized in Table 17.3; recent guidelines for diagnosis have been formulated [65].

Glucagonoma syndrome

The association of a dermatitis well termed *necrolytic migratory erythema* with stomatitis, weight loss, diabetes mellitus, anemia, and a glucagon-secreting α-cell tumor of the pancreas is noteworthy [66]. The first patient was described by Becker and associates [67] in 1942 in a 45-year-old housewife. However, despite the postulation of an underlying pancreatic neoplasm, it was not until 1966 that McGavran and associates [67] described a patient with a "bullous and eczematoid dermatitis of the hands, feet and

Table 17.3 Neurofibromatosis (von Recklinghausen's disease): essential features

Birth incidence: 1 in 2500
Autosomal dominant; half new mutations
Café-au-lait spots, peripheral neurofibromas, Lisch nodules
NF-1 gene on chromosome 17, encodes for neurofibromin
Neurofibromas, neurofibrosarcomas
Gliomas, astrocytomas, pheochromocytomas, Wilms' tumor
Childhood nonlymphocytic leukemia
Other tumors: malignant fibrous histiocytomas, rhabdomyosarcomas, etc.

legs," mild diabetes mellitus, and anemia in whom they demonstrated a glucagon-secreting α-cell carcinoma of the pancreas. Skin and oral changes may be the only manifestations of the glucagonoma syndrome [68], which is probably still underdiagnosed.

The skin eruption is clinically and histologically distinctive [66]. It begins as erythematous patches that develop superficial blisters. They expand with healing after crust formation centrally (Fig. 17.5), whereas the edges progress to form a well-demarcated circinate pattern that evolves from vesicle formation through crusting to resolution. The latter may be associated with hyperpigmentation. The whole sequence evolves within a 2-week time frame, with new lesions developing while others

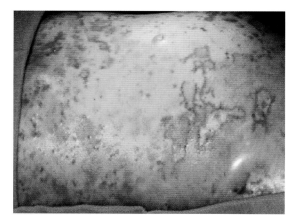

Fig. 17.5 Glucagonoma syndrome with characteristic rash (necrolytic migratory erythema), which remitted after excision of the underlying pancreatic tumor.

heal. The eruption is often widespread and most commonly appears on the lower abdomen, groin, and intertriginous regions, and circumorally. A tendency toward koebnerization has been observed, with new lesions appearing at sites of trauma. Microscopically, a good correlation with the gross pathology was observed, with early lesions showing necrosis of the granular and upper malpighian layers resulting in subcorneal vesiculation and older ones showing only the changes of a nonspecific subacute dermatitis [69]. The former is noteworthy microscopically; there are no acantholytic or dyskeratotic features to augment the clinical resemblance of the rash to benign familial pemphigus or pemphigus foliaceus and no evidence of large collections of polymorphonuclear leukocytes as might be seen in generalized pustular psoriasis and subcorneal pustular dermatosis. In fact, the area of separation is quite specific for this syndrome; in the staphylococcal "scalded skin syndrome," the level of separation is higher up, and in toxic epidermal necrosis (nonstaphylococcal scalded skin syndrome; severe erythema multiforme), the separation is much lower, at the dermal epidermal junction.

This syndrome tends to affect people between 19 and 73 years of age at the time of diagnosis, is more common in women (60% women), and most often affects the tail of the pancreas [70]. However, it can occur anywhere in the pancreas, and although it is usually solitary, multiple small tumors may be rarely found. It tends to metastasize late, so the tumor may still be localized and resectable when the cutaneous eruption develops. Regrettably, the syndrome is usually undiagnosed for years. Sometimes, there is no cutaneous involvement. This may explain why most cases appear to be sporadic in nature, despite the possibility that this is an autosomal dominant disorder. Impressive is a family study in which four of nine relatives of the proband with glucagonoma syndrome were without skin or other symptoms yet had hyperglucagonemia [71]. One of these patients also had a medullary carcinoma of the thyroid; another had chemical evidence suggestive of a pheochromocytoma.

The association of glucagonoma with multiple endocrine adenomatosis was noted in two other patients, although it appeared to be part of the type

I syndrome rather than the type IIa syndrome of medullary thyroid carcinoma and pheochromocytoma. Accordingly, it would seem wise to carefully consider an investigation of family members of patients with the glucagonoma syndrome and to evaluate the patients and possibly their families for other endocrine dysfunctions. This is especially important because metastases from this slow-growing tumor were noted in 64% of patients by the time of diagnosis. These metastases were mainly to the liver [70]. Surgical resection of a localized tumor may result in complete reversal of cutaneous and systemic signs and symptoms and be associated with a return of plasma glucagon levels to normal. Thus, it is imperative to detect the glucagonoma early.

Ultrasonography, CT, and selective celiac axis arteriography are usually accurate in localizing the tumor, although in at least one patient they were all negative [70]. Glucagonoma may have high uptake on FDG-PET, making this an important test to consider [72,73]. The total blood immunoreactive glucagon level is not sufficient for diagnosis. Other conditions with elevated plasma glucagon levels are cirrhosis, chronic renal failure, and diabetes mellitus [70]. One should evaluate both the elevation of 3500-Da "true glucagon" and the 9000- and 160,000-Da fractions. Two families have been described with autosomal dominant inheritance of hyperglucagonemia due to a large molecular weight glucagon, predominately of 160,000 Da [70,71]. An arginine intravenous infusion test may be useful for diagnosis.

A number of patients have been described in whom the skin findings of this syndrome were not associated with a pancreatic tumor [66,74–76]. Pseudo-glucagonoma syndrome patients may have a variety of disorders, including malnutrition, liver cirrhosis, hepatitis B, celiac sprue, chronic pancreatitis, small bowel syndrome, jejunal adenocarcinoma, and diabetes mellitus. However, glucagon-secreting tumors may also occur in the kidney, duodenum, and lung as well as from liver metastases from a pancreatic glucagonoma [66,77,78].

The etiology of the skin lesions has been debated. The original report of Becker and associates [67] suggested a deficiency state and noted improvement on a vitamin-reinforced diet. Although deficiencies of zinc or essential fatty acids have been considered, the best postulation is that the cutaneous eruption is to the result of an amino acid deficiency. Amino acid levels in a number of patients have been shown to be low, as one might expect with an increased serum glucagon level. Correction of this amino acid deficiency may or may not be associated with resolution of the cutaneous lesions [79]. Other catabolic effects of glucagon probably account for the anemia and weight loss noted in these patients; an increase in serum glucagon increases the serum glucose level, so it is not surprising that these patients have a mild diabetic state.

Virtually all patients in whom determinations were made had elevated glucagon levels in the plasma or in the tumor, with plasma glucagon levels between 0.3 and 96 ng/mL (normal, <0.2 ng/mL) [70]. Glucagon with a molecular weight of 9000 Da usually represents less than 18% of the total serum glucagon; the elevation of this possible prohormone in patients with a glucagonoma has been noted, with the suggestion that elevations of this fraction may indicate an underlying glucagonoma. With these islet cell tumors, glucagon alone may be produced or it may be seen in association with insulin and gastrin or extra-pancreatic hormones such as corticotropin.

Surgical cure with complete eradication of the anemia, hyperglycemia, hyperglucagonemia, weight loss, stomatitis, and cutaneous lesions may be achieved. Laparoscopic resection of a pancreatic glucagonoma is safe and feasible in selected patients [80]. However, some tumors may be beyond any type of surgical resection, prompting chemotherapy regimens or the use of a somatostatin analogue [81]. Essential features of glucagonoma syndrome are summarized in Table 17.4.

Florid cutaneous papillomatosis

Florid cutaneous papillomatosis (FCP) is characterized by the sudden eruption of wartlike papillomas on the trunk and extremities (Fig. 17.6) [82–85]. It is often seen before or concurrent with malignant acanthosis nigricans or the sign of Leser-Trélat. In fact, these three signs of internal cancer may occur together and may be viewed as part of a continuum.

Table 17.4 Glucagonoma syndrome

Mild diabetes mellitus
Stomatitis
Weight loss
Anemia
Necrolytic migratory erythema
Glucagon-secreting a-cell tumor of pancreas
Surgically curable, with complete reversal of symptoms

In 1891, Pollitzer [86] noted "striking . . . peculiar flat warts on the arms of recent onset" and numerous papillomas of the side of the lips. Other reports noted "acanthosis nigricans with discrete warts" [87] or the sudden appearance of warty papules on the trunk and extremities with lanugo hairs, and then later, malignant acanthosis nigricans [88] or generalized wartlike lesions with acanthosis nigricans [89]. As noted, FCP may appear with acquired hypertrichosis lanugosa, another sign of internal cancer. The usual underlying cancer in patients with FCP is an adenocarcinoma of the gastrointestinal tract. The essential features of FCP are summarized in Table 17.5.

The sign of Leser-Trélat

The sign of Leser-Trélat is the sudden appearance and rapid increase in size and number of discrete seborrheic keratoses in association with an underlying

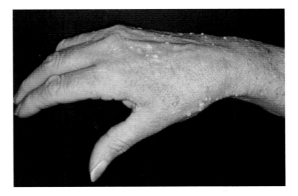

Fig. 17.6 Florid cutaneous papillomatosis, showing wartlike lesions on the hand in patient with underlying gastric adenocarcinoma.

Table 17.5 Florid cutaneous papillomatosis: essential features

Fulminant onset of wartlike lesions on trunk and
   extremities
Hyperkeratosis of palms
May occur together with downy lanugo hair
May occur before malignant acanthosis nigricans
May occur before sudden appearance of seborrheic
   keratoses
Internal malignancy is usually of gastrointestinal tract

Table 17.6 Sign of Leser-Trélat: essential features

Sudden eruption of multiple seborrheic keratoses
Credited to two European surgeons (Leser and Trélat)
Pruritus may be only symptom
May be associated with malignant acanthosis nigricans
Underlying malignancy is adenocarcinoma in two thirds
   of patients
In other one third, usually lymphoma or leukemia

malignancy [90]. The abruptness of the eruption of seborrheic keratoses is striking and should not be confused with generalized seborrheic keratoses of gradual onset. Each seborrheic keratosis appears distinct, with its warty stuck-on morphology and brownish black coloration that is characteristic clinically of a seborrheic keratosis.

This sudden eruption of seborrheic keratoses may occur with other signs of internal malignancy, such as acanthosis nigricans, acquired hypertrichosis, tylosis, acquired ichthyosis, FCP, Cowden's disease, and acrokeratosis of Bazex [91,92]. Malignant acanthosis nigricans is seen in up to half of patients with the sign of Leser-Trélat. Pruritus may be the only symptom accompanying the sign of Leser-Trélat. The lesions are typical seborrheic keratoses histologically.

With the sign of Leser-Trélat, most patients have an adenocarcinoma, most commonly of the stomach and colon [90]. Figure 17.7 illustrates a patient seen in consultation with an adenocarcinoma of the bile duct and the sign of Leser-Trélat [93]. However, about 40% of patients reported in the literature have a lymphoma or leukemia rather than an adenocarcinoma [90], in my opinion reflecting a bias to publish the apparently unusual association rather than the typical one. This diagnosis makes a thorough evaluation for underlying malignancy mandatory. The distribution of underlying cancer shows a similar distribution to that noted with malignant acanthosis nigricans; that is, adenocarcinomas, especially of the stomach and colon, predominate. A polypeptide such as or similar to epidermal growth factor (EGF) may be a good candidate for producing the sign of Leser-Trélat. Essential characteristics of the sign of Leser-Trélat are summarized in Table 17.6.

Acanthosis nigricans

With acanthosis nigricans, there is hyperpigmented, velvety thickening of the skin on any part of the body but typically on the nape and sides of the neck and in the axillae and groin [94]. The eruption itself is never malignant but rather when associated with a malignancy, is referred to as "malignant acanthosis nigricans." In that case, acanthosis nigricans has a sudden and rapid onset (Figs. 17.8 and 17.9). The name *acanthosis nigricans* was first employed in 1881 to describe a woman with "widespread pigmentation and papillary hypertrophy." By 1909, the same author, Pollitzer [95], described 50 patients with acanthosis nigricans, and an

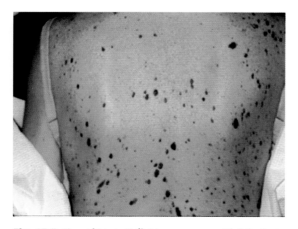

Fig. 17.7 Sign of Leser-Trélat in a woman with bile duct adenocarcinoma.

association in adult patients with highly malignant abdominal cancer became clear.

"Benign" acanthosis nigricans may be evident at birth, puberty, or early adulthood, although it may occur at any age [94]. Acanthosis nigricans with cancer appears in the older "cancer-prone" age group but may occur in patients as young as 17 years [96]. Benign acanthosis nigricans may occur as part of a syndrome.

Acanthosis nigricans is a reaction of the skin to different stimuli. In some patients, the cutaneous changes appear before, after, or concomitantly with the onset of an internal malignancy or an endocrine disorder. Other people have a familial tendency to develop acanthosis nigricans. In the obese person, an undiscovered endocrinopathy may be responsible for the skin lesions. No single cause accounts for all cases of acanthosis nigricans. Factors associated with malignancies, endocrine disease, and genetic predisposition may produce acanthosis nigricans. Acanthosis nigricans may be caused by release of a peptide similar to EGF from either the pituitary gland or a nonpituitary neoplasm. However, no such polypeptide has as yet been identified. The association of acanthosis nigricans with insulin resistance encourages speculation that acanthosis nigricans might result from endogenous (e.g., autoantibodies, adenoma elaborated or carcinoma elaborated) or exogenous (e.g., nicotinic acid or diethylstilbestrol) substances acting at the cell receptor level.

Acanthosis nigricans is characterized by a dark, velvety thickening of the skin in any location. The verrucous lesions, small or large, are situated symmetrically, with a predilection for the axillae, neck, genitalia, groin, perineum, face, knuckles of the hands, and intertriginous surfaces of the elbows, knees, thighs, and breasts (Fig. 17.8).

The first cutaneous change is hyperpigmentation, followed by an intensification of skin markings and varying degrees of hypertrophy of the epidermis without induration. Ordinarily brown, they may be yellow, gray, or black. The dark color, representing melanin deposition in the skin, fades at the margin. Soft papillomas and warty nodules may stud the affected surface. Hair loss on the scalp and eyebrows has been noted. The nails may be striated and brittle.

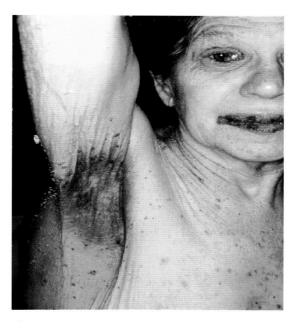

Fig. 17.8 A sudden fulminant eruption of malignant acanthosis nigricans.

The palms and soles may show a diffuse thickening with prominence of the creases and a yellowish hue, especially when acanthosis nigricans is associated with malignancy. This epidermal thickening may be so exuberant as to produce a rugose appearance with deep sulci labeled "tripe palms" [97]. Periorificially and on the mucosa, especially of the oral cavity, thickening and papillation without hyperpigmentation may occur. These mucosal and periorificial lesions may be prominent and extensive (Fig. 17.9). Hyperkeratosis of the nipple and areola is also noted in patients with acanthosis nigricans but may occur alone, as may hyperkeratosis of the palms and soles. Diethylstilbestrol, a medication that may produce acanthosis nigricans, may alone induce these nipple and areola changes.

Acanthosis nigricans beginning early in life was noted to display an irregular autosomal dominant pattern of inheritance. When associated with obesity, acanthosis nigricans is usually obesity dependent and may appear at any age, regressing with weight loss. Acanthosis nigricans may also be induced by steroids, nicotinic acid, and diethylstilbestrol. A number of dark-skinned patients have been

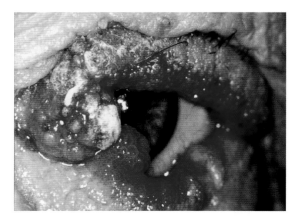

Fig. 17.9 Malignant acanthosis nigricans with extensive periorificial involvement.

Table 17.7 Malignant acanthosis nigricans: essential features

Rapid onset and sudden spread of dark, velvety skin
  thickening
Usual sites are sides of neck, axillae, and groin
Underlying malignancy is usually adenocarcinoma
Should be distinguished from other types of acanthosis
  nigricans

noted to have velvety hyperkeratosis of the dorsum of the hands and feet, an acral variant of benign acanthosis nigricans called acral acanthotic anomaly [98,99].

Acanthosis nigricans has been reported to be associated with a large number of syndromes [94]. The syndromes of insulin resistance and acanthosis nigricans are of tremendous interest. These may be classified into a type A syndrome, which occurs in younger women with signs of virilization or accelerated growth, and a type B syndrome, which is seen in older women with signs of autoimmune disease, including circulating antibodies to the insulin receptor. Acanthosis nigricans may occur with Alström's, Crouzon's, Capozucca's, Rud's, and Bloom's syndromes; pituitary basophilism; other pituitary tumors; gigantism; acromegaly; streak gonads; familial hypertrophy of the pineal body; and many other syndromes. Lupoid hepatitis, lupus erythematosus, dermatomyositis, and scleroderma are also reported in association with acanthosis nigricans, possibly related by multiple autoantibody production, including antibodies to insulin receptors. Malignant acanthosis nigricans may coexist with other cutaneous markers of internal malignancy, including the sign of Leser-Trélat, florid cutaneous papillomatosis, and pachydermoperiostosis.

In Curth's [100] classic review, cancers were preceded by malignant acanthosis nigricans in 17% of patients, occurred simultaneously in 61%, and were followed by the onset of acanthosis nigricans in 22%. If the diagnosis of malignant acanthosis nigricans is made, a vigorous effort should be performed to identify the responsible cancer. Acanthosis nigricans usually regresses when the tumor responsible is excised; acanthosis nigricans may sometimes recur with metastatic disease. When acanthosis nigricans does not change after a cancer is completely excised, one should consider the possibility of a second cancer. Unfortunately, the cancer producing acanthosis nigricans is extremely aggressive, with many of the patients dying within a year after the onset of the acanthosis nigricans.

The skin lesions of acanthosis nigricans are histologically identical in the presence or absence of internal malignancy, endocrinopathy, and obesity. Microscopically, the plaques show hyperkeratosis and papillary hypertrophy, correlating well with the clinical findings. The epidermis may be thick or thin with alternating areas of acanthosis and atrophy. Some increase in melanin pigmentation is seen in the stratum corneum and within histiocytes located in the upper corium. No malignant changes are present. The mucous membranes, when involved, show parakeratosis and papillary hypertrophy without pigmentation. The essential features of malignant acanthosis nigricans are summarized in Table 17.7.

Cutaneous radiation damage overlying the thyroid, breasts, and other sites

The association between x-ray exposure and cancer is not new [101,102]. Although it has been well accepted with regard to thyroid cancer, Mackenzie [101] in 1965 first observed a patient with

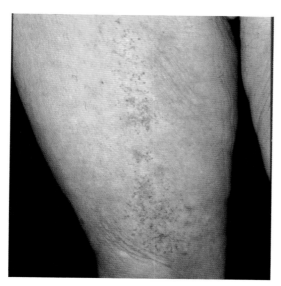

Fig. 17.10 Chronic cutaneous radiation damage after x-ray therapy for generalized hirsutism.

upper outer quadrant breast cancer and overlying cutaneous radiation damage. In this Nova Scotia tuberculosis sanitarium study, 40 women with breast cancer were identified who had received multiple fluoroscopic examinations 14 to 15 years earlier. In the 1950s, the method employed for fluoroscopic examination in bilateral artificial pneumothorax therapy resulted in skin and breast areas receiving considerable amounts of unfiltered x-rays.

Ionizing radiation is clearly carcinogenic in humans. Its stigmata is "radiation dermatitis," which is not a true dermatitis but rather chronic radiation damage characterized by telangiectasia, atrophy, and mottled pigmentary changes (Fig. 17.10).With the 20- to 50-year carcinogenic lag, patients treated appropriately years ago are now at risk of developing a number of cancers, both cutaneous and extracutaneous postradiation. In addition, exposure to radiation is often cryptic, and a thoughtful history must be taken with regard to such exposure to treat tinea capitis, postpartum mastitis, acne vulgaris, hirsutism, tonsillitis, retinoblastomas, hemangiomas, and other "birth marks." The TrichoSystem, a franchised arrangement of allegedly harmless x-ray therapy leased to beauty parlor operators and others from the 1920s through the 1950s, is another

example of cryptic and harmful exposure, employed mainly to treat excessive body hair [103]. The latent period for skin cancer after x-ray exposure ranges from 7 weeks to 56 years, varying inversely with dosage [104].

Although good epidemiologic evidence linking x-ray exposure to skin and visceral cancer is probably lacking except for thyroid, the breast is very sensitive to radiation and clinical observation has preceded good epidemiologic studies before. Unfortunately, much of the x-ray exposure we now see today occurred at a time when measurements were not made, because non-physicians often employed it. Clearly, sites overlying areas of chronic cutaneous radiation damage should be viewed askance because a number of reports of patients with appendageal carcinoma and sarcomas have been made. For example, a number of patients have developed sebaceous carcinoma after radiation therapy for retinoblastoma [105]. Similarly, radiation-induced angiosarcoma has been well described as a sequela of radiotherapy for breast cancer [106].

I consider cutaneous findings of chronic radiation exposure to be a marker of possible underlying cancer at or adjacent to the site (Fig. 17.11A,B), and warn my patients to report any nearby alteration promptly for evaluation. The essential features of cutaneous radiation damage are summarized in Table 17.8.

Acute neutrophilic dermatosis

The association of skin findings suggestive of pyoderma gangrenosum and malignancy has been of much interest [107–110]. Jablonska and associates [111] described two patients with pyoderma gangrenosum and myeloma. Pyoderma gangrenosum has been linked to leukemia in so-called bullous pyoderma gangrenosum [112]. The typical lesion of pyoderma gangrenosum is an elevated papule or plaque with aggressive and spreading central necrosis of tissue as it expands, leaving a bluish necrotic border surrounded by a bright erythematous halo. It may be associated with ulcerative colitis, rheumatoid arthritis, or no underlying disorder. However, the lesions of "bullous pyoderma gangrenosum" are more superficial and thus less destructive, appearing

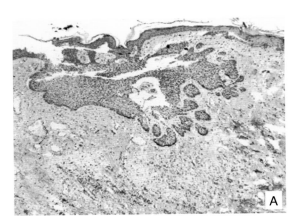
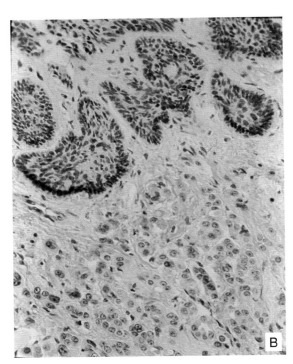

Fig. 17.11 Skin biopsy in the woman described in Fig. 17.10, who also had chronic cutaneous radiation damage over the breasts and a basal cell carcinoma overlying a breast adenocarcinoma. *A*, Lower power. *B*, Higher power.

as concentric bullous inflammatory erosions spreading peripherally (Fig. 17.12). The surrounding area has a bluish gray hue rather than the bright reddish halo of typical pyoderma gangrenosum.

Some of these patients had been reported as having acute febrile neutrophilic dermatosis (Sweet's syndrome) with underlying malignancy. There is certainly a close resemblance of this atypical or bullous pyoderma gangrenosum to Sweet's syndrome. These neutrophilic dermatoses are part of

Table 17.8 Cutaneous radiation damage over thyroid, breast, other sites: essential features

---

Telangiectasia, subcutaneous fibrosis, mottled
  pigmentary changes, alopecia (not a dermatitis)
Cryptic exposure
Long latent period, up to >50 years
Multiple skin cancers, mainly basal cell carcinomas
Possible angiosarcomas, sebaceous carcinomas, breast
  and thyroid cancer

---

the same spectrum, often without fever or neutrophilia, hence the unifying name *acute neutrophilic dermatosis*, as the histologic pattern in these patients consistently displays an extensive diffuse dermal infiltrate of neutrophils, often with leukocytoclasia.

Acute neutrophilic dermatosis is usually detected months after the onset of the myeloproliferative disease, although in some patients they have been observed simultaneously. In a few of these patients, it was the first sign of the underlying malignancy [112]. The course of the skin lesions tends to parallel that of the leukemia, with the original observation of the rapid demise. Acute neutrophilic dermatosis has also been reported in association with cervical cancer, embryonal testicular cancer, breast cancer, adenocarcinoma of unknown origin, myeloma, T-cell lymphoma, and histiocytic lymphoma [110,113,114].

Systemically, fever and neutrophilia may or may not be present [107]. There may also be a nondeforming asymmetric large joint arthritis,

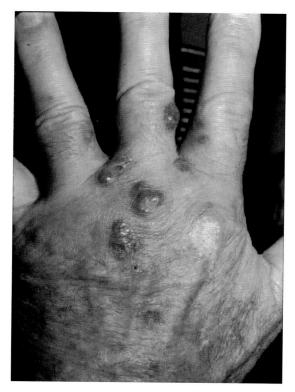

Fig. 17.12 Acute neutrophilic dermatosis (Sweet's syndrome, bullous pyoderma gangrenosum) in a 56-year-old man with lymphoma.

conjunctivitis, episcleritis, albuminuria, anemia, and an elevated erythrocyte sedimentation rate [115]. A high-grade fever and pulmonary infiltrates may be seen [116].

Histologically, acute neutrophilic dermatosis shows a picture dissimilar from pyoderma gangrenosum, the latter displaying a nonspecific reaction pattern corresponding to the clinical morphology, with necrosis, an impressive acute inflammatory infiltrate in the upper dermis with a mixed chronic one in the deep dermis, and fibrocystic reaction in resolving lesions. Acute neutrophilic dermatosis shows a dense dermal infiltrate of neutrophils often with a normal epidermis. However, there may be spongiosis and intraepidermal vesiculation.

The differential diagnosis of acute neutrophilic dermatosis includes secondary syphilis and

Table 17.9 Acute neutrophilic dermatosis: essential features

Spreading annular superficial necrosis with bulla formation
After this morphology, myelogenous leukemia is detected
May be same as "Sweet's syndrome" with malignancy
Often fever and polymorphonuclear (PMN) leukocytosis
Histology: massive PMN infiltrate

neutrophilic eccrine hidradenitis [117,118]. The latter is particularly noteworthy because it is evident as inflammatory nodules in patients with acute leukemia and Hodgkin's disease and may be associated with hyperpyrexia and a cutaneous neutrophilic infiltrate. However, the infiltrate is around eccrine glands, which degenerate. This represents a reaction to chemotherapeutic agents. The essential features of acute neutrophilic dermatosis are summarized in Table 17.9.

Acquired ichthyosis

Ichthyosis vulgaris is a common genetic disorder in which there is a generalized scaling eruption most prominent on the arms and legs, sparing the face, flexural areas, and palms and soles [119,120]. Each scale is characterized by a rhomboidal morphology with free edges, resembling fish scales (Fig. 17.13). In the genetic form, the inheritance pattern is autosomal dominant. However, it may occur later in life,

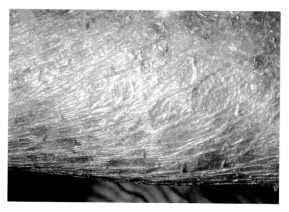

Fig. 17.13 Acquired ichthyosis.

as a marker for internal malignancy. Lately, I have seen it in a number of our intravenous drug-abusing AIDS patients with no evidence of Kaposi's sarcoma or other malignancy; it has also been observed with AIDS and Kaposi's sarcoma as well as in association with traditional Kaposi's sarcoma [121,122].

Historically, acquired ichthyosis has been linked with Hodgkin's disease, usually seen after the cancer is diagnosed, although sometimes before [123]. It may be the first sign of a myeloproliferative disease [124]. Other associations include malignancies of the breast, lung, and cervix [120]. Acquired ichthyosis has been described in a patient with the sign of Leser-Trélat and an underlying lymphoma [125]. The course of the ichthyosis parallels that of the underlying malignancy. Acquired ichthyosis is also associated with leprosy, tuberculosis, anorexia nervosa, graft-versus-host disease, sarcoidosis, thyroid disease, systemic lupus erythematosus, dermatomyositis, nutritional disorders, and certain medications [120,126,127].

Acquired ichthyosis must be distinguished from xerotic eczema. The latter disorder may be mild or severe, in which case the patient displays a fine scale and roughened erythematous fissures, called erythema craquelé. Unlike ichthyosis, in xerosis there is no hyperkeratosis with decreased or absent granular layer; xerosis is a subacute dermatitis with a lymphohistiocytic dermal infiltrate.

The irregular reticular dry fissuring of erythema craquelé is common in hospitalized patients, but as a generalized eruption resistant to topical steroids and emollients, it is uncommon. A report associated generalized erythema craquelé as part of the presentation in two patients who were later diagnosed as having Hodgkin's disease [128]. A similar widespread eruption was reported in a 20-year-old man who was undergoing evaluation for lymphadenopathy, which was diagnosed as angioimmunoblastic lymphadenopathy [128]. In addition, pityriasis rotunda, an eruption of circular disciform patches, may be a localized form of acquired ichthyosis, serving as a cutaneous marker for hematologic malignancies or for hepatoma [129,130]. Essential features of acquired ichthyosis are summarized in Table 17.10.

Table 17.10 Acquired ichthyosis: essential features

Diffuse fish-scale eruption resembling inherited form
Usually follows diagnosis of Hodgkin's disease
May be associated with breast, cervical, and lung cancer, leiomyosarcoma
Course parallels fluctuations in underlying malignancy
Histology: hyperkeratosis with reduced granular layer

Hypertrichosis lanuginosa acquisita

Hypertrichosis lanuginosa acquisita refers to the eruption in an adult of lanugo—extremely fine, soft, usually unmedullated hairs, normally seen in fetal life between the third and seventh months. Embryologically, lanugal hairs are followed by similar but shorter vellus hairs, then by thick medullated terminal hairs.

Sometimes thick terminal hair may revert to vellus hairs, as occurs to produce male pattern baldness. Rarely, lanugo hairs are seen after birth, either as the inherited strikingly diffuse hirsutism giving affected individuals dog- or monkey-like faces (as in the circus "monkey-men") or in an acquired form (Fig. 17.14). The latter represents a reversion from terminal to fetal hairs. Acquired hypertrichosis may be induced by medication, especially diazoxide used in treating children with leucine-sensitive hypoglycemia. However, this hypertrichosis is of terminal hairs rather than of vellus or lanugo ones. Likewise, terminal hair hypertrichosis may be seen in a number of diseases such as porphyria cutanea tarda or secondary to medications such as phenytoin or to physical agents such as psoralen–ultraviolet-A (PUVA) therapy. True acquired lanugo hypertrichosis, especially in those of middle age or older, is almost always associated with an advanced internal malignancy [131–135] However, autoimmune hepatitis was also recently associated with it [136].

About fifty cases have been described to date [137]; in almost all cases, the patient either had visceral cancer or did not undergo a complete evaluation to exclude that possibility. Most patients have been older than 40 years, although some have been

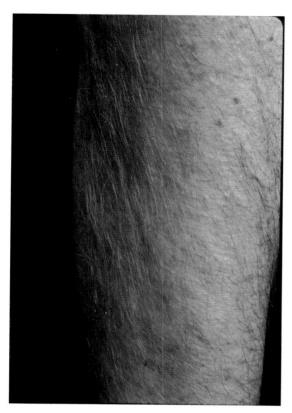

Fig. 17.14 Hypertrichosis lanuginosa acquisita in a patient with villous adenocarcinoma of the cecum. Note the normal terminal black hair in contrast to the wispy lanugal hairs.

Table 17.11 Acquired hypertrichosis lanuginosa: essential features

Sudden appearance of soft, fine, unmedullated fetal hair
Associated with underlying malignancies, mainly of gut and respiratory tract, but many other cancers also
May antedate or occur together with symptoms of malignancy
Autosomal dominant trait, the circus "dog-faced man"
When inherited, appears in childhood or adolescence

[88]. Essential features of acquired hypertrichosis lanuginosa are summarized in Table 17.11.

Conclusion

There are a number of other associations with internal cancer. For example, herpes zoster, both as shingles and as chickenpox, may be seen—often in fulminant form—in cancer patients with Hodgkin's disease and solid tumors on chemotherapy [140]. In addition, chemotherapy itself may produce a number of cutaneous eruptions. We have already alluded to neutrophilic eccrine hidradenitis in the discussion of acute neutrophilic dermatitis. Muehrcke's lines may also be seen as an apparent result of chemotherapy [141].

considerably younger. In a number of patients, the hypertrichosis was noted months to years before the cancer was diagnosed [131–133]. Those noted without an internal malignancy should be followed carefully in case one develops.

Most of the associated malignancies are colon, rectal, or lung carcinomas [133]. Other possible malignancies include breast [135], bladder, ovary, gall bladder, metastatic melanoma [138], prostate [139], pancreas, lymphoma, cervix [132], and extraskeletal Ewing's sarcoma [120,131]. I have seen a patient in consultation with this syndrome and villous adenocarcinoma of the cecum. Some patients also had a glossitis, and one had the sudden eruption of multiple seborrheic keratoses (the sign of Leser-Trélat)

References

1 Jeghers H, McKusick VA, Katz KH. Generalized intestinal polyposis and melanin spots of the oral mucosa, lips and digits; a syndrome of diagnostic significance. N Engl J Med 1949;241:1031–6.

2 Gungor B, Bektas A, Anadol AZ, et al. Endoscopy-assisted resection for multiple polyps of the small intestine in Peutz-Jeghers syndrome: a father and daughter story. J Laparoendosc Adv Surg Tech A 2006;16:41–4.

3 Giardiello FM, Trimbath JD. Peutz-Jeghers syndrome and management recommendations. Clin Gastroenterol Hepatol 2006;4:408–15.

4 Dai YC, Song YG, Xiao B, et al. [Clinical classification of Peutz-Jeghers syndrome]. Nan Fang Yi Ke Da Xue Xue Bao 2006;26:79–81.

5 Pelizzo G, Martelossi S, Popoiu MC, et al. Laparoendoscopically assisted endoscopic small bowel polypectomy in a patient with Peutz-Jeghers

syndrome. J Laparoendosc Adv Surg Tech A 2007;17:140–2.

6 von Herbay A, Arens N, Friedl W, et al. Bronchioloalveolar carcinoma: a new cancer in Peutz-Jeghers syndrome. Lung Cancer 2005;47:283–8.

7 de Leng WW, Westerman AM, Weterman M, et al. Nasal polyposis in Peutz-Jeghers syndrome: a distinct histopathologic and molecular genetic entity. J Clin Pathol 2006;60:392–6.

8 Lefevre H, Bouvattier C, Lahlou N, et al. Prepubertal gynecomastia in Peutz-Jeghers syndrome: incomplete penetrance in a familial case and management with an aromatase inhibitor. Eur J Endocrinol 2006;154:221–7.

9 Song SH, Lee JK, Saw HS, et al. Peutz-Jeghers syndrome with multiple genital tract tumors and breast cancer: a case report with a review of literatures. J Korean Med Sci 2006;21:752–7.

10 Gibbon DG. Conservative management of sex cord tumors with annular tubules of the ovary in women with Peutz-Jeghers syndrome. J Pediatr Hematol Oncol 2005;27:630–2.

11 Brichard B, Chantrain C, Wese F, et al. Peutz-Jeghers syndrome and bilateral ovarian tumors in a 14-year-old girl. J Pediatr Hematol Oncol 2005;27:621–3.

12 Ayadi-Kaddour A, Bouraoui S, Bellil K, et al. Colonic adenocarcinoma and bilateral malignant ovarian sex cord tumor with annular tubules in Peutz-Jeghers syndrome. Pathologica 2004;96:117–20.

13 Hearle N, Schumacher V, Menko FH, et al. Frequency and spectrum of cancers in the Peutz-Jeghers syndrome. Clin Cancer Res 2006;12:3209–15.

14 Conneely JB, Kell MR, Boran S, et al. A case of bilateral breast cancer with Peutz-Jeghers syndrome. Eur J Surg Oncol 2006;32:121–2.

15 Kara C, Kutlu AO, Tosun MS, et al. Sertoli cell tumor causing prepubertal gynecomastia in a boy with Peutz-Jeghers syndrome: the outcome of 1-year treatment with the aromatase inhibitor testolactone. Horm Res 2005;63:252–6.

16 Thakur N, Reddy DN, Rao GV, et al. A novel mutation in STK11 gene is associated with Peutz-Jeghers syndrome in Indian patients. BMC Med Genet 2006;7:73.

17 Zaheri S, Chong SK, Harland CC. Treatment of mucocutaneous pigmentation in Peutz-Jeghers syndrome with potassium titanyl phosphate (KTP) laser. Clin Exp Dermatol 2005;30:710–2.

18 Torre D. Multiple sebaceous tumors. Arch Dermatol 1968;98:549–51.

19 Muir EG, Bell AJ, Barlow KA. Multiple primary carcinomata of the colon, duodenum, and larynx associated with kerato-acanthomata of the face. Br J Surg 1967;54:191–5.

20 Schwartz RA, Flieger DN, Saied NK. The Torre syndrome with gastrointestinal polyposis. Arch Dermatol 1980;116:312–4.

21 Schwartz RA, Torre DP. The Muir-Torre syndrome: a 25-year retrospect. J Am Acad Dermatol 1995;33:90–104.

22 Lynne-Davies G, Brown J. Multiple sebaceous gland tumours associated with polyposis of the colon and bony abnormalities. Can Med Assoc J 1974;110:1377–9.

23 Bitran J, Pellettiere EV. Multiple sebaceous gland tumors and internal carcinoma: Torre's syndrome. Cancer 1974;33:835–6.

24 Cohen PR, Kohn SR, Kurzrock R. Association of sebaceous gland tumors and internal malignancy: the Muir-Torre syndrome. Am J Med 1991;90:606–13.

25 Arnold A, Payne S, Fisher S, et al. An individual with Muir-Torre syndrome found to have a pathogenic MSH6 gene mutation [published online ahead of print on February 24, 2007]. Fam Cancer. PMID: 17323113.

26 Mangold E, Rahner N, Friedrichs N, et al. MSH6 mutation in Muir-Torre syndrome: could this be a rare finding? Br J Dermatol 2007;156:158–62.

27 Ponti G, Losi L, Pedroni M, et al. Value of MLH1 and MSH2 mutations in the appearance of Muir-Torre syndrome phenotype in HNPCC patients presenting sebaceous gland tumors or keratoacanthomas. J Invest Dermatol 2006;126:2302–7.

28 Levi Z, Hazazi R, Kedar-Barnes I, et al. Switching from tacrolimus to sirolimus halts the appearance of new sebaceous neoplasms in Muir-Torre syndrome. Am J Transplant 2007;7:476–9.

29 Paghdal KV, Schwartz RA. Sirolimus (rapamycin): from the soil of Easter Island to a bright future [published online ahead of print on June 19, 2007]. J Am Acad Dermatol. PMID: 17583372.

30 Schwartz RA, Whitworth JM, Janniger CK, et al. The Muir-Torre syndrome. Chron Dermatol (Roma) 1996;6:845–52.

31 Yohay K. Neurofibromatosis types 1 and 2. Neurologist 2006;12:86–93.

32 Crawford AH, Schorry EK. Neurofibromatosis update. J Pediatr Orthop 2006;26:413–23.

33 Walker L, Thompson D, Easton D, et al. A prospective study of neurofibromatosis type 1 cancer incidence in the UK. Br J Cancer 2006;95:233–8.

34 Szudek J, Birch P, Riccardi VM, et al. Associations of clinical features in neurofibromatosis 1 (NF1). Genet Epidemiol 2000;19:429–39.

35 Hsueh YP. Neurofibromin signaling and synapses [published online ahead of print on March 17, 2007]. J Biomed Sci.

36 Lee MJ, Stephenson DA. Recent developments in neurofibromatosis type 1. Curr Opin Neurol 2007;20:135–41.

37 Crowe FW, Schull WJ. Diagnostic importance of cafe-au-lait spot in neurofibromatosis. AMA Arch Intern Med 1953;91:758–66.

38 Whitehouse D. Diagnostic value of the cafe-au-lait spot in children. Arch Dis Child 1966;41:316–9.

39 Lee JS, Kim YC. Sclerosing segmental neurofibromatosis. J Dermatol 2005; 32: 303–5.

40 Benedict PH, Szabo G, Fitzpatrick TB, et al. Melanotic macules in Albright's syndrome and in neurofibromatosis. Jama 1968;205:618–26.

41 De Schepper S, Boucneau J, Vander Haeghen Y, et al. Café-au-lait spots in neurofibromatosis type 1 and in healthy control individuals: hyperpigmentation of a different kind? Arch Dermatol Res 2006;297:439–49.

42 Slater C, Hayes M, Saxe N, et al. Macromelanosomes in the early diagnosis of neurofibromatosis. Am J Dermatopathol 1986;8:284–9.

43 Crowe FW. Axillary freckling as a diagnostic aid in neurofibromatosis. Ann Intern Med 1964;61:1142–3.

44 Richetta A, Giustini S, Recupero SM, et al. Lisch nodules of the iris in neurofibromatosis type 1. J Eur Acad Dermatol Venereol 2004;18:342–4.

45 Riccardi VM. Neurofibromatosis and Albright's syndrome. Dermatol Clin 1987;5:193–203.

46 Khosrotehrani K, Bastuji-Garin S, Riccardi VM, et al. Subcutaneous neurofibromas are associated with mortality in neurofibromatosis 1: a cohort study of 703 patients. Am J Med Genet A 2005;132:49–53.

47 Dabski C, Reiman HM Jr, Muller SA. Neurofibrosarcoma of skin and subcutaneous tissues. Mayo Clin Proc 1990;65:164–72.

48 Riccardi VM, Powell PP. Neurofibrosarcoma as a complication of von Recklinghausen neurofibromatosis. Neurofibromatosis 1989;2:152–65.

49 Ferner RE, Lucas JD, O'Doherty MJ, et al. Evaluation of (18)fluorodeoxyglucose positron emission tomography ((18)FDG PET) in the detection of malignant peripheral nerve sheath tumours arising from within plexiform neurofibromas in neurofibromatosis 1. J Neurol Neurosurg Psychiatry 2000;68:353–7.

50 Solomon SB, Semih Dogan A, Nicol TL, et al. Positron emission tomography in the detection and management of sarcomatous transformation in neurofibromatosis. Clin Nucl Med 2001;26:525–8.

51 Ferner RE. Neurofibromatosis 1. Eur J Hum Genet 2007;15:131–8.

52 King AA, Debaun MR, Riccardi VM, et al. Malignant peripheral nerve sheath tumors in neurofibromatosis 1. Am J Med Genet 2000;93:388–92.

53 Brenner W, Friedrich RE, Gawad KA, et al. Prognostic relevance of FDG PET in patients with neurofibromatosis type-1 and malignant peripheral nerve sheath tumours. Eur J Nucl Med Mol Imaging 2006;33:428–32.

54 Czyzyk E, Jozwiak S, Roszkowski M, et al. Optic pathway gliomas in children with and without neurofibromatosis 1. J Child Neurol 2003;18:471–8.

55 Lama G, Esposito Salsano M, Grassia C, et al. Neurofibromatosis type 1 and optic pathway glioma. A long-term follow-up. Minerva Pediatr 2007;59:13–21.

56 Sharif S, Moran A, Huson S, et al. Women with neurofibromatosis 1 (NF1) are at a moderately increased risk of developing breast cancer and should be considered for early screening [published online ahead of print on March 16, 2007]. J Med Genet. PMID: 17369502.

57 Stay EJ, Vawter G. The relationship between nephroblastoma and neurofibromatosis (von Recklinghausen's disease). Cancer 1977;39:2550–5.

58 Oguzkan S, Terzi YK, Guler E, et al. Two neurofibromatosis type 1 cases associated with rhabdomyosarcoma of bladder, one with a large deletion in the NF1 gene. Cancer Genet Cytogenet 2006;164:159–63.

59 Shin HT, Harris MB, Orlow SJ. Juvenile myelomonocytic leukemia presenting with features of hemophagocytic lymphohistiocytosis in association with neurofibromatosis and juvenile xanthogranulomas. J Pediatr Hematol Oncol 2004;26:591–5.

60 Bader JL, Miller RW. Neurofibromatosis and childhood leukemia. J Pediatr 1978;92:925–9.

61 Lew JI, Jacome FJ, Solorzano CC. Neurofibromatosis-associated pheochromocytoma. J Am Coll Surg 2006;202:550–1.

62 Bausch B, Borozdin W, Neumann HP. Clinical and genetic characteristics of patients with neurofibromatosis type 1 and pheochromocytoma. N Engl J Med 2006;354:2729–31.

63 Coffin CM, Cassity J, Viskochil D, et al. Non-neurogenic sarcomas in four children and young adults with neurofibromatosis type 1. Am J Med Genet A 2004;127:40–3.

64 Sorensen SA, Mulvihill JJ, Nielsen A. Long-term follow-up of von Recklinghausen neurofibromatosis. Survival and malignant neoplasms. N Engl J Med 1986;314:1010–5.

65 Ferner RE, Huson SM, Thomas N, et al. Guidelines for the diagnosis and management of individuals with neurofibromatosis 1. J Med Genet 2007;44:81–8.

66 Schwartz RA. Glucagonoma and pseudoglucagonoma syndromes. Int J Dermatol 1997;36:81–9.

67 Becker SW, Kahn D, Rothman S. Cutaneous manifestations of internal malignant tumors. Arch Dermatol Syphilol 1942;45:1069–80.

68 Kovacs RK, Korom I, Dobozy A, et al. Necrolytic migratory erythema. J Cutan Pathol 2006;33:242–5.

69 Kheir SM, Omura EF, Grizzle WE, et al. Histologic variation in the skin lesions of the glucagonoma syndrome. Am J Surg Pathol 1986;10:445–53.

70 Montenegro-Rodas F, Samaan NA. Glucagonoma tumors and syndrome. Curr Probl Cancer 1981;6:1–54.

71 Boden G, Owen OE. Familial hyperglucagonemia— an autosomal dominant disorder. N Engl J Med 1977;296:534–8.

72 Nishiguchi S, Shiomi S, Ishizu H, et al. A case of glucagonoma with high uptake on F-18 fluorodeoxyglucose positron emission tomography. Ann Nucl Med 2001;15:259–62.

73 Fernandez-Represa JA, Fernandez Rodriguez D, Perez Contin MJ, et al. Pancreatic glucagonoma: detection by positron emission tomography. Eur J Surg 2000;166:175–6.

74 Nakashima H, Komine M, Sasaki K, et al. Necrolytic migratory erythema without glucagonoma in a patient with short bowel syndrome. J Dermatol 2006;33:557–62.

75 Kitamura Y, Sato M, Hatamochi A, et al. Necrolytic migratory erythema without glucagonoma associated with hepatitis B. Eur J Dermatol 2005;15:49–51.

76 Bak H, Ahn SK. Pseudoglucagonoma syndrome in a patient with malnutrition. Arch Dermatol 2005;141:914–6.

77 Pavelic K, Popovic M. Insulin and glucagon secretion by renal adenocarcinoma. Cancer 1981;48:98–100.

78 Wood SM, Bloom SR. Glucagon and gastrin secretion by a pancreatic tumour and its metastases. J R Soc Med 1982;75:42–4.

79 Alexander EK, Robinson M, Staniec M, et al. Peripheral amino acid and fatty acid infusion for the treatment of necrolytic migratory erythema in the glucagonoma syndrome. Clin Endocrinol (Oxf) 2002;57:827–31.

80 Pierce RA, Spitler JA, Hawkins WG, et al. Outcomes analysis of laparoscopic resection of pancreatic neoplasms. Surg Endosc 2007;21:579–86.

81 Appetecchia M, Ferretti E, Carducci M, et al. Malignant glucagonoma. New options of treatment. J Exp Clin Cancer Res 2006;25:135–9.

82 Singhi MK, Gupta LK, Bansal M, et al. Florid cutaneous papillomatosis with adenocarcinoma of stomach in a 35 year old male. Indian J Dermatol Venereol Leprol 2005;71:195–6.

83 Schwartz RA, Burgess GH. Florid cutaneous papillomatosis. Arch Dermatol 1978;114:1803–6.

84 Schwartz RA. Florid cutaneous papillomatosis. Clin Dermatol 1993;11:89–91.

85 Gheeraert P, Goens J, Schwartz RA, et al. Florid cutaneous papillomatosis, malignant acanthosis nigricans, and pulmonary squamous cell carcinoma. Int J Dermatol 1991;30:193–7.

86 Pollitzer S. Acanthosis nigricans. In: Pollitzer S, editor. International atlas of rare skin diseases. London: K Lewis & Co; 1890. p. 1–3.

87 Forman L. Acanthosis nigricans with discrete warts and marked mucous membrane changes in a patient with vitiligo. Proc Roy Soc Med 1943;36:611.

88 Dingley ER, Marten RH. Adenocarcinoma of the ovary presenting as acanthosis nigricans. J Obstet Gynaecol Br Emp 1957;64:898–900.

89 White H. Acanthosis nigricans and wart-like lesions associated with metastatic carcinoma of the stomach. Cutis 1976;17:931–3.

90 Schwartz RA. Sign of Leser-Trelat. J Am Acad Dermatol 1996;35:88–95.

91 Rubisz-Brzezinska J, Zebracka T, Musialowicz D. [Coexistence of 2 paraneoplastic syndromes— acrokeratosis bazex and Leser-Trelat syndrome—in a case of squamous-cell laryngeal cancer]. Przegl Dermatol 1983;70:205–8.

92 Schwartz RA. Acanthosis nigricans, florid cutaneous papillomatosis and the sign of Leser-Trelat. Cutis 1981;28:319–22, 26–7, 30–1 passim.

93 Schwartz RA, Helmold ME, Janniger CK, et al. Sign of Leser-Trelat with a metastatic mucinous adenocarcinoma. Cutis 1991;47:258–60.

94 Schwartz RA. Acanthosis nigricans. J Am Acad Dermatol 1994;31:1–19; quiz 20–2.

95 Pollitzer S. Acanthosis nigricans. A symptom of a disorder of the abdominal sympathetic. J Am Med Assoc 1909;53:1369–73.

96 Sinha S, Schwartz RA. Juvenile acanthosis nigricans [published online ahead of print on June 23, 2007]. J Am Acad Dermatol. PMID: 17592743.

97 Kebria MM, Belinson J, Kim R, et al. Malignant acanthosis nigricans, tripe palms and the sign of Leser-Trélat, a hint to the diagnosis of early stage ovarian cancer: a case report and review of the literature. Gynecol Oncol 2006;101:353–5.

98 Schwartz RA. Acral acanthotic anomaly (AAA). J Am Acad Dermatol 1981;5:345–6.

99 Schwartz RA. Acral acanthosis nigricans (acral acanthotic anomaly). J Am Acad Dermatol 2007;56:349–50.

100 Curth HO. Malignant acanthosis nigricans. Arch Dermatol 1965;91:412.

101 Mackenzie I. Breast cancer following multiple fluoroscopies. Br J Cancer 1965;19:1–8.

102 Schwartz RA, Burgess GH, Milgrom H. Breast carcinoma and basal cell epithelioma after x-ray therapy for hirsutism. Cancer 1979;44:1601–5.

103 Lapidus SM. The tricho system: hypertrichosis, radiation, and cancer. J Surg Oncol 1976;8:267–74.

104 Mole RH. Radiation induced tumours—human experience. Br J Radiol 1972;45:613.

105 Howrey RP, Lipham WJ, Schultz WH, et al. Sebaceous gland carcinoma: a subtle second malignancy following radiation therapy in patients with bilateral retinoblastoma. Cancer 1998;83:767–71.

106 Tahir M, Hendry P, Baird L, et al. Radiation induced angiosarcoma a sequela of radiotherapy for breast cancer following conservative surgery. Int Semin Surg Oncol 2006;3:26.

107 Walling HW, Snipes CJ, Gerami P, et al. The relationship between neutrophilic dermatosis of the dorsal hands and sweet syndrome: report of 9 cases and comparison to atypical pyoderma gangrenosum. Arch Dermatol 2006;142:57–63.

108 Brodkin RH, Schwartz RA. Sweet's syndrome with myelofibrosis and leukemia: partial response to interferon. Dermatology 1995;190:160–3.

109 Sharma PK, Schwartz RA, Janniger CK, et al. Sweet's syndrome with acute leukemia. Cutis 1991;47:249–52.

110 Schwartz RA, French SW, Rubenstein DJ, et al. Acute neutrophilic dermatosis with diffuse histiocytic lymphoma. J Am Acad Dermatol 1984;10:350–4.

111 Jablonska S, Stachow A, Dabrowska H. [Relationships between pyoderma gangrenosum and myeloma]. Ann Dermatol Syphiligr (Paris) 1967;94:121–32.

112 Fox LP, Geyer AS, Husain S, et al. Bullous pyoderma gangrenosum as the presenting sign of fatal acute myelogenous leukemia. Leuk Lymphoma 2006;47:147–50.

113 Culp L, Crowder S, Hatch S. A rare association of Sweet's syndrome with cervical cancer. Gynecol Oncol 2004;95:396–9.

114 Teng JM, Draper BK, Boyd AS. Sweet's panniculitis associated with metastatic breast cancer. J Am Acad Dermatol 2007;56: S61–2.

115 Vignon-Pennamen MD, Juillard C, Rybojad M, et al. Chronic recurrent lymphocytic Sweet syndrome as a predictive marker of myelodysplasia: a report of 9 cases. Arch Dermatol 2006;142:1170–6.

116 Petrig C, Bassetti S, Passweg J, et al. Acute respiratory failure due to sweet syndrome. Am J Med Sci 2006;331:159–61.

117 Morice A, Penven K, Comoz F, et al. [Neutrophilic eccrine hidradenitis in a healthy patient]. Ann Dermatol Venereol 2005;132:686–8.

118 Belot V, Perrinaud A, Corven C, et al. [Adult idiopathic neutrophilic eccrine hidradenitis treated with colchicine]. Presse Med 2006;35:1475–8.

119 Patel N, Spencer LA, English JC 3rd, et al. Acquired ichthyosis. J Am Acad Dermatol 2006;55:647–56.

120 Schwartz RA, Williams ML. Acquired ichthyosis: a marker for internal disease. Am Fam Physician 1984;29:181–4.

121 Nobre V, Guedes AC, Martins ML, et al. Dermatological findings in 3 generations of a family with a high prevalence of human T cell lymphotropic virus type 1 infection in Brazil. Clin Infect Dis 2006;43:1257–63.

122 Young L, Steinman HK. Acquired ichthyosis in a patient with acquired immunodeficiency syndrome and Kaposi's sarcoma. J Am Acad Dermatol 1987;16:395–6.

123 Rizos E, Milionis HJ, Pavlidis N, et al. Acquired icthyosis: a paraneoplastic skin manifestation of Hodgkin's disease. Lancet Oncol 2002;3:727.

124 Tsochatzis E, Vassilopoulos D, Deutsch M, et al. Myelodysplastic syndrome presenting as acquired ichthyosis. Eur J Intern Med 2006;17:368–9.

125 Safai B, Grant JM, Good RA. Cutaneous manifestation of internal malignancies (II): the sign of Leser-Trelat. Int J Dermatol 1978;17:494–5.

126 Sparsa A, Boulinguez S, Le Brun V, et al. Acquired ichthyosis with pravastatin. J Eur Acad Dermatol Venereol 2007;21:549–50.

127 Huang J, Pol-Rodriguez M, Silvers D, et al. Acquired ichthyosis as a manifestation of acute cutaneous graft-versus-host disease. Pediatr Dermatol 2007;24:49–52.

128 Barker DJ, Cotterill JA. Generalized eczema craquele as a presenting feature of lymphoma. Br J Dermatol 1977;97:323–6.

129 Etoh T, Nakagawa H, Ishibashi Y. Pityriasis rotunda associated with multiple myeloma. J Am Acad Dermatol 1991;24:303–4.

130 Berkowitz I, Hodkinson HJ, Kew MC, et al. Pityriasis rotunda as a cutaneous marker of hepatocellular carcinoma: a comparison with its prevalence in other diseases. Br J Dermatol 1989;120:545–9.

131 Perez-Losada E, Pujol RM, Domingo P, et al. Hypertrichosis lanuginosa acquisita preceding extraskeletal Ewing's sarcoma. Clin Exp Dermatol 2001;26:182–3.

132 Sanchez-Estella J, Yuste M, Santos JC, et al. [Acquired paraneoplastic hypertrichosis lanuginosa]. Actas Dermosifiliogr 2005;96:459–61.

133 Toyoki Y, Satoh S, Morioka G, et al. Rectal cancer associated with acquired hypertrichosis lanuginosa as a possible cutaneous marker of internal malignancy. J Gastroenterol 1998;33:575–7.

134 Worret WI, Mayerhausen W, Emslander HP. Hypertrichosis lanuginosa acquista associated with florid cutaneous papillomatosis. Int J Dermatol 1993;32:56–8.

135 Farina MC, Tarin N, Grilli R, et al. Acquired hypertrichosis lanuginosa: case report and review of the literature. J Surg Oncol 1998;68:199–203.

136 Roh MR, Chung HJ, Cho YH, et al. Hypertrichosis lanuginosa acquisita associated with autoimmune hepatitis. J Dermatol 2006;33:574–6.

137 Bauer HI, Kaatz M, Elsner P. [Circumscribed hypertrichosis lanuginosa in acute myeloid leukemia]. Dtsch Med Wochenschr 2001;126:845–6.

138 Begany A, Nagy-Vezekenyi K. Hypertrichosis lanuginosa acquisita. Acta Derm Venereol 1992;72:18–9.

139 Wyatt JP, Anderson HF, Greer KE, et al. Acquired hypertrichosis lanuginosa as a presenting sign of metastatic prostate cancer with rapid resolution after treatment. J Am Acad Dermatol 2007;56:S45–7.

140 Schwartz RA, Jordan MC, Rubenstein DJ. Bullous chickenpox. J Am Acad Dermatol 1983;9:209–12.

141 Schwartz RA, Vickerman CE. Muehrcke's lines of the fingernails. Arch Intern Med 1979;139:242.

CHAPTER 18

Early oral and oropharyngeal cancer diagnosis and management

Arthur Mashberg and Robert A. Schwartz

It has been estimated that 22,560 cases of oral cavity squamous cell carcinoma (SCC), excluding lip, will occur in the United States in 2007 [1]. Pharyngeal cancers (including oropharyngeal and hypopharyngeal) will probably account for 11,800 additional new cases. Appreciation of the predominance of SCC in head and neck cancer is essential because it represents more than 90% of all upper aerodigestive malignancies. Other aerodigestive SCCs (e.g., larynx, esophagus, and lung), which probably share a common etiology with oral and pharyngeal cancer, frequently coexist as synchronous or metachronous second primaries.

There is general agreement that the stage of disease at the time of diagnosis influences survival more than any other parameter. It has been stated that "No lethal disease is easier to cure than oral cancer less than 1 cm in diameter" [2]. Unfortunately, clinical size and symptomatology are directly related, with the result that most lesions are detected only after they become symptomatic and, in some cases, excessively large (Figs. 18.1 and 18.2). Although oral cavity/oropharyngeal (OC/OP) SCCs are easily accessible for visual examination and high-risk populations—drinkers and smokers— have long been identified in multitudes of studies, early diagnosis has not been forthcoming, resulting in a lack of significant increase in 5-year survival rates when compared with cancers of other sites. Paradoxically, even though the mucosa of the colon/rectum is internal and requires endoscopic examination for evaluation, 39% of these cancers are localized as compared with 33% of OC/OP cancers [1]. They are overwhelmingly SCCs, which

at diagnosis are usually large, in some cases demonstrating extensive lymphadenopathy [1] (Fig. 18.3). Although lymphadenopathy may not be visualized, as compared to the obvious necrotic node shown in Fig. 18.3, careful palpation usually reveals positive nodes. It is not surprising that the majority of oral cancers are well advanced when detected, because the primary concern of many clinicians appears to be the management of symptomatic SCC demonstrating induration, ulceration, bleeding, and so forth, rather than the detection of early ones [3]. Surgery, radiotherapy, and chemotherapy have increased the quality of survival following treatment, in the United States, but the 5-year survival rate for these cancers was documented in 2002 at 62%, slowly rising from 55% in 1975 [1]. Although statistically significant, there has not been much change for a cancer that should be diagnosed in its early stages, when the survival rate could be in the 90% range. Worldwide survival is less than 50% [4].

Oral cavity/oropharyngeal SCC should be particularly favorable for early diagnosis because it appears to be a disease with identifiable risk factors [5–8], a detectable asymptomatic phase [9,10], and an efficient screening method [11–13]. However, even well-intentioned attempts at early diagnosis have resulted in poor yields, probably because of failure to focus on specific high-risk populations and high-risk sites of occurrence, use of inadequate criteria for the clinical recognition of early disease, and reliance on equivocal diagnostic modalities [3]. We concur with Mignogna and Fedele's [4] admonition "5 minutes to save a life!"

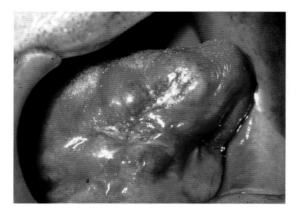

Fig. 18.1 T3 (>4 cm) carcinoma of tongue—ulcerated and indurated; primarily endophytic with surface invagination.

Groups at high risk and etiology

In the United States and western Europe, OC/OP SCC appears to be a disease of men in the 50 to 70–year age group, related to the risk factors of cigarette smoking and alcohol consumption [7]. Recent studies support this concept once again [14]. In addition, a multitude of studies over the past 40 years have revealed a similar risk for other sites of the aerodigestive tract, to be discussed later [8,15–17]. SCCs of other areas, including upper aerodigestive tract (oral cavity, pharynx, larynx, esophagus) and lung, prob-

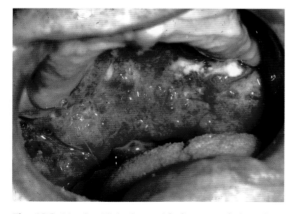

Fig. 18.2 Massive T4 (>4 cm with deep muscle invasion) of the soft palate with extension to the hard palate. Total replacement of normal mucosa by tumor.

ably share a common etiology with oral and pharyngeal cancer and frequently coexist as second primaries. Specific mechanisms are being investigated. The role of immunocompetence, human papilloma virus [18], and genotypes [19] warrants scrutiny.

There are no experimental studies to our knowledge that suggest a specific mechanism that indict alcohol, but case-control studies have shown that carcinoma of the upper aerodigestive tract bears a definite relationship to alcohol intake. Although tobacco has been shown to be a carcinogen and cancer of the respiratory tract has been directly related to cigarette smoking, both alcohol and cigarette smoking are factors in these anatomic areas [7]. Feldman and Hazan [15] demonstrated that nondrinking smokers have two to four times the risk of developing carcinoma as do abstainers of alcohol and tobacco. Heavy-drinking smokers have a risk six to 15 times greater than that of abstainers. Mashberg and colleagues [8] confirmed the synergistic effect of alcohol and tobacco and also suggested an independent role for alcohol in oral cancer. Their data indicate that for someone who smokes and drinks, doubling the alcohol consumption leads to much greater risk of OC/OP SCC than does doubling cigarette consumption (Table 18.1). This study also suggested that imbibing beer or wine is more significant than whiskey.

Tuyns and associates [16] conducted a retrospective case-control study in France of 200 male patients with esophageal cancer and 778 controls. When the adjusted relative risks were calculated for various levels of alcohol and tobacco consumption, the effects of drinking and smoking appeared to be independent of each other. When alcohol and tobacco intake were considered together, the risks observed were consistent with a multiplicative model.

In the western world, other forms of tobacco have also been indicated as etiologic factors in the development of oral carcinoma. Although not as prevalent as cigarette smoking or drinking, habitual use of cigars and pipes does contribute to the frequency of cases. The sites of occurrence and clinical manifestations of such SCCs appear quite different from those related to cigarette smoking and alcohol consumption. Significantly, lesions related to cigars and pipes appear to develop at specific sites, primarily

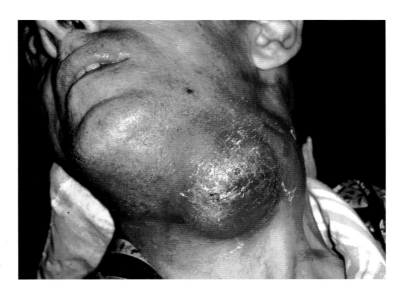

Fig. 18.3 Cervical lymphadenopathy with central necrosis. Metastases from pharyngeal carcinoma.

buccal mucosa, in response to direct contact with the oral mucosa. There is considerable disagreement as to the role of "smokeless tobacco." Many believe that unburned tobacco is carcinogenic [18,20]. Nitrosamines in tobacco are considered a possible source of carcinogenicity. Citing shammah or the betel nut quid as producing leukoplakia and SCC without explaining the role of carbonate of lime and other substances, which are part of the quid, is problematic. In the United States, an epidemiologic study by Winn and coworkers [21] found an increased risk for snuff dipping among white women older than 60 years at the site of placement. Concerns arise as to the confounding effect of the alcohol and tobacco. An evaluation of mortality incidence raises significant questions [22,23]. These substances produce keratinized lesions at the site of placement, which are then identified as leukoplakia, a questionable precursor of SCC. This paradigm, which is in great contention, will be discussed shortly. The concept of the carcinogenicity of smokeless tobacco is supported by government, media, and medical and dental groups, although we are not aware of any adequate prospective longitudinal or case-control studies, similar to those of alcohol and tobacco, that document it as a significant risk factor. It is hoped that research in this area will be attempted in the future.

Squamous cell carcinoma, despite its local manifestations, is most likely a regional disease process that becomes clinically significant only when the patient's immunologic capacity is altered. Cellular atypia, carcinoma in situ, and/or microinvasive carcinoma probably exist in the mucosa for a prolonged time before they become clinically evident.

Chronic irritation from dentures, irregular or sharp teeth, hot or spicy foods, and various other physical agents have been implicated as factors in the development of intraoral SCCs. However, evidence has not supported this idea. Physical irritation plays little or no part in the natural history of oral carcinoma. The most traumatized areas of the mouth (lips, tip of tongue, gingiva, cheeks, and hard palate) have the lowest incidence of squamous malignancies. Additionally, it is difficult to accept the concept that trauma will induce the nuclear changes responsible for the development of carcinoma.

Associations between cancer and syphilis or vitamin deficiencies have been stressed in the past but are not given much credence today. Environmental factors, especially exposure to ultraviolet light, appear to affect the incidence of lip cancer but probably exert negligible effect on the intraoral distribution of SCC. Oral lichen planus, especially the erosive form, has also been associated with oral SCC [24,25]. A retrospective analysis of 1028 Swedish

Table 18.1 Summary of relative risks by smoking and drinking habits

	Relative risks			
	Cases	Controls	Crude	Adjusted
Drinking Habits				
Minimal drinking	10	206	1.0	1.0
<6 WEs/day[a]	23	106	4.5	3.3
6–9 WEs/day	47	52	18.6	15.2
≥10 WEs/day	101	133	15.6	10.6
Total	181	497		
Smoking Habits				
Minimal smoking	14	173	1.0	1.0
Cigar/pipe	14	41	4.2	4.1
10–19 cigarettes/day	16	48	4.1	3.2
20–39 cigarettes/day	82	150	6.8	4.5
≥40 cigarettes/day	55	85	8.0	5.0
Total	181	497		

Note: Relative risks by smoking habits are adjusted for drinking habits and age; relative risks by drinking habits are adjusted for smoking habits and age.
[a] One WE = 1 oz of 86 proof whiskey or 4 oz of dry wine (11% to 12%) or 12 oz of beer.
Source: Mashberg et al. [8].

oral lichen planus patients confirmed an incidence of oral SCC higher than expected; there is a small but increased risk for oral SCC in these patients [24]. Further studies are necessary to establish a clear relationship. Unfortunately, concern arises when an initial histologic misdiagnosis of oral lichen planus is in reality severe dysplasia or in situ change, which subsequently develops into an SCC.

High-risk intraoral sites

Geographic and regional differences in the intraoral distribution of SCC are recognized. Environmental carcinogens, actinic exposure, and local customs each probably contribute to the site distribution pattern for any given population. Lesions related to cigar and pipe smoking are often found in the buccal mucosa and are characteristically "keratotic." Cancers related to alcohol and cigarette smoking, the predominant risk factors in the United

States and Europe, are also localized to distinct sites within the oral cavity. Although the hard palate, buccal mucosa, gingiva, floor of the mouth, soft palate, and tongue once were considered sites commonly involved with SCC, studies by Moore and Catlin [26] and Mashberg and Meyers [9] clearly demonstrated that three specific intraoral oropharyngeal sites are predisposed to develop SCC. The floor of the mouth, ventrolateral tongue, and soft palate complex (soft palate proper, lingual aspect of the retromolar trigone, and anterior tonsillar pillar) should be regarded as high-risk sites (Fig. 18.4).

In Mashberg's prospective study [9] of 222 asymptomatic, randomly diagnosed SCCs (excluding 15 lip lesions) in 146 drinking cigarette smokers, 201 lesions (97%) were found in three locations: 101 (48.8%) in the floor of the mouth, 36 (17.2%) in the ventral or lateral tongue, and 64 (30.9%) in the soft palate complex. Of the 101 lesions in the floor of the mouth, 73 (72.3%) occurred in the anterior portion, with 33 (32.7%) involving the papilla at the orifice of Wharton's duct. These anatomic sites were identified as "high-risk" sites of occurrence. Significantly, only one SCC was found in the hard palate, three in the alveolar gingiva, and two in the buccal mucosa (Fig. 18.5).

The small number of hard palate, buccal mucosa, and alveolar asymptomatic SCCs, 82% of which were 2 cm or less and 42% of which were 1 cm or less in diameter, suggests that the traditional sites described in the literature of comparatively larger symptomatic SCCs may have been points of termination or extension rather than sites of origin. It is rare to find studies, prospective or retrospective, of such small lesions. For example, a symptomatic SCC (T2 or T3) in the floor of the mouth, extending to or invading the alveolus, may be documented erroneously as an alveolar or gingival lesion. Similarly, a large soft palate SCC that extends to the hard palate and necessitates a maxillectomy may be mistakenly described as a hard palate malignancy. It is rare to find studies, prospective or retrospective, of SCCs of such minimal size as described here.

In a study by Lederman [27], most carcinomas of the upper aerodigestive tract occurred in specific locations. These sites comprised a portion of the lateral

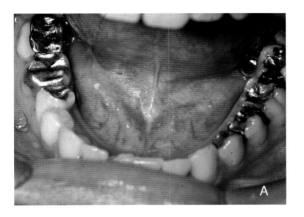
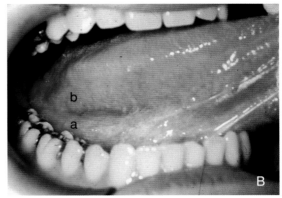
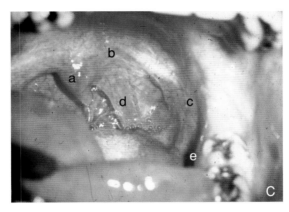

Fig. 18.4 High-risk sites. *A*, Anterior floor of the mouth, the most common site for development of oral squamous carcinoma in drinking cigarette smokers. *B*, Ventrolateral tongue and posterior floor of the mouth. Sites *a* and *b* are of particular concern. Unless tongue retraction to the contralateral side is adequate, visualization is poor. *C*, soft palate complex: (*a*) uvula, (*b*) posterior soft palate, (*c*) anterior tonsillar pillar, (*d*) posterior tonsillar pillar, (*e*) lingual aspect retromolar trigone and junction of the tongue and anterior pillar.

food channels and the sphincters controlling the volume of food passing through those channels. In addition, involvement of "reservoir systems," which act to pool food and prevent the bolus from inundating the air passage, was described. Such "reservoirs" may collect dissolved or concentrated carcinogens, permitting more prolonged contact with the mucosa. Because the anterior floor of the mouth is the most dependent part of the oral cavity, alcohol may remain in prolonged contact with the mucosa and act as a carcinogen. Although the soft palate and posterolateral tongue are not dependent reservoirs, it is possible that inhaled tobacco smoke, directed to these areas, has a similar carcinogenic effect. In an analysis [28] of Mashberg's continuing prospective study of 359 US veterans with 24 OC/OP SCCs, it was found that tobacco smoking was more strongly associated with soft palate cancers than with SCCs of anterior sites and that patients with cancers of the floor of the mouth and oral tongue had higher odds ratios for alcohol consumption than did subjects with cancers of other sites, tending to support the hypothesis of the carcinogenic effect of tobacco smoke and alcoholic beverages on the mucosa through direct contact. The greater risk relationship between alcohol and esophageal cancer and smoking and laryngeal cancer further supports the concept.

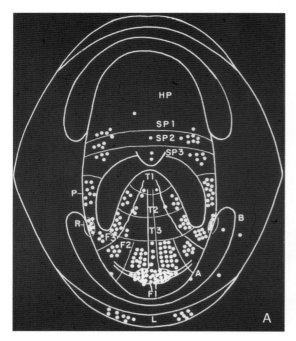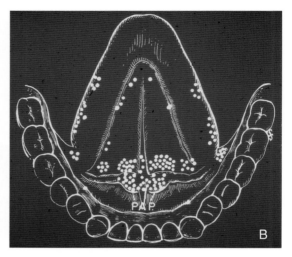

Fig. 18.5 Scattergrams. *A*, Scattergram of subdivided sites of 222 asymptomatic lesions. T, ventrolateral tongue; F, floor of mouth; SP, soft palate trigone (1, 2, and 3 refer to anterior, middle, and posterior thirds, respectively); L, lip; A, alveolus; B, buccal; and HP, hard palate. *B*, Detailed scattergram of the floor of the mouth and ventrolateral tongue. Note the concentration of lesions in the anterior floor of the mouth, especially at PAP (papilla), at the exit of Wharton's duct (submaxillary gland). (Reprinted from Mashberg and Meyers [9].)

The histologic similarity of the tissues in the high-risk areas also may be significant. Tissues at high-risk sites have a thin epithelium relatively devoid of keratin and a submucosa that contains fat and glands. In contrast, the tissues of low-risk areas are more richly keratinized or highly specialized, specifically the dorsum of the tongue, the hard palate, and buccal mucosa. The high-risk sites, unprotected by keratin or specialized structures, may be more subject to the local effects of carcinogens.

Intraoral examination

The high-risk sites require careful scrutiny in an effective oncologic examination of the oral cavity. These areas are difficult to evaluate without adequate lighting. Standard dental lights and some fiberoptic light systems appear to be best for detection of early lesions. Head mirrors and lamps do not

have sufficient intensity or color balance to allow an appreciation of minute mucosal alterations.

A dental or laryngeal mirror facilitates adequate visualization of areas that cannot be seen directly. Use of a wooden tongue depressor as a retractor does not permit viewing of all pertinent intraoral mucosal surfaces because light cannot be directed or reflected with the instrument. In addition, the mirror is more rigid and better tolerated by patients, further facilitating the examination.

For inspection of the anterior and middle thirds of the floor of the mouth and the anteroventral two thirds of the tongue, the mandible should be horizontal when the mouth is open. The tip of the tongue should be extended upward, contacting the hard palate posteriorly. Examination of the posterior floor of the mouth, retromolar trigone, and posterior ventrolateral aspect of the tongue (including the area of the foliate papillae) necessitates grasping the anterior third of the tongue with a 2 × 2-inch gauze sponge, distracting it to the contralateral labial commissure, and withdrawing it from the oral cavity as far as possible. External pressure in the area of the submandibular gland on the ipsilateral side permits the posterior floor of the mouth to be elevated and its contiguous structures to be visualized. At the same time, the mirror should be employed to view, indirectly, the lingual aspect of the retromolar trigone. With the tongue still hyperextended, the anterior pillar (glossopalatine fold) may also be evaluated. The soft palate, uvula, and posterior pillars may be seen directly by depressing the middle third of the tongue and having the patient say "ah" or take a deep breath.

Although palpation is an important part of head and neck examination, direct visualization of mucosal surfaces is more significant in detecting early lesions, which usually have little mass and minimal depth. Mirror examination should be employed for lesions in the base of the tongue and vallecula, because these areas are not accessible for direct viewing.

Early lesions: erythroplasia versus leukoplakia

A diagnosis of advanced SCC is not difficult to establish. Symptomatic cancers, characterized by ulceration, bleeding, pain, or induration, are usually at least stage II lesions (T2 or larger). Complaints of intraoral pain and dysfunction, extraoral swelling, or cervical lymphadenopathy impel the clinician to evaluate the oral cavity, nasopharynx, oropharynx, and hypopharynx for a primary SCC. Early cancers, however, are frequently asymptomatic and differ markedly from symptomatic ones in their appearance and clinical presentation. Unfortunately, the former frequently remain undetected.

In attempts to diagnose early carcinomas of the oral cavity, leukoplakia has often been regarded as the most common "precancerous" lesion of the oral cavity. The paradigm is presented as "white patch or plaque of unknown etiology = leukoplakia = precancer = eventually cancer." There is a tendency to describe mucosal aberrations with a keratotic part as white lesions or "leukoplakias" and to disregard

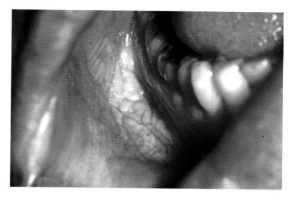

Fig. 18.6 Benign keratosis, "leukoplakic" lesion, in buccal sulcus. Frequently related to smokeless tobacco.

other components. Thus, clinicians often respond reflexively to whiteness in documenting the appearance of these lesions when submitting a biopsy specimen to a pathologist. However, in past studies it was noted that only 0.13 to 6.05 of leukoplakias develop into SCC over a prolonged period [29–37]. The color composition of those leukoplakias is rarely described. Despite evidence that leukoplakia is overrated as a clinically significant pathologic entity and has only a low malignant potential, the paradigm *leukoplakias of the oral mucosa are precancerous or early carcinoma* still abounds in the literature and in teaching institutions (Figs. 18.6 and 18.7). In employing

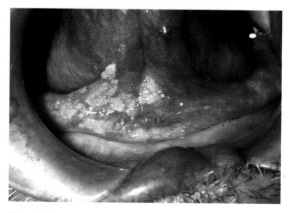

Fig. 18.7 Carcinoma in situ in the floor of the mouth. Pebbly, heaped-up keratin with slight inflammation increases the index of suspicion in such leukoplakic lesions.

Table 18.2 Color characteristics of asymptomatic intraoral SCC

Color Component	Number	Percent
Erythroplasia (red) only	69	33.3
Erythroplasia with white	124	60.0
White only	10	4.8
Other or not stated	4	1.9
Total	207	100.0

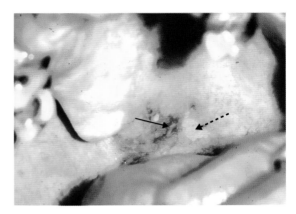

Fig. 18.8 Asymptomatic invasive carcinoma of the soft palate. *Solid arrow* points to diffuse inflammation erythroplasia with associated areas of keratin; *dashed arrow* indicates that keratin patch biopsy of the keratinized area is frequently unrevealing, whereas biopsy of the erythroplastic site is usually diagnostic.

terms such as *homogenous leukoplakia, speckled leukoplakia,* and *nodular leukoplakia,* the implied significance of leukoplakia persists.

However, studies of Mashberg have considerably altered the significance of this paradigm. The "innocuous"-appearing red inflammatory or erythroplastic (erythroplasia of Queyrat) mucosal changes related to early cancer, not precancer, were proposed by the early 1970s and have proved to be the most common presentation of early cancer [38]. In a prospective study by Mashberg and associates [10,39], areas of mucosal erythroplasia were the most usual appearance of early carcinomas, not rare as had been previously believed, especially in high-risk drinkers and smokers. Most of these asymptomatic SCCs were less than 2 cm in diameter, predominately red, with or without a white component, and smooth, granular, or minimally elevated. Approximately 33% of 207 asymptomatic intraoral carcinomas were entirely erythroplastic (red), 4.9% were all white, and 60% were mixed [40]. Significantly, in the mixed lesions, erythema (red) was the predominant component (Table 18.2). Further studies by Mashberg and Feldman [41] continued to corroborate these findings. In one recent retrospective study of 269 lesions in 236 patients, Holmstrup and associates [37] showed nonhomogenous leukoplakia accounted for the highest frequency of malignant development, about 20%, whereas only 3% of the homogenous leukoplakias developed carcinomas, supporting our findings. Thomson's recent report also confirms these results [42].

Unfortunately, most retrospective studies leave much to be desired. The term *nonhomogenous* or *speckled leukoplakia* continues to reinforce the leukoplakia paradigm because no mention is made of the appearance of the mucosa that is speckled. It is true that leukoplakia, a white plaque, is more common than erythroplasia, a red one. However, in considering the earliest sign of cancer, the reverse is true. It is essential that when the practitioner documents a lesion, it be described by its actual color composition and morphology, not a substitute clinical term that introduces bias.

There are two distinct types of erythroplastic lesions that suggest carcinoma. The first is granular and red velvety with stippled or patchy areas of keratin within or peripheral to it (Figs. 18.8 and 18.9). The keratinized areas appear to be lying on a red, inflamed mucosal surface. Usually, the mucosa is not ulcerated but may be "heaped up." The other type is smooth and nongranular, primarily red with minimal or no keratosis (Figs. 18.10 to 18.12). The mucosal surface, however, is not like that of a nonspecific inflammatory lesion in that it seems atrophic and "worn." These smooth, nongranular lesions may wax and wane. Frequently, their appearance changes from one day to the next; the degree of inflammation may also vary. Ulceration, bleeding, induration, and exophytic growth (<1 mm) are uncommon (Table 18.3).

Significant areas of mucosal abnormality frequently are not well defined. Many are irregular,

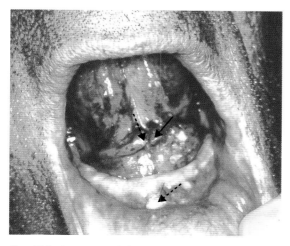

Fig. 18.9 Asymptomatic invasive carcinoma of the floor of the mouth. *Dashed arrow* indicates keratinized salivary papilla. *Solid arrow* on the contralateral papilla identifies the erythroplastic area. This site is indicated for biopsy: see Fig. 18.13. *Dashed arrow* on the labial aspect of the alveolus indicates a benign keratinized lesion.

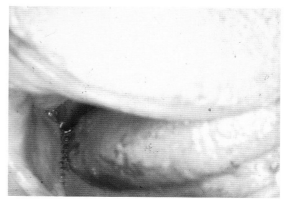

Fig. 18.11 Irregular erythroplastic asymptomatic carcinoma on the lateral aspect of the mid-tongue. The mucosal surface is atrophic.

with a blending of inflamed and normal mucosa. Some contain islands of normal mucosa, entrapped by the growth and coalescence of separate erythroplastic areas. Although these islands appear white or gray, they are not truly keratotic.

Because their appearance is altered by saliva, the mucosal surface should be dried gently before examination. Lesions, when dry, often are more granular or slightly abraded. There are no reliable clinical signs that differentiate in situ from invasive SCC, although textural changes, such as roughness or granularity, greatly increase the probability that a lesion is invasive. Cervical lymph node metastases are rare at this stage.

Although the mucosal changes in early cancer often resemble the tissue responses associated with

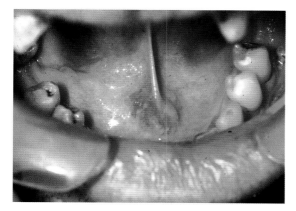

Fig. 18.10 Asymptomatic erythroplastic invasive carcinoma of the floor of the mouth—red and velvety smooth. Surrounding paler areas are islands of normal mucosa.

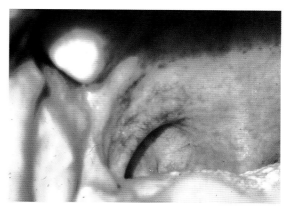

Fig. 18.12 Asymptomatic carcinoma of the anterior tonsillar pillar. The only change noted is diffuse redness of the entire pillar.

Table 18.3 Surface characteristics of asymptomatic intraoral SCC

Characteristic	Carcinoma in situ[a]		Invasive SCC[b]	
	Number	Percent	Number	Percent
Surface texture				
Granular	15	32.6	54	48.2
Smooth	26	56.5	37	33.1
Rough	1	2.2	12	10.7
Crusting	4	8.7	9	8.0
Elevation				
None	30	65.3	47	42.0
Slight	14	30.4	43	38.3
1 mm	2	4.4	22	19.6
Ulceration				
No	42	91.3	96	85.7
Yes	4	8.7	16	14.3
Bleeding				
No	45	97.8	110	98.2
Yes	1	2.2	2	1.8
Induration				
No	46	100.0	101	90.2
Yes	—	—	11	9.8

[a] Carcinoma in situ: 46 lesions represent 29.1% of 158 total lesions.
[b] Invasive SCC: 112 lesions represent 70.9% of 158 total lesions.

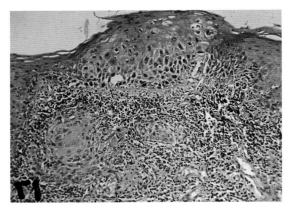

Fig. 18.13 Microscopic section of erythroplastic area in Fig. 18.9. Note dysplasia, nests of squamous carcinoma, and inflammatory barrier below the basement membrane.

candidiasis, histoplasmosis, or local tissue injury of a physical, chemical, or thermal nature, diagnostic distinctions can be made. SCCs are usually discrete entities located in the high-risk areas of the mouth, are not associated with a specific etiology, and persist despite removal of local factors. Occasionally, there may be more than one primary neoplasm, multicentricity, as the result of field cancerization, a concept originally proposed by Slaughter [43]. Non-neoplastic inflammatory lesions, localized or diffuse, can usually be attributed to a specific etiology or event and typically subside within 14 days following elimination of local factors. If lesions persist beyond this 2-week observation period, biopsy is mandatory [39]. In this analysis, 80% of the erythroplastic lesions (red component) persistent

after 2 weeks were found to be invasive SCC. Their erythematous character appears to be related to a reactive inflammatory barrier (submucosal vascular and lymphohistiocytic infiltrate) associated with the malignant squamous cells. This infiltrate may be present in SCCs that are primarily white, but not visualized on the surface, obscured by the keratin. Microscopic specimens of early cancer invariably demonstrate such an inflammatory reaction below the basement membrane, probably reflecting angiogenesis and/or immune response to the developing cancer (Fig. 18.13). The presence of keratin (the identity factor in leukoplakia) appears to be a response not to the cancer per se but to many forms of irritation, including carcinogens.

Because 90% of early oral SCCs are not palpable, meticulous visual examination of high-risk patients, with particular attention to asymptomatic areas of erythroplasia in high-risk sites, facilitates the discovery of early cancers. Approximately 75% of early asymptomatic erythroplastic cancers documented were 2 cm or less; about half of these were 1 cm or smaller [10]. Obviously, minimal size does not preclude invasiveness. Lymphadenopathy was rarely demonstrated. Such localized SCCs usually can be managed with minimal residual deformity, negligible loss of function, and optimal 5-year survival of greater than 90%.

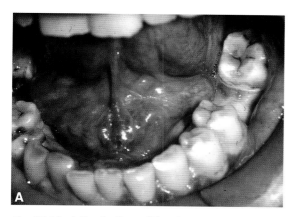 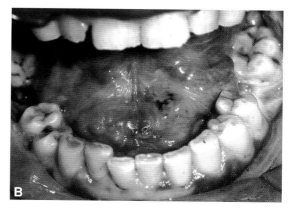

Fig. 18.14 *A*, Barely discernible minute area of erythroplasia in the floor of the mouth, of questionable significance, which persisted. *B*, Same area after staining application. Biopsy of stained area revealed SCC.

Vital staining

It is believed that toluidine blue, a basic metachromatic dye, stains the nuclear material of SCCs, but not that of normal mucosa. The nuclei of malignant cells manifest increased DNA synthesis, theoretically resulting in increased toluidine blue pickup [11,12]. Alternately, it has been suggested that uptake by nuclear material may not account for the deep-blue hue of malignant lesions but rather diffusion through three to four layers of haphazardly arranged tumor cells allowing for deeper penetration of the dye [44]. A third concept (unpublished)

suggests that attachment to the DNA of mitochondria is responsible for the staining. Further studies are indicated to determine the mechanism.

The use of toluidine blue has been advocated by many to detect oral malignancies [11,44–46]. Mashberg's prospective studies [12,13,47] reveal conclusively that all or part of malignant lesions (carcinoma or carcinoma in situ) stain dark blue with topical application (Figs. 18.14 and 18.15). Staining of severe dysplasia is inconclusive.

Although appreciation of the staining characteristics of early mucosal cancers is more objective than the clinical impressions before staining, some

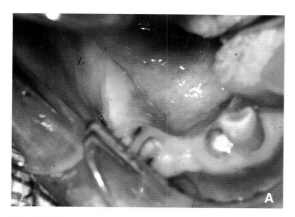 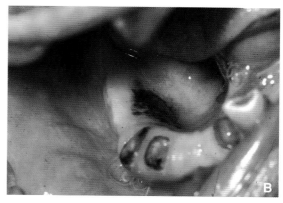

Fig. 18.15 *A*, Granular erythroplastic area at the junction of the alveolus and floor of the mouth in a patient with lupus erythematosus. *B*, Site stained by toluidine blue application. Biopsy revealed SCC.

degree of familiarity with stain interpretation is desirable. If an entire lesion or a portion of it stains dark blue in a solid or stippled pattern, malignancy must be considered. Occasional circumscribed light blue equivocal stains must also be considered positive.

Normal tissue does not absorb stain, but small areas of intense, mechanically retained stain may be observed. These may be removed by gently swabbing the area with acetic acid. Larger regions of extraneous stain also may occur, especially in the dorsum of the tongue, areas coated with surface debris or exfoliated keratin, and gingival crevices. Retention in these areas is usually of little concern because asymptomatic oral cancers arise infrequently in these sites. Occasionally, a film of stain from the dorsum of the tongue may be transferred to portions of the posterior soft palate during swallowing. Here, the stain is not well circumscribed but appears diffuse and amorphous. A light blue film may also be observed over a large area of mucosa as a result of dye-tinged saliva. These variants should not be misconstrued as positive or equivocal results.

Lesions with limited dysplasia or atypia do not stain consistently. Correlation between the staining impression and the pathologic diagnosis is tenuous at best in these cases. However, the typical early erythroplastic carcinoma associated with alcohol consumption and cigarette smoking usually stains dark blue. These lesions are often stippled or patchy because of areas of interspersed keratin. Neoplasia below the mucosal surface and normal mucosa do not pick up stain.

Areas of inflammation may occasionally yield false-positive results. However, as a rule, they do not persist for more than 14 days. If a lesion stains dark blue after a 14-day waiting period, the probability of malignancy is greatly increased. Topical application alone results in a 6.7% false-negative rate [12]. When erythroplastic criteria are used as a prime factor in suspicion, before topical application of toluidine blue, results produce less than a 2.0% false-negative rate. False positives or overdiagnosis occurs in about 8% if the 14-day waiting period is observed.

Staining is a simple, expeditious office procedure that does not require an intermediary. The great value of toluidine blue staining lies in its immediate reinforcement of the clinical impression, its control over false-negative clinical findings, and its ability to detect additional SCCs. It must be stressed that a high level of clinical suspicion mandates biopsy regardless of staining outcomes. Although a lesion meets the visual criteria for early cancer, persists beyond the 2-week observation period, and stains with toluidine blue, the diagnosis of carcinoma can be established only by biopsy.

In vivo staining is superior to cytologic study because the information obtained is immediate and specific. Oral cytology has been advocated as a screening modality for evaluation of intraoral lesions. Although cytology has validity in other anatomic locations, its routine use in intraoral cancer detection is questionable. The need to have the smears evaluated by an intermediary and the subjective nature of interpretation reduce the validity of cytologic diagnoses. The development of well-defined visual criteria, the accessibility of OC/OP surfaces, and the absence of significant morbidity make toluidine blue the screening procedure of choice. Suspicious lesions should be stained in preference to smearing.

Toluidine blue also serves as a guide to biopsy by localizing tumor cells within the area of erythroplasia. Obtaining multiple random samples from the entire area of involvement is not always a reliable diagnostic procedure. Early cancers often consist of islands of normal mucosa interspersed with tumor and/or areas of keratin. Small foci of cells may be missed. Selection of the most representative biopsy site should not be left to chance. Because only the neoplastic or dysplastic mucosa will stain, biopsy of areas of dye retention is most likely to demonstrate invasive cancer on microscopy.

Occasionally, minute carcinomas that stain may not be confirmed microscopically. The area of uptake may be so small that it is missed on histologic sectioning. Biopsy specimens taken of minute areas of stain should be small to increase the probability that histologic sectioning will involve the pathologic entity.

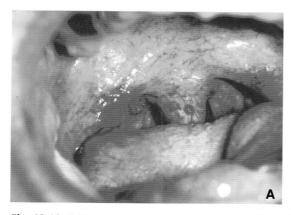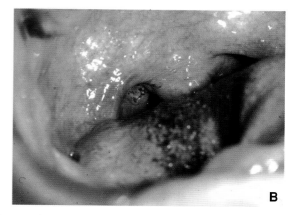

Fig. 18.16 *A*, Vague area on the right posterior tonsillar pillar, not observed during a clinical examination of a patient with carcinoma of the left tonsillar fossa. *B*, Unsuspected carcinoma stained in a stippled manner by toluidine blue rinse.

The technique of application is as follows:
1 Rinse the mouth with water twice, for about 20 seconds each time, to remove debris.
2 Rinse the mouth well with 1% acetic acid for 20 seconds to remove ropy saliva.
3 Gently dry the area with gauze. Do not abrade the tissue.
4 Apply 1% toluidine blue solution to the lesion and swab high-risk areas.
5 Rinse with 1% acetic acid (approximately 150 mL) for 1 minute to clear excess stain.
6 Rinse with water.

Various modifications and different staining techniques have been advocated [44–46]. Mashberg [13,47] has employed a rinse modality that is all encompassing for the oral mucosa, showing 7.4% false positives (Fig. 18.16).

In conclusion, the topical application of toluidine blue to suspicious lesions serves as a diagnostic "control" over the subjective impression of the clinician. If screening procedures are desired, a toluidine blue rinse may be used for those at high risk (drinkers and smokers and those who have had a prior upper aerodigestive SCC) to include all the high-risk sites. Lesions not detected during a visual examination may be revealed by the stain.

Methylene blue staining in the diagnosis of oral cancer was evaluated in 58 patients, with a reported sensitivity of 90% and a specificity of only 69%

[48]. Direct fluorescence visualization of clinically occult high-risk oral premalignant lesions using a simple handheld device has been described [49]. Tissue showing loss of autofluorescence would then be biopsied. Much more experience is needed to evaluate the value of this technique.

Workup of suspicious lesions

A standardized protocol should be employed when an asymptomatic lesion is detected. Probable sources of acute or chronic irritation should be removed if possible; attempts should be made to curtail the use of alcohol and tobacco. The patient should have a reappointment for observation in 10 to 14 days. Inflammatory lesions, resulting from trauma or chronic irritation, usually will be markedly improved or resolved, especially if the inciting etiology—that is, dentures or chemical or physical factors—has been eliminated. Lesions persisting without apparent cause should be considered malignant until proven otherwise by biopsy.

A complete medical history is obtained and evaluated to rule out other mucosal entities. The oral cavity, hypopharynx, pharynx, and supraglottic larynx should be evaluated by visual examination, palpation, indirect mirror visualization, or direct endoscopic inspection. Careful palpation of the neck for cervical adenopathy before biopsy must also be performed, because lymphoid hyperplasia related to the biopsy cannot be clinically differentiated from tumor involvement with certainty. The patient may be subjected to unnecessary surgery or radiotherapy unless the status of the neck nodes is established definitively before biopsy. Special attention should be directed to the size, location, texture, mobility, and presence or absence of tenderness in any nodes that are appreciated. Soft, freely mobile, tender nodes suggest inflammatory reaction. Nodes that are firm or hard, not freely mobile, or nontender are more suggestive of tumor involvement. The presence of clinically positive cervical or supraclavicular nodes associated with an asymptomatic early lesion suggests the possible existence of a second primary SCC in the upper aerodigestive tract, most commonly of the lung.

Biopsy

Biopsy diagnosis of an SCC is an absolute requirement before therapy can be initiated. Although visual criteria and techniques for the clinical detection of asymptomatic intraoral cancers have been refined, severe dysplasia, carcinoma in situ, or invasive carcinoma can be demonstrated only histologically, the only valid method for diagnosis.

The biopsy specimen must be a representative one. Adequate depth, through the epithelium and dermis into connective tissue, is necessary to determine the integrity of the basement membrane and to search for invasive tumor cells. Inclusion of a zone of adjacent, clinically normal tissue is not required for the pathologist to recognize malignant changes. However, when necrosis or ulceration is present, including some clinically involved peripheral tissue in the specimen usually assures a representative sample of active tumor, rather than nondiagnostic necrosis.

Incisional biopsy is the procedure of choice for microscopic diagnosis of suspected malignant intraoral lesions. Intentional excisional biopsy is generally not indicated in the diagnosis of oral cancer. Total removal of all abnormal tissue for diagnostic purposes is justifiable only when the lesion is almost certainly benign on clinical grounds or when the suspect lesion is small so that total removal (at least

1 cm in all dimensions) assures a positive prognosis without compromising function.

If a lesion is considered highly suspicious for malignancy, a negative biopsy report should not be accepted as the final word. Microscopic diagnoses of early lesions may be subjective; reevaluation of the original sections and re-cut ones from the paraffin-embedded block are sometimes indicated. In some instances, the original specimen may not have been representative or adequate for diagnosis. Well-founded clinical suspicion, even in the face of negative histologic reports, mandates repeat biopsy and reevaluation.

Microscopic findings

Leukoplakia has been defined by the World Health Organization as a clinical term describing a white patch or plaque that cannot be characterized, clinically or pathologically, as any other disease. It has no histologic significance. However, by implication, it is thought to be a lesion involving dysplastic cells with malignant potential and is termed a *precancer*. This ambiguity has generated much confusion. Patient management would probably be improved by deleting the term altogether in any discussion of malignancy. The term *premalignancy* is also misleading because it implies a potential toward malignant change in benign lesions where usually none exists. The concept that benign oral leukoplakias progress to malignancy more often than normal tissue has not been corroborated by controlled studies.

Cellular atypia (dysplasia) describes alterations in the relationships of cells and in the size, shape, and staining characteristics of their nuclei. Predominant microscopic features that indicate dysplastic cellular activity include (1) increased or abnormal mitoses, (2) changes in nuclear/cytoplasmic ratio, (3) hyperchromatic nuclei, (4) loss of cell polarity, (5) pleomorphism, and (6) loss of cellular adhesion with increased intercellular space. Although individual atypical cells on occasion may be found randomly throughout the thickness of the epithelium, generally the presence of a group of these cells arising in the basal layer may be considered a "lesion."

Dysplastic changes that involve increasing proportions of the epithelium are reported as mild,

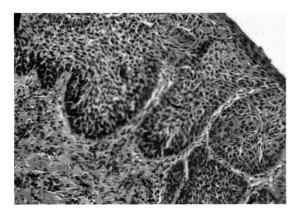

Fig. 18.17 Squamous cell carcinoma in situ—cellular atypia or dysplasia occupying the full thickness of epithelium. Note the questionable interruption of the basement membrane (*upper left*).

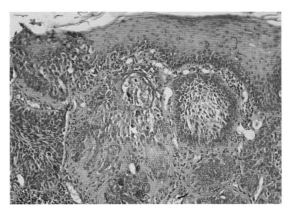

Fig. 18.18 Invasive SCC with an inflammatory barrier and increased vascularity.

moderate, or severe dysplasia, or are expressed as percentages (i.e., 10% to 90% atypia). Treatment for dysplasias depends on degree. A diagnosis of mild dysplasia usually represents a simple inflammatory lesion and is not highly indicative of an early malignant process. It should be observed periodically to rule out further clinical change. Moderate dysplasias are best conservatively excised. Severe atypia should be treated as carcinoma in situ.

When the epithelial lining in a particular microscopic field is replaced with atypical cells throughout its entire thickness from basement membrane to surface, the diagnosis is carcinoma in situ (Fig. 18.17). Oral carcinoma in situ should be regarded as significant and aggressively managed, because untreated it will likely progress to invasive carcinoma. In addition, because areas of carcinoma in situ are frequently present within invasive SCCs, it is possible that a biopsy diagnosis of carcinoma in situ does not accurately reflect the nature of the entire lesion. Significantly, the subjective impressions of the pathologist may vary. One pathologist may report severe dysplasia, whereas another, viewing the same specimen, may diagnose it as microinvasive carcinoma and a third may report moderate dysplasia. Clinicians should be aware of this phenomenon when treating patients with these early lesions.

Clinical correlation with the pathologist may be indicated. When nests or sheets of abnormal cells disrupt the basement membrane and extend into the underlying connective tissue, the diagnosis of invasive SCC is established (Figs. 18.13 and 18.18).

The degree of microscopic differentiation demonstrated by an individual SCC may correlate with its aggressiveness or relative radiosensitivity. Well-differentiated carcinomas, which closely resemble squamous epithelium, are generally considered less aggressive than poorly differentiated ones, seen microscopically as amorphous masses of highly dysplastic cells with little order or uniformity. It should be appreciated that the clinical behavior of an individual tumor is unpredictable. A well-differentiated SCC may be aggressive because of a host's inadequate immune response. The degree of differentiation cannot be determined clinically.

Mohit-Tabatabai and colleagues [50] evaluated the histologic thickness or depth of 84 stage I and II oral SCCs, a high percentage of which were early asymptomatic ones, and correlated development of nodal metastases after treatment. They reported that only one of 57 patients with SCCs less than 1.5 mm thick developed cervical metastases after treatment. This incidence increased to four of 12 patients when the SCC was 1.6 to 3.5 mm thick and to nine of 15 for those thicker than 3.6 mm, suggesting that tumor thickness plays a significant role in prognosis. Further studies support this observation [51].

Invariably, a submucosal vascular reaction and lymphohistiocytic cell infiltrate (Fig. 18.13), which appears to be an angiogenic and/or immune response to a developing SCC, are found beneath areas of carcinoma in situ and early invasive SCC on microscopy. This inflammatory barrier is extremely significant in the clinical appearance and detection of asymptomatic SCCs and in the subsequent prognosis. A minimal response bodes a poorer prognosis.

Dissemination of squamous cell carcinoma

The spread of SCC of the head and neck region occurs primarily via direct tumor extension into adjacent tissues and, later in the disease process, by metastases to regional lymph nodes and direct invasion of the overlying skin. Cervical node involvement in head and neck cancer is relatively orderly and usually follows a predictable course, depending on the primary SCC site and size. As Mohit-Tabatabai's [50] study indicates, early asymptomatic SCCs rarely demonstrate metastases at the time of diagnosis. In later stages, dissemination to the ipsilateral submandibular and jugulodigastric nodes is common, with subsequent spread to additional neck node groups. Contralateral or bilateral nodal metastases may be present, especially late in the clinical course or when midline oral structures are involved. Occasionally, expected node groups are skipped and noncontiguous adenopathy is appreciated.

When lymph node or remote bone and organ metastases are associated with an early oral primary cancer, a second primary upper aerodigestive or lung tumor may be present. Documentation of widely disseminated disease arising from a tumor in the head and neck region is most typically a postmortem finding. Death occurs in most head and neck cancer cases because of recurrence at the primary site or the cervical region, before distant metastases are clinically significant.

Staging of squamous cell carcinoma

Head and neck cancers are staged clinically to correlate treatment outcomes and survival with the extent of disease initially diagnosed. Results from one patient to another or one institution to another may then be compared to determine, on a percentage basis, which modalities of treatment are most effective for a particular site or extent of tumor involvement.

Staging for OC/OP SCC varies as far as the tumor size (T), detected lymph nodes (N), and distant metastasis (M), as published in the sixth edition of the *American Joint Committee on Cancer Staging Manual* [52]. It is important to recognize that wide variation may exist among identically staged cancers at the same primary site. For example, a nonpalpable 0.5-cm erythroplasia of minimal thickness and a 1.9-cm palpable indurated ulcer in the floor of the mouth are both classified as T1 lesions. One of us (AM) has repeatedly suggested to the American Joint Committee on Cancer that palpability, which implies thickness, be included as a subset of T.

Treatment

Surgical excision is the preferred treatment modality for early intraoral squamous carcinoma without associated lymphadenopathy. In most cases, local excision of a tumor with a 1.0- to 1.5-cm margin of clinically uninvolved tissue in all dimensions, including depth, yields optimal 5-year survival rates. This treatment approach is particularly suitable for SCCs in the anterior floor of the mouth and the posterolateral oral tongue, especially when excision is performed with electrosurgery and only the mobile portions of the tongue are sutured. Contracture of the floor of the mouth is negligible, and functional deformity is minimal, although transient salivary outflow obstruction may be problematic. Transplantation of Wharton's duct at the time of excision usually ameliorates this problem. When these tumors lie in close proximity to bone or have invaded periosteum, step resection or resection of the adjacent cortex may be necessary to assure adequate margins. This can be performed en bloc with local excision and results in minimal deformity.

Squamous cell carcinomas of the soft palate also can be locally excised as early soft palate lesions. However, the requirement for adequate surgical margins in an SCC with depth often mandates through-and-through resection of the palate, producing postoperative velopharyngeal incompetence with voice changes and nasal reflux. The surgical morbidity associated with excision of soft palate carcinomas and the diffuse field cancerization support application of radiotherapy as a primary treatment modality for many SCCs in this location. Xerostomia, radiation caries, risks of osteoradionecrosis, and limited ability to apply additional radiation treatment for subsequent tumors are, in some cases, associated with radiotherapy.

Laser surgery has been advocated for premalignant and early oral cancer [53]. To us, it is a questionable technique because there is no specimen to evaluate microscopically to determine margins, especially depth, and complete removal. Some stage I lesions are small; others are 1.99 cm with considerable depth. Wide local excision allows for evaluation of depth and margins. Radiotherapy, although there is no final specimen, at least encompasses a field much greater than the stage I SCC, so it may be effective. However, we believe that excisional surgery is best.

Associated lesions of the upper aerodigestive tract

Squamous cell carcinoma, despite its local manifestations, appears to be a regional disease of the squamous epithelium of the upper aerodigestive tract that possibly becomes clinically established only when the patient's immunologic capacity is altered. Cellular atypia (dysplasia), carcinoma in situ, and microinvasive carcinoma probably exist in the squamous mucosal field for indeterminant intervals before they become clinically evident.

Oral cavity/oropharyngeal SCC is often associated with additional primary squamous cancers of the lung, larynx, pharynx, and esophagus. The concept of field cancerization is important to consider when evaluating oral cancer patients. The incidence of multiple primary SCCs reported in the literature has ranged between 1% and 20%. In addition, in a recent population-based series of 3092 first primary oral and pharyngeal cancers, the cumulative risk of second SCCs 15 years after diagnosis of the first one approached 22% in men and 17% in women [54].

An evaluation of 981 patients with OC/OP cancer showed a total of 9.2% of the patients were affected by a second cancer, 1.5% from tertiary cancer and 0.2% from quaternary cancer [55]. Of the multiple cancers, 27.8% were synchronous and 72.2% metachronous. Thus, the presence of an SCC in the upper aerodigestive tract enhances the risk of having or developing another cancer in the same anatomic region [55]. This phenomenon of "field cancerization," in which dysplastic changes occur over a wide epithelial field in high-risk patients (i.e., heavy smokers and drinkers), indicates that the appearance of the initial SCC heralds a general susceptibility to carcinomas related to squamous epithelium [42,56,57].

It was reported that male and female patients who developed multiple primary SCCs within 5 years after an index cancer consumed significantly more alcohol per day than a control group [58]. The relative risk of multiple primary cancers in men and women exposed to the equivalent of 40 or more cigarettes and three or more whiskey equivalents per day for at least 30 years was 3.9 times that of patients exposed to the equivalent of zero to 19 cigarettes and zero to two whiskey equivalents per day.

In a continuous prospective study of a group of 101 heavy drinkers and smokers with asymptomatic index OC/OP SCCs, Mashberg [17] found that 33 of 101 patients (32.7%) with an oral carcinoma had a second primary SCC of the oropharynx (4), hypopharynx (10), larynx (7), esophagus (3), and lung (9). Of these cases, 23 (70%) were synchronous, occurring within 1 year of diagnosis of the original oral one. Seven (21%) of these were diagnosed more than a year later, and three (9%) were discovered at least 1 year before the oral primary SCC (Table 18.4).

It is not uncommon for a patient followed for a treated index carcinoma without recurrence to be confronted with a second, symptomatic primary esophageal or lung SCC 3 or 4 years later. This small sample suggests an even greater incidence of second primaries of the upper aerodigestive tract and lung in patients with an index oral carcinoma than has been reported in the literature. We believe that continued surveillance would have produced an increased number of metachronous SCCs. Detection

Table 18.4 Other primaries of the upper aerodigestive tract and lung in 101 patients with asymptomatic oral carcinoma

Location	>1 Year prior	Synchronous[a]	>1 Year later
Hypopharynx (10)	—	8	2
Pharynx (4)	—	3	1
Larynx (7)	2	5	—
Lung (9)	1	4	4
Esophagus (3)	—	3	—
Total (33)	3 (9.1%)	23 (69.7%)	7 (21.2%)

[a] Within 1 year of oral lesion.

of oral cancers identifies individuals at very high risk for upper aerodigestive and lung SCCs.

It is incumbent on all specialties to recognize the fact that treatment of the first cancer carries with it the responsibility to evaluate patients for other primary ones and to conduct close and careful surveillance (endoscopy and chest radiography) of the upper aerodigestive tract (oral cavity, pharynx, larynx, esophagus) and lungs every 6 months to 1 year.

Summary

1 Drinkers and cigarette smokers are at very high risk for upper aerodigestive tract and lung SCC.
2 The floor of the mouth, ventrolateral tongue, and soft palate complex are high-risk sites within the oral cavity and oropharynx.
3 Mucosal erythroplasia rather than leukoplakia is the earliest visual sign of oral and pharyngeal carcinoma.
4 Areas of mucosal abnormality, especially redness or inflammation in high-risk sites, persisting for more than 14 days without obvious etiology or resolution should be biopsied.
5 Asymptomatic lesions with erythroplastic components should not be regarded merely as precancerous changes. The evidence indicates that these lesions in high-risk sites should be considered invasive carcinoma or, at the very least, carcinoma in situ, unless proven otherwise by biopsy.
6 Toluidine blue staining serves as a useful diagnostic adjunct, especially to rule out false-negative

clinical impressions. It may also be used as a cancer screening rinse in patients at high risk to encompass the entire oral mucosa after a negative clinical examination and as a guide to improve biopsy yields.
7 If an oral or pharyngeal cancer is identified, evaluations of the larynx, hypopharynx, esophagus, and lungs should be performed to rule out second primary SCCs. After satisfactory treatment of the index cancer, yearly aerodigestive surveillance is indicated.

References

1 Jemal A, Siegel R, Ward E, et al. Cancer statistics, 2007. CA Cancer J Clin 2007;57:43–66.
2 Moore C. Education and oral cancer. Washington, DC: US Government Printing Office; 1966.
3 Mashberg A. Diagnosis of early oral and oropharyngeal squamous carcinoma: obstacles and their amelioration. Oral Oncol 2000;36:253–5.
4 Mignogna MD, Fedele S. Oral cancer screening: 5 minutes to save a life. Lancet 2005;365:1905–6.
5 Wynder EL, Bross IJ, Feldman RM. A study of the etiological factors in cancer of the mouth. Cancer 1957;10:1300–23.
6 Seixas FA. Alcohol, a carcinogen? CA Cancer J Clin 1975;25:62–5.
7 Mashberg A, Boffetta P, Winkelman R, et al. Tobacco smoking, alcohol drinking, and cancer of the oral cavity and oropharynx among US veterans. Cancer 1993;72:1369–75.
8 Mashberg A, Garfinkel L, Harris S. Alcohol as a primary risk factor in oral squamous carcinoma. CA Cancer J Clin 1981;31:146–55.
9 Mashberg A, Meyers H. Anatomical site and size of 222 early asymptomatic oral squamous cell carcinomas: a continuing prospective study of oral cancer. II. Cancer 1976;37:2149–57.
10 Mashberg A, Morrissey JB, Garfinkel L. A study of the appearance of early asymptomatic oral squamous cell carcinoma. Cancer 1973;32:1436–45.
11 Pabiszczak M, Wierzbicka M, Wasniewska E, et al. [Toluidine blue in monitoring of recurrences and second primary tumors in patients treated for oral cavity and pharynx cancer]. Otolaryngol Pol 2006;60:691–5.
12 Mashberg A. Reevaluation of toluidine blue application as a diagnostic adjunct in the detection of asymptomatic oral squamous carcinoma: a continuing prospective study of oral cancer. III. Cancer 1980;46:758–63.

13 Mashberg A. Tolonium (toluidine blue) rinse—a screening method for recognition of squamous carcinoma. Continuing study of oral cancer. IV. JAMA 1981;245:2408–10.

14 Kim HY, Elter JR, Francis TG, et al. Prevention and early detection of oral and pharyngeal cancer in veterans. Oral Surg Oral Med Oral Pathol Oral Radiol Endod 2006;102:625–31.

15 Feldman JG, Hazan M. A case-control investigation of alcohol, tobacco, and diet in head and neck cancer. Prev Med 1975;4:444–63.

16 Tuyns AJ, Pequignot G, Jensen OM. [Esophageal cancer in Ille-et-Vilaine in relation to levels of alcohol and tobacco consumption. Risks are multiplying]. Bull Cancer 1977;64:45–60.

17 Mashberg A, Samit A. Current concepts in the diagnosis and treatment of asymptomatic squamous cancer. In: De Michelis B, editor. XX Congresso Nationale Societa Italiana Di Odontostomatologia e Chirurgia Maxillo-facciale. St. Vincent, Italy; 1985.

18 Tsantoulis PK, Kastrinakis NG, Tourvas AD, et al. Advances in the biology of oral cancer. Oral Oncol 2007;43:523–34.

19 Majumder M, Sikdar N, Paul RR, et al. Increased risk of oral leukoplakia and cancer among mixed tobacco users carrying XRCC1 variant haplotypes and cancer among smokers carrying two risk genotypes: one on each of two loci, GSTM3 and XRCC1 (codon 280). Cancer Epidemiol Biomarkers Prev 2005;14:2106–12.

20 Scheifele C, Nassar A, Reichart PA. Prevalence of oral cancer and potentially malignant lesions among shammah users in Yemen. Oral Oncol 2007;43:42–50.

21 Winn DM, Blot WJ, Shy CM, et al. Snuff dipping and oral cancer among women in the southern United States. N Engl J Med 1981;304:745–9.

22 Bouquot JE, Meckstroth RL. Oral cancer in a tobacco-chewing US population—no apparent increased incidence or mortality. Oral Surg Oral Med Oral Pathol Oral Radiol Endod 1998;86:697–706.

23 Rodu B, Jansson C. Smokeless tobacco and oral cancer: a review of the risks and determinants. Crit Rev Oral Biol Med 2004;15:252–63.

24 Rodstrom PO, Jontell M, Mattsson U, et al. Cancer and oral lichen planus in a Swedish population. Oral Oncol 2004;40:131–8.

25 Mignogna MD, Fedele S, Lo Russo L, et al. Immune activation and chronic inflammation as the cause of malignancy in oral lichen planus: is there any evidence? Oral Oncol 2004;40:120–30.

26 Moore C, Catlin D. Anatomic origins and locations of oral cancer. Am J Surg 1967;114:510–3.

27 Lederman M. The anatomy of cancer, with special reference to tumours of the upper air and food passages. J Laryngol Otol 1964;78:181–208.

28 Boffetta P, Mashberg A, Winkelmann R, et al. Carcinogenic effect of tobacco smoking and alcohol drinking on anatomic sites of the oral cavity and oropharynx. Int J Cancer 1992;52:530–3.

29 Einhorn J, Wersall J. Incidence of oral carcinoma in patients with leukoplakia of the oral mucosa. Cancer 1967;20:2189–93.

30 Malaovalla AM, Silverman S, Mani NJ, et al. Oral cancer in 57,518 industrial workers of Gujarat, India: a prevalence and followup study. Cancer 1976;37:1882–6.

31 Gupta PC, Mehta FS, Daftary DK, et al. Incidence rates of oral cancer and natural history of oral precancerous lesions in a 10-year follow-up study of Indian villagers. Community Dent Oral Epidemiol 1980;8:283–333.

32 Silverman S Jr. Observations on the clinical characteristics and natural history of oral leukoplakia. J Am Dent Assoc 1968;76:772–7.

33 Roed-Petersen B, Gupta PC, Pindborg JJ, et al. Association between oral leukoplakia and sex, age, and tobacco habits. Bull World Health Organ 1972;47:13–9.

34 Mehta FS, Shroff BC, Gupta PC, et al. Oral leukoplakia in relation to tobacco habits. A ten-year follow-up study of Bombay policemen. Oral Surg Oral Med Oral Pathol 1972;34:426–33.

35 Banoczy J. Follow-up studies in oral leukoplakia. J Maxillofac Surg 1977;5:69–75.

36 Pindborg JJ. Clinical relevance of precancerous lesions of oral mucosa. Recent Results Cancer Res 1994;134:9–16.

37 Holmstrup P, Vedtofte P, Reibel J, et al. Long-term treatment outcome of oral premalignant lesions. Oral Oncol 2006;42:461–74.

38 Shedd DP. Clinical characteristics of early oral cancer. JAMA 1971;215:955–6.

39 Mashberg A. Erythroplasia vs. leukoplasia in the diagnosis of early asymptomatic oral squamous carcinoma. N Engl J Med 1977;297:109–10.

40 Mashberg A, Meyers H, Garfinkel L. Criteria for the diagnosis of asymptomatic oral squamous cell carcinoma. In: Third International Symposium on Detection and Prevention of Cancer, 1976. Abstract No. 622.

41 Mashberg A, Feldman LJ. Clinical criteria for identifying early oral and oropharyngeal carcinoma: erythroplasia revisited. Am J Surg 1988;156:273–5.

42 Thomson PJ, Hamadah O. Cancerisation within the oral cavity: the use of 'field mapping biopsies' in clinical management. Oral Oncol 2007;43:20–6.

43 Slaughter DP, Southwick HW, Smejkal W. Field cancerization in oral stratified squamous epithelium; clinical implications of multicentric origin. Cancer 1953;6:963–8.

44 Strong MS, Vaughan CW, Incze JS. Toluidine blue in the management of carcinoma of the oral cavity. Arch Otolaryngol 1968;87:527–31.

45 Niebel HH, Chomet B. In vivo staining test for delineation of oral intraepithelial neoplastic change: preliminary report. J Am Dent Assoc 1964;68:801–6.

46 Shedd DP, Hukill PB, Bahn S. In vivo staining properties of oral cancer. Am J Surg 1965;110:631–4.

47 Mashberg A. Final evaluation of tolonium chloride rinse for screening of high-risk patients with asymptomatic squamous carcinoma. J Am Dent Assoc 1983;106:319–23.

48 Chen YW, Lin JS, Fong JH, et al. Use of methylene blue as a diagnostic aid in early detection of oral cancer and precancerous lesions [published online ahead of print on October 31, 2006]. Br J Oral Maxillofac Surg.

49 Poh CF, Ng SP, Williams PM, et al. Direct fluorescence visualization of clinically occult high-risk oral premalignant disease using a simple hand-held device. Head Neck 2007;29:71–6.

50 Mohit-Tabatabai MA, Sobel HJ, Rush BF, et al. Relation of thickness of floor of mouth stage I and II cancers to regional metastasis. Am J Surg 1986;152:351–3.

51 O'Brien CJ, Lauer CS, Fredricks S, et al. Tumor thickness influences prognosis of T1 and T2 oral cavity cancer—but what thickness? Head Neck 2003;25:937–45.

52 Greene FL, Page DL, Fleming ID, et al. American Joint Committee on Cancer staging manual. 6th ed. New York: Springer; 2002.

53 Tewari M, Rai P, Singh GB, et al. Long-term follow-up results of Nd: YAG laser treatment of premalignant and malignant (stage I) squamous cell carcinoma of the oral cavity. J Surg Oncol 2007;95:281–5.

54 Levi F, Te VC, Randimbison L, et al. Second primary oral and pharyngeal cancers in subjects diagnosed with oral and pharyngeal cancer. Int J Cancer 2006;119:2702–4.

55 Kramer FJ, Janssen M, Eckardt A. Second primary tumours in oropharyngeal squamous cell carcinoma. Clin Oral Investig 2004;8:56–62.

56 Berg JW, Schottenfeld D, Ritter F. Incidence of multiple primary cancers. III. Cancers of the respiratory and upper digestive system as multiple primary cancers. J Natl Cancer Inst 1970;44:263–74.

57 Mashberg A, Samit A. Early detection, diagnosis and management of oral and oropharyngeal cancer. CA Cancer J Clin 1989;39:67–8.

58 Schottenfeld D, Gantt RC, Wyner EL. The role of alcohol and tobacco in multiple primary cancers of the upper digestive system, larynx and lung: a prospective study. Prev Med 1974;3:277–93.

CHAPTER 19

Histopathologic considerations in the management of skin cancer

Mark R. Wick

As the treatment of skin cancers continues to evolve and become more sophisticated, the necessity for accurate pathologic assessment of tissue specimens is increasingly more crucial to optimal clinical management. A diversity of surgical procedures and adjuvant treatments is currently recommended for the wide range of malignant epithelial and mesenchymal neoplasms that may arise in the skin, and evaluations of the ultimate efficacy of each modality of therapy depend on the validity of tissue diagnoses.

This chapter briefly presents pathologic aspects of both common and uncommon cutaneous malignancies. Variant forms of each neoplasm are discussed, whenever they relate to differing therapeutic approaches or prognoses, or in instances in which they may create diagnostic confusion for the pathologist. With respect to the latter point, those neoplasms that usually require special studies for a definitive diagnosis are also enumerated, along with specific recommendations for their pathologic evaluation. Finally, the skin tumors discussed in this chapter are grouped according to their biologic behaviors, and in relation to modalities of therapy that are currently recommended for them.

Procurement of pathologic specimens

Proper collection and processing techniques by the dermatologic surgeon may be critical to good pathologic evaluation in selected cases. Enzyme histochemistry, immunocytochemistry, and electron microscopy may be necessary in these instances to obtain a firm diagnosis. Because the clinician may not be able to anticipate these eventualities before a biopsy is performed, he or she should follow a preset routine in the handling of *all* tissue specimens.

A cardinal tenet to be followed relates to the minimization of procedure-related artifacts. As little compression, shearing motion, and traction as possible must be exerted in punch biopsy or excisional biopsy techniques. Cautery excision should not be employed. The pathologic specimen should be divided into at least two portions with a sharp scalpel blade and gentle dissection, and macroscopic inspection must be done to assure that each contains tissue that is representative of the tumor concerned.

After this step, immersion of the specimens in appropriate fixative solutions should follow immediately, to avoid drying artifacts and autolysis. One exception to the latter statement concerns cases in which cutaneous lymphoma is included among clinical diagnostic considerations. In this circumstance, touch preparations are recommended, for cytologic and cytochemical evaluation. These may be obtained by lightly touching a portion of the excised specimen to glass slides, in four or five areas of each slide. A total of six slides usually suffices; these should be placed in 95% ethanol, before staining. Other recommended fixatives include 10% neutral-buffered formalin for conventional microscopy and immunohistochemistry, and 2% glutaraldehyde for electron microscopy. Tissue should be placed in the latter fixative only after it has been minced gently into 1- to 2-mm cubes. Liquid nitrogen is

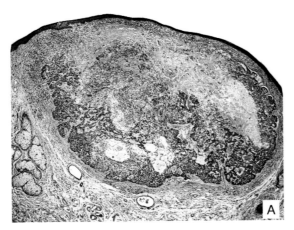 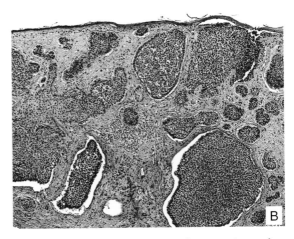

Fig. 19.1 *A,* Nodular BCC demonstrating a cohesive proliferation of basaloid cells in the dermis with connection to the basal epidermis. (Hematoxylin-eosin [H&E], ×60.) *B,* The tumor cell groups exhibit artifactual retraction from the adjacent dermal stroma. (H&E, ×160.)

suitably employed in preparation for frozen-section immunocytochemistry; tissue may be suspended in this vehicle by securing a length of suture to it and using a small thermos bottle container.

If a hematopoietic proliferation is suspected, flow cytometry may be desirable. In that instance, no fixation at all should be undertaken and the specimen is optimally submitted rapidly in saline or in a transport solution such as Michel's medium.

An obvious yet often-omitted step in the submission of tissue to the dermatopathology laboratory concerns the inclusion of appropriate clinical information on accompanying request forms. The patient's age, the history of present illness, a brief description of the lesions that were biopsied, and a listing of clinical differential diagnoses facilitate optimal handling of tissue by the pathologist and help in avoiding clinicopathologic miscorrelations.

Specific types of cancer of the skin

Epithelial neoplasms
Basal cell carcinoma

Basal cell carcinoma (BCC) is the most frequently seen malignancy in dermatologic practice. Most clinicians and pathologists are thoroughly familiar with its classic histopathologic features, including an attachment to the basal epidermis; an organoid growth pattern; its composition by small, polygonal cells with high nucleocytoplasmic ratios; peripheral nuclear palisading within cell nests; fibromyxoid stroma with artifactual detachment from tumor cell clusters; and the presence of stromal amyloid in a sizable proportion of cases (Fig. 19.1). Several distinctive variants are also well known, such as adenoid BCC, basosebaceous BCC, morpheaform BCC, and metatypical BCC, among others [1]. Those subtypes are characterized by a pseudoglandular cellular arrangement, focal sebaceous differentiation, densely sclerotic stroma and compressed cellular nests, and exclusively squamoid cytologic attributes, respectively.

Basal cell carcinoma is a locally aggressive tumor, with only rare instances of true metastases [2]. The latter have most often occurred in large, clinically neglected lesions. Nonetheless, the morbidity associated with BCC may be great, sometimes necessitating mutilating surgery to effect extirpation. Because of this fact, specific clinicopathologic indicators of potentially aggressive behavior are of interest. Jacobs and colleagues [3] found that ulcerative, infiltrative, or morpheaform growth patterns, a "spiky" appearance of tumor cell nests (Fig. 19.2), loss of nuclear palisading, invasion of subcutaneous tissue, nuclear pleomorphism or spindling, and hyalinization of tumoral stroma were correlated with adverse

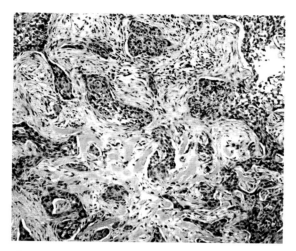

Fig. 19.2 Infiltrative, adverse histology–type BCC showing angular cell groups in the dermis. (H&E, ×200.)

clinical behavior of BCC. Neoplasms showing such features were more common in men, and were most often located in the nasal, ocular, or malar skin. Conversely, BCCs with multifocal-superficial or nonulcerative and nodular growth patterns, and with typical cytologic features, were associated with a high rate of cure following conventional local excision.

Squamous cell carcinoma

Although it has a propensity to arise in sun-damaged skin, squamous cell carcinoma (SCC) may occur anywhere on the body surface. Again, the histopathologic findings in usual SCC should be familiar to most dermatologic surgeons. These include transepidermal epithelial atypia ("bowenoid change"), abnormal nucleocytoplasmic ratios, nuclear hyperchromasia, nucleolar prominence, mitotic activity, cytoplasmic eosinophilia, and the formation of keratin "pearls." Actinic dermal elastosis is a frequent concurrent observation. A range of histologic grades is seen in squamous carcinomas, ranging from grade 1 (well differentiated; Fig. 19.3) to grade 4 (Fig. 19.4; poorly differentiated) [4]. This scheme refers to the degree of nuclear anaplasia and the level of organoid growth seen in the tumor, and shows a direct correlation with adverse clinical behavior.

Tumors at the extremes of this spectrum of differentiation pose the greatest diagnostic challenges for the pathologist. Well-differentiated SCC may be almost indistinguishable from pseudoepitheliomatous hyperplasia associated with prior trauma or underlying dermatoses. In such cases, a thorough description of the clinical history of the lesion is invaluable in reaching an accurate tissue diagnosis.

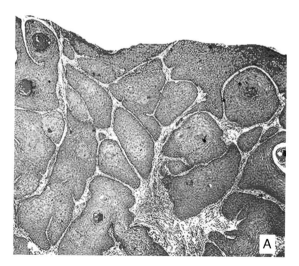
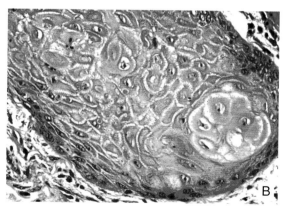

Fig. 19.3 *A*, Well-differentiated SCC manifesting irregularly invasive nests of obviously keratinizing squamous epithelial cells. (H&E, ×60.) *B*, The tumor cells show intercellular "bridges" and form small keratin "pearls." (H&E, ×350.)

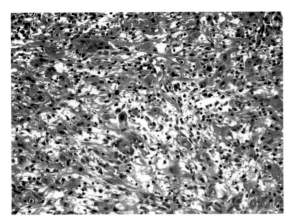

Fig. 19.4 Poorly differentiated SCC comprising epithelial cells with widely variable sizes and shapes. There is little tendency for them to form cohesive clusters. (H&E, ×200.)

Immunostaining for filaggrin [5] and β_2-microglobulin [6] in a squamous proliferative lesion has been claimed by some to equate with benignancy, but my experience has not substantiated this contention [7]. At the other extreme, poorly differentiated SCC may simulate small cell neuroendocrine carcinoma (Merkel cell carcinoma) [8], or, if composed of pleomorphic and spindled tumor cells (Fig. 19.5), may imitate amelanotic melanoma, or atypical fibroxanthoma and other cutaneous sarcomas. In these circumstances,

electron microscopy or immunohistology (IHL) is often necessary for a correct diagnosis. Even high-grade SCC retains a capacity for the formation of cytoplasmic tonofilaments (keratin filaments) and shows intercellular desmosomal attachments ultrastructurally, in contrast to the other neoplasms to be considered in differential diagnosis. In addition, virtually all squamous carcinomas are immunoreactive for high molecular weight (64- to 68-kDa) keratin and p63 protein, whereas Merkel cell carcinoma and mesenchymal tumors are not [9]. Rather, the latter two lesions commonly stain positively for keratin-20 or PAX-5 [10] and vimentin content, respectively. Positivity for epithelial membrane antigen (EMA), cytokeratin, p63, and MOC-31 distinguish spindle cell SCC from atypical fibroxanthoma and sarcomas of the skin, which lack those determinants [9,11].

Immunohistochemistry is also useful in separating another variant, "adenoid" SCC (Fig. 19.6), from sweat gland carcinoma or angiosarcoma, which it may imitate in some instances. Adenoid SCC manifests a pseudoglandular growth pattern, and was formerly known as "adenoacanthoma" [12]. Its behavior is like that of conventional SCC, grade for grade, and differs from the biologic properties of cutaneous adnexal malignancies. Carcinoembryonic antigen (CEA) is demonstrable in sweat gland carcinoma in 75% of cases by immunostaining, but it is absent in adenoid SCC [12,13]. This finding

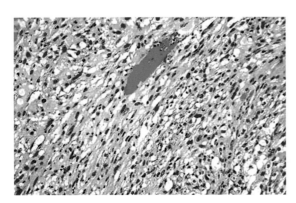

Fig. 19.5 Spindle cell SCC showing neither clustered growth nor obvious keratinocytic differentiation. (H&E, ×200.)

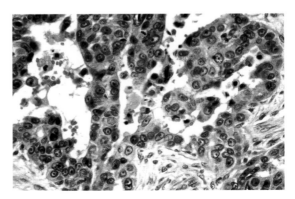

Fig. 19.6 Adenoid (acantholytic) SCC in which the neoplastic cells have lost cohesion and form pseudoglandular spaces. (H&E, ×350.)

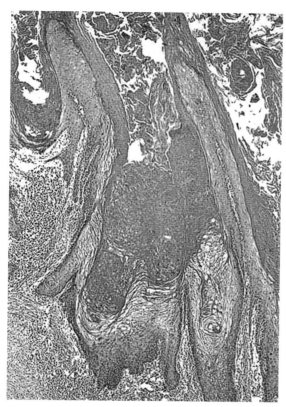

Fig. 19.7 Verrucous SCC demonstrating a sharply papilliform surface and irregular infiltration of the dermis by broad "tongues" of well-differentiated squamous cells. (H&E, ×60.)

is also useful in the separation of intraepidermal adnexal carcinoma (extramammary Paget's disease [EPD]) from pagetoid Bowen's disease (intraepidermal SCC) [14]. With regard to "pseudovascular" adenoid SCC, which resembles angiosarcoma, CD31 reactivity is expected in the latter but not the former of those two neoplasms, whereas the converse applies to staining for p63 [9].

Two forms of SCC that show a high level of cellular differentiation behave in distinctive, yet opposite, fashions. These are verrucous carcinoma (Fig. 19.7; "giant condyloma acuminatum of Buschke and Löwenstein," "epithelioma cuniculatum"), which occurs most often in the perineal or perianal skin and on the distal extremities [15,16], and "Marjolin's ulcer," or well-differentiated SCC

arising in areas of chronic injury such as burn scars and osteomyelitis tracts [17].

Histologically, verrucous carcinoma is composed of a broadly papilliform proliferation of squamous cells with little nuclear atypia, and with "pushing" borders. It is best treated by wide excision and rarely metastasizes if not irradiated [15]. Hence, radiotherapy is generally contraindicated in the management of this tumor. Misdiagnoses of squamous papilloma, verruca, or condyloma are easily avoided by supplying clinical information to the pathologist.

Marjolin's ulcer–type SCC commonly simulates pseudoepitheliomatous hyperplasia in that it is composed of deeply penetrating tongues of bland squamous cells in the dermis, with associated chronic inflammation. Clinical information on the gross features of such lesions, which are usually obviously malignant clinically, is crucial to correct histopathologic diagnosis. The latter point is more important than one might assume, based on the cytologically innocuous appearance of the neoplastic cells in Marjolin's SCC; a significant proportion (13% to 15%) of such tumors will metastasize and may be responsible for death [17].

Evans and Smith [18] considered the significance of depth of invasion by spindled and pleomorphic cell squamous tumors; they found that those neoplasms that extended no deeper than the subcutis were associated with a favorable prognosis, whereas others involving muscle or bone behaved aggressively. In addition, the origin of such tumors in previously irradiated skin carried a poor prognosis. Immerman and colleagues [19] observed a similar correlation between depth of invasion and behavior for cutaneous squamous carcinomas in general, because the rate of metastasis increased dramatically in cases involving the deep dermis and subcutaneous fat.

Cutaneous adnexal carcinomas

Carcinomas of the skin that show cellular differentiation toward sweat glands or pilosebaceous units are uncommon, and thus are discussed only briefly herein. The scope of their histologic appearances is too great to be covered in depth in this chapter, and likewise is referenced for the interested reader [20,21].

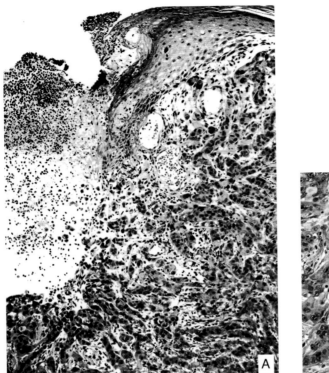
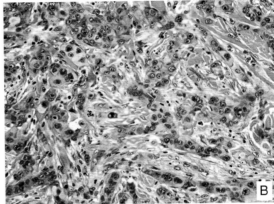

Fig. 19.8 *A,* Ductal eccrine adenocarcinoma in which solid cords of poorly differentiated epithelial cells are present in the dermis. Only rudimentary lumen formation is apparent. (H&E, ×100.) *B,* Metastatic ductal adenocarcinoma of the breast involving the skin; the histologic image of this tumor is essentially identical to that shown in part *A.* (H&E, ×300.)

Perhaps of greater importance to the dermatologic surgeon are the neoplasms with which adnexal cutaneous carcinomas may be confused. Sweat gland carcinomas (SGCs) commonly resemble metastases to the skin from carcinomas of the breasts (Fig. 19.8), lungs, kidneys, gastrointestinal tract, and salivary glands [20]. Electron microscopy and IHL are currently of limited use in separating those diagnostic considerations. Hence, the surgeon is usually ultimately responsible for the final diagnosis of a primary tumor of the skin, after careful clinical evaluation has failed to reveal evidence of neoplasia elsewhere. Another problem with respect to the pathologic features of SGCs is that their histopathologic attributes do not correlate consistently with their biologic behavior. Some tumors that appear to be well differentiated may metastasize widely whereas others showing a high level of anaplasia fail to do so [20]. Local recurrence of this class of neoplasms is common (40% to 60%) and is helpful in confirming a tentative diagnosis, although not a desirable event clinically.

Current recommendations for therapy of SGC include wide excision and removal of obviously metastatically-involved regional lymph nodes; however, there is little evidence that prophylactic node dissection improves survival. Radiotherapy appears to offer little benefit in management, and insufficient data are available to make definite recommendations on the use of adjuvant chemotherapy [22].

One form of cutaneous adnexal neoplasia has already been mentioned, namely EPD. Jones and associates [23] have provided convincing evidence

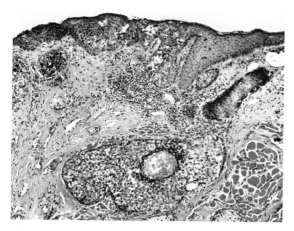

Fig. 19.9 Sebaceous carcinoma showing pagetoid involvement of the epidermis by finely vacuolated tumor cells as well as cohesive nests of similar cellular elements in the dermis. (H&E, ×160.)

that most cases of EPD represent intraepidermal sweat gland tumors and that an associated invasive dermal component is seen only infrequently. Nevertheless, EPD should be excised with frozen-section–directed margins to avoid subsequent recurrence due to clinical underestimation of its peripheral extent [24]. In addition, specific comments on the presence or absence of dermal invasion should be made because it may be associated with aggressive clinical behavior [25].

Sebaceous carcinomas (Fig. 19.9) are usually seen in the oculocutaneous adnexa, with relatively rare reports of such neoplasms in other skin areas [26]. Differential diagnoses include sebaceous adenoma, BCC with sebaceous differentiation, "balloon cell" malignant melanoma, and cutaneous metastases from carcinomas of the breasts, kidneys, and female genital tract [27]. This group of tumors is associated with a diversity of prognoses, and therefore adequate distinction between them is clearly indicated. Sebaceous adenoma and BCC with sebaceous differentiation are adequately definable on morphologic grounds alone for the experienced dermatopathologist. Immunohistochemical studies are useful in excluding metastatic breast and gynecologic carcinomas, because these stain positively for CEA and CA-125, respectively [9], but sebaceous carcinoma

shows neither of those antigens. The S-100 protein immunopositivity of balloon cell melanoma is not shared by sebaceous carcinoma. Lipophilic stains such as oil red O may be applied to frozen sections for the characterization of sebaceous carcinoma, which is uniformly positive [26]. Although metastatic renal cell carcinoma contains intracellular lipid as well, it is also strongly reactive with the period acid-Schiff (PAS) stain in contrast to sebaceous carcinoma.

A review of the literature [28] and our own experience indicates that extraocular sebaceous carcinoma has a definite potential for metastasis, in spite of previous assertions that it did not. Therefore, it would seem wise to approach the treatment of this tumor in a manner similar to that recommended for sweat gland carcinomas.

Pilar carcinomas are rare. Pilomatrix carcinoma [29,30] (Fig. 19.10) and carcinoma arising in proliferating trichilemmal cysts (malignant proliferating pilar tumors) [31] appear to represent the principal forms of malignant pilar neoplasia. The histopathologic characteristics of these tumors are clear cut, and differential diagnostic considerations are consequently academic. Although rare examples of metastasizing pilar carcinomas have been reported [29,31], their behavior is generally like that of low-grade SCC. Thus, adequate primary excision is usually curative.

Malignant tumors of specialized epithelioid cutaneous cells
Malignant melanoma
Few individuals who regularly deal with cancer of the skin would dispute the contention that malignant melanoma is the most lethal among all primary malignant cutaneous tumors. For this reason, early diagnosis and adequate treatment of this neoplasm is critical to minimize its mortality. In the past, substantial effort was expended to subclassify malignant melanoma into superficial spreading, nodular, and lentiginous variants histologically (Fig. 19.11). These growth patterns are of relatively little importance with respect to the prognostic and behavioral characteristics attending malignant melanomas [32]. Rather, the growth phase (radial vs. vertical) and depth of invasion are the

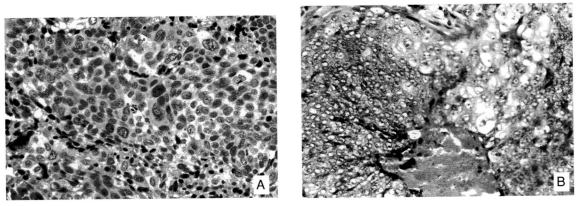

Fig. 19.10 Pilomatrix carcinoma. *A*, The area of the tumor simply has the image of an anaplastic large cell carcinoma. (H&E, ×160.) *B*, However, the focus exhibits ghost cell keratinization. (H&E, ×250.)

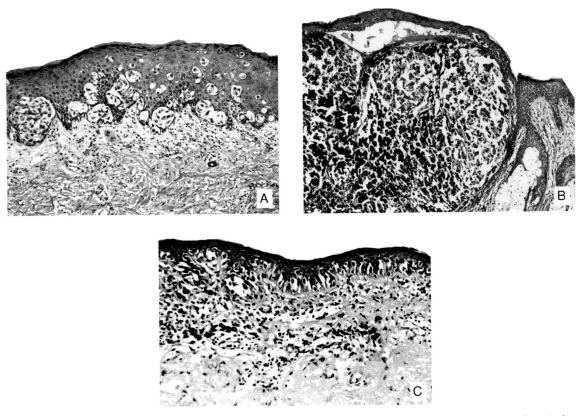

Fig. 19.11 Malignant melanoma. *A*, Superficial spreading variant demonstrating a "buckshot" distribution of atypical melanocytes throughout the epidermis. (H&E, ×160.) *B*, Nodular type showing a cohesive spherical tumor invading the dermis, with little if any junctional melanocytic proliferation. (H&E, ×100.) *C*, Lentiginous variant demonstrating confluent proliferation of atypical melanocytes at the base of an atrophic epidermis with superficial invasion of the dermis. (H&E, ×100.)

most valuable criteria for the prediction of an aggressive clinical course and risk of metastasis. Malignant melanomas that are infiltrative into the dermis and subcutaneous tissue and that have a thickness of 1 mm or greater are the most likely to behave badly [33].

Two histologic types of malignant melanoma continue to challenge the dermatopathologist. These are amelanotic nodular melanoma, which is not associated with a lateral junctional component, and nevus-like melanoma. In the first instance, confusion with anaplastic SCC or sweat gland carcinoma may be encountered. A metastatic neoplasm may also be considered in differential diagnosis. In such circumstances, electron microscopy will demonstrate cytoplasmic premelanosomes in the tumor cells of melanoma [34], in contrast to the features of squamous carcinoma or adenocarcinoma. In addition, IHL for the expression of S-100 protein, MART-1, tyrosinase, and PNL2 shows positivity for those antigens in melanocytic tumors [9,35,36]. S-100 protein may be observed in some carcinomas, but only concurrently with keratin, which is absent in melanomas. In nevus-like melanomas, special pathologic studies are of no assistance in their separation from atypical nevi. Histologic criteria such as irregular lateral extension of the lesion at the dermoepidermal junction, asymmetry of the dermal elements, transepidermal "migration" of atypical melanocytes, nuclear hyperchromasia and pleomorphism, finely granular intracellular melanin pigment, and lack of dermal "maturation" of melanocytic cells favor an interpretation of malignancy [37]. Nevertheless, clinicians will continue to receive such diagnoses as "atypical (or biologically indeterminate) melanocytic neoplasm" in cases in which those features are equivocal. Complete surgical removal is indicated in such circumstances, with adequately uninvolved margins of excision.

Still other subtypes of malignant melanoma are capable of causing histodiagnostic uncertainty. Spindle cell melanoma is, as the name suggests, composed exclusively of elongated tumor cells and may resemble mesenchymal neoplasms of the skin [38]. If the stroma of these tumors is fibrous, individual cells or narrow cords of them

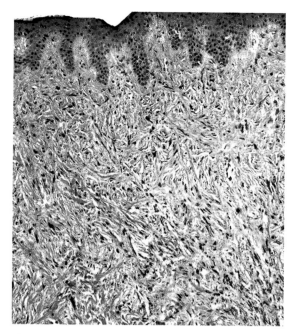

Fig. 19.12 Desmoplastic melanoma comprising modestly atypical amelanotic spindle cells in the dermis, with marked stromal fibroplasia. (H&E, ×100.)

may be entrapped within collagen bundles [39]. The latter melanoma variant is called "desmoplastic" melanoma (Fig. 19.12). Both spindle cell and desmoplastic malignant melanoma are often observed in association with lentiginous melanoma in situ [40]. Surgical margins of excision are notoriously difficult to assess on frozen-section examination of desmoplastic melanomas, so the surgeon must exercise special care to widely remove these tumors [41]. More than occasionally, spindle cell melanoma exhibits neurotropic growth within the dermis and subcutis [42]. This peculiarity further contributes to uncertainty in defining surgical margins.

Spindle cell SCC enters into differential diagnosis with spindled malignant melanoma, but the former entity is easily separated from melanoma on immunohistologic grounds. Melanoma is negative for EMA, p63, and keratin but is immunoreactive for S-100 protein, even in areas of desmoplasia [43].

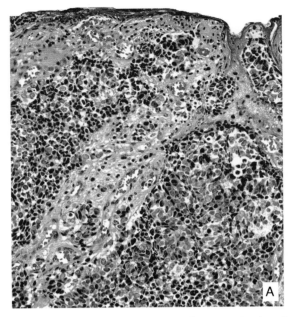
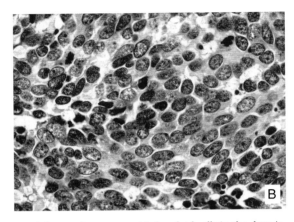

Fig. 19.13 *A*, Merkel cell carcinoma demonstrating broad nests and sheets of monomorphic basaloid cells in the dermis. (H&E, ×100.) *B*, The neoplastic cells have uniformly shaped nuclei with dispersed chromatin and numerous mitotic figures. (H&E, ×400.)

These findings are the converse of those seen in association with spindle cell SCC [44]. In addition, the two neoplasms differ ultrastructurally.

Small cell melanoma is an uncommon entity that may mimic poorly differentiated basaloid squamous carcinoma or Merkel cell carcinoma [45]. EMA and keratin are detectable in the latter two tumors, but not in melanoma; conversely, among these three possibilities, only melanoma labels for S-100 protein, MART-1, and PNL2 [9].

Primary cutaneous neuroendocrine carcinoma

Since its description under the name *trabecular carcinoma* in 1972 [46], primary cutaneous neuroendocrine carcinoma (PCNC), or Merkel cell carcinoma, has been the object of continued study. This tumor is composed of uniform small lymphocyte-like cells, which are arranged in medullary or organoid growth patterns in the dermis [47,48] (Fig. 19.13). Nuclear chromatin is evenly dispersed, mitoses are numerous, and nucleoli are inconspicuous.

Ultrastructurally, the tumor cells show intracellular junctions, cytoplasmic neurosecretory (dense-core) granules (Fig. 19.14), and perinuclear whorls of intermediate filaments [49,50].

With respect to differential diagnostic considerations, the most common problems in dealing with PCNC center on its resemblance to cutaneous lymphoma and metastatic small cell carcinoma of visceral origin. The first possibility may be excluded by electron microscopy, because lymphomas do not display the presence of cell-to-cell junctions. Immunocytochemistry demonstrates staining for leukocyte common antigen (LCA; CD45) in virtually all cases of lymphoma cutis [51], whereas PCNC lacks such reactivity [52]. Conversely, all PCNCs display EMA or keratin or both, but lymphomas do not [47]. Difficulties in separating PCNC from secondary neuroendocrine carcinomas of the skin are not resolved quite as easily. The two most helpful immunostains in this context are CEA and thyroid transcription factor-1, both of which are seen in metastatic pulmonary small cell neuroendocrine

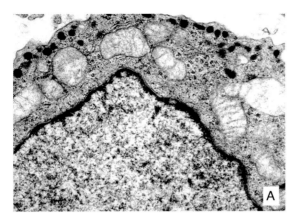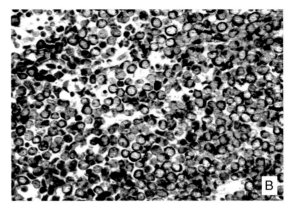

Fig. 19.14 *A*, Electron micrograph of Merkel cell carcinoma showing a peripherocellular accumulation of dense-core neurosecretory granules. (Uranyl acetate and lead citrate, ×11,700.) *B*, An immunostain of the same tumor shows diffuse reactivity for pankeratin, with perinuclear accentuation, corresponding to accumulations of intermediate filaments in the same location as seen by electron microscopy. (Keratin immunostain, ×200.)

carcinoma but not PCNC [9]. Despite that knowledge, the clinician must thoroughly investigate the possibility of occult, visceral, neuroendocrine neoplasia—particularly in the lungs—before accepting a diagnosis of PCNC as final.

The similarities between PCNC and small cell SCC or small cell malignant melanoma have already been discussed. Again, electron microscopy and IHL are valuable in the separation of those entities.

One distinctive variant of PCNC is that which is associated with concomitant or previous SCC in the same skin area. Gomez and colleagues [53] and others [54] have shown that such neoplasms are aggressive biologically, often metastasizing within a short time after diagnosis.

In general, PCNC displays indolent growth, with a propensity for local recurrence. However, long-term follow-up indicates that this tumor is behaviorally tenacious, with systemic spread and mortality reaching 35% to 40% at 10 years because of the delayed growth of metastases [55]. Suggestions for the management of PCNC include wide local excision; removal of regional lymph nodes for tumors greater than 2 cm in diameter or with a mitotic rate of 10 or more per single 400× microscopic field; and postoperative irradiation [56]. Multiagent chemotherapy should be employed in cases with

metastases, but, currently, that modality appears to be only palliative [57].

Tumors with nonlymphoreticular mesenchymal differentiation
Selected vascular neoplasms: Kaposi's sarcoma and angiosarcoma

Although it was previously rare in the western hemisphere, Kaposi's sarcoma (KS) has come to the forefront of attention in dermatopathology because of its association with the acquired immunodeficiency syndrome [58]. KS has two basic histopathologic forms, which often merge together, depending on the time of biopsy after the onset of growth. The first appears deceptively bland and is composed of dilated capillary- and venule-sized blood vessels in the reticular dermis—this has been called "patch stage" KS [59] (Fig. 19.15). The pathologist must rely heavily on clinical information in reaching a diagnosis of this lesion, because it may be mimicked by angiomas and reactive processes microscopically. However, clues to a correct interpretation of patch stage KS that have been useful in our experience are a tendency for the neoplastic blood vessels to cluster around sweat gland units in the deep dermis and the formation of new vascular channels around preexisting ones, yielding profiles resembling

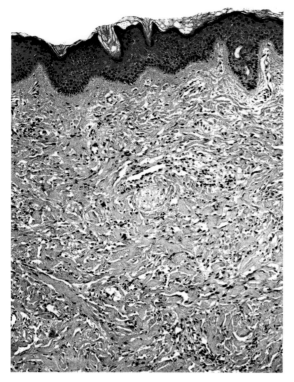

Fig. 19.15 "Patch" stage KS showing an irregular and somewhat subtle proliferation of neovascular channels in the dermis. (H&E, ×160.)

"promontories." These features are not shared by the other lesions just mentioned. The second histologic variant of KS is the nodular form, in which aggregates of spindle cell fascicles are observed in the dermis [60] (Fig. 19.16).

Cytoplasmic vacuolization may be seen in the spindle cells, and numerous extravasated erythrocytes are typically admixed with them. Hemosiderin pigment is also common within the lesions. "Hyaline bodies" (Fig. 19.17), which are small (3- to 5-µmol) globules in the cytoplasm of tumor cells, may aid in making a diagnosis of KS, because they are infrequently seen in other vascular proliferations [61]. These structures have been thought to represent red blood cell fragments. They stain positively with the PAS method, both with and without diastase digestion. Endothelial markers such as CD31, CD34, factor VIII–related antigen (FVIIIRAg), and thrombomodulin are consistently present in the patch stage of KS, but only inconsistently in the nodular variant [60]. Similarly, electron microscopy has failed to demonstrate cytoplasmic Weibel-Palade bodies (specific endothelial cell inclusions) in most cases of spindle cell–predominant KS [62]. Fortunately, a recent addition to the IHL armamentarium—namely, an antibody to the human herpesvirus-8 latent nuclear antigen-1

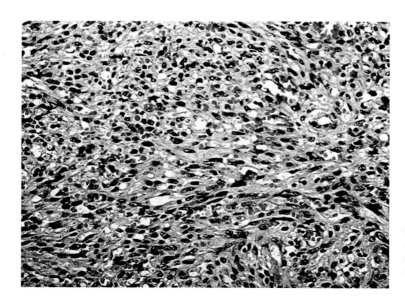

Fig. 19.16 Nodular KS comprising aggregates of spindle cells with cytoplasmic vacuolization and extravasated erythrocytes. (H&E, ×200.)

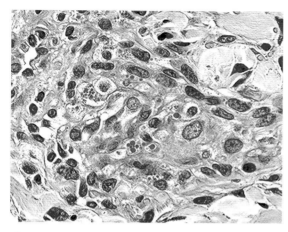

Fig. 19.17 Hyaline globules are present in the tumor cell cytoplasm of this KS. They likely represent degenerated erythrocytes. (H&E, ×300.)

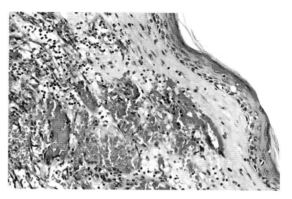

Fig. 19.18 Cutaneous angiosarcoma demonstrating an irregular proliferation of interanastomosing vascular channels in the dermis. (H&E, ×160.)

[63]—is reactive in approximately 85% of KS cases, regardless of histologic subtype. Other vascular proliferations in the skin are consistently negative for that marker.

Angiosarcoma most often arises de novo in the skin of the face and neck in elderly patients [60,64] or as a complication of longstanding lymphedema of the extremities (Stewart-Treves syndrome) [65]. Histologically, this tumor is typified by a proliferation of neovascular channels, which "dissect" dermal collagen and commonly destroy appendages (Fig. 19.18). Neoplastic endothelial cells lining such channels show nuclear atypia, and nuclei are often polarized in the luminal portions of the cells, imparting a "hobnail" appearance to them. Commonly, the intravascular neoplastic cells are arranged in a piled-up or papillary fashion [60] (Fig. 19.19). Mitotic figures are variably prominent [66].

In some cases, angiosarcoma assumes a spindle cell or pleomorphic cellular appearance, with compressed vascular lumina [66]. In these instances, other pleomorphic sarcomas and metastatic sarcomatoid carcinomas enter the histopathologic differential diagnosis.

Electron microscopy and IHL are helpful in resolving diagnostic uncertainties. Angiosarcoma cells show an external lamina, pinocytosis, intercellular junctions, and cytoplasmic intermediate filaments in almost all cases [67], unlike the ultrastructural features of most other sarcomas. They do not express EMA as seen in metastatic carcinomas, and virtually all will label for CD31, CD34, or thrombomodulin. Only 15% to 30% contain FVIIIRAg [9].

The usual clinical course of angiosarcoma is unfavorable, with death being caused by repeated cutaneous recurrences and metastasis. The first of these problems may be minimized through frozen-section–directed primary excision or, even better, by peripheral "mapping" of the lesion preoperatively using several peripheral punch biopsies. Those measures are necessary because of the common

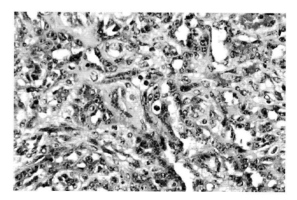

Fig. 19.19 The tumor cells in angiosarcoma are overtly atypical and often project into vascular channels in a "hobnail" fashion, as shown here. (H&E, ×250).

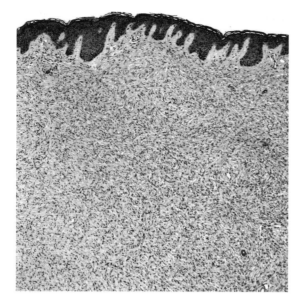

Fig. 19.20 Dermatofibrosarcoma protuberans composed of storiform arrays of monomorphic spindle cells that efface the dermis. The tumor extends into the subcutaneous fat. (H&E, ×100.)

Dermatofibrosarcoma protuberans is familiar to dermatologists as a raised, nodular, nonulcerated neoplasm usually seen on the trunk or proximal extremities. Histologically, it is typified by a dense proliferation of uniform spindle cells with fusiform nuclei, arranged in a storiform or "cartwheel" pattern (Fig. 19.20). Mitotic activity is variable. DFSP usually does not involve the epidermis but extends deeply into the subcutis or underlying fascia and muscle. Variants showing intracellular pigment ("Bednar tumors") [70] have been reported, as have others with myxoid stroma [71] or "fibrosarcomatous" transformation [72]. The last of those subtypes is felt to be more aggressive biologically. All forms of DFSP manifest immunoreactivity for CD34, making them unique in this family of mesenchymal tumors [73].

Atypical fibroxanthoma is a cytologically bizarre, pleomorphic, mitotically active tumor of the dermis, usually occurring in sun-damaged skin areas [74]. Atypical tumor giant cells are admixed with spindled, fibroblast-like, and xanthoma cells in AFX (Fig. 19.21). This lesion is poorly circumscribed, but

underestimation of tumor growth by surgeons, and consequent suboptimal removal of the lesion. Radiotherapy and chemotherapy do not appear to alter the outcome of angiosarcoma cases significantly. However, Holden and associates [68] identified a subgroup of patients with a longer survival; they tended to be elderly men with peripheral facial angiosarcoma. Histologically, the neoplasms in such individuals do not destroy dermal appendages and are associated with a marked peritumoral lymphoid response.

Specialized fibroblastic and "fibrohistiocytic" neoplasms

The group of malignant cutaneous tumors that is thought to show specialized fibroblastic and facultative "fibrohistiocytic" differentiation includes dermatofibrosarcoma protuberans (DFSP), atypical fibroxanthoma (AFX), and superficial malignant fibrous histiocytoma (MFH). Substantiation for this nosologic scheme is based on shared immunocytochemical and ultrastructural features of such neoplasms [69,70].

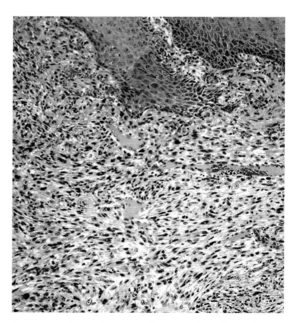

Fig. 19.21 Atypical fibroxanthoma, a dermal neoplasm comprising atypical spindle cells and large pleomorphic elements. (H&E, ×160.)

it is confined to the reticular dermis in classic examples.

Superficial MFH has a microscopic appearance similar to that of AFX, and, in fact, we consider the two to be essentially synonymous. By definition, however, superficial MFH is centered more deeply than AFX in the skin, in the lower dermis and subcutaneous fat [73]. Mitoses are numerous, often with pathologic shapes.

It is our belief that all three of these tumors should be regarded as at least low-grade malignancies, although their potential for metastasis varies. DFSP and AFX are usually associated with local recurrence if inadequately excised, but examples of distant metastasis are few. Those features contrast with the behavior of superficial MFH, which metastasizes in 10% to 20% of all cases [75]. The major factor accounting for this difference in behavior appears to be depth of tumor growth. It is well known that repeated recurrence of DFSP is associated with progressively deeper invasion of the subcutis and underlying tissue, and with a greater risk of metastasis. In addition, Helwig and May [76] observed that metastases of AFXs most often occurred in cases that infiltrated fascia and striated muscle.

Wide excision is the treatment of choice for fibrohistiocytic malignancies of the skin. Radiotherapy and chemotherapy are of unproven benefit in such cases.

Leiomyosarcoma and fibrosarcoma

Though leiomyosarcoma (LMS) and fibrosarcoma are tumors with dissimilar lines of differentiation, they will be discussed together because of similarities in their clinical features and biologic behavior. Both neoplasms are uncommon as true cutaneous lesions, and, in particular, involvement of the skin by fibrosarcoma more often represents secondary invasion by a more deeply seated tumor of the soft tissues. Cutaneous LMS and fibrosarcoma share a tendency to occur on the extremities of adult patients; both have been seen in association with prior cutaneous injury [77,78].

Leiomyosarcoma is composed of spindle cells with blunt-ended, cigar-shaped nuclei and fibrillar eosinophilic cytoplasm, arranged in intertwining fascicles (Fig. 19.22). Mitotic activity varies considerably, with an average of one to two division figures per 10 400× fields. When fascicles of tumor cells are cut transversely, a characteristic (though artifactual) perinuclear clear zone may be observed. Rare examples of LMS display gross nuclear anaplasia, with hyperchromatic tumor giant cells. An apparent origin from blood vessel walls or erector pilorum muscles may be observed occasionally.

In contrast, the cells of cutaneous fibrosarcoma—a rare lesion—do not possess fibrillar cytoplasm and are arranged in a "herringbone" fascicular pattern (Fig. 19.23). Nuclei have more tapered poles than those of LMS, but mitotic activity is comparable. Difficulty may be encountered in separating high-grade fibrosarcoma from MFH or transformed DFSP, but this issue is of academic interest only and does not affect treatment or prognosis.

Differential diagnostic considerations include other spindle cell malignancies of the skin, including sarcomatoid SCC and malignant melanoma, and fibrohistiocytic sarcomas. Immunohistochemical evaluation is the most helpful ancillary pathologic study in the separation of these entities. LMS and fibrosarcoma lack keratin and EMA, and S-100 protein, in contrast to SCC and malignant melanoma, respectively [9]. Like MFH, AFX, and DFSP, LMS and fibrosarcoma are vimentin positive, but LMS exhibits myogenous markers including desmin, actins, and caldesmon [79]. It lacks CD34, unlike DFSP. Electron microscopy also makes a diagnostic contribution in this setting.

Both LMS and fibrosarcoma will recur predictably if a suboptimal excision is performed; in cases in which the tumors involve the skin around joints, or deep fascia and skeletal muscle, amputation may be necessary. Metastasis will occur in 20% to 40% of cases of either LMS or fibrosarcoma [77,78]. Adjuvant irradiation and chemotherapy may be of benefit for recurrent or metastatic disease.

Sarcomas with epithelioid features

As pathologic techniques improved, some primary tumors of soft tissue and skin that were originally classified as sarcomas were found to possess epithelial characteristics. Most notable among these lesions is epithelioid sarcoma [80,81]. Conversely, another epithelioid superficial soft tissue tumor—clear cell sarcoma—shows substantial melanocytic differentiation [82].

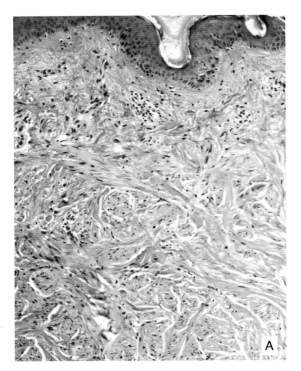

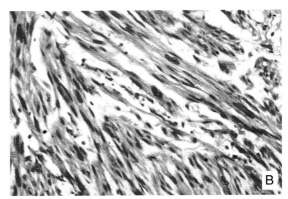

Fig. 19.22 Leiomyosarcoma of the skin showing a deep dermal proliferation of atypical spindle cells (*A*), which demonstrate cigar-shaped nuclear contours and cytoplasmic fibrillation (*B*). (Part *A*: H&E, ×160; part *B*: H&E, ×250.)

Of these two tumors, epithelioid sarcoma is most likely to involve the skin in a primary sense, usually on the extremities. It is composed of polygonal

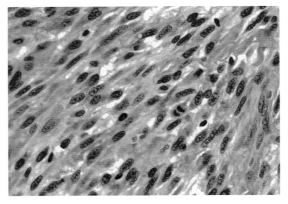

Fig. 19.23 Fibrosarcoma in the dermis, showing roughly parallel arrays of atypical spindle cells with a collagenized stroma. (H&E, ×250.)

cells with eosinophilic cytoplasm and variably atypical nuclei, arranged in clusters or cords (Fig. 19.24). Mitotic activity is usually notable in epithelioid sarcoma, but it is not marked. A peculiar feature of this neoplasm is its tendency to undergo spontaneous necrosis, resulting in an appearance that simulates that of palisading granulomas [81]. Indeed, many examples of epithelioid sarcoma are still misdiagnosed as deep granuloma annulare or rheumatoid nodule. These lesions are easily separated by electron microscopy and IHL. Epithelioid sarcoma shows intercellular junctional complexes and cytoplasmic intermediate filaments [83], whereas the histiocytic cells of granulomas do not. In addition, the former lesion manifests reactivity for keratins [81,84], CD34, and EMA, in contrast to negativity for those antigens in true granulomas [9,85,86].

Clear cell sarcoma tends to occur in fascia or tendons but may involve the skin early by direct extension and thus present to the dermatologist.

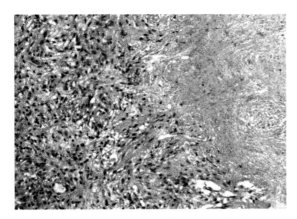

Fig. 19.24 Epithelioid sarcoma of the deep dermis showing a central zone of necrobiosis (*right*) mantled by atypical epithelioid and bluntly spindled tumor cells. (H&E, ×200.)

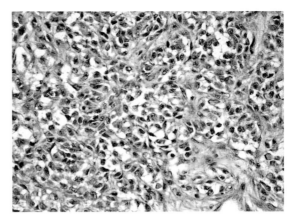

Fig. 19.25 Clear cell sarcoma of the superficial soft tissue comprising small nests of epithelioid cells with clear cytoplasm and nuclear atypia. (H&E, ×250.)

This tumor comprises organoid arrays of spindled or polygonal cells containing oval nuclei with prominent nucleoli, and optically clear or slightly eosinophilic cytoplasm (Fig. 19.25). Its morphologic resemblance to amelanotic melanoma is represented by the ultrastructural presence of premelanosomes and expression of S-100 protein, MART-1, and PNL2 [87].

Both epithelioid sarcoma and clear cell sarcoma require wide excision for adequate control, and amputation may be necessary, depending on the location of the tumor. Radiotherapy and chemotherapy may be effective in cases showing metastasis, which occurs in 40% to 50% of all cases of either neoplasm [80,81,88].

Lymphoreticular tumors

Special pathologic techniques designed to determine the lineage of lymphoid proliferations and their clonality have contributed significantly to the analysis of cutaneous lymphoreticular lesions. It is in these cases that procurement of fresh tissue specimens and touch preparations may be important for definitive diagnosis.

Although malignant lymphoma most commonly involves the skin only after systemic dissemination, 5% of cases present with cutaneous lesions [89] (Fig. 19.26). Small cell B-lymphocytic tumors

demonstrate surface-immunoglobulin monoclonality, which distinguishes them from reactive lymphoid infiltrates. However, paraffin-embedded tissue is a poor substrate for detection of that feature. T-cell lymphomas, such as mycosis fungoides and

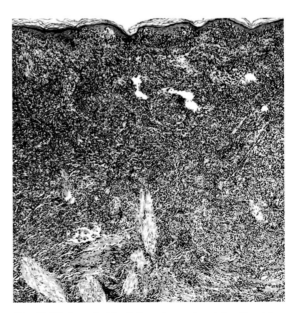

Fig. 19.26 Lymphoblastic lymphoma involving the skin and effacing the dermis and subcutis. (H&E, ×60.)

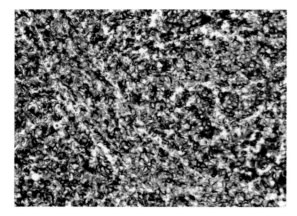

Fig. 19.27 Diffuse immunoreactivity for CD45 in cutaneous lymphoblastic lymphoma. (CD45 immunostain, ×250.)

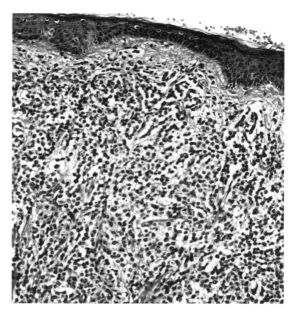

Fig. 19.28 Granulocytic sarcoma of the skin (extramedullary myeloid tumor), demonstrating a sheet of atypical lymphocyte-like cells in the dermis. (H&E, ×200.)

Sézary's tumor, are often diagnosable on conventional microscopy, providing that sufficient clinical information is given to the pathologist. In cases in which additional pathologic confirmation of these diagnoses is desirable, the most helpful technique is probably that of genotypic analysis [90,91]. This method assesses the presence of rearranged immunoglobulin heavy-chain genes or T-cell receptor genes in the constituent lymphoid cells, and can be applied to either fresh tissue or paraffin blocks.

Large cell lymphoma of the skin sometimes closely resembles anaplastic carcinoma, from which it may usually be distinguished by its LCA immunoreactivity (Fig. 19.27) [92]. Further categorization into B-cell proliferations can be accomplished if there is labeling for CD20, CD79a, or PAX-5. On the other hand, staining for CD2, CD3, CD5, CD7, or CD43 is typical of T-cell lesions [9]. A special variant of cutaneous large cell lymphoma demonstrates positivity for CD30; it paradoxically shows slow clinical evolution and prolonged localization to the skin, despite its anaplastic histologic image [93].

Even though leukemia cutis is usually an obvious clinical diagnosis, nonlymphocytic leukemia may sometimes present with diffuse or localized skin involvement in the absence of peripheral blood or bone marrow abnormalities (extramedullary myeloid tumor; granulocytic sarcoma) [94] (Fig. 19.28). A microscopic clue to this diagnosis is

the presence of immature eosinophilic leukocyte precursors admixed in a dermal mononuclear cell infiltrate. Cytochemical and immunohistologic confirmation of leukemia cutis of the FAB-M1 through M4 subtypes may be accomplished with the chloracetate (Leder) and myeloperoxidase stains [95].

Establishing the diagnosis of a lymphoreticular tumor in the skin has two important consequences. The first is that the clinician is thereby alerted to perform staging evaluations for the extent of disease, before instituting therapy. Second, even in patients with obviously disseminated lymphoma or leukemia, skin biopsy represents a relatively noninvasive means of obtaining specific cell typing, so correspondingly specialized treatment regimens may be effectively employed.

Current classification schemes of the malignant lymphomas have become complex and are beyond the scope of this review. The interested reader is referred to several excellent resources elsewhere [96–99], including Chapter 15 of this book.

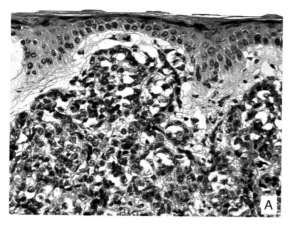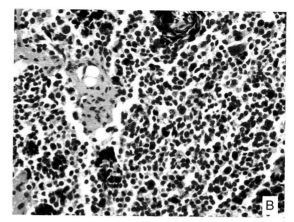

Fig. 19.29 *A*, Metastatic adenocarcinoma of the lung involving the skin. The tumor bears a strong resemblance to primary sweat gland carcinoma, as shown in Fig. 19.8A. (H&E, ×200.) *B*, Metastatic pulmonary small cell neuroendocrine carcinoma manifesting virtual histologic synonymity with Merkel cell carcinoma (see Fig. 19.13). (H&E, ×160.)

Metastatic carcinomas

Selected visceral carcinomas have a tendency to secondarily involve the skin. Such behavior may be the initial clinical manifestation of disease. In these cases, cutaneous metastases tend to be multiple and synchronous, and are often grouped near the primary visceral lesion topographically [100,101]. However, occasional patients have solitary secondary tumors and may not demonstrate symptoms and signs referable to an occult neoplasm. Thus, differential diagnostic possibilities usually include sweat gland carcinoma, PCNC, and malignant melanoma, among others. As we have mentioned previously, the safest course of action in such cases is to recommend extensive clinical evaluation for a possible visceral tumor. It is unfortunately true that no absolutely sensitive and determinative markers of carcinomas that commonly seed the skin—those in the breast (Fig. 19.8), lung (Fig. 19.29), gastrointestinal tract, and kidney—are currently available for application in immunohistochemistry [102].

Overview of specialized techniques in the evaluation of malignant skin tumors

Throughout this chapter, I have mentioned instances in differential diagnosis in which adjunctive pathologic studies are desirable. By way of brief recapitulation, ultrastructural data are useful in assessment of the following problems:

1 Small cell SCC versus PCNC versus small cell malignant lymphoma

2 Sarcoma versus spindle cell SCC versus spindle cell melanoma

3 Angiosarcoma versus primary or metastatic carcinoma

4 EPD versus pagetoid Bowen's disease versus melanoma

5 Epithelioid sarcoma versus granuloma

6 Adenoid BCC or SCC versus cutaneous adnexal carcinoma

7 Sebaceous carcinoma versus metastatic mammary or gynecologic carcinomas

Discriminating immunohistochemical findings are presented in Figs. 19.30 through 19.33.

Therapeutic considerations

Similarly, recommended treatment approaches are given for most tumors included herein, in the text of the previous discussion. These are grouped according to the following protocol, in Table 19.1:

1 Conservative excision

2 Conservative excision with frozen-section–directed margins

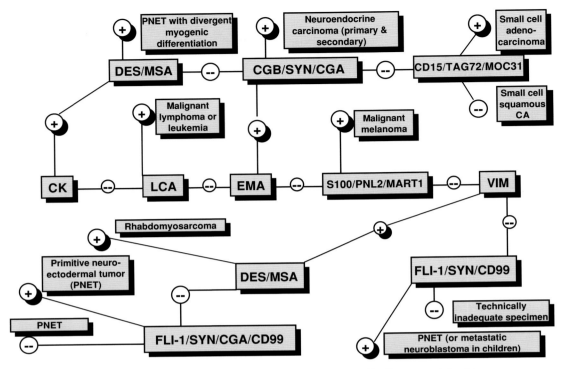

Fig. 19.30 Algorithm for immunohistologic diagnosis of undifferentiated small cell tumors of the skin.

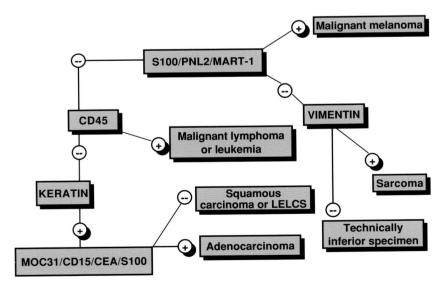

Fig. 19.31 Algorithm for immunohistologic diagnosis of undifferentiated epithelioid cell tumors of the skin. LELCS, lymphoepithelioma-like carcinoma of the skin.

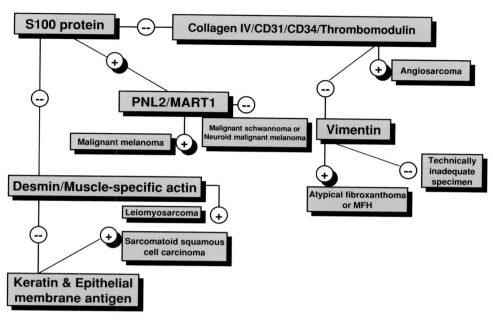

Fig. 19.32 Algorithm for immunohistologic diagnosis of undifferentiated spindle cell and pleomorphic tumors of the skin.

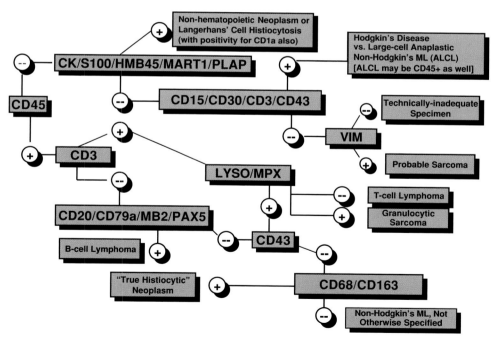

Fig. 19.33 Algorithm for immunohistologic diagnosis of hematopoietic tumors of the skin. ALCL, anaplastic large cell lymphoma; ML, malignant lymphoma.

Table 19.1 Therapeutic categories pertaining to cutaneous neoplasms

Group 1: Conservation Excision
Classic BCC
Classic SCC
Adenoid BCC
Adenoid SCC
Verrucous SCC
Bowen's disease

Group 2: Conservative Excision with Frozen-Section–Directed Margins
BCC with unfavorable histology (see text)
Extramammary Paget's disease
Pilar carcinomas
Kaposi's sarcoma
Atypical fibroxanthoma

Group 3: Wide Excision with Frozen-Section–Directed Margins
All localized malignant melanomas
Marjolin's ulcer SCC
Small cell SCC
Pleomorphic and spindle cell SCC
Sweat gland carcinomas
Sebaceous carcinomas
Angiosarcoma
Dermatofibrosarcoma protuberans
Malignant fibrous histiocytoma
Leiomyosarcoma
Fibrosarcoma
Primary anaplastic carcinoma NOS

Group 4: Wide Excision with Adjuvant Chemo- or Radiotherapy
Malignant melanomas with metastases
Primary cutaneous neuroendocrine carcinoma
Epithelioid sarcoma
Clear cell sarcoma

Group 5: Biopsy Only with Aggressive Radio- or Chemotherapy
Lymphoma and leukemia cutis
Metastatic carcinomas

NOS, not otherwise specified.

3 Wide excision with frozen-section–directed margins
4 Wide excision with adjuvant radiotherapy/chemotherapy
5 Biopsy only, with primary radiation treatment or chemotherapy

References

1 Raasch BA, Buettner PG, Garbe C. Basal cell carcinoma: histological classification and body site distribution. Br J Dermatol 2006;155:401–7.
2 Farmer ER, Helwig EB. Metastatic basal cell carcinoma: a clinicopathologic study of seventeen cases. Cancer 1980;46:748–57.
3 Jacobs GH, Rippey N, Altini M. Prediction of aggressive behavior in basal cell carcinoma. Cancer 1982;49:533–7.
4 Broders AC. Carcinoma: grading and practical applications. Arch Pathol 1926;2:376–81.
5 Klein-Szanto AP, Barr RJ, Reiners N, Mamrack MD. Filaggrin distribution in keratoacanthomas and squamous cell carcinoma. Arch Pathol Lab Med 1984;108:888–90.
6 Holden CA, McKee PH, MacDonald DM. Epidermal B2M labeling in verrucous carcinoma, viral warts, and pseudoepitheliomatous hyperplasia. In: MacDonald DM, editor. Immunodermatology. London: Butterworth; 1984. p 53–4.
7 Wick MR. Immunocytochemical markers of benignancy and malignancy: do they exist? Arch Pathol Lab Med 1986;110:180–1.
8 Matsuo K, Sakamoto A, Kawai K, et al. Small cell carcinoma of the skin, non-Merkel-cell type. Acta Pathol Jpn 1985;35:1029–36.
9 Wick MR, Swanson PE, Patterson JW. Immunohistology of skin tumors. In: Dabbs DJ, editor. Diagnostic immunohistochemistry. 2nd ed. New York: Churchill-Livingstone; 2006. p. 404–41.
10 Dong HY, Liu W, Cohen P, et al. B-cell-specific activation protein encoded by the PAX-5 gene is commonly expressed in Merkel cell carcinoma and small-cell carcinomas. Am J Surg Pathol 2005;29:687–92.
11 Kuwano H, Hashimoto H, Enjoji M. Atypical fibroxanthoma distinguishable from spindle cell carcinoma in sarcoma-like skin lesions. Cancer 1985;55:172–80.
12 Nappi O, Pettinato G, Wick MR. Adenoid (acantholytic) squamous cell carcinoma of the skin. J Cutan Pathol 1989;16:114–21.

13 Penneys NS, Nadji N, Ziegels-Weissman J, Ketabchi M, Morales AR. Carcinoembryonic antigen in sweat gland carcinomas. Cancer 1982;50:1608–11.

14 Helm KF, Goellner JR, Peters MS. Immunohistochemical stains in extramammary Paget's disease. Am J Dermatopathol 1992;14:402–7.

15 Kraus FT, Perez-Mesa C. Verrucous carcinoma. Cancer 1966;19:26–38.

16 Balazs M. Buschke-Loewenstein tumour: a histologic and ultrastructural study of six cases. Virchows Arch (Pathol Anat) 1986;410:83–92.

17 Barr LH, Menard JW. Marjolin's ulcer: the LSU experience. Cancer 1983;52:173–5.

18 Evans HL, Smith JL. Spindle cell squamous carcinomas and sarcoma-like tumors of the skin: a comparative study of 38 cases. Cancer 1980;45:687–97.

19 Immerman SC, Scanlon EF, Christ M, Knox KL. Recurrent squamous cell carcinoma of the skin. Cancer 1983;51:1537–40.

20 Cooper PH. Carcinomas of sweat glands. Pathol Annu 1987;22 Part 1:83–124.

21 Ackerman AB, Reddy VB, Soyer HP. Neoplasms with follicular differentiation. 2nd ed. New York: Ardor Scribendi; 2001.

22 Chintamani SR, Badran R, Singhal V, et al. Metastatic sweat gland adenocarcinoma: a clinicopathological dilemma. World J Surg Oncol 2003;1:13.

23 Jones RE Jr, Austin C, Ackennan AB. Extramammary Paget's disease: a critical reexamination. Am J Dermatopathol 1979;1:101–32.

24 Pitman GH, McCarthy JG, Perzin KH, Herter FP. Extramammary Paget's disease. Plast Reconstr Surg 1982;69:238–44.

25 Wick MR, Goellner JR, Wolfe JT 3rd, Su WPD. Vulvar sweat gland carcinomas. Arch Pathol Lab Med 1985;109:43–7.

26 Pereira PR, Odashiro AN, Rodrigues-Reyes AA, et al. Histopathological review of sebaceous carcinoma of the eyelid. J Cutan Pathol 2005;32:496–501.

27 Rulon DB, Helwig EB. Cutaneous sebaceous neoplasms. Cancer 1974;33:82–102.

28 Moreno C, Jacyk WK, Judd MJ, Requena L. Highly aggressive extraocular sebaceous carcinoma. Am J Dermatopathol 2001;23:450–5.

29 Gould E, Kurzon R, Kowalczyk AP, Saldana M. Pilomatrix carcinoma with pulmonary metastasis: report of a case. Cancer 1984;54:370–372.

30 Manivel JC, Wick MR, Mukai K. Pilomatrix carcinoma: an immunohistochemical comparison with benign pilomatrixoma and other benign cutaneous lesions of pilar origin. J Cutan Pathol 1986;13:22–9.

31 Ye J, Nappi O, Swanson PE, et al. Proliferating pilar tumors: a clinicopathological study of 76 cases with a proposal for definition of benign and malignant variants. Am J Clin Pathol 2004;122:566–74.

32 Maize JC. Primary cutaneous malignant melanoma: an analysis of the prognostic value of histologic characteristics. J Am Acad Dermatol 1983;8:857–63.

33 Breslow A. Tumor thickness, level of invasion, and node dissection in stage I cutaneous melanoma. Ann Surg 1975;182:575–85.

34 Mazur MT, Katzenstein ALA. Metastatic melanoma: the spectrum of ultrastructural morphology. Ultrastructural Pathol 1980;1:337–56.

35 Smoller BR. Immunohistochemistry in the diagnosis of melanocytic neoplasms. Pathology 1994;2:371–83.

36 Yaziji H, Gown AM. Immunohistochemical markers of melanocytic tumors. Int J Surg Pathol 2003;11:11–15.

37 Magro CN, Crowson AN, Mihm MC. Unusual variants of malignant melanoma. Mod Pathol 2006;19 Suppl 2:S41–70.

38 McGovern VI, McPeak C, Reed RJ, Sugarbaker EV. Malignant melanoma: a clinical and pathologic symposium. Pathol Annu 1982;17:361–83.

39 Conley J, Lattes R, Orr W. Desmoplastic malignant melanoma (a rare variant of spindle-cell melanoma). Cancer 1971;28:914–36.

40 Lens MB, Newton-Bishop JA, Boon AP. Desmoplastic malignant melanoma: a systematic review. Br J Dermatol 2005;152:673–8.

41 Busam KJ. Cutaneous desmoplastic melanoma. Adv Anat Pathol 2005;12:92–102.

42 Su LD, Fullen DR, Lowe L, et al. Desmoplastic and neurotropic melanoma. Cancer 2004;100:598–604.

43 Lim E, Browning J, MacGregor D, et al. Desmoplastic melanoma: comparison of expression of differentiation antigens and cancer testis antigens. Melanoma Res 2006;16:347–55.

44 Dotto JE, Glusac EJ. p63 is a useful marker for cutaneous spindle-cell squamous cell carcinoma. J Cutan Pathol 2006;33:413–417.

45 Hanson IM, Banerjee SS, Menasce LP, Prescott RJ. A study of eleven cutaneous malignant melanomas in adults with small-cell morphology: emphasis on diagnostic difficulties and unusual features. Histopathology 2002;40:187–95.

46 Toker C. Trabecular carcinoma of the skin. Arch Dermatol 1972;105:107–10.

47 Llombart B, Monteagudo C, Lopez-Guerrero JA, et al. Clinicopathological and immunohistochemical analysis of 20 cases of Merkel cell carcinoma in search of

prognostic markers. Histopathology 2005;46:622–34.

48 Mott RT, Smoller BR, Morgan MB. Merkel cell carcinoma: a clinicopathologic study with prognostic implications. J Cutan Pathol 2004;31:217–23.

49 Sibley RK, Dehner LP, Rosai J. Neuroendocrine (Merkel cell?) carcinoma of the skin: I. Clinicopathologic and ultrastructural study of 43 cases. Am J Surg Pathol 1985;9:95–108.

50 Wick MR, Goellner JR, Scheithauer BW, Thomas JR 3rd, Sanchez NP, Schroeter AL. Primary neuroendocrine carcinomas of the skin (Merkel cell tumors): a clinical, histologic, and ultrastructural study of 13 cases. Am J Clin Pathol 1983;79:6–13.

51 Kurtin P, Pinkus GS. Leukocyte common antigen—a diagnostic discriminant between hematopoietic and nonhematopoietic neoplasms in paraffin sections using monoclonal antibodies: correlation with immunologic studies and ultrastructural localization. Hum Pathol 1985;16:353–365.

52 Wick MR, Kaye VN, Sibley RK, Tyler R, Frizzera G. Primary neuroendocrine carcinoma and small-cell malignant lymphoma of the skin: a discriminant immunohistochemical comparison. J Cutan Pathol 1986;13:347–58.

53 Gomez LG, DiMaio S, Silva EG, Mackay B. Association between neuroendocrine (Merkel cell) carcinoma and squamous carcinoma of the skin. Am J Surg Pathol 1983;7:171–7.

54 Tang C-K, Toker C, Nedwich A, Zaman ANF. Unusual cutaneous carcinoma with features of small-cell (oat-cell-like) and squamous cell carcinomas: a variant of malignant Merkel cell neoplasm. Am J Dermatopathol 1982;4:537–48.

55 Skelton HG, Smith KJ, Hitchcock CL, et al. Merkel cell carcinoma: analysis of clinical, histologic, and immunohistologic features of 132 cases with relation to survival. J Am Acad Dermatol 1997;37:734–9.

56 Silva EG, Mackay B, Goepfert H, et al. Endocrine carcinoma of the skin (Merkel cell carcinoma). Pathol Annu 1984;19 Part 2:1–30.

57 Pectasides D, Pectasides M, Economopoulos T. Merkel cell cancer of the skin. Ann Oncol 2006;17:1489–95.

58 Gottlieb GJ, Ackerman AB. Kaposi's sarcoma: an extensively disseminated form in young homosexual men. Hum Pathol 1982;13:882–92.

59 Schwartz RA, Burgess GH, Hoshaw RA. Patch-stage Kaposi's sarcoma. J Am Acad Dermatol 1980;2:505–12.

60 Hunt SJ, Santa Cruz DJ. Vascular tumors of the skin: a selective review. Semin Diagn Pathol 2004;21:166–218.

61 Fukunaga M, Silverberg SG. Hyaline globules in Kaposi's sarcoma: a light microscopic and immunohistochemical study. Mod Pathol 1991;4:187–90.

62 Templeton AC. Kaposi's sarcoma. Pathol Annu 1981;16 Part 1:315–36.

63 Patel RM, Goldblum JR, Hsi ED. Immunohistochemical detection of human herpesvirus-8 latent nuclear antigen-1 is useful in the diagnosis of Kaposi's sarcoma. Mod Pathol 2004;17:456–60.

64 Maddox JC, Evans HL. Angiosarcoma of skin and soft tissue: a study of forty-four cases. Cancer 1981;48:1907–21.

65 Roy P, Clark MA, Thomas JM. Stewart-Treves syndrome: treatment and outcome in six patients from a single centre. Eur J Surg Oncol 2004;30:982–6.

66 Morgan MB, Swann M, Somach S, et al. Cutaneous angiosarcoma: a case series with prognostic correlation. J Am Acad Dermatol 2004;50:867–74.

67 Rosai J, Sumner HW, Kostianovsky M, Perez-Mesa C. Angiosarcoma of the skin: a clinicopathologic and fine structural study. Hum Pathol 1976;7:83–109.

68 Holden CA, Spittle MF, Wilson-Jones E. Angiosarcoma of the face and scalp: prognosis and treatment. Cancer 1987;59:1046–57.

69 DuBoulay CEH. Demonstration of alpha-1-antitrypsin and alpha-l-antichymotrypsin in the fibrous histiocytomas using the immunoperoxidase technique. Am J Surg Pathol 1982;6:559–64.

70 Dupree WB, Langloss LM, Weiss SW. Pigmented dermatofibrosarcoma protuberans (Bednar tumor): a pathologic, ultrastructural, and immunohistochemical study. Am J Surg Pathol 1985;9:630–9.

71 Frierson HF, Cooper PH. Myxoid variant of dermatofibrosarcoma protuberans. Am J Surg Pathol 1983;7:445–50.

72 Abbott JJ, Oliveira AM, Nascimento AG. The prognostic significance of fibrosarcomatous transformation in dermatofibrosarcoma protuberans. Am J Surg Pathol 2006;30:436–43.

73 Oliveira-Soares R, Viana L, Vale E, et al. Dermatofibrosarcoma protuberans: a clinicopathological study of 20 cases. J Eur Acad Dermatol Venereol 2002;16:441–6.

74 Kempson RL, McGavran MH. Atypical fibroxanthomas of the skin. Cancer 1964;17:1463–71.

75 Weiss SW, Enzinger FM. Malignant fibrous histiocytomas: an analysis of 200 cases. Cancer 1978;41:2250–66.

76 Helwig EB, May D. Atypical fibroxanthoma of the skin with metastasis. Cancer 1986;57:368–76.

77 Dahl I, Angervall L. Cutaneous and subcutaneous leiomyosarcoma: a clinicopathologic study of 47 patients. Pathol Eur 1974;9:307–15.

78 Stevanovic DV. Fibrosarcoma of the skin. Dermatol Monatsschr 1979;165:104–15.

79 Jensen ML, Jensen OM, Michalski W, et al. Intradermal and subcutaneous leiomyosarcoma: a clinicopathological and immunohistochemical study of 41 cases. J Cutan Pathol 1996;23:458–63.

80 Chase DR, Enzinger FM. Epithelioid sarcoma: diagnosis, prognostic indicators, and treatment. Am J Surg Pathol 1985;9:241–63.

81 Miettinen M, Fanburg-Smith JC, Virolainen M, et al. Epithelioid sarcoma: an immunohistochemical analysis of 112 classical and variant cases with a discussion of the differential diagnosis. Hum Pathol 1999;30:934–42.

82 Swanson PE, Wick MR. Clear cell sarcoma: an immunohistochemical analysis of six cases and comparison with other epithelioid neoplasms of soft tissue. Arch Pathol Lab Med 1989;113:55–60.

83 Miettinen M, Lehto V-P, Vartio T, Virtanen I. Epithelioid sarcoma: ultrastructural and immunohistologic features suggesting a synovial origin. Arch Pathol Lab Med 1982;106:620–3.

84 Chase DR, Enzinger FM, Weiss SW, Langloss JM. Keratin in epithelioid sarcoma: an immunohistochemical study. Am J Surg Pathol 1984;8:435–41.

85 Modlin RL, Vaccaro SA, Gottlieb B, et al. Granuloma annulare: identification of cells in the cutaneous infiltrate by immunoperoxidase techniques. Arch Pathol Lab Med 1984;108:379–82.

86 Wick MR, Manivel JC. Epithelioid sarcoma and isolated necrobiotic granuloma: a comparative immunohistochemical study. J Cutan Pathol 1986;13:253–60.

87 Rochaix P, Lacroix-Triki M, Lamant L, et al. PNL2, a new monoclonal antibody directed against a fixative-resistant melanocyte antigen. Mod Pathol 2003;16:481–90.

88 Jacobs IA, Chang CK, Guzman G, Salti GI. Clear cell sarcoma: an institutional review. Am Surg 2004;70:300–3.

89 Evans HL, Winkelmann RK, Banks PM. Differential diagnosis of malignant and benign cutaneous lymphoid infiltrates: a study of 57 cases in which malignant lymphoma had been diagnosed or suspected in the skin. Cancer 1979;44:699–717.

90 Chen M, Deng A, Crowson AN, et al. Assessment of T-cell clonality via T-cell receptor-gamma rearrangements in cutaneous T-cell-dominant infiltrates using polymerase chain reaction and single-stranded DNA conformational polymorphism assay. Appl Immunohistochem Molec Morphol 2004;12:373–9.

91 Ritter JH, Wick MR, Adesokan PN, et al. Assessment of clonality in cutaneous lymphoid infiltrates by polymerase chain reaction analysis of immunoglobulin heavy chain gene rearrangement. Am J Clin Pathol 1997;108:60–8.

92 Goodlad JR, Krajewski AS, Batstone PJ, et al. Primary cutaneous diffuse large B-cell lymphoma: prognostic significance of clinicopathological subtypes. Am J Surg Pathol 2003;27:1538–45.

93 Kempf W. CD30+ lymphoproliferative disorders: histopathology, differential diagnosis, new variants, and simulators. J Cutan Pathol 2006;33 Suppl 1:58–70.

94 Paul TR, Sundaran C, Gayathri K, et al. Extramedullary myeloid cell tumors: the NIMS experience. Indian J Pathol Microbiol 2005;48:318–21.

95 Menasce LP, Banerjee SS, Beckett E, Harris M. Extramedullary myeloid tumor (granulocytic sarcoma) is often misdiagnosed: a study of 26 cases. Histopathology 1999;34:391–8.

96 Burg G, Kempf W, Cozzio A, et al. WHO/EORTC classification of cutaneous lymphomas 2005: histological and molecular aspects. J Cutan Pathol 2005;32:647–74.

97 Cerroni L. Lymphoproliferative lesions of the skin. J Clin Pathol 2006;59:813–26.

98 Campo E, Chott A, Kinney MC, et al. Update on extranodal lymphomas: conclusions of the workshop held by the EAHP and the SH in Thessaloniki, Greece. Histopathology 2006;48:481–504.

99 Assaf C, Steinhoff M, Gellrich S, Sterry W. Classification of primary cutaneous lymphomas. Front Radiat Ther Oncol 2006;39:25–37.

100 Brownstein MH, Helwig EB. Metastatic tumors of the skin. Cancer 1972;29:1298–307.

101 Rosen T. Cutaneous metastases. Med Clin North Am 1980;64:885–900.

102 Saeed S, Keehn CA, Morgan MB. Cutaneous metastases: a clinical, pathological, and immunohistochemical appraisal. J Cutan Pathol 2004;31:419–30.

CHAPTER 20

Historical survey: methods used to treat skin cancer

Sharyn A. Laughlin and Denis K. Dudley

Fellow citizens, we cannot escape history.

—Abraham Lincoln

History is bunk.

—Henry Ford

The very ink with which all of history is written is merely fluid prejudice.

—Mark Twain

It is probable that every skin cancer could be cured at one time by the application of the end of a freshly extinguished wooden match.

—Anonymous

We are intrigued forever by physicians who are incapable of seeing that there is more than one way to treat a patient with skin cancer. The literature on the treatment of skin cancer is full of enthusiasts for one particular mode of therapy. History is the road map to the future and a historical survey of treatment methods used for skin cancer. It provides a useful perspective, particularly because current therapy is a blend of old and new. New methods, such as the use of immune response modifiers (IRMs), are based on principles of immunotherapy first applied in cutaneous medicine by Edmund Klein just over 40 years ago.

Methods of diagnosis

The diagnosis of skin cancer over the last 100 years must first be reviewed briefly. A study of the living gross pathology was the primary diagnostic test used before it became routine to confirm the clinical diagnosis by histologic examination of fixed and stained tissue. The use of the microscope has clearly increased diagnostic accuracy, especially for small basal and squamous cell carcinomas, small malignant melanomas, and other rare skin cancers. However, one must not underestimate the ability of those trained in living gross pathology to make an accurate diagnosis, especially when the natural course of the lesion is also studied. A biopsy shows only one area of the tumor at one stage of its development. As well, histologic criteria of malignancy are not necessarily the same as biologic criteria. This is illustrated by keratoacanthomas and melanoma.

The basic concept of a keratoacanthoma is clinical [1]: a neoplasm, at times histologically indistinguishable from a squamous cell carcinoma (SCC), that disappears by itself without treatment. Once this clinical fact was established, histopathologists tried, with some success, to define microscopic criteria. Melanoma is another area in which living gross pathology led the way. Trapl and colleagues [2] in 1964 developed the biologic concept of different growth patterns for melanomas based on clinical findings. The distinctive work of Clark and associates [3] clarified the various histologic types of malignant melanoma, but the original observations were clinical.

Topical applications

Caustics

Many different chemicals have been used as caustics to treat skin cancer. The three principal chemicals have been zinc chloride ($ZnCl_2$), potassium hydroxide (KOH), and arsenious acid (As_2O_3).

Zinc chloride was used quite extensively at the turn of the 20th century [4]. It destroyed healthy and diseased tissue with a mummifying action. Any intact skin over the cancer was softened by the brief application of 5% to 10% caustic potash (KOH). Pure zinc chloride was rarely used. It was mixed into a paste with flour (1:3), and 5% to 20% cocaine from a saturated solution of cocaine hydrochlorate was added for analgesia. The paste was spread on a cloth and applied to the cancer, extending slightly beyond the border. The neoplasm destroyed was usually equal to two to three times the thickness of the layer of paste. The plaster was removed after 24 to 28 hours. If the destruction was insufficient, the mummified tissue was pared or curetted away and a fresh application made. The "slough" required 5 to 20 days to separate. Zinc chloride was useful if the tumor was over a large vessel, as the mummifying action helped prevent hemorrhage. The curetting performed there was not a primary treatment procedure; it was meant to remove the tissue shriveled by the paste. Mohs chemosurgery fixed-tissue technique used a 50% solution of zinc chloride to fix the tissue before it was removed for histologic examination to determine whether any residual tumor was left [5].

Potassium hydroxide (caustic potash, potash, potassa fusa, KOH) is a powerful caustic that acts rapidly [6]. Vienna paste was made from a mixture of potassium hydroxide and calcium hydroxide (5:6) [7]. It was mixed to a fine powder, stored securely in a bottle, then made into a paste with 10% alcohol before use. London paste was made from a mixture of calcium oxide and sodium hydroxide in equal parts, prepared in the same way as Vienna paste [7]. One application was sufficient, and this caustic was painful. These preparations were used for small early skin cancers, particularly when the patient could remain under observation for only a short time. They could be used as a thick, saturated solution or as a paste. Any overlying crust was first removed and the adjacent skin protected by petrolatum. Small and superficial lesions required only 1 to 2 minutes of potash application, after which vinegar was applied.

Arsenic trioxide (arsenous oxide, arsenious oxide, arsenic, white arsenic, arsenious anhydride,

arsenious acid, As_2O_3) is a potent caustic, as are other inorganic and organic arsenicals [7]. Darier [8] may be quoted on the use of arsenious acid:

> The most convenient and most desirable caustic, which has yielded the largest number of durable and good esthetic results in my experience is arsenious acid . . . After the epidermised surfaces have been scraped, or freshened or burned with the galvanocautery, they are painted with a brush dipped in a supersaturated solution of arsenic (arsenious acid, 1 part; water and 90% alcohol, $\overline{aa}$ [i.e., equal parts of each] 50 parts): they are then left to dry and are covered with a pledget of cotton. At the end of 5 to 8 days, the crust should be removed: if the subadjacent surface is white, it is practically certain that the entire neoplasm has been destroyed; If it is mottled with gray and red, another series of cauterizations should be applied until a perfect result is obtained. This progressive plan of operating provides great security and spares the healthy tissues to the greatest possible degree: the pain is rarely very severe and does not last long. (p. 688)

Except for the use of a microscope to confirm the presence or absence of residual tumor, it is striking how similar the procedure described above is to Mohs chemosurgical technique [5]. Arsenic pastes were not used over large areas and, despite Darier's assurances, it was a painful procedure.

The turn of the last century probably represented the time when caustics were the most widely used. By 1920, x-ray was the preferred treatment, although texts of that time still include instructions for the preparation and use of caustics [6,8].

The use of caustic pastes as "quack" cancer remedies continued long after their general use by medical practitioners had stopped. In the Ottawa River Valley, cancer pastes were used up to the late 1950s. Dickie and Hughes [9] reviewed the history of the nonmedical use of caustic pastes in Ireland in the previous 25 years. They reported on 25 patients treated by them after nonmedical use of cancer pastes. Thirteen required treatment for the resulting deformity and eight for recalcitrant ulcers, but only four required treatment for persistent cancer. So 21 of 25 patients were cured by this treatment. The contents of these pastes were closely guarded secrets, and few have been analyzed in detail. Most appeared to contain various inorganic and organic arsenicals and zinc chloride, both described previously as potent agents that cause necrosis and sloughing.

Other topical agents

Podophyllin in 1950 [10] and demecolcine in 1959 [11] are examples of many other topical agents that have been studied. Falkson and Schulz [12] in 1962 reported on the disappearance of actinic keratoses in patients receiving systemic 5-fluorouracil (5-FU) for carcinomatosis. This disappearance occurred following one exposure to sunlight and was associated with a marked perilesional erythema. Klein and colleagues [13] and Dillaha and associates [14] followed this up with studies on the effects of the topical use of 5-FU. This agent is now used as monotherapy in a limited role for the treatment of basal cell carcinoma (BCC), when surgery is contraindicated or for difficult anatomic sites. Its efficacy as combination therapy with surgery, cryotherapy, or curettage and electrodesiccation (CED) is still being evaluated. Its use is limited by severe local effects and cure rates lower than those for other methods of treating skin cancer.

Dr. Douglas J. Grant, a medical resident on the service of Dr. J. R. Haserick in Cleveland, suggested the topical use of nitrogen mustard for mycosis fungoides in 1959 [15]. It quickly became one of the mainstays of the therapy for early stages of this disease.

Surgery

Bennett [16] reviewed the historical background of the surgical treatment of rodent ulcer (basal cell carcinoma). Daviel in 1755 was the first to recommend excision, although this was not widely practiced for many years. There was an increase in excisional surgery for rodent ulcers in the first half of the 19th century that coincided with the development of plastic surgery procedures. The lack of general anesthesia probably deterred many because of the additional pain needed to excise a tumor or raise or rotate a flap. Spencer Wells in 1854 used a direct advancement flap to close the defect after excision of a rodent ulcer on the infraorbital area. Hutchinson in 1860 used a forehead flap slit into two parts for a

rodent ulcer involving the medial one half of the upper and lower eyelids and medial canthus. In 1869, Reverdin introduced the free skin graft; in 1875, Wolfe in Glasgow described the full-thickness skin graft.

From the surgical perspective, there has been little new added to the treatment of small well-localized BCC and SCC since the turn of the 20th century. There are certainly more surgeons better trained in these procedures. Modern anesthesia and other life support facilities have made the procedure safer and less traumatic to the patient. Melanoma, however, is a very different matter. The surgical principle of extensive, wide, deep local excision with contiguous removal of the nearest anatomic group of lymph nodes was laid down in 1907 by Handley [17] and in 1908 by Pringle [18] (Fig. 20.1). Pringle based his findings on two patients with malignant melanoma. He admitted in 1937 that they were "the only two on whom I have operated for melanoma" [19]. Handley described a detailed postmortem study on one patient who died of disseminated melanoma. From the spread pattern of secondary tumor deposits in the femoral lymph nodes, he concluded that the tumor dispersed by direct centrifugal invasion of the lymphatics, with late or terminal hematogenous dissemination. Therefore, it seemed logical to him that the more tissue and lymph nodes one could excise, the better the outcome. This naive concept had a profound and persistent effect on the surgery of malignant melanoma, especially as medical advances allowed more extensive surgery to be performed.

Another pervasive surgical principle was the idea that cauterizing a mole could change it into a malignant melanoma that would immediately metastasize. A typical paper condemning electrocoagulation is by Amadon [20]. He reported a series of 27 cases of malignant melanoma treated by electrocoagulation, all of which recurred locally "with early regional and generalized metastases in the majority of cases." Electrocoagulation was felt to have this effect by:

1 Stimulating the cells to malignant change
2 Releasing melanin, which is a chemical irritant and may cause cancer
3 Causing bubbles of "tissue steam" in the lymphatics and venules that push the tumor cells along

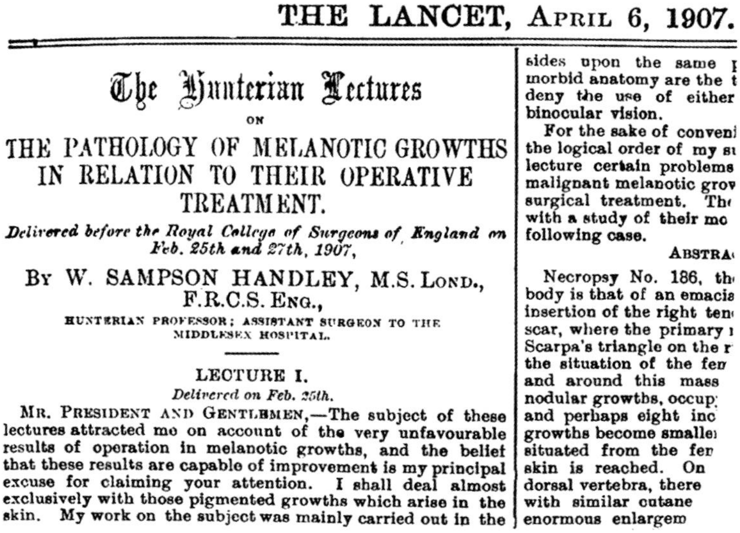

THE LANCET, APRIL 6, 1907.

The Hunterian Lectures

ON

THE PATHOLOGY OF MELANOTIC GROWTHS IN RELATION TO THEIR OPERATIVE TREATMENT.

Delivered before the Royal College of Surgeons of England on Feb. 25th and 27th, 1907,

BY W. SAMPSON HANDLEY, M.S. LOND., F.R.C.S. ENG.,

HUNTERIAN PROFESSOR; ASSISTANT SURGEON TO THE MIDDLESEX HOSPITAL.

LECTURE I.

Delivered on Feb. 25th.

MR. PRESIDENT AND GENTLEMEN,—The subject of these lectures attracted me on account of the very unfavourable results of operation in melanotic growths, and the belief that these results are capable of improvement is my principal excuse for claiming your attention. I shall deal almost exclusively with those pigmented growths which arise in the skin. My work on the subject was mainly carried out in the

sides upon the same p
morbid anatomy are the t
deny the use of either
binocular vision.
For the sake of conveni
the logical order of my su
lecture certain problems
malignant melanotic grow
surgical treatment. The
with a study of their mo
following case.

ABSTRA

Necropsy No. 186, the
body is that of an emacia
insertion of the right ten
scar, where the primary
Scarpa's triangle on the r
the situation of the fem
and around this mass
nodular growths, occup
and perhaps eight inc
growths become smalle
situated from the fem
skin is reached. On
dorsal vertebra, there
with similar cutane
enormous enlargem

Fig. 20.1 Handley's paper on the spread of melanoma.

The logical follow-up of these principles of "no touch" and wide excision and en bloc regional lymph node excision led to some startling events and statements. Cameron [21] in 1968 reported, "I have removed the great toe deliberately for a subungual simple [i.e., nonmalignant] mole; and frequently removed wide skin areas and applied skin grafts in simple [i.e., nonmalignant] cases."

Ewing and Powell [22] reported that a 19-year-old girl, who was shortly to be married, presented with a bleeding black lesion 2.0 cm in diameter on the anterior aspect of the left thigh. The lesion had recurred after local surgical removal. A biopsy was not done. Based on the clinical findings, a radial local excision with a radical in-continuity inguinal and femoral lymph node dissection was performed. The histology examination showed a hemorrhagic ulcerated angioma. The authors reported that it was "distressing to leave this young woman with a disfiguring scar and troublesome recurrent edema of the foot and ankle." Inevitably, forequarter and hindquarter amputations and even hemipelvectomy were performed in an effort to get rid of all the cancer [23]. Fortner and coworkers [24] in 1964 reported on 220 patients treated from 1931 to 1956 by groin dissections; 33 had superficial groin dissections, and 14 had bilateral superficial or radical groin dissections. There were also 31 groin dissections secondary to hemipelvectomy or hip joint amputation. Five of the 31 showed "negative nodes" (i.e., no evidence of malignant melanoma). It is not clear from this report whether these patients did have malignant melanoma in the skin or subcutaneous tissue at the time of operation.

Fortunately, dissenting voices were raised. In 1955, Lund and Ihnen [25] asked, "Is prophylactic lymph node dissection indicated?" Block and Hartwell [26] stated that "we disagree with the dogma of Pack, that elective or prophylactic lymphadenectomy must be done routinely to adequately treat malignant melanoma."

X-rays and radium

The discovery of ionizing radiation was announced to the world by William Conrad Roentgen, professor of physics at the Royal University of Wurzburg on December 28, 1896, to the Physico-Medical Society of Wurzburg [27]. Johan Thor Stenbac opened the Roentgen Institute of Stockholm in 1896 and was treating skin cancer by 1900. In 1901, Sequeira [28] reported on the response of 12 patients with rodent ulcers treated by "the X-Rays." Radium was discovered by Madame Marie Curie-Skłodowska in

1898 from pitchblende [27]. Radium therapy began with the famous "Becquerel burn." In 1901, Antoine-Henri Becquerel placed a tube of radium in the pocket of his waistcoat, where it remained for several hours. A week or two later, Besnier examined this dermatitis and expressed the belief that it was the result of to the radium. Becquerel loaned radium to Danlos of the Hospital St. Louis, where it was used to treat skin diseases in 1902.

After the discovery of x-ray, the flood gates were opened. Up to 1906, x-rays were used for everything and anything, using very crude and uncalibrated machinery. This was the era of the "radiomaniac." From 1906 to 1912, there was an era of pessimism as the side effects became obvious, and the response to treatment was not miraculous. X-ray sequelae on the skin were seen very early and reported by J. C. White of Boston and C. A. Codman. The Coolidge electron tube was introduced in 1914. Many further advances continued. In 1940, Cipollaro and Mutscheller [29] reported on roentgen radiation absorption curves in the skin, showing depth dosage as modified by voltage and filtration.

In 1944, Strandqvist reported his famous curves, showing the time–dose relationship between the death of normal and cancerous tissue [30,31]. Different recovery rates between normal and cancerous tissues were the basis for fractional dose therapy, in which normal tissue recovers faster than malignant tissue from each treatment. Strandqvist used prolonged clinical study with a series of carefully controlled cases to determine the best degree of fractionation or combination of protraction and fractionation.

From 1934 to 1941, he treated 280 cases of carcinoma of the skin and lip with x-rays. Minimum tumor dose was calculated. Based on clinical follow-up of 5 years or more, he divided his series into three groups:

1 Patients with recurrence or continuing disease
2 Those who were well, with no complications
3 Those without disease but with late radiation damage

He then plotted the position of each on a time–dose basis. His charts showed a narrow zone where recurrences and damage were equally likely to occur. This was considered the zone for correct dosage, and the proper change in total dose related to total treatment time could be determined.

Smithers [32] indicated the degree of sophistication achieved by 1946 with the following quote from his text:

> If a certain method of treatment proves successful in 85 percent of cases of basal cell carcinomas, then the chief point of interest is not that this is a satisfactory method or that this figure is 5 percent higher than was obtained in some previously published report, but why this method failed in 15%. It is important to know what peculiarities the tumors which failed to respond possessed, whether they would have responded to the same or even lower dose given in another way, whether they required a higher dose, whether they were not suitable for radiotherapy at all, and how to recognize them before starting treatment in future. What is required, in fact, is to know the best method of treating each individual patient and not merely to evolve a method that is successful in a good proportion of all the cases seen. Each patient requires a special treatment, each tumor presents a new problem; standard doses and standard methods are not enough. (pp. iv–v)

Kindel [33] in 1957 reported in detail on the clinical and experimental use of different types of x-rays, applying them to lesions at various levels of the skin, and Kalz [34] reported in 1959 on the effect of Grenz rays (very low kilovoltage) on the skin. Radiotherapy continues to be used for therapy of skin cancer but became established firmly after 1958 when Wrong [35] and Fitzpatrick and colleagues [36] published similar results.

To place radiotherapy in perspective as a treatment modality, two quotations are presented. One is in Sutton's text [37], which reads as follows:

> Radiation in Treatment of Neoplasms—There are analogies between the application of radiation and the application of a caustic paste. In either case cure, if cure results, depends on destruction. In either case one does not know what the exact boundary of the destruction is going to be, and in either case one does not command this boundary but simply intends that it will be sufficient. Except in palliation and under uncommon combinations of circumstances I prefer surgical

attack if it is feasible, where with a single procedure one takes definitive steps to destroy that tissue which in one's judgment ought to be destroyed and leaves healthy that which one does not wish damaged. The surgical scar is not an x-ray burn. (p. 90)

Friedman and associates [38] further observed:

The relative values of the factors influencing radiation cures are: the biologic nature and extent of the tumour—60%; the skill and experience of the therapists—30% and the modality—10%. (p. 10)

A detailed historical, clinical, and histologic review of chronic roentgen ray dermatoses was published in 1925 by Cole [39] in describing six physicians who developed cutaneous SCC. Pack and Davis [40] reported 59 cases of radiation cancer of the skin. Radiotherapy by the monoenergetic electron beam has been used extensively for lymphomas involving the skin [41]. It has now been replaced in the early phase of mycosis fungoides by the topical use of nitrogen mustard (*quod vide*).

After 1951, cobalt-60 teleradiotherapy techniques were successfully employed in the treatment of difficult cases of carcinoma of the skin in accessible areas such as the ears, nose, and penis [42]. Radium has never been a big favorite for treating skin cancer, except in certain localized areas, such as the southwestern United States [43]. A book titled *Radium Recipes for Cutaneous Cancer* [44] indicated that radium was still being used in 1972 in the treatment of skin cancer.

Electrosurgery

Electrocautery (galvanocautery)

Despite the simplicity of the equipment required and the results obtainable by proper use, electrocautery (or "hot poker" treatment) has never had a high degree of popularity. It was and may be used in two separate ways. The cancer may be burned out (after biopsy), or an "en bloc" removal may be performed [37,45,46]. Paquelin's thermocautery (1876; Fig. 20.2) and Post cautery (Fig. 20.3) were favorite early models. In many of these cauteries, the wire tip was made red hot electrically. Unna's microburner was a platinum needle around which

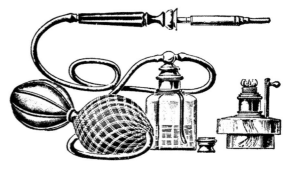

Fig. 20.2 Paquelin's thermocautery. (Reprinted with permission from Ahlswede E. Practical treatment of skin disease with special reference to technique. New York: Paul B. Hoeber; 1932.)

a heating wire was coiled. The platinum needle, which did not get as hot as the heating wire, was used for treatment. Much of the literature on the use of cautery is written by surgeons. Head and neck tumors, breast cancer, and carcinoma of the uterus and cervix are among the lesions that have been

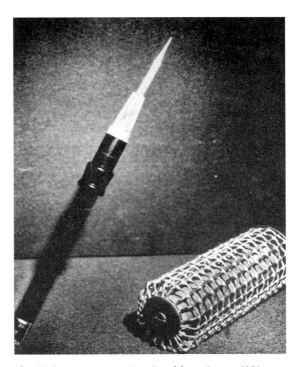

Fig. 20.3 Post cautery. (Reprinted from Sutton [37], courtesy of Richard L. Sutton, Jr., MD.)

Table 20.1 Brief outline of the historical development of electrosurgery

Date	Author	Event
1146	Masschewbrock	Leyden Jar
1821	Oersted	Electromagnetic induction
1842	Henry	Leyden Jars discharge oscillatory vibrators
1881	Morton	Oscillation current of 100,000,000/sec produced by static induction
1884	Hertz	Vibratory waves pass from a generator to a distant receiver without tangible electrical connections
1891	d'Arsonval	High-frequency currents (10,000/sec) of high tension could be passed through living tissue without pain or muscular contraction
1891	Tesla	d'Arsonval's coarse spiral enclosed in a fine wire coil of many turns to step up current
1893	d'Arsonval	Induction coil used to a powerful current with a spark from 5–15 mm long in air
1893	Oudin	Added a special variable resonator to the free end, to which is fixed the electrode, which is applied to the patient
1900	Riviére	By using increased current with a small electrode, destructive effects were obtained; "indolent" ulcer on back of hand of musician successfully treated
1906–1907	Cook	Treated warts, moles, acne pustules, infected tonsils. and hemorrhoids
1908	Beer	Destruction of bladder tumors through a cystoscope
1908	De Forrest	Obtained a cutting current from the vacuum tube apparatus; electrocutting "radio-knife"
1909	de Keating–Hart and Pozzi	Used term *fulguration* and treated accessible tumors
1909	Doyen	Used biterminal connections that concentrated the current to destroy cancerous tissue to a depth of 1–2 cm; no spark used
1910	Nagelschmidt	Coined term *electrocoagulation*
1923	Wyeth	Practical cutting current apparatus developed
1924	Clark et al.	Increased amperage of both unilateral and biterminal currents and made currents more smooth; also studied histopathologic changes; used term *electrodesiccation*
1928	Bovie	Cutting and coagulating current combined to produce a machine versatile enough for neurosurgical procedures

Sources: Elliott [48] and Ward [49].

treated. The cautery designed by Percy was widely used for these purposes [47].

Electrodesiccation, electrocoagulation, and electrosection

The history of the development of these techniques is tied in general with the development of electrical equipment. Based on the excellent reviews of Elliott [48] and Ward [49], the list in Table 20.1 outlines the historical background. The practical use of the various methods has been discussed in some detail by Ward [50], Kovacs [51], and Fritsch [52]. The popularity of these forms of therapy in comparison with other modalities is discussed later, as is the incidental use of electrosurgery and curettage.

Cryosurgery

A. Campbell White [53] first introduced the use of liquid air in medicine and surgery in 1899. He obtained his liquid air from Professor Charles E. Triples of Columbia University. It was initially swabbed on by a cotton-tipped stick that had been dipped in liquid air or sprayed on from a Dewar (double-glass) bulb. In 1905, Juliusberg [54] reported a method of spraying carbon dioxide on the skin lesion being treated. In 1907, Pusey [55] used shaped cylinders to apply carbon dioxide snow to varying-sized skin lesions. Liquid air was not used in cryosurgery after 1910 because of its high cost and limited availability. Irvine and Turnacliffe [56] described the use of liquid oxygen in 1929.

Liquid nitrogen replaced liquid oxygen in the 1940s because liquid nitrogen was not flammable. Allington [57] popularized the use of the swab method using liquid nitrogen in 1950. In 1961, Cooper and Lee [58] reported their closed-system liquid nitrogen apparatus for use in neurosurgical cryosurgery. In 1966, Zacarian and Adham [59,60] introduced the use of solid copper cylinder disks, which were immersed in liquid nitrogen until their temperature was noted and then were applied to the skin lesion.

Over the past 40 years, Torre [61] developed and refined a cryosurgical system that produces a spray of varying size or cools a cryoprobe to be applied to a particular skin tumor. Thermocouple-tipped needles are required to measure the depth of freezing. Kuflik [62] summarized the various techniques and his results.

Curettage

Curettage is the use of a small spoon-like instrument to scrape away morbid tissue. The basic premise of curettage is that the instrument traverses diseased tissue with little resistance and that the texture of the tissue is characteristic of the tumor. A BCC imparts a smooth, gelatinous feel to the operator; an SCC seems slightly more gritty; and both separate easily compared with the firm resistance of normal skin. The silent abrasion and smooth consistency of diseased tissue are associated with pooling of blood, which gives way to rough resistance, a scratching sound, and pinpoint hemorrhage when the instrument breaches the fibrous tissue of normal skin. Therefore, one can feel with the curette when all the cancer has been removed. Visual inspection may also help decide when the treatment is

sufficient. The curettes used do not have a knifelike or cutting edge (i.e., the tumor is scraped away, not excised).

Curettes come in all sizes and shapes. Varying-sized oval, solid, or fenestrated (ring) curettes have been most commonly used. Volkmann is credited with the early medical use of curettes for skin diseases. Others who have described their use or proposed modifications in size or shape are Duhring, Besnier, Squire, Fox, Vidal, Piffard, and Schamberg. Burns [63] made note of the value of a small curette.

In surveying the literature on the use of curettage as a method of treatment of skin cancer, one is reminded of the comment of de Saint Exupery, the philosopher and pilot: "...perfection is finally attained not when there is no longer anything to add, but when there is no longer anything to take away..." [64]. Curettage has had four stages in its evolution: its use with caustics, its use with ionizing radiation, its use with electrodesiccation, and finally its use alone. Each stage is discussed in the following paragraphs.

The Sherwell technique was described in 1908 [65]. Sherwell's procedure was "thorough, deep and efficient" curettage followed by immediate and just as thorough application of 60% solution of acid nitrate of mercury. This caustic was neutralized by sodium carbonate. Sherwell openly admitted "neither entire novelty as to method or absolute perfection as to result." His relapse rate was "very much less than 10 per cent." He did not exclude the use of surgical excision or "the wonderful and potential dynamic action of the x-ray, and radium...." He suggested the use of dermal curettes of differing sizes; the large curette is to remove the bulk of the tumor. "The smaller curettes can then be used in all sinuses and anfractuosities, and as I have said before with energy. Do not fear hurting the sound tissue. The normal skin is a pretty tough proposition."

The use of curettage and ionizing radiation was well described by Elliott and Welton in 1946 [66]. They gave 12 references to other papers using the same therapy from 1906 to 1938. This method is essentially the Brocq-Belot technique first used in 1903 [67]. Reporting on patients treated between 1919 and 1941, they stated:

We do not treat all of our patients by any one method, but, briefly, the method we have employed most frequently is, first, thorough curettage of all the abnormal tissue followed by electrodesiccation or coagulation of the new surface. Then the area thus treated, plus a peripheral margin of normal skin, is exposed to 600 to 800r unfiltered roentgen rays. This exposure is repeated at four to seven day intervals until a total of 3000r or more has been given. We believe that this method of administering roentgen rays produces results superior to those when the same total dose is given at one sitting. The time required for healing ranges from five to seven weeks, depending on the original size and depth of the lesion.

In reports on the use of curettage with caustics and ionizing radiation, it is hard to ascertain how significant the curettage was in actually curing the cancer. In some reports, the description indicates that the curettage was the main treatment and the caustics or radiation were added for insurance. In others, the curettage was used mainly to remove the bulk of the tumor and later on probably to obtain a biopsy specimen.

In 1954, Osborne [68] stated that "in my opinion in the majority of malignant cutaneous lesions, the use of thorough curettage followed by electrothermic destruction is favoured whenever possible over all other methods." Other reports on electrodesiccation and curettage in the 1950s were by Lamb [69], Cipollaro [70], Epstein [71], King [72], and Pillsbury and coauthors [73]. In the 1960s, electrodesiccation and curettage became firmly established in the world's tumor literature by reports from authors such as Knox in the United States [74,75], Sweet in England [76], and Williamson and Jackson in Canada [77]. The major advance of these and other articles was that detailed statistics were included, giving a scientific basis to the procedure. All these articles also show that the therapeutic emphasis is on the curettage and the electrodesiccation was used to destroy small peripheral, invisible, superficial deposits and to control bleeding. Finally, Reymann [78] reported favorably on the use of curettage alone.

The retrospective literature is not able to claim better efficacy for any method of treatment, including Mohs micrographic surgery (MMS), in the overall management of nonmelanoma skin cancer (NMSC). CED is still favored by most dermatologists. Surgically trained dermatologists, plastic surgeons, and physicians trained in MMS may prefer surgical excision for most NMSCs, such as BCC and SCC. The premise that surgical techniques produce better cosmetic results than CED has never been proven by large randomized prospective studies. In experienced hands, curettage followed by light and delicate electrodesiccation achieves excellent cosmetic outcome, if larger lesions on convex surfaces are excluded from treatment. A multidisciplinary approach is optimal for metastatic cancer. After 1970, it became obvious that combined therapy was also a consideration for the various types of NMSC. Table 20.2 is a chronologic summary of methods used to treat BCC in the past 100 years. Table 20.3 lists those for SCC and is a notably shorter list, for the likely reason that the greater risk of invasion and morbidity encouraged caution and less experimentation. Both lists have been extended to include recent information but were derived from other sources [79,80].

More recent developments

After 1850, the use of surgery and various caustic preparations persisted for almost 70 years until the introduction of radiotherapy around 1920. For the next 50 years, curettage and various methods of electrosurgery were added to the clinical menu in wide use, which still included surgery and radiation. The development of Mohs chemosurgery eventually represented a shift in the approach to the treatment of skin cancer. It was within the past 40 years that a number of alternative therapies were introduced. Some were based on the development of new concepts, but others were really new or refined versions of old strategy. A chronologic summary is given in Table 20.4, which does not attempt to include every approach, particularly the increasing use of combination therapy.

Topical chemo- and immunotherapy
The pioneering use of topical 5-FU began by Edmund Klein in the early 1960s, but more recent

Table 20.2 Treatment of BCC as reported at various times

Author	Year	Treatment	Lesions, no.
Sequeira	1901	X-rays	236
Williams CM	1906	X-rays	16
Bisserie	1906	X-rays	186
Williams	1907	X-rays	53
Pusey	1907	X-rays	111
Stem	1907	X-rays	85
Hahn	1908	X-rays	509
Sherwell	1910	Surgery and acid nitrate of mercury	
Williams & Ellsworth	1913	Radium	181
Hahn	1919	Scalpel excision	64
Simpson	1922	Radium	1000
Morrow & Taussig	1923	Radium	322
Quigley	1923	Radium	593
Hazen & Whitmore	1925	X-rays	244
Dolloway	1926	X-rays	153
MacKee	1927	X-rays	644
Montgomery	1928	Scalpel excision	18
Archambault & Maisin	1930	Curettage and x-rays	21
Archambault & Maisin	1930	Surgical diathermy	32
Falchi	1930	Surgical diathermy	21
Halberstaedter & Simons	1931	Interstitial radium	302
Belot	Many	Curettage and x-rays	6000
Zeisler	1933	Curettage, x-rays, and surgical diathermy	359
Shelmire & Fox	1936	Radium needles	66
Warren & Lulenskie	1941	Surgery	164
		Irradiation	110
		Combined	80
Elliott & Welton	1946	Mainly curettage followed by x-rays	1742
Churchill-Davidson & Johnson	1954	X-rays	711
Knox et al.	1960	CED	287
		Surgery	63
		Irradiation	40
Sweet	1963	Curettage	511
Knox et al.	1964	CED	755
Mitchell & Hardie	1965	CED	148
Helm & Klein	1965	Trenimon	110
Lauritzon et al.	1965	Surgery	2900
Gooding et al.	1965	Surgery	1197
Tromovitch	1965	CED	75
Shigematsu et al.	1966	X-rays	831
Knox et al.	1966	Irradiation	120
		Surgery	281
		CED	881

(*Continued*)

Table 20.2 (*Continued*)

Author	Year	Treatment	Lesions, no.
Shanoff et al.	1967	Excision	550
Klein et al.	1968	5-FU	6
Monhallin	1968	Radiotherapy	663
Jackson	1969	CED	330
		Surgery	80
		Irradiation	25
Grabb et al.	1969	CED	327
		Surgical excision	196
		Radiation	95
		Mohs chemosurgery	32
		Combined	3
Frame	1970	X-rays	1348
Reyman	1971	Curettage	338
Torre	1973	Cryosurgery (both BCC & SCC)	800
Zacarian	1975	Cryosurgery	2000
Mohs	1976	Chemosurgery	935
Pennington et al.	1988	Photodynamic therapy	
Beutner et al.	1999	Topical 5% imiquimod	35

Table 20.3 Pivotal studies on the treatment of SCC

Author	Year	Treatment	Lesions, no.
Halberstaedter & Simons	1931	Radium mostly; no surgical diathermy	556
Zeisler	1933	Surgery, electrosurgery, and radiation	102
Schreiner	1933	Surgery, electrosurgery, and radiation	164
Traub & Tolmach	1933	Electrosurgery and radiation	26
Knox et al.	1960	CED	315
Klein et al.	1962	5-FU for keratoacanthoma	3
Williamson & Jackson	1964	CED	53
		Surgery	23
		Irradiation	31
Knox et al.	1966	Irradiation	80
		Surgery	23
		CED	495
Shigematsu et al.	1966	Irradiation	214
Klein et al.	1968	In situ SCC	20
Frame	1970	X-rays	595
Mohs	1978	Chemosurgery	3302
Robins et al.	1981	MMS—15-year experience	414
Mackenzie-Wood et al.	2001	Imiquimod 5% for Bowen's disease ≥1 cm	16
Leibovitch et al.	2005	MMS	1263

Table 20.4 Primary methods of skin cancer treatment for each decade from 1850 to 2000

Year	Treatments Commonly Used	Other Treatments
1850	Surgery, caustics	
1900	Surgery, caustics	
1920	X-rays, surgery, caustics	
1930	X-rays, surgery, electrosurgery	
1940	X-rays, surgery, electrosurgery	Extended radical melanoma surgery, Mohs chemosurgery
1950	X-rays, surgery, curettage, CED	MMS
1960	Surgery, curettage, CED, x-rays	MMS, topical nitrogen mustard for mycosis fungoides
1970	Surgery, curettage, CED, x-rays	MMS, cryosurgery, topical 5-FU
1980	Surgery, MMS, curettage, CED, x-rays	Topical 5-FU, cryosurgery, PDT, intralesional interferon
1990	Surgery, MMS, curettage, CED, x-rays	Topical imiquimod, topical 5-FU, cryosurgery, PDT, intralesional interferon
2000	Surgery, MMS, curettage, CED, 5% imiquimod	Topical 5-FU, cyrosurgery, PDT

PDT, photodynamic therapy.

studies have refined its use as a monotherapy in selected cases and attempted to define precise benefits from combining this agent with surgery or CED. The use of IRMs is a promising new direction in the area of immunotherapy begun by Klein [81], who first reported in 1968 on the use of the effects of specific cell-mediated immunity (delayed hypersensitivity) on skin cancer. He found that an immune reaction of the delayed hypersensitivity type could cure superficial premalignant and malignant cutaneous lesions, with minimal or no effects on adjacent normal tissue. The initial sensitizer used was triethylene-imino-benzoaquinone (TEIM). Klein also worked with other nonspecific agents and introduced the use of lymphokines for treatment of accessible tumors [82]. After introducing local immunotherapy for curing cutaneous premalignant and cancerous neoplasms, Klein was recognized as the father of modern immunotherapy. He also devised the low-dose vinblastine therapy for Kaposi's sarcoma in the 1960s.

From a historical perspective, it is necessary to give a concise review of the new therapeutic methods being investigated and to identify their appropriate role in contemporary practice.

Light-based methods
Laser therapy
In 1963, Leon Goldman, the father of laser medicine, used a ruby laser to treat malignant melanoma [83]. BCC was also treated with laser therapy around the same time [84], but the use of laser radiation for the treatment of skin cancer remains limited to a few defined areas. It is permissible to use a carbon dioxide laser for excisional surgery in the same way that electrosection is used as an alternative to cold knife incision. Shave biopsy followed by carbon dioxide laser ablation provides a practical and useful method to treat superficial multifocal or extensive skin cancer. This laser has also been used as an alternative to electrodesiccation after curettage.

Photodynamic therapy
The principle of photodynamic therapy (PDT) uses a foreign substance or photosensitizer to destroy tissue after light activation, which produces molecular oxygen intermediates that are cytotoxic. The ideal photosensitizer is absorbed more rapidly by atypical cells than normal skin and concentrates within the target tissue. The absorbed photosensitizer is activated with a color of laser or nonlaser light that is preferentially absorbed by the specific agent. The concept and the essence of PDT originated more than 100 years ago when Raab observed that *Paramecium* cells died at a faster rate when exposed to light in the presence of acridine orange. In 1904, Von Tappeiner and Jodblauer described fluorescence in protozoa using aniline dyes as a "photodynamic effect" that consumed oxygen.

In 1905, Jesionek and Von Tappeiner used topical 5% eosin to treat NMSC and other benign conditions. PDT languished until 1948 when Figge and colleagues [85] confirmed that hematoporphyrin was selectively concentrated by embryonic, neoplastic, and injured skin. PDT has emerged to play an important role in the spectrum of modern therapy. Dougherty [86,87] published a series of papers between 1974 and 1987 that established a role for PDT in treatment for skin cancer. Since that time, 5-aminolevulinic acid (ALA) has replaced the original porphyrin derivatives used by Dougherty, because it is associated with a lower risk of photosensitivity. ALA is a precursor that is concentrated by abnormal skin and converted to active protoporphyrin. A variety of light sources are now used to activate ALA depending on the condition being treated. ALA-PDT is used for the cosmetic treatment of photodamage and acne but is also used in the management of actinic keratoses, BCC, and Bowen's disease.

Various types of nonablative therapy have been investigated for the treatment of actinic keratoses, BCC, and Bowen's disease [88]. This type of therapy is generally not considered for SCC, which carries a greater risk for invasion and morbidity. Perilesional injection of interferon-α-2b shows promising efficacy as another nonsurgical treatment for BCC but is not widely used. Many new compounds are being evaluated for chemoprevention of cancer, but the accepted therapy of skin cancer with topical agents is focused on the use of 5-FU and imiquimod.

Surgical excision

A surgical approach has been the most enduring method in the treatment of skin cancer. Excisional techniques by scalpel or electrosection were traditionally the forte of general or plastic surgeons. Radiation was performed by the radiotherapist, and all other nonsurgical methods for treating skin cancer were generally the province of the dermatologist. In contemporary practice, the role of the dermatologist in the area of excisional surgery has increased. Most residency programs now offer formal training in cutaneous surgery. MMS is generally regarded as a subspecialty technique for use by dermatologists.

Standard excision

Toward the end of the 20th century, many dermatologists started to perform surgical excision of appropriate skin cancers using the basic elliptical or fusiform incision followed by primary closure. Techniques such as M-plasty and the use of flaps were transplanted from plastic surgery. In current practice, surgical excision using controlled margins is a technique performed by dermatologists and plastic surgeons, which meets most of the objectives of MMS. It is a useful alternative when micrographic surgery is not feasible or available. The introduction and evolution of MMS after its introduction in 1941 was the most important change in the surgical approach to occur for almost a century [89].

Mohs micrographic surgery

Frederic Mohs was a medical student at the University of Wisconsin. He worked at a cancer research laboratory in the early 1930s and observed that tissue injected with 20% zinc chloride had fixed histologic features suitable for examination on the microscope. He proposed the idea of excising cancers under microscopic control, and the concept of micrographic chemosurgery was pioneered. Mohs went on to train as a general surgeon and in 1941 reported his technique for a microscopically controlled method of cancer excision [89]. Eventually, fixation with zinc chloride was eliminated and real-time observations with the microscope achieved the principle of controlled margins. The technique was initially treated with skepticism and resistance. The use of wide surgical margins was considered essential to prevent metastatic spread. The theory that serial sections through disease tissue would increase the risk of dissemination was contradicted by the high cure rates reported for the procedure [90]. A recent review by Brodland and colleagues [91] traces the history and evolution of this novel technique to reach its current position as the treatment of choice for certain types of skin cancer.

Current trends in treatment

It is evident from Table 20.4 that many methods of treatment have shown noticeable longevity in the treatment of skin cancer. Surgery and x-ray therapy have been around since 1920. CED entered the clinical landscape in the 1950s, and is still the most widely used method for the treatment of uncomplicated NMSC. In most instances, a particular method is sustained in clinical practice only if it consistently achieves optimal results. The use of one method as the preferred standard of care at a certain time or by one group of physicians results from a complex interplay of factors. It is still not possible to develop an evidence-based approach comparing all these treatment methods, as there are very few controlled studies designed to address relevant issues. In the last century, clinical standards were driven by medical societies, market forces, and even social attitudes. In current practice, patients in a user-pay system generally receive more expensive treatments. Physicians are still accused of favoring procedures for which they receive more remuneration. (George Bernard Shaw addresses this issue adroitly in *The Doctor's Dilemma*, in which he opines that the physician who decides whether or not an operation is necessary is not the one who should be financially rewarded for doing it.)

Commentary

A historian is a prophet in reverse.

—Friedrich von Schlegel

In 1988, Robert Jackson made an interesting observation in an earlier review of this subject [92]: "We had hoped to present a dramatic change in the treatment of skin cancer in the last 125 years. Really, while there have been changes, they have been slow and undramatic, which is probably the way it should be." He also stated, "Immunotherapy is both the way of the past and that of the future." Jackson, astute clinician and historian that he is, gave credence to the corollary of von Schlegel's quotation "A prophet is a historian in reverse." In this decade, cutaneous medicine is on the threshold of a new area, where immunotherapy offers the potential to replace all existing modes of therapy for skin cancer and numerous dermatologic conditions. When the change arrives, it will likely be dramatic and at a faster tempo than the preceding 125 years.

The history of skin cancer treatment should consider prevention efforts, as "prevention is better than cure." Any discussion of preventive measures for NMSC begins with the controversy of whether actinic keratosis is an early change in the spectrum of SCC, a continuing controversy. From a therapeutic and cosmetic perspective, the authors suggest that it is irrelevant whether actinic keratosis is a form of SCC in situ (with the potential to develop into the invasive cancer) or a separate entity that coexists as another effect of ultraviolet damage. Historically, the discovery and use of chemical peels, retinoids, dermabrasion, laser resurfacing, imiquimod, 5-FU, and ALA-PDT are all potentially useful and thus important, particularly for extensive multifocal disease in patients in whom there is very likely a field defect. Chemoprevention has been one focus of research. It is defined as the oral or topical use of dietary or pharmacologic agents to inhibit or reverse the development of cancer [93]. The discovery of toll-like receptors as an important component of the innate immune system, and their regulatory role for the proper function of adaptive and host immune responses, is another exciting part in the field of immunotherapy [94]. Additional recent history includes the development of protein kinase inhibitors and the promise of molecular targeted therapy [95]—because uncontrolled protein kinase activity occurs in human cancer, leading to limitless cell proliferation and tumor survival [96,97].

References

1 Ereaux LP, Schopflocher P, Fournier C. Keratocanthomata. Arch Dermatol 1955;71:73–9.
2 Trapl J, Palacek L, Ebel J, Kucera M. Origin and development of skin melanoblastoma on the basis of 300 cases. Acta Derm Venereol (Stockh) 1964;44:377–80.
3 Clark WH Jr, From L, Bernardino EA, Mihm MC. The histogenesis and biologic behaviour of primary malignant melanoma of the skin. Cancer Res 1969;29:705–26.
4 Stelwagon HW. Treatment of skin cancers without operation. JAMA 1900;35:1547–52.
5 Mohs FE. Chemosurgery in cancer, gangrene and infections. Springfield, IL: Charles C. Thomas; 1956.

6 Stelwagon HW. Diseases of the skin. 8th ed. Philadelphia: WB Saunders; 1918.

7 Martindale W. The extra pharmacopeia. 25th ed. London: Pharmaceutical Press; 1967.

8 Darier J. A text-book of dermatology. (Translated with notes by S. Pollitzer.) Philadelphia: Lea & Febiger; 1920.

9 Dickie WR, Hughes NC. Caustic pastes: their survival as quack cancer remedies. Br J Plast Surg 1961;14:97–109.

10 Smith LM, Garrett HD. Resin of podophyllin in treatment of cancerous and precancerous conditions of skin: Effect on basal cell epithelioma and seborrheic, senile and radiation keratoses. Arch Dermatol Syphilol 1950;61:946–56.

11 Jackson R. Histological findings in normal skin and superficial epitheliomatosis treated with an ointment containing demecolcine. Dermatologica 1959;119:20–30.

12 Falkson G, Schulz EJ. Skin changes in patients treated with 5 fluorouracil. Br J Dermatol 1962;74:229–36.

13 Klein E, Milgrom H, Helm F, et al. Tumors of the skin: I. Effects of local use of cytostatic agents. Skin 1962;1:81–7.

14 Dillaha CJ, Jansen GT, Honeycutt WM, Bradford AC. Selective effect of topical 5-fluorouracil. Arch Dermatol 1963;88:247–256.

15 Haserick JR, Richardson JH, Grant DJ. Remission of lesions in mycosis fungoides following topical application of nitrogen mustard. Cleve Clin Q 1959;26:144–47.

16 Bennett JP. From noli-me-tangere to rodent ulcer: the recognition of basal cell carcinoma. Br J Plast Surg 1974;27:144–54.

17 Handley WS. Pathology of melanotic growths in relation to their operative treatment. Lancet 1907;1:927–33.

18 Pringle JH. Method of operation in cases of melanotic tumours of skin. Edinb Med J 1908;23:496–99.

19 Pringle JH. Cutaneous melanoma: two cases alive thirty and thirty-eight years after operation. Lancet 1937;1:508–9.

20 Amadon PD. Electrocoagulation of the melanoma and its dangers. Surg Gynecol Obstet 1933;56:943–46.

21 Cameron JR. Melanoma of skin: clinical account of series of 209 malignant melanomas of skin. J R Coll Surg Edinb 1968;13:233–54.

22 Ewing MR, Powell T. Some observations on the diagnosis of clinically pigmented skin tumours. Br J Surg 1951;38:442–54.

23 McNeer G, Das Gupta T. Life history of melanoma. Am J Roentgen Ther Nuclear Med 1965;93:686–94.

24 Fortner JG, Booher RJ, Pack GT. Results of groin dissection for malignant melanoma in 220 patients. Surgery 1964;55:485–94.

25 Lund RH, Ihnen M. Malignant melanoma. Clinical and pathologic analysis of 93 cases. Is prophylactic lymph node dissection indicated? Surgery 1955;38:652–59.

26 Block GE, Hartwell SW. Malignant melanoma: a study of 217 cases: part 11. Treatment effect. Ann Surg 1961;154 Suppl:88–101.

27 MacKee G, Cipollaro AC. X-rays and radium in the treatment of disease of the skin. 4th ed. Philadelphia: Lea & Febiger; 1946.

28 Sequeira JH. A preliminary communication on the treatment of rodent ulcer by the x-rays. Br Med J 1901;Feb 9:332–34.

29 Cipollaro AC, Mutscheller A. Absorption of roentgen rays by the skin. Arch Dermatol Syphilol 1940;41:87–97.

30 Strandqvist M. Studein ober die kumulative Wirkung der Røntgenstrahlen bei Fraktionierung. Acta Radio1 1944;55 Suppl:1–300.

31 Goodwin PN, Quimby EH, Morgan RH. Physical foundations of radiology. 4th ed. New York: Harper & Row; 1970.

32 Smithers WD. The x-ray treatment of accessible cancer. London: Edward Arnold; 1946.

33 Kindel DJ. The clinical and experimental use of different types of x-rays, applying them to various levels of the skin. In: Hellerstrom S, Wikstrom K, Hellerstrom A-M, editors. Acta Derm Venereol (Stockh) Proc 11th Int Congr Dermatol 1957;2:392–403.

34 Kalz F. Observations of Grenz ray reactions: I. The response of normal human skin to Grenz rays. II. The effect of over-dosage. Dermatologica 1959;118:357–71.

35 Wrong NM. Treatment of carcinomas of the alae nasi by fractional doses of x-rays. Arch Dermatol 1958;77:73–78.

36 Fitzpatrick PJ, Allt WEC, Thompson GA. Cancer of the eyelids: their treatment by radiotherapy. Can Med Assoc 1972;106:1215–7.

37 Sutton RL Jr. Diseases of the skin, 11th ed. St. Louis: CV Mosby; 1956.

38 Friedman M, Brucer M, Anderson E, Roentgens rads and riddles. Washington, DC: US Government Printing Office; 1959.

39 Cole HN. Chronic roentgen-ray dermatoses as seen in the professional man. JAMA 1925;84:865–74.

40 Pack GT, Davis J. Radiation cancer of the skin. Radiology 1965;84:436–41.

41 Hare HF, Fromer JL, Trump JG, et al. Cathode ray treatment for lymphomas involving the skin. Arch Dermatol Syphilol 1953;68:635–42.

42 Smith IH, Fetterly JCM, Scott J, et al. Cobalt 60 teletherapy: a handbook for the radiation therapist and physicist. New York: Hoebner Medical Divisions, Harper & Row; 1964.

43 Lehman CF, Pipkin JL. Radium in malignant cutaneous disease. JAMA 1954;154:4–8.

44 Howell JB. Radium recipes for cutaneous cancer: the Manchester method. Springfield, IL: Charles C. Thomas; 1972.

45 Epstein E. Cautery excision. In: Epstein E, editor. Skin surgery. 3rd ed. Springfield, IL: Charles C. Thomas; 1970. p. 268–74.

46 Hazen HH. The electric cautery in cutaneous surgery. J Cutan Dis 1917;35:590–93.

47 Jacobson HP, Alcorn DN. Actual cautery surgery in dermatology. Arch Dermatol Syphilol 1950;61:842–52.

48 Elliott JA. Electrosurgery: its use in dermatology, with a review of its development and technologic aspects. Arch Dermatol 1966;94:340–50.

49 Ward GE. Electricity in medicine: electrosurgery. Am J Surg 1932;17:86–93.

50 Ward GE. Value of electrothermic methods in the treatment of malignancy. JAMA 1925;84:660–66.

51 Kovacs R. Minor electrosurgery. Med Rec 1942;155:163–65.

52 Fritsch WC. Electrosurgical excision. Cutis 1971;7:265–69.

53 White AC. Liquid air in medicine and surgery. Med Rec NY 1899;56:109–14.

54 Juliusberg M. Getrierhandlung bei hautkrankheiten. Berl Klinische Wochenschr 1905;10:260.

55 Pusey WA. The use of carbon dioxide snow in treatment of nevi and other skin lesions. JAMA 1907;49:1354–9.

56 Irvine HG, Turnacliffe DP. Liquid oxygen in dermatology. Arch Dermatol Syphilol 1929;19:270–280.

57 Allington HV. Liquid nitrogen in the treatment of skin diseases. Calif Med 1950;72:153–5.

58 Cooper IS, Lee AS. Cryostatic coagulation: a system for producing a limited controlled region of cooling or freezing of biologic tissues. J Nerv Ment Dis 1961;133:259.

59 Zacarian SW, Adham MI. Cryotherapy of cutaneous malignancy. Cryobiology 1966;2:212–8.

60 Zacarian S. Cryosurgery of skin cancer. In: Epstein E, editor. Skin surgery. 3rd ed. Springfield, IL: Charles C. Thomas; 1970. p. 571–7.

61 Torre D. Cutaneous cryosurgery: current state of the art. J Dermatol Surg Oncol 1985;11:292–3.

62 Kuflik EG, Gage AA. Cryosurgical treatment of skin cancer. New York: Igaku-Shoin; 1990.

63 Burns RE. The little curette—a useful adjunct in the treatment of epithelioma. Arch Dermatol 1961;84:662–3.

64 de Saint Exupery A. Wind, sand and stars. New York: Harcourt, Brace & Co; 1940. p. 66.

65 Sherwell S. The technic of an efficient operative procedure for the removal and cure of superficial malignant growths. NY State J Med 1908;8:304–8.

66 Elliott JA, Welton DG. Epithelioma—report on 1742 treated patients. Arch Dermatol Syphilol 1946;53:307–32.

67 Brodeur P. Brocq-Belot's technique in treatment of superficial skin cancers. Can Med Assoc J 1943;49:109–10.

68 Osborne ED. Treatment of malignant cutaneous lesions. JAMA 1954;154:1–4.

69 Lamb JH. Role of the dermatologist in therapy of cancer of the skin. JAMA 1953;153:509–12.

70 Cipollaro AC. Electrosurgery for the treatment of cutaneous neoplasms. Arch Phys Med 1953;34:621.

71 Epstein NN. Electrodesiccation and curettage. In: Epstein E, editor. Skin surgery. Philadelphia: Lea & Febiger; 1956. p. 157–63.

72 King AD. Treatment of epithelioma by modified Sherwell technique: review of 271 cases. Del Med J 1956;28:7–8.

73 Pillsbury DM, Shelley WB, Kligman AM. Dermatology. Philadelphia: WB Saunders; 1956.

74 Knox JM, Lyles TW, Shapiro EM, Martin RG. Curettage and electrodesiccation in the treatment of skin cancer. Arch Dermatol 1960;82:197–204.

75 Freeman RA, Knox JM, Heaton CL. The treatment of skin cancer. Cancer 1964;17:535–8.

76 Sweet RD. The treatment of basal cell carcinoma by curettage. Br J Dermatol 1963;75:137–48.

77 Williamson GS, Jackson R. Treatment of basal cell carcinoma by electrodesiccation & curettage. Can Med Assoc J 1962;86:855–62.

78 Reymann F. Treatment of basal cell carcinoma of the skin with curettage. Arch Dermatol 1971;103:623–7.

79 MacKee GM, Cipollaro AC. X-rays and radium in the treatment of diseases of the skin. 4th ed. Philadelphia: Lea & Febiger; 1946.

80 Proceedings of the 16th Clinical Conference on Selected Aspects of Skin Cancer. Toronto, Ontario: Ontario Cancer Treatment and Research Foundation; 1970.

81 Klein E. Tumors of the skin X-immunotherapy of cutaneous and mucosal neoplasms. NY State J Med 1968;68:900–11.

82 Klein E, Schwartz RA, Solomon J, et al. Accessible tumors. In: LoBuglio AF, editor. Clinical immunotherapy. New York: Marcel Dekker; 1980. p. 31–71.

83 Goldman L, Silver VE, Blaney D. Laser therapy of melanomas. Surg Gynecol Obstet 1967;124:49–56.

84 McGuff PE. Laser radiation for basal cell carcinoma. Dermatologica 1966;133:379–83.

85 Figge FH, Weiland GS, Manganiello LD. Cancer detection and therapy: affinity of neoplastic embryonic and traumatized tissue for porphyrins and metalloporphyrins. Proc Soc Exp Biol Med 1948;68:640.

86 Dougherty TJ. Activated dyes as antitumor agents. J Nat Cancer Inst 1974;52:1333–6.

87 Dougherty TJ. Photosensitizers: therapy and detection of malignant tumors. Photochem Photobiol 1987;45:879–89.

88 Beumer KR, Geisse JK, Helman 0, Fox TL, Ginkel A, Owens ML. Therapeutic response of basal cell carcinoma to the immune response modifier imiquimod 5% cream. J Am Acad Dermatol 1999;41:1002–7.

89 Mohs FE. Chemosurgery: a microscopically controlled method of cancer excision. Arch Surg 1941;42:279.

90 Thissen MR, Neumann MH, Schouten LJ. A systematic review of treatment modalities for primary basal cell carcinomas. Arch Dermatol 1999;135:1177–83.

91 Brodland DG, Amonette RA, Hanke CW, et al. The history and evolution of Mohs micrographic surgery. Dermatol Surg 2000;26:303–7.

92 Jackson R, Laughlin S. Historical survey of methods of treatment of skin cancer. In: Schwartz RA, editor. Skin cancer: recognition and management. New York: Springer-Verlag; 1988. p. 276–91.

93 Wright TI, Spencer JM, Flowers FP. Chemoprevention of nonmelanoma skin cancer. J Am Acad Dermatol 2006;54:933–46.

94 Kang SS, Kauls LS, Gaspari AA. Toll-like receptors: applications to dermatologic disease. J Am Acad Dermatol 2006;54:951–83.

95 Kondapalli L, Soltani K, Lacouture ME. The promise of molecular targeted therapies: Protein kinase inhibitors in the treatment of cutaneous malignancies. J Am Acad Dermatol 2005;53:291–302.

96 Easty DJ, Bennett DC. Protein tyrosine kinases in malignant melanoma. Melanoma Res 2000;10:401–11.

97 Sawyers CL. Opportunities and challenges in the development of kinase inhibitor therapy for cancer. Genes Dev 2003;17:2998–3010.

CHAPTER 21

Curettage and electrodesiccation

Sharyn A. Laughlin, Denis K. Dudley, and Robert A. Schwartz

Curettage and electrodesiccation (CED) is a popular technique employed to treat small skin cancers and precancers [1–4]. It is favored by most dermatologists. Some surgically trained physicians may prefer excision for most nonmelanoma skin cancers (NMSCs), such as basal cell carcinoma (BCC) and squamous cell carcinoma (SCC). However, CED remains an effective modality in properly selected patients.

The curette's semi-sharp edge allows easy distinction and removal of friable malignant tissue with minimal sacrifice of adjacent normal healthy tissue. Electrodesiccation is a type of electrosurgery that is only superficially destructive. It generates electrical energy to destroy tumor cells beyond the reach of the curette, aids in hemostatis, and seals lymphatics [1].

Curettage

The use of a small instrument to remove abnormal tissue by abrasion, or curettage, arose in the 19th century. In 1876, Wigglesworth [5] credited Volkmann of Halle, Germany, for its introduction into dermatologic practice and enthusiastically endorsed the curettage as advantageous when compared with excision or the use of caustics, with healing time and treatment expense lowered and cosmesis improved. In 1870, Piffard [6] introduced the dermal curette in New York; George Henry Fox [7] in 1902 devised a variation on the Piffard curette with a more delicate handle. This small curette with a round head and rectangular handle is still used today. The head contains a thin, sharp side and a dull, thicker side. There is an oval version of this curette and other specialty curettes with thinner handles and angulated heads. Newer instruments may have an open head that allows the exit of debraded material. Most dermatologists use curettes within the 1- to 7-mm range.

Electrodesiccation

Electrodesiccation is the effect produced by a high-frequency (500,000- to 1,000,000-Hz) alternating electrical current of comparatively high voltage ($\geq$2000 V) and low amperage (100 to 1000 mA) using one active electrode [1,3]. The oscillations are damped; that is, the intensity of the voltage rapidly diminishes with each oscillation followed by a gap when there is no voltage, the cycle then being repeated. The two main types of oscillating circuits used to produce electrodesiccation are spark gap (Fig. 21.1) and solid-state devices, the latter largely superseding the former. The active or operating electrode is placed in direct contact with the tissue.

Electrofulguration is the same as electrodesiccation except that the active or operating electrode is held at a slight distance from the tissue, causing a sparking without touching the target tissue. Both terms are often used interchangeably. Both produce superficial tissue damage in contrast to electrocautery, which causes deep destructive tissue injury, with or without coagulation. The dispersive electrode on the patient gives biterminal, low-voltage, high-amperage current, with low or no damping, to cause deep destructive tissue injury.

Procedure and technique
(Figs. 21.1 and 21.2)

Precautions
Caution is advised in the patient with a demand or unshielded pacemaker; digital hearing aids should

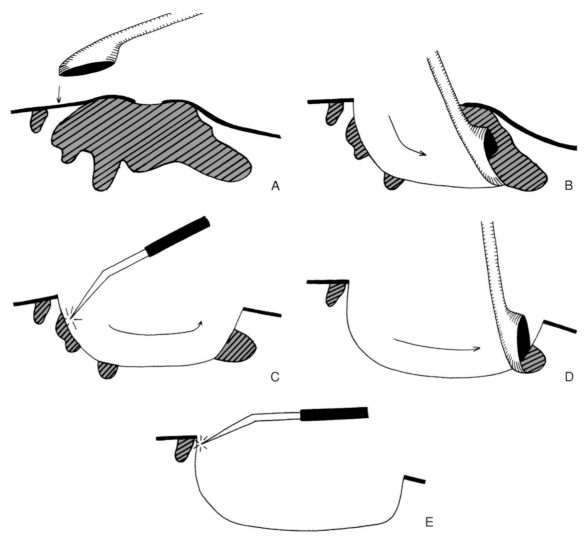

Fig. 21.1 Schematic representation of the technique of removing a BCC by electrodessication and curettage. *Striped areas* represent tumor. *A*, Irregularly shaped tumor with outpouchings. *B*, Anesthetized neoplasm is curetted. *C*, The electrode is applied to the base and edges, so thermal injury can destroy tumor cells beyond the area of curettage. *D*, Repeat curettage. *E*, Electrodesiccation is performed until no visible or curettable tumor is evident.

be removed during any electrosurgery. The procedure should not be performed in the vicinity of flowing oxygen because of the potential for explosion. If employing a reusable needle electrode, care must be taken so there is no transfer of hepatitis B virus or HIV [1]. The patient should be educated in advance about potential complications. Aspirin or warfarin

may predispose to hematologic complications, but this is uncommon. Bleeding can be managed by 10 minutes of firm pressure to facilitate hemostasis.

Morphologic assessment

Inspection and palpation with lit magnification (optical or surgical loupes) facilitates macroscopic

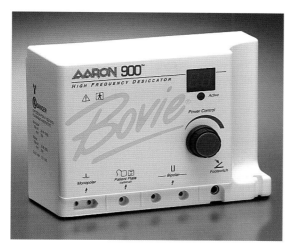

Fig. 21.2 A modern electrosurgical unit used for electrodesiccation, fulguration, and coagulation. (Courtesy of Bovie Aaron Medical, St. Petersburg, Florida.)

diagnosis. Experienced clinicians can often recognize a morpheaform BCC, which has the typical appearance of a flattened sclerotic nodule, similar to a scar, and is unsuitable for CED. Gross examination usually distinguishes small well-defined SCCs from larger invasive ones unsuitable for CED. Obviously, the art of morphologic diagnosis is not foolproof, but facilitates proper selection of neoplasms amenable to CED.

Delineation of clinical margin

Delineate the clinical margin with a skin marker. This assists the operator to insure that the margin of resection by CED extends 2 to 4 mm beyond the clinical border. Outline the tumor with a dark pen or skin marker because the margins are blurred by the local anesthetic, particularly if epinephrine is used.

Antiseptic cleansing of the operative field

The skin is prepared with the antiseptic of choice, avoiding those tinctures with an alcohol base. Flammable solutions, such as alcohol, should not be used to clean the operative field. For lesions on the scalp or face, it is important to inquire whether the patient has applied flammable aftershave, skin care,

or hairspray products. In these instances, it may be necessary to have the patient wash the entire face and hair with a detergent soap solution.

Local anesthetic

With a 27- to 30-gauge needle, local anesthetic is introduced intradermally into uninvolved skin. The choice of ring block, local infiltration, or regional block depends on the size and site of the tumor. Lidocaine with or without epinephrine is used with a suitable technique based on the size and anatomic location of the tumor.

Shave biopsy

A specimen should always be taken, either by shave, punch, or wedge biopsy technique. We usually prefer the shave biopsy. Punch biopsies make curettage more difficult by penetrating the subcutis, so the curette cannot distinguish deep tumor extension from an iatrogenic tract. Punch biopsies may also leave a larger scar. Others suggest that routine biopsy is not necessary before curettage or CED. However, tissue specimens obtained by curettage are inferior to those obtained by shave or punch biopsy. In these litigious times, the prudent physician should rely on a biopsy free from crush artifact for histologic confirmation.

Adequate or firm curettage

Two popular approaches to curettage are the pen and the potato peeler techniques. In the former, the surgeon holds the curette between the thumb, index, and middle fingers, as one would a pen, while the lesion is stabilized by three-point traction. This method is useful for the delicate removal of small to medium-sized tumors. It is always easier to immobilize the skin on the trunk or extremities as compared with that on the ears, eyelids, or lip margins. The curette is held at a 45° angle and is drawn from one margin of the lesion to the other. The second technique uses the curette in a manner similar to that of a potato peeler, by placing the curette between the fold of the index finger, supported by the remaining fingers in a bent position. The thumb from the hand bearing the curette is used with fingers of the other hand to stabilize the lesion by countertraction. Curettage should be performed with the tissue under stretch.

Observation of sensory cues

The basic premise of curettage is that the instrument traverses malignant tissue with little resistance. The texture of the tissue may be indicative of the type of tumor. For example, a BCC imparts a smooth, gelatinous feel to the operator, whereas an SCC may seem slightly more gritty. Both types are easily distinguishable from the firm resistance of normal skin. The silent abrasion and smooth consistency of diseased tissue is associated with pooling of blood, which gives way to rough resistance, a scratching sound, and pinpoint hemorrhage when the instrument breaches the fibrous tissue of normal skin. Match the size of the curette to the lesion to start the process. Once the lesion is essentially abraded, use smaller curettes to probe the base and borders for micro-extensions of tumor. A small curette may be used for the final curettage to locate any tiny pseudopods of tumor that might have been missed. Persistent bleeding is a reliable sign of residual tumor.

Light electrodesiccation

The needle or electrode is applied to the base and edges of the crater until an adequate margin of skin beyond the clinical border is ablated. Thermal injury extends beyond the desiccated zone, and heat transfer probably destroys tumor cells beyond the area of curettage. This produces efficient hemostasis and likely seals the lymphatics and tissue spaces to reduce dissemination of abnormal cells. Electrodessication is employed at a setting that just achieves hemostasis and is used instead of electrofulguration or electrosection with coagulation (electrocautery).

Repeat procedure

Repeat CED for a minimum of two cycles. CED should be performed three times or until there is no visible or curettable tumor. The use of one cycle, presumably in the interest of better cosmesis, is associated with an increased incidence of recurrence. Cure should always take priority over any other objective. The need for additional cycles is appreciated by the experienced clinician from the feel of the previous curettage. If subcutaneous fat is reached, the procedure should be halted and surgical excision used to complete removal of the tumor. As recurrences are common at the periphery, the wound borders should be extended 1 to 2 mm beyond the tumor to insure adequate destruction of pseudopods or small separate tumor foci. The final result is a dry carbonized eschar. The crust will detach within 2 to 6 weeks.

Further management

The wound should be cleansed with a mild soap solution or hydrogen peroxide. It may be kept dry or be treated with a topical antibiotic ointment under occlusion for faster wound healing. At this time, the possible complications of CED should be reviewed again with the patient:
1 Delayed hemorrhage (rarely occurs)
2 Recurrent disease
3 Scarring (atrophic, hypertrophic, or keloidal) and dyschromia
Follow-up examinations should be recommended.

Patient selection

Tumor selection for the curettage and electrodesiccation technique depends on the size, type, and location of the lesion. A balanced approach based on the individual patient should be used. Morpheic or infiltrative BCCs may be suspected midprocedure, when sclerotic stroma produces the resistant consistency of normal dermis. In that case, the area should be sealed by electrodesiccation and abandoned for a surgical approach.

Suitable candidates for CED or curettage alone include those with the following:
• Basal cell carcinomas:
  1 Types: superficial or nodular BCC.
  2 Lesions involving the low-risk locations (trunk, neck, and extremities) measuring less than 1 to 2 cm. An experienced clinician may consider CED for well-defined lesions larger than 2 cm on the trunk or extremities, particularly if surgical expertise is difficult to access.
  3 Lesions on the head measuring less than 1 cm on the intermediate-risk areas (scalp, forehead, pre- and postauricular areas, and the malar prominences).

4 In the high-risk anatomic areas of the eyelids, periorbital area, nose, and nasolabial folds, CED is preferred for small lesions, less than 0.6 cm.
5 Large superficial-multicentric BCC in which surgical excision is fraught with technical and cosmetic problems. CED avoids removing dermis because these tumors are usually very superficial and confined to the epidermis.
• Squamous cell carcinomas: Primary, well-differentiated SCC less than 1 to 2 cm in diameter in areas exposed to the sun are ideal for CED, with the same location and neoplasm size admonitions noted above for BCC.

For the SCC, CED is best avoided in high-risk anatomic sites and for an SCC in which there is a good chance of invasive involvement. The latter category includes SCCs derived from Bowen's disease, inflammatory ulcers or sinuses, and areas of prior radiation or thermal injury, High-risk areas for recurrent SCC include the ear, nose, eyelids, lips, scalp, and regions with no solar exposure—the perineum, sacrum, plantar aspect of the feet, and mucosal surfaces. SCCs that exceed 2 cm have higher recurrence rates and a greater risk of metastasis over smaller ones. These recommendations provide an intuitive basis for avoiding CED in favor of surgical excision or Mohs micrographic surgery. The authors agree that CED is to be discouraged for these clinical situations but is not absolutely contraindicated. Bowen's disease may be better treated by other means as the abnormal cells distribute along the hair follicle and may be missed by CED, although some suggest that treatment with CED is appropriate [4,8].

Lesions usually unsuitable for this treatment include:
1 Large BCCs or SCCs (i.e., >2 cm)
2 Unfavorable histologic subtype: morpheic, micronodular, or metatypical and infiltrative BCC or SCC when invasive or poorly differentiated
3 Lesions involving the nasolabial fold, oral commissures, external auditory canal, and inner canthus of the eye
4 Bowen's disease: the abnormal cells distribute along the hair follicle and may be missed, a relative but not absolute contraindication

5 Tumors that extend into subcutaneous tissue or are deeply invasive
6 SCC associated with inflammatory ulcers or sinuses or prior radiation or thermal injury, in which there is a greater chance of invasive involvement
7 Recurrent or ill-defined tumors
8 Melanomas (excisional biopsy with either an electrocuting instrument or cold-knife surgery is preferable)
9 Postirradiation recurrences

Advantages

The advantages of CED include the following:
• Scars improve with time in contrast to scars from x-ray therapy
• The procedure may be performed in the office quickly and easily without lengthy preparation and is rapid and cost-effective
• Elderly and infirm patients can be treated without hospitalization
• It is a tissue-sparing technique and an appropriate approach for multiple tumors
• In experienced hands, curettage followed by light and delicate electrodesiccation achieves excellent cosmetic outcome (assuming larger lesions on convex surfaces are excluded)
• Recurrences are rare and easily recognized
• There is a low rate of infection with the application of topical antibiotics
• Oral analgesics are not necessary

Disadvantages

The disadvantages of CED include the following:
• Healing depends on the site, size, and depth of the wound, as well as the age of the patient.
• Granulation tissue occasionally develops, is friable, bleeds easily, and may resemble tumor. Application of 75% silver nitrate ($AgNo_3$) stick or removal by electrodesiccation and curettage with biopsy may be necessary.
• Scars show individual variation in size and shape and are also affected by race and tumor site. Punched-out scars are common on the nose. Stellate scars occur in areas that are relatively bound

down. The deltoid and shoulder area, anterior chest, and neck are more prone to development of hypertrophic scars or keloids. This complication may be helped by intralesional corticosteroids. Wound contractures from lesions removed around the eyelid margins or upper lip may result in scars that distort the normal architecture of the face (i.e., ectropions and elevation of lip margins). Multiple small white scars, on a background of dermatoheliosis, are obvious.

• Infection may occasionally develop. Signs of infection include erythema, purulent discharge, and pain. Secondary infection tends to occur in areas that are difficult to keep dry or following prolonged occlusion if the patient insists on covering the wound. A recent prospective study of wound infections in dermatologic surgery in the absence of prophylactic antibiotics found curettage had a 0.73% infection rate (three of 412 procedures) [9].

Variations

Although CED is widely used to treat BCC, the value of electrodesiccation itself is uncertain. Reymann [10] reported that curettage without electrodesiccation, followed by occlusive surgical dressing, results in more rapid healing, better cosmetic results, and the same recurrence rate as for patients treated with CED. Others have had similar experiences [2,11]. A retrospective records review of patients treated with curettage alone at 5-year follow-up or longer showed a 5-year cure rate of 96% [2]. The complications were minimal, mainly hypopigmentation and scarring. Tumors involving more than 50% of the deep edge of the shave biopsy specimen had an increased risk of recurrence. Thus, for nonaggressive BCC, curettage alone may have a cure rate similar to the published rates for CED. Curettage-cryosurgery is another alternative, safe, and inexpensive therapy for selected NMSCs [12,13]. Carefully selected patients receive a thorough curettage followed by freezing with liquid nitrogen in a double-freeze–thaw cycle. Curettage and cautery may be employed for Bowen's disease [8]. One study found it superior to cryotherapy in the treatment of Bowen's disease, especially for lesions on the lower leg.

We recommend consideration of a carbon dioxide laser instead of electrodesiccation after curettage, both of which produce excellent cosmesis. Furthermore, we believe that topical 5% imiquimod after CED also results in improved cosmesis, and possibly a lower rate of recurrence. A pilot study of imiquimod 5% cream once daily for a month as adjunctive therapy to CED for nodular BCC found substantially reduced frequency of residual tumor and improved cosmesis as compared with CED alone [14]. Another pilot study examining the efficacy of curettage alone followed by imiquimod 5% cream for the treatment of primary nodular BCC found primary nodular BCCs on the trunk and limbs were cured, with a favorable cosmetic outcome [15]. The prior curettage provided significant reduction in volume and/or pigmentation of lesions. A similar idea may be employed to optimize photodynamic therapy, using curettage to debulk NMSC and facilitate improved clinical results [16].

Curettage with electrodesiccation may also be performed before excision of BCC and SCC. The intent is to better define the extent of the cancer and thus make its excision more likely to include the entire tumor. By using preoperative curettage, the frequency of incomplete excision, as measured by cancer at the margins after excision, was lower for BCC but not for SCC in one series [17]. Thus, this variation may be beneficial in treating selected skin cancer patients.

A cure is of utmost importance. Scar revision is always possible after adequate follow-up of at least 12 months.

Commentary

Curettage and electrodessication remains the most widely used method of treatment for NMSCs. A balanced appraisal supports the observation that CED is comparable to surgical excision in treating many NMSCs [18]. Dermatologists with training and experience in CED achieve 5-year cure rates around 95% in properly selected patients with BCC and SCC [19,20]. Reported recurrence rates vary from 1.3% to 18.8% [2].

The literature has framed the assessment of risk based on the recurrence rates for anatomic areas

[21,22]. Low-risk sites include the neck, trunk, and extremities, with about 50% less recurrence than on high-risk areas, such as the eyelids and periorbital region, nose, paranasal area, ears, chin, and jaw area. Relatively high recurrence rates occur with SCCs on the pinnae of ears, regardless of therapeutic modality [13]. The unique anatomy of the pinnae, with its lack of adipose tissue or its lymphatic drainage, or both, lends itself to early dissemination or inadequate treatment. In addition, these tumors may be biologically more aggressive. Moderate-risk sites include the other areas on the head: scalp, forehead, and cheeks. Small lesions at any location do well with CED; a 95% cure at 5 years was attained for cancers less than 0.6 cm at high-risk anatomic sites and less than 1 cm at intermediate ones [21]. Physician experience may play a role in outcome, as it has been observed that faculty in clinics or private practices obtain significantly lower recurrence rates than do residents in clinic settings [1,3].

Salasche [23] reported that the nose and nasolabial folds, because of local anatomic peculiarities, were high-risk areas for the recurrence of BCCs treated by electrodesiccation and curettage. He studied electrodesiccation and curettage by the Mohs technique after tumor removal. He was able to demonstrate residual tumor in 30% of cases on the nose and nasolabial fold compared with only 12% of lesions located elsewhere on the head and neck.

Despite these findings, recurrence rates in these special areas are still not 30%. There has been much speculation as to why all cancers do not recur [23,24]. Reactive fibrosis may choke out the blood supply to remaining tumor cells. Insufficient tumor cells may survive to proliferate. An autoimmune regression of remaining cells may occur as the result of release of tumor antigen into the circulation at the time of surgery, with subsequent antibody formation. The surviving cells may be destroyed by a treatment-induced inflammatory response. A combination of these factors may be operative.

The size of tumors being seen today is often much smaller than it was 20 to 30 years ago. Thus, simple methods such as CED may be used more frequently. Larger tumors should be dealt with by a multidisciplinary approach. A plastic surgeon, radiotherapist,

and dermatologist, with a pathologist available for consultations, should contribute their expertise in their approach to management of these patients.

Numerous uncontrolled retrospective studies have been published, some with favorable 5-year recurrence rates: 4% or less for CED [25–27] and up to 10.1% for curettage alone [11]. McDaniel [11] reported a lower recurrence rate of 4.7% in a study of 644 tumors treated by curettage, using life-table analysis to correct for patients lost to follow-up. Proponents of surgical excision emphasize retrospective literature showing higher 5-year recurrence rates, up to 6% to 26% for CED compared with 3% to 10% for surgical excision or radiation [19,20]. Two large reviews were reported by Crissey [28] and by Rowe and colleagues [29], with 5-year recurrence rates of 7.4% and 7.7%, respectively. The latter group reviewed all studies after 1947 and reported combined 5-year recurrence rates of 7.7% (274/3573) for CED, 10.1% for excision, 7.5% for cryotherapy, 8.7% for radiation, and the lowest rate of 1% for Mohs micrographic surgery. More recent studies confirm the trend that CED compares favorably with excision—3% versus 1%, respectively [18]—and curettage alone achieves a 96% cure rate at 5 years [2]. High 5-year cure rates can also be obtained after CED of primary nonfibrosing BCCs of medium- and high-risk facial areas [30].

The essential skill required for CED is a tactile phenomenon facilitated by visual and auditory signals [21,22,31,32]. Tumor detaches easily, with a smooth consistency, and is replaced by the coarse resistance of normal fibrous tissue. The "feel" transmitted to the experienced dermatologist by the curette is associated with visual and audible changes. During abrasion of abnormal tissue, there is a relative silence and a pooling or oozing of blood that is replaced by a scraping sound and pinpoint bleeding as the curette traverses normal tissue. Critics dispute this concept as subjective and nebulous. However, it should be emphasized that this skill or "feel" is real and is easily learned.

Proponents of surgical excision claim that higher recurrence, scarring, and dyschromia should restrict the use of CED in current dermatologic practice. A recent quality-of-life outcomes study of patients with NMSC found similar results after excision and

Mohs surgery, with both therapies having better outcomes than CED [33]. However, the fact that it has survived for 100 years with excellent results suggests that CED is an effective treatment in properly selected patients that can be employed with confidence.

References

1 Sheridan AT, Dawber RP. Curettage, electrosurgery and skin cancer. Australas J Dermatol 2000;41:19–30.

2 Barlow JO, Zalla MJ, Kyle A, et al. Treatment of basal cell carcinoma with curettage alone. J Am Acad Dermatol 2006;54:1039–45.

3 Jackson R, Laughlin S. Electrosurgery: a review. Dermatol Clin 1984;2:233–44.

4 Goldman G. The current status of curettage and electrodesiccation. Dermatol Clin 2002;20:569–78, ix.

5 Wigglesworth E. The curette in dermal therapeutics. Bost Med Surg J 1876;94:143–6.

6 Piffard HG. Histological contribution. Am J Syphilol Dermatol 1870;1:217.

7 Fox GH. Photographic atlas of the diseases of the skin in four volumes. New York: Kettles Publishing Co; 1905.

8 Ahmed I, Berth-Jones J, Charles-Holmes S, et al. Comparison of cryotherapy with curettage in the treatment of Bowen's disease: a prospective study. Br J Dermatol 2000;143:759–66.

9 Dixon AJ, Dixon MP, Askew DA, et al. Prospective study of wound infections in dermatologic surgery in the absence of prophylactic antibiotics. Dermatol Surg 2006;32:819–26; discussion 826–7.

10 Reymann F. 15 years' experience with treatment of basal cell carcinomas of the skin with curettage. Acta Derm Venereol Suppl (Stockh) 1985;120:56–9.

11 McDaniel WE. Therapy for basal cell epitheliomas by curettage only. Further study. Arch Dermatol 1983;119:901–3.

12 Dixon AJ. Multiple superficial basal cell carcinomata—topical imiquimod versus curette and cryotherapy. Aust Fam Physician 2005;34:49–52.

13 Nordin P, Stenquist B. Five-year results of curettage-cryosurgery for 100 consecutive auricular non-melanoma skin cancers. J Laryngol Otol 2002;116:893–8.

14 Spencer JM. Pilot study of imiquimod 5% cream as adjunctive therapy to curettage and electrodesiccation for nodular basal cell carcinoma. Dermatol Surg 2006;32:63–9.

15 Wu JK, Oh C, Strutton G, et al. An open-label, pilot study examining the efficacy of curettage followed by imiquimod 5% cream for the treatment of primary nodular basal cell carcinoma. Australas J Dermatol 2006;47:46–8.

16 Souza CS, Neves AB, Felicio LA, et al. Optimized photodynamic therapy with systemic photosensitizer following debulking technique for nonmelanoma skin cancers. Dermatol Surg 2007;33:194–8.

17 Chiller K, Passaro D, McCalmont T, et al. Efficacy of curettage before excision in clearing surgical margins of nonmelanoma skin cancer. Arch Dermatol 2000;136:1327–32.

18 Werlinger KD, Upton G, Moore AY. Recurrence rates of primary nonmelanoma skin cancers treated by surgical excision compared to electrodesiccation-curettage in a private dermatological practice. Dermatol Surg 2002;28:1138–42; discussion 1142.

19 Dubin N, Kopf AW. Multivariate risk score for recurrence of cutaneous basal cell carcinomas. Arch Dermatol 1983;119:373–7.

20 Thissen MR, Neumann MH, Schouten LJ. A systematic review of treatment modalities for primary basal cell carcinomas. Arch Dermatol 1999;135:1177–83.

21 Williamson GS, Jackson R. Treatment of basal cell carcinoma by electrodesiccation and curettage. Can Med Assoc J 1962;86:855–62.

22 Kopf AW, Bart RS, Schrager D, et al. Curettage-electrodesiccation treatment of basal cell carcinomas. Arch Dermatol 1977;113:439–43.

23 Salasche SJ. Curettage and electrodesiccation in the treatment of midfacial basal cell epithelioma. J Am Acad Dermatol 1983;8:496–503.

24 Jackson R. Why do basal cell carcinomas recur (or not recur) following treatment? J Surg Oncol 1974;6:245–51.

25 Tromovitch TA. Skin cancer; treatment by curettage and desiccation. Calif Med 1965;103:107–8.

26 Knox JM, Freeman RG, Duncan WC, et al. Treatment of skin cancer. South Med J 1967;60:241–6.

27 Spiller WF, Spiller RF. Treatment of basal cell epithelioma by curettage and electrodesiccation. J Am Acad Dermatol 1984;11:808–14.

28 Crissey JT. Curettage and electrodesiccation as a method of treatment for epitheliomas of the skin. J Surg Oncol 1971;3:287–90.

29 Rowe DE, Carroll RJ, Day CL Jr. Long-term recurrence rates in previously untreated (primary) basal cell carcinoma: implications for patient follow-up. J Dermatol Surg Oncol 1989;15:315–28.

30 Rodriguez-Vigil T, Vazquez-Lopez F, Perez-Oliva N. Recurrence rates of primary basal cell carcinoma in facial risk areas treated with curettage and electrodesiccation. J Am Acad Dermatol 2007;56:91–5.

31 Zalla MJ. Basic cutaneous surgery. Cutis 1994;53:172–86.

32 Adam JE. The technic of curettage surgery. J Am Acad Dermatol 1986;15:697–702.

33 Chren MM, Sahay AP, Bertenthal DS, et al. Quality-of-life outcomes of treatments for cutaneous basal cell carcinoma and squamous cell carcinoma. J Invest Dermatol 2007;127:1351–7.

CHAPTER 22
Cryosurgery

Emanuel G. Kuflik

Cryosurgery is generally used to some degree by all dermatologists. It is useful as a primary or as an alternate form of treatment for cutaneous malignancies. The word *cryotherapy* is often used interchangeably with *cryosurgery*, although the latter is more descriptive. Actinic and other keratoses and skin cancers can be treated with it.

Cryobiology

Although cryosurgery is relatively simple to perform, one should have an understanding of the cryobiological effects and tissue reactions that occur after deep freezing of tissue. This knowledge along with selection of a suitable patient and proper technique can bring about successful treatment.

The goal of cryosurgery is to cause selective necrosis of tissue. The extent of destruction depends on the type, size, and depth of the lesion and the volume of freezing that is needed. Tissue alterations are caused by reduction of the skin temperature and consequent freezing of the cells [1]. The rate of heat transfer is a function of the temperature difference between the skin and the heat sink (liquid nitrogen). Because the difference is great, rapid heat transfer occurs.

The tissue response to freezing of tissue ranges from an inflammatory reaction to mild destruction, and to complete necrosis, as is needed for eradication of malignant lesions [2–4]. The mechanisms of injury in cryosurgery may be attributed to the direct effects of freezing tissue and to vascular stasis. The former results in intracellular and extracellular ice crystal formation, disruption of cell membrane integrity, pH changes, impairment of multiple homeostatic functions, and thermal shock. This damage

is enhanced during subsequent thawing of the tissue by the development of vascular stasis, which leads to failure of the local microcirculation. Slow cooling produces extracellular ice, but this is not as damaging as rapid cooling that produces intracellular ice formation. Therefore, rapid cooling of the target tissue is imperative, whereas the rate of rewarming, or thawing, should proceed slowly. With repeated freeze–thaw cycles, maximum destructive effects are produced. The tissue reactions that ensue after deep freezing are predictable. The underlying stroma provides a structural framework for wound repair.

Liquid nitrogen is the coldest cryogenic agent ($-196°C$ boiling point) with the greatest freezing capability. Other cryogenic agents are available, including nitrous oxide, carbon dioxide, and fluorinated hydrocarbons, but they are not recommended for skin cancer, rather for lesions that require lesser degrees of freezing. Modern cryosurgery uses an apparatus that employs liquid nitrogen in a closed system that permits continuous and rapid extraction of heat from tissue. The dominant apparatus for dermatologic use is a handheld unit that can be used either with a spray-tip accessory or with a closed cryoprobe (also known as contact therapy). Although the same equipment is used for various types of neoplasms, the technique of treatment, the volume of liquid nitrogen, the duration of cooling, and the amount of tissue being frozen may vary.

Indications and contraindications

Cryosurgery is good for actinic keratoses, Bowen's disease, and selected basal and squamous cell malignant carcinomas. The indications are related to

Table 22.1 Indications for cryosurgery

Lesion selection
Actinic keratoses
Other premalignant keratoses
Bowen's disease
Basal cell carcinomas
Squamous cell carcinomas

Patient selection
No age limitation
High-risk surgical patient
Pacemaker, blood coagulopathy
Limited mobility, debilitated
Where other methods are contraindicated, impractical
Patients fearful of surgery

the nature of the lesion and to the type of patient (Table 22.1). The advantages of cryosurgery are numerous and are listed in Table 22.2.

Different types of basal cell carcinomas (BCCs) and squamous cell carcinomas (SCCs) may be treated, as well as actinic and other keratoses, Bowen's disease, Kaposi's sarcoma, and skin metastases [5]. Lesions most amenable to treatment have well-delineated borders, but they may be of any size. Cryosurgery is suitable for difficult tumors, especially for patients who are elderly, are debilitated, or

Table 22.2 Advantages of cryosurgery

Versatility
Treatment of any area of the body
Palliative therapy for inoperable tumors
Excellent cosmetic results
Suitable for office, nursing home, or outpatient facility
Low cost
No general anesthesia
Local anesthesia optional
Operative suite not required
Safe and relatively simple procedure
No restriction of work or sports
Useful in pregnancy
For patients who are fearful of undergoing surgery
For poor surgical risk patients
No age limitations—excellent for the very elderly
Suitable for wheelchair and stretcher patients

have limited mobility. It is useful for patients with pacemakers or coagulopathies, for lesions located within psoriatic plaques, or when other methods of treatment are impractical or undesirable. Any area of the body may be treated, including the eyelids.

Cryosurgery may also be effective in selected recurrent tumors and ones that are fixed to cartilage or bone [6]. It may be used for inoperable tumors or for cases in which the goal of therapy is palliation—for example, to relieve pain, reduce tumor bulk, or facilitate nursing care.

There are few contraindications to cryosurgery. Patients who have cold urticaria, cold intolerance, cryofibrinogenemia, or cryoglobulinemia are best treated by other means. Tumors with indistinct or ill-defined borders (e.g., morpheaform or infiltrative histologic subtypes) as well as deeply penetrating and very aggressive lesions are not suitable candidates. Cryosurgery is not considered to be a standard treatment for malignant melanoma. The operator should be aware that in patients with darkly pigmented skin, freezing may result in hypopigmentation. Undertreatment of malignancies should be avoided, for it may lead to inadequate destruction or recurrence. Caution should be observed when treating lesions that lie superficially over nerves, such as those on the fingers or ulnar fossa, and the free margin of the ala nasi should be carefully treated because scarring or retraction of the tissue may occur. The physician should also be aware of treating cancers located at the inner canthus and the auditory canal, because tumors may invade deeply or unwanted tissue damage may occur. Also, lesions in which treatment might lead to functional alterations or an unsightly cosmetic appearance are best treated by other means. Patients may opt for another form of treatment when faced with the prospect of a long healing period.

Practical considerations

In planning treatment, consideration should be given to the characteristics of the cancers, which technique of cryosurgery to employ, and the expected results. An explanation of the procedure and the expected response of the tissue to freezing—for example, exudation, crusting, re-epithelialization, and healing time—should be discussed with the patient.

When tissue is frozen, the surface freezing and extension of the ice ball is visible, yet the depth of freeze cannot be seen. Therefore, the amount of freezing and the temperature reached beneath and surrounding the lesion must be determined by the surgeon. This is referred to as the depth dose. It consists of measuring certain clinical factors (observation, palpation, freeze time, thaw time, and lateral spread of freeze) as well as the tissue temperature. The proper depth dose estimation is achieved when clinical observations and the tissue temperature, if measured, have reached the desired end point [7].

Treatment factors

Freeze time

The *freeze time* refers to the duration of cooling. It is longer for a malignancy than it is for a premalignant lesion. For example, 4 to 10 seconds with the open spray technique is sufficient for an actinic keratosis, whereas 45 seconds may be required for a small BCC. For large tumors, a proportionately longer freeze time is needed. The freeze time may be altered by the thickness of the lesion and by the amount of liquid nitrogen being emitted from the spray tip. When the cryoprobe technique is used, the freeze time is approximately two to three times longer than the open spray technique. After freezing, the tissue is permitted to thaw spontaneously and the thaw time is usually two to three times longer than the freeze time.

Lateral spread of freeze

The *lateral spread of freeze* refers to the freezing of the tissue beyond the margins of the lesion. For BCCs and SCCs, the lateral spread of freeze should extend at least 3 to 5 mm or more around the tumor.

Freeze–thaw cycle

A *freeze–thaw cycle* refers to the actual cooling and thawing of the lesion. A single cycle is usually sufficient for benign and premalignant conditions, whereas a double freeze–thaw cycle is recommended for malignant lesions. This is done to ensure greater lethality to cancerous cells.

Temperature at the base of the tissue

To supplement the clinical estimations, one can measure the temperature at the base of a malignancy with the use of a thermocouple that is mounted in the tip of a 25- to 30-gauge needle. It is inserted into the skin at a 25° to 30° angle, from a point lateral to the lesion, with the tip coming to lie beneath the lesion. This is useful for lesions that lie more than 3 mm below the skin surface and for medicolegal reasons. Because the temperature recorded is very localized, more than one thermocouple may need to be inserted for a large lesion. The recommended temperature to be reached at the base of a malignancy is between −50°C and −60°C.

Description of techniques

There are four techniques of cryosurgical treatment for malignancies. The choice of which one to use depends on the lesion and the preference of the operator. The cotton-tip applicator method is not recommended for malignant lesions.

Open spray and cotton-tip application

The open spray method is the most frequently used technique and employs a cryosurgical unit, liquid nitrogen, and spray-tip attachments. A fine spray of liquid nitrogen is directed at the lesion from a distance of approximately 1 to 2 cm. A cotton-tip applicator may also be used for actinic keratoses, as will be described in the section on actinic keratoses. An intermittent spray of liquid nitrogen is desirable when malignant lesions are treated to ensure that there is complete conversion of the nitrogen to the gaseous phase. The duration of freezing may range between 30 and 60 seconds, for a small lesion, and proportionately longer times for larger ones.

Cryoprobe

The cryoprobe technique, also known as contact therapy, employs a cryosurgical unit and consists of application of a flat, precooled metal tip that is placed firmly onto the lesion. It is useful for round lesions and those on flat surfaces. The freeze time may range up to several minutes for malignancies.

Confined spray

The confined spray technique is a variation of the open spray in which the spray is directed into a cone that is held against the skin, thereby confining its effect. The freeze time is the same as for the open spray technique.

Closed cone

The freeze time is half that of the open spray technique because the liquid nitrogen is very concentrated to a focal area of skin. The closed cone technique also confines the spray by an accessory that is attached to the cryosurgical unit at one end and open at the other. It is held against the skin, enabling it to rapidly freeze the lesion.

Treatment of BCC and SCC

Treatment is carried out after determination of the type of lesion and selection of the technique of treatment. During the past two decades, there has been an increased use of colder temperatures, greater use of debulking techniques, and a trend toward more aggressive treatment for BCCs and SCCs. For malignant lesions, the same volume of tissue must be destroyed by freezing that would have been removed by conservative local excision if that had been the chosen procedure. Several preoperative biopsy specimens may be obtained to delineate the margins of a tumor.

The target site is cleaned, and a local anesthetic is generally injected. Thermocouple needles may be implanted at this time. The entire tumor is usually frozen in one session using a double freeze–thaw cycle. The aforementioned clinical factors are observed, and through palpation, one can ascertain the extent of the ice ball. The recommended temperature is between −50°C and −60°C at the base of the tumor, and the freeze time approximately 45 seconds for a 1-cm lesion (Table 22.3). At the conclusion of treatment, a dry gauze dressing is applied and instructions given to the patient concerning postoperative care.

The author reported a 5-year cure rate of 99% for 522 new cancers [8]. The overall 30-year cure rate was 98.6% for 4406 BCCs, SCCs, and basosquamous cell carcinomas. Other investigators

Table 22.3 Recommendations

Temperature goals: −50°C to −60°C
Debulking
Aggressive therapy
Experience with cryosurgical techniques

obtained results similar to those of conventional surgery [9,10]. Graham [11] had a combined cure rate of 98% for 3593 new BCCs using mostly the open spray technique. Holt [12] reported a 5-year cure rate of 97% in 395 nonmelanoma skin cancers. Zacarian [13] reported an 18-year cure rate of 97.4% in the treatment of 4228 carcinomas. A 5-year follow-up study by Nordin and colleagues[14] of 50 patients with large primary BCCs on the nose resulted in only one recurrence. The cure rate for recurrent BCCs was found to be lower (88.4%) [15].

After treatment of a malignancy, the tissue responds in a predictable manner that leads to healing of the wound by second intention. The reactions that ensue after freezing include erythema, edema, exudation, and sloughing. Malignant lesions on the face, eyelids, nose, ears, and neck generally heal between 4 and 6 weeks (Figs. 22.1 to 22.4). Large

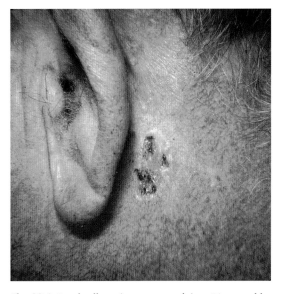

Fig. 22.1 Basal cell carcinoma on neck in a 64-year-old man.

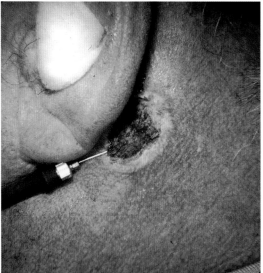

Fig. 22.2 Cryosurgery to entire tumor.

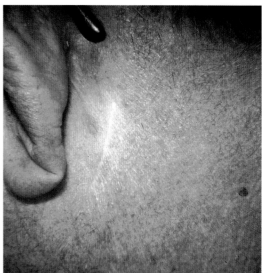

Fig. 22.4 The area is completely healed 2.5 years after treatment.

tumors and those on the trunk and extremities take longer to heal, sometimes up to 14 weeks (Figs. 22.5 to 22.8). The cosmetic results after cryosurgery are often equal or superior to those achieved by other modalities. Wounds reapproximate natural skin contours, and keloid formation does not occur. Cryosurgery is advantageous for tumors on the ears and nose because cartilage is relatively resistant to freezing damage and the architecture of the structure is preserved. Lesions on the eyelids and in the vicinity of the lacrimal duct are good candidates for cryosurgery because the

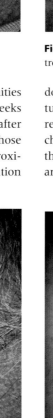

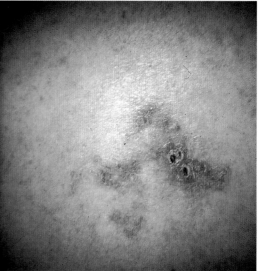

Fig. 22.3 Exudative reaction 1 week after treatment.

Fig. 22.5 Large BCC on chest of a 70-year-old woman.

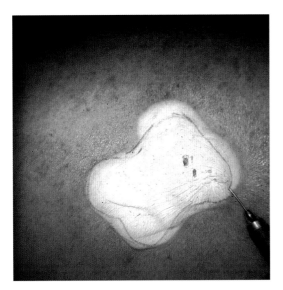

Fig. 22.6 Cryosurgery to entire tumor. Thermocouple needle is in place.

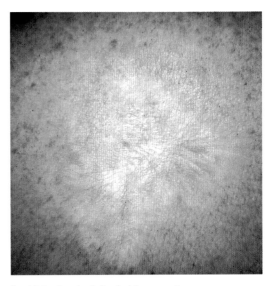

Fig. 22.8 The site is healed 2 years after treatment.

likelihood of ectropion is small and damage to the lacrimal outflow system is rare [16,17] (Figs. 22.9 to 22.13).

Variations and unusual situations

If a lesion is thick or bulky, it is beneficial to reduce it to a shallow one with a curette, scissors, or electrosurgery. This is done because the mass is detrimental to proper treatment, either by hindering the advancement of the ice ball, misjudging the placement of thermocouple needles, or prevention of proper assessment of the lateral margins and base of the lesion. After debulking, hemostasis must be obtained before proceeding with cryosurgery.

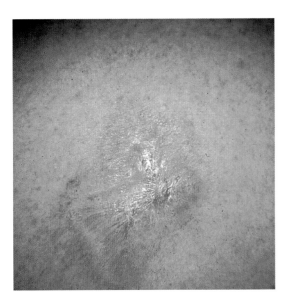

Fig. 22.7 Healing 14 weeks after treatment.

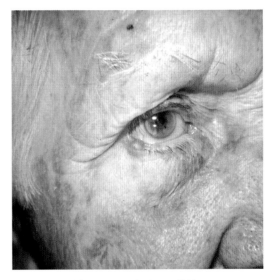

Fig. 22.9 Nodular BCC on the lower lid in an 82-year-old woman.

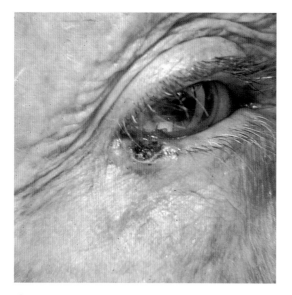

Fig. 22.10 Target site after biopsy.

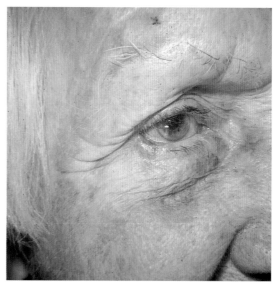

Fig. 22.12 Healed site 5 weeks after treatment.

It is sometimes beneficial to inject lidocaine for the purpose of lifting a lesion away from underlying tissue or nerves that lie superficially. Examples include the treatment of lesions on the hands, head, neck, and scalp.

Selected large BCCs or SCCs are amenable to cryosurgery using segmental treatment [18]

(Figs. 22.14 to 22.16). A lesion is treated in stages after being divided and can be treated either on the same day or at subsequent visits. Each section is treated according to its characteristics and depth. Wound healing is not hindered by overlapping treatment at the margins.

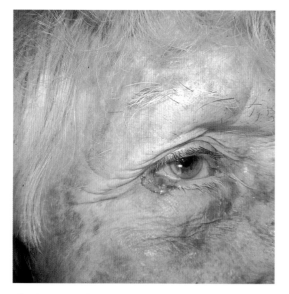

Fig. 22.11 Exudative reaction 1 week after treatment.

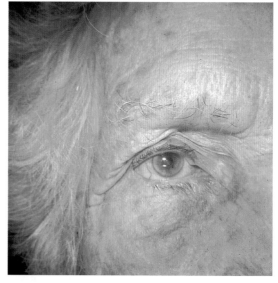

Fig. 22.13 Healed site 2 years after treatment.

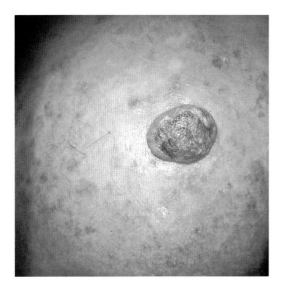

Fig. 22.14 Nodular SCC on scalp in an 80-year-old woman.

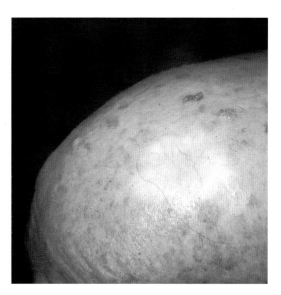

Fig. 22.16 The area is completely healed 1 year after treatment.

Postoperative care

Extensive exudation begins within 24 hours and diminishes in an orderly manner as the wound heals and re-epithelializes. The wound is washed with soap and water four times daily in the exudative

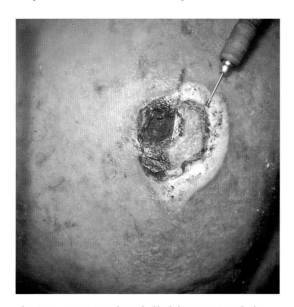

Fig. 22.15 Freezing of one half of the tumor, with the lateral spread of freeze visible.

stage and less often during the granulating period. A dry gauze dressing is initially applied, and as the wound begins to heal, an antibiotic ointment is used. In some instances, oral antibiotics are beneficial, such as for cancers on the legs and ears, or where otherwise indicated. Bullae may form at the periphery of a large lesion but are not a complication. The bullae are simply drained, and healing proceeds as normal. Edema, particularly periorbital, can be minimized or ameliorated with open wet compresses, corticosteroid cream, or a short course of systemic corticosteroids. The author reported using an intramuscular injection of 4 mg betamethasone sodium phosphate, 1 mL 30 minutes before treatment, and followed by oral prednisone, 20 mg/day for 3 days [19].

Complications

The incidence of complications after cryosurgery is low. They can be divided into temporary or permanent complications. However, it is important to distinguish between expected sequelae and untoward results. A complication may arise as an unexpected event (e.g., infection), as an unsatisfactory cosmetic result (e.g., hypertrophic scarring), or as a more pronounced response of the tissue to freezing than had been anticipated (e.g., residual hypopigmentation).

Temporary complications that may develop during the healing stage or after completion of treatment generally resolve spontaneously. Some examples include edema of the eyelids or ears and hypertrophic scarring. Occasionally, hypertrophic scarring may develop, particularly after treatment of a large lesion, but this always improves and resolves with time, usually within months. If desired, intralesional injection of a corticosteroid suspension may hasten resolution. Uncommon reactions include delayed bleeding, headache, paresthesia, neuropathy, secondary infection, syncope, nitrogen gas insufflation (gas bubbles in skin), milia, hyperpigmentation, and pyogenic granuloma.

Permanent complications include retraction of tissue, (e.g., lips, eyebrows, ala nasi), tissue defect, depigmentation, notching, ectropion, alopecia, and contour defects. Improvement in some may occur, often in an elderly patient, as a result of skin laxity.

Treatment of actinic keratoses and other neoplasms

Cryosurgery is a treatment of choice for actinic keratoses and other keratoses and may be effective for Bowen's disease, Kaposi's sarcoma, actinic cheilitis, and skin metastases [2]. For actinic keratoses, some use a cotton-tip applicator, dipping the applicator stick into liquid nitrogen and then onto the lesion. But the open spray technique, spraying a lesion for approximately 4 to 10 seconds, is a better choice because it is more consistent and reliable. It produces a shallow crust that falls off within 2 weeks. The freeze time for actinic cheilitis ranges between 10 and 20 seconds. Bowen's disease responds well to cryosurgery but the freeze time may vary depending on the size of the lesion. Small Kaposi's sarcoma lesions and metastatic ones can be similarly treated.

References

1 Kuflik EG, Gage AA. Cryobiology. In: Cryosurgical treatment for skin cancer. New York: Igaku-Shoin; 1990. p. 35–51.

2 Kuflik EG. Cryosurgery updated. J Am Acad Dermatol 1994;31:925–44.

3 Yamada S, Tsubouchi S. Rapid cell death and cell population recovery in mouse skin epidermis after freezing. Cryobiology 1976;13:317–27.

4 Giuffrida TJ, Jimenez G, Nouri K. Histologic cure of basal cell carcinoma treated with cryosurgery. J Am Acad Dermatol 2003;49:483–6.

5 Kuflik EG, Gage AA. Cryosurgical treatment for skin cancer. New York: Igaku-Shoin; 1990.

6 Kuflik EG, Gage AA. Recurrent basal cell carcinoma treated with cryosurgery. J Am Acad Dermatol 1997;37:82–4.

7 Torre D. Depth dose in cryosurgery. J Dermatol Surg Oncol 1983;9:219–25.

8 Kuflik EG. Cryosurgery for skin cancer: 30-year experience and cures rates. Dermatol Surg 2004;24:297–300.

9 Bernardeau K, Derancourt C, Cambie M, et al. Cryosurgery of basal cell carcinoma: a study of 358 patients. Ann Dermatol Venereal 2000;127:175–9.

10 Jaramillo-Ayerbe F. Cryosurgery in difficult to treat basal cell carcinoma. Int J Dermatol 2000;39:223–9.

11 Graham GF. Cryosurgery. Clin Plast Surg 1993;20:131–47.

12 Holt P. Cryotherapy for skin cancer: results over a 5-year period using liquid nitrogen spray cryotherapy. Br J Dermatol 1998;119:231–40.

13 Zacarian SA. Cryosurgery of cutaneous carcinomas: an 18-year study of 3022 patients with 4228 carcinomas. J Am Acad Dermatol 1983;9:947–56.

14 Nordin P, Larko O, Stenquist B. Five-year results of curettage—cryosurgery of selected large basal cell carcinomas on the nose: an alternative treatment in a geographical area underserved by Mohs' surgery. Br J Dermatol 1997;136:1.

15 Kuflik EG, Gage AA. Cryosurgical treatment for skin cancer. New York: Igaku-Shoin; 1990. p. 243–54.

16 Kuflik EG. Cryosurgery for carcinomas of the eyelids: a 12-year experience. J Dermatol Surg Oncol 1985;11:243–6.

17 Buschmann W. A reappraisal of cryosurgery for eyelid basal cell carcinomas. Br J Ophthalmol 2002;86:453–7.

18 Kuflik EG. Cryosurgical treatment of large basal cell carcinomas on the trunk. J Dermatol Surg Oncol 1983;9:226–30.

19 Kuflik EG, Webb W. Effects of systemic corticosteroids on post-cryosurgical edema and other manifestations of the inflammatory response. J Dermatol Surg Oncol 1985;11:464–8.

CHAPTER 23
Excision of skin cancer

Daniel M. Siegel and Jeffrey I. Ellis

Basal cell carcinomas (BCCs) and squamous cell carcinomas (SCCs) comprise the bulk of skin cancers. These neoplasms may start out asymptomatic and inconsequential looking, but if improperly treated, may be very destructive to the host and, even more ominously, incurable. Their cure is accomplished either by destroying or removing all malignant cells. There are several means of achieving this goal. The skill of the therapist is perhaps more important than the means. The best treatment is one that cures the patient with minimal discomfort and has the best long-term cosmetic result.

Excision provides a means not only of removing a cancer, but also of providing an intact specimen for microscopic evaluation. Excision specimens are typically examined in a "bread loaf" fashion, a suboptimal method that is often adequate for small tumors [1]. Microscopic control of surgical margins by Mohs technique can maximize both success and cosmesis.

When excision is selected as the method of treatment, the following factors have an immediate bearing on a successful result:

1 Microscopic characteristics of the cancer: A good biopsy is essential in most cancer therapy. Excision is likely to be successful when the histology shows a compact lesion. Infiltrative and sclerotic neoplasms have a higher risk of recurrence. To minimize this risk, it is often appropriate to widen surgical margins when excising such a tumor, or to use Mohs micrographically controlled surgery.

2 Location: Ideal areas for excision are those where skin is loose enough to allow adequate margins while permitting linear repairs. In areas where the skin is tightly bound, as the nose and ears, or func-

tional, as in the eyelids, reconstruction may become more complex.

3 Size of the lesion: The smaller the lesion, the easier it is to treat, especially in the difficult areas mentioned above.

4 Age of the neoplasm: Cancers are not static; they may grow unpredictably. As they age, both wider and deeper invasion often occurs. Wider margins or Mohs micrographically controlled excisions may become necessary. Thus, over time, reconstruction of defects becomes more complex.

5 Previous treatment: Unsuccessful therapy may alter the architecture of a skin cancer. Scar tissue may hide residual tumor, increasing the likelihood of incomplete excision and recurrence with each subsequent treatment. Recurrent tumors are often best treated with Mohs micrographically controlled surgery.

The mechanics of excisional surgery are facilitated by:

1 An assistant trained in operative procedures: Such an assistant can prepare the patient, take preoperative photographs, inject local anesthetic, set up instruments on a Mayo stand, sponge out a bloody field, apply pressure as needed, apply the cautery electrode to forceps to coagulate bleeders, cut sutures after tying, retract incision margins, and in many ways aid in making the surgery faster and more efficient. An able aide or nurse can be trained to do this work in about 6 to 8 weeks. It is important to include as part of training tips related to safety. An excellent review of safety tips can be found in an article by Trizna and Wagner titled "Surgical pearl: preventing self-inflicted injuries to the dermatologic surgeon" [2].

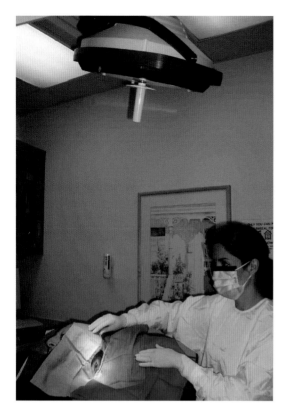

Fig. 23.1 Good surgical lighting and an adjustable table are essential in a well-equipped operating room.

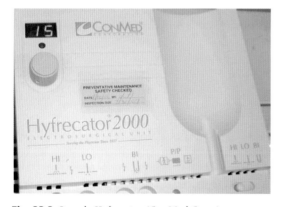

Fig. 23.2 Sample Hyfrecator (ConMed Corp.).

2 A well-equipped operating room: This should include a good light, adjustable operating table, Mayo stand, an electrodesiccator, electrosurgical or radiofrequency surgical unit, and an electric suction apparatus. See Figs. 23.1 to 23.3.

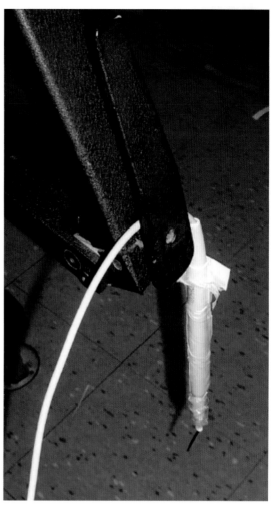

Fig. 23.3 The hyfrecator handpiece may be conveniently draped over the headrest table lock.

3 High-quality stainless steel instruments: A satisfactory basic surgical pack may include (see Fig. 23.4):

Needle holder: 5 to 5.5 inches
Forceps: Adson 2-1 (two teeth on one tip, one on the other)
Siegel scalpel handle with #15 blades and #10 blades
Scissors: suture cutting
Curved iris (fine and medium)
Undermining (Kilner type)

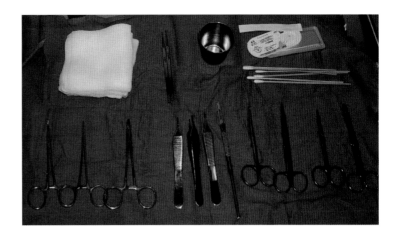

Fig. 23.4 A sample surgical pack.

Bandage (Lister)

Skin hooks

Mosquito clamps (straight and curved)

Towel clamp

4 General surgical supplies, including:

Gauze: 3 × 3, or 4 × 4

Hyfrecator sterile sleeves

Medicine glass

Sutures: a satisfactory variety includes 2-0, 3-0, 4-0, 5-0, 6-0 Vicryl, nylon, and Prolene on 3/8-circle reverse cutting needle or half-circle reverse cutting needle in a variety of sizes dictated by the surgeon's preferences. 5-0 and 6-0 fast-absorbing gut sutures are also quite useful for surface closures where there is minimal tension on the wound [3].

Suture removal scissors and forceps

Adhesive reinforcing strips

Adhesive tape for postoperative bandaging

Syringes and 30-gauge needles for anesthesia

5 Emergency supplies: These should also be available in a suitable container in or near the operating room. A suggested list includes:

Spirits of ammonia

Airway

3-mL syringes with 26-gauge 0.5-inch needles

Epinephrine (1:1000)

Oxygen, with demand valve, mask, and bag

These emergency supplies, including the pressure of the oxygen tank, should be checked on a regular schedule. In addition, staff should have routine basic life support training. Advanced cardiac life support training might also be of value. Most critically, a plan to contact local emergency services, usually by dialing 911 in the United States, and to support the patient until their arrival is invaluable. A vasovagal episode should be followed up by an electrocardiogram, as it may represent a silent posterior wall myocardial infarction.

Instruments are best prepared by washing and scrubbing with a brush with or without ultrasonic cleansing. Some lubricate with "instrument milk" before packing and sterilization. Sterilization by autoclave is most common in the office setting, but some opt for dry heat or gas sterilization. Several basic surgical packs can be kept available for immediate use when desired. Instruments used less frequently should be kept sterilized and individually wrapped, to be opened as needed for complex cases.

Procedure

Before surgery, a careful history is taken and the procedure discussed with the patient. It is essential to know if there are allergies, particularly to local anesthetics and antibiotics. True lidocaine allergies are extremely rare. The authors have sent patients claiming these for allergy prick testing and

have never seen a positive confirmation. Most reactions that patients describe are the result of the
epinephrine, though patients may be allergic to
amide anesthetics or the preservative. "Epinephrine
allergy" itself does not exist, but rather reflects
a history of inadvertent intravascular infusion of
epinephrine containing local anesthetic, often during a dental procedure. An allergist may be helpful
if a true allergy to anesthetic is suspected. General
conditions, such diabetes mellitus, hypertension,
bleeding tendencies, anticoagulant therapy, and
cardiac arrhythmia should be checked and noted.
Patients should also be asked about pacemakers,
defibrillators, artificial valves, or other implanted
hardware, and appropriate antibiotic prophylaxis,
if indicated, should be prescribed. It is useful to capture this on a standardized form that forces staff to
specifically inquire about these items. The discussion should include an explanation of the planned
operation, alternative methods of therapy, and
expected cosmetic results. The patient should also
be made aware of risks, complications, and the possibility that further treatment may be required. The
consent form should be written in language under-
standable to the patients and their lawyers. A well-
informed patient is often more cooperative and may
accept a suboptimal result more readily than would
a less prepared patient.

Before starting the procedure, the patient should
be given an opportunity to empty his or her bladder.
Preoperative antibiotics, when indicated, should
also be given before the procedure. The patient is
then placed on the operating table in a comfort-
able position and grounded to the electrosurgical or
radiofrequency surgical devices, if appropriate. The
area to be operated on is then well exposed and the
neoplasm marked.

Usually no premedication is given, and many patients return to work after surgery if the operative
site is not compromised by doing so. If mild preoperative sedation is needed, sublingual diazepam, 2.5
to 10 mg, or similar agents 30 minutes before the
procedure may be helpful. The patient receiving sedation must be accompanied by someone who can
drive him or her home.

A careful examination of the biopsy slide or
pathology report at this time will assist the surgeon

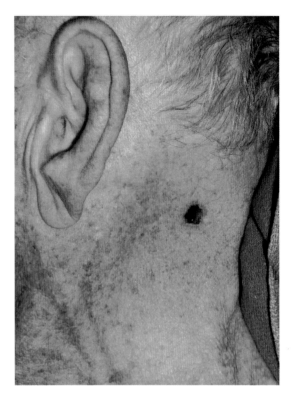

Fig. 23.5 Surgical site before marking.

in deciding on adequate margins. Sometimes tumor margins are clinically distinct, and other times
they are ill defined (Fig. 23.5). Successfully removing all the malignant tissue at the time of initial
surgery depends on precisely defining the borders
of the carcinoma. If the skin is dampened with alcohol or water, stretched, and studied carefully with a
good binocular loupe of at least 5-diopter strength,
borders can often be identified. (The use of dermoscopy with a device such as the DermLite [3Gen,
LLC] may also be valuable in elucidating poorly defined margins.) Margins are dotted with 0.5% aqueous gentian violet or other suitable marker, such as
the Sharpie permanent black marker. When complete, the dots are connected, outlining the clinical
margins of the tumor (Fig. 23.6). Outside of this,
an additional line of dots is placed to indicate the
planned border of normal tissue to be included in
the excision (Figs. 23.7 to 23.9). The area to be
anesthetized is also marked with several dots (see

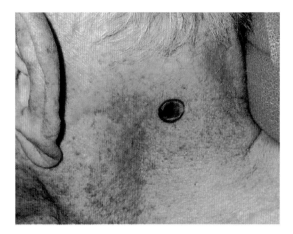

Fig. 23.6 The clinically evident cancer is marked.

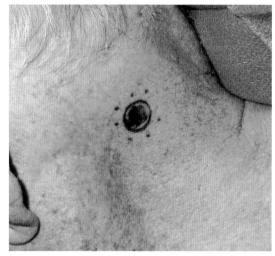

Fig. 23.8 The margin is marked with dots.

Fig. 23.13). For BCCs less than 2 cm in diameter, a minimum margin of 4 mm is expected to clear the tumor in more than 95% of cases [4]. Surgical margins for primary cutaneous SCCs range from 4 to 6 mm, depending on anatomic and histopathologic factors [5]. All marks should be done before anesthesia is injected (see Figs. 23.15 and 23.16), as this will change the color and texture enough to make evaluation of tumor margins more difficult.

The tissue is then pinched lightly (Figs. 23.10 and 23.11). The patient is asked to wrinkle and move the site. This will help to determine the best orientation for the line of closure and may be drawn in if desired. In some cases, the drawing of lines par-

allel to relaxed skin tension lines may help in designing the excision. Where this is obvious, the initial excision may be fusiform (Fig. 23.12). It may additionally be useful to draw in anatomic landmarks or anticipated locations of important structures (Fig. 23.14). In cases in which the best line

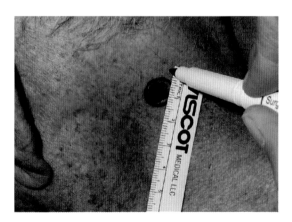

Fig. 23.7 The appropriate margin is measured.

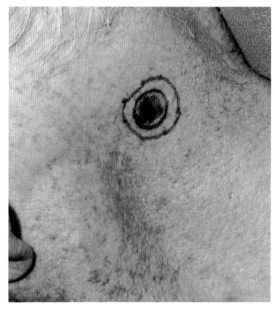

Fig. 23.9 The dots are connected.

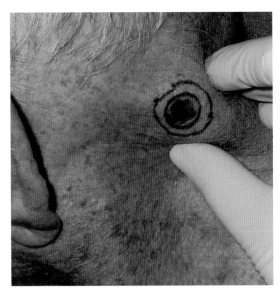

Fig. 23.10 The area is pinched to determine the best line of closure.

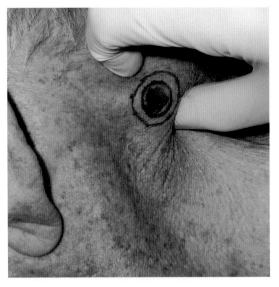

Fig. 23.11 The area is pinched in an alternative orientation to determine the best line of closure.

of closure is difficult to determine before excision, the neoplasm may be removed as a disk in the shape of the tumor plus the planned margin of normal tissue (Fig. 23.17). Once this disk

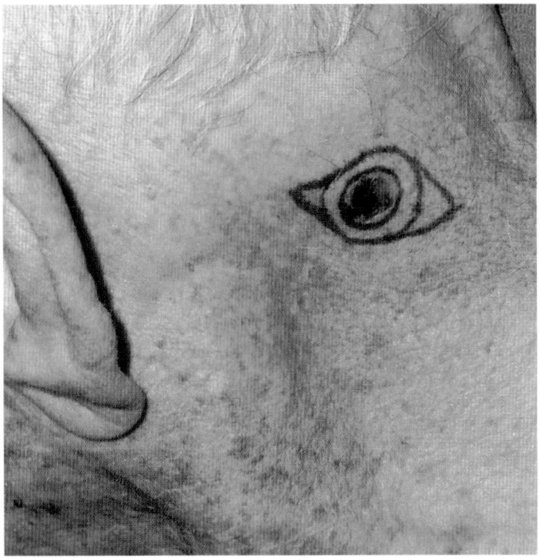

Fig. 23.12 A fusiform is outlined in the chosen orientation of closure.

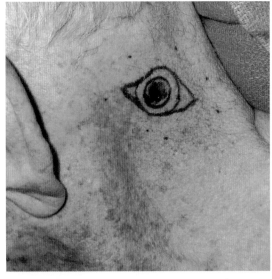

Fig. 23.13 The area that will need local anesthesia is identified with dots.

has been removed, the margins of the defect can be pressed together (Figs. 23.18 to 23.20) until it becomes apparent which direction will give the most satisfactory closure (Fig. 23.20), and

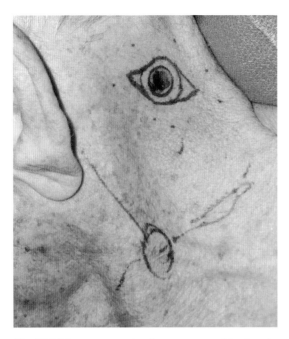

Fig. 23.14 Important anatomic structures and landmarks are outlined.

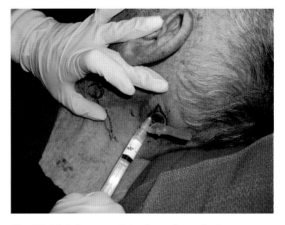

Fig. 23.16 Subsequent injections of anesthesia are administered into areas that are already anesthetized to minimize patient discomfort.

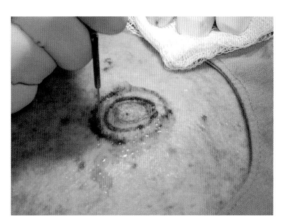

Fig. 23.17 A cancer with margin is excised as a disk.

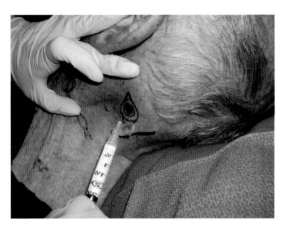

Fig. 23.15 Anesthesia is administered.

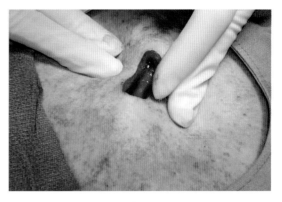

Fig. 23.18 The area is pinched in several orientations to determine the best line of closure.

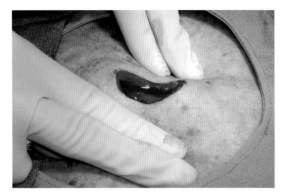

Fig. 23.19 An alternative orientation for wound closure.

standing cones are then removed if necessary to create a fusiform defect (Fig. 23.21).

In addition to visual assessment, another means of determining the tumor borders is by careful curettage. Friable malignant tissue may be curetted out to a firm, healthy base. The "feel" of the curette aids in discovering nonvisible extensions of the carcinoma. The resulting defect, which may actually be tumor-free, can then be outlined and the defect plus a margin of "normal" tissue excised in the usual manner for microscopic evaluation. This procedure provides a means for discovering extensions of tumor that are not clinically visible, and may result in a lower likelihood of recurrence.

The main disadvantage of this method is that the architecture of the tumor in relation to the margins of excision is lost. However, if the initial biopsy was adequate, all that need be seen on excisional pathology is residual scar with surrounding disease-

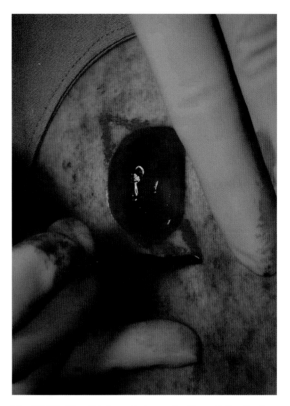

Fig. 23.21 The disk is made into a fusiform defect in the orientation chosen.

free tissue to be reassured of a successful operation. Both methods may be tried; experience will indicate to the surgeon which one he or she finds preferable.

After marking, the area is ready for anesthesia. Lidocaine with or without epinephrine is an excellent local anesthetic. The authors use 10 parts lidocaine, 1% with epinephrine 1:100,000 buffered in the bottle with 1 part 8.4% sodium bicarbonate solution (10 mL of anesthetic to 1 mL of buffer), which eliminates the sting of the anesthetic without affecting efficacy or shelf life [6]. Some find it convenient to use steel dental syringes with glass carpules, though drawing 3-mL syringes from a 30-mL vial of 1% lidocaine with epinephrine is more cost-effective. Carpules are available without preservative, without epinephrine, and with a variety of ester anesthetics as needed.

For larger lesions, or in patients in whom hemostasis is a concern, tumescent anesthesia is

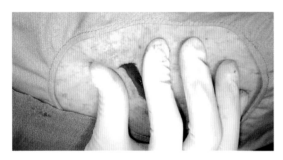

Fig. 23.20 Another option to consider for wound closure.

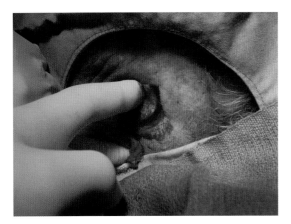

Fig. 23.22 The island of tissue moves freely.

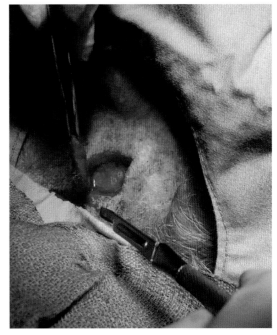

Fig. 23.23 The base of the tumor island is dissected.

often useful. Preparations are easily made by diluting one part 1% lidocaine with epinephrine with 10 parts normal saline. For example, 25 mL of 1% lidocaine with epinephrine would be injected into a 250-mL bag of normal saline. For patient comfort, the saline bag should be slightly warmer than room temperature. An 18-gauge needle attached to a 30- to 60-mL syringe may then be used to rapidly inject the tumescent mixture, passing through areas of the skin that have received small amounts of undiluted lidocaine superficially. To allow for maximal hemostasis, at least 30 to 45 minutes should be allowed to pass before beginning any procedure in which the patient is anesthetized via the tumescent technique.

After marking and anesthetizing the planned excision, a thorough surgical preparation is done, including the area of excision and a wide zone around it. PHisoHex, Betadine, and Hibiclens all work well. Betadine is our preferred preparation, as it is safe around the eye and ear and is not teratogenic.

If 10 to 20 minutes are allowed after injection when standard anesthesia is employed, excellent hemostasis will usually be obtained. This markedly cuts down bleeding during surgery. Before starting the operation, the surgeon should test by needle pricking to confirm that the anesthesia is working. The patient who feels no pain is usually much calmer and completes the procedure in much better condition than if there is discomfort.

Using the previous guidelines, an incision is made through the full thickness of the skin to the subcutaneous fatty tissue. If the depth is sufficient, considerable gaping will take place between the block of tissue containing the carcinoma and the adjacent skin. The island of tissue should move freely, giving a good indication that the cancer has not invaded deeper to bind it down (Fig. 23.22).

If deep tethering is noted, the entire underlying subcutaneous fat should be removed in continuity with the overlying tumor.

As soon as this has been determined, one edge of this island is grasped with toothed Adson forceps and cut free of its base with scissors or a knife (Figs. 23.23 and 23.24). A suture or hemostat is then placed for orientation (Figs. 23.25 and 23.26). To reduce confusion and chance of error, this suture is usually placed at the superior or most proximal portion of the specimen. The specimen should be oriented on a piece of suture packet paper to further diminish the risk of misorientation.

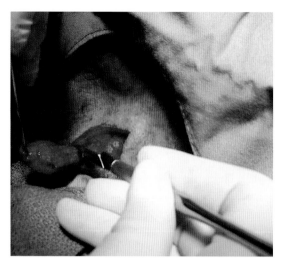

Fig. 23.24 The base of the tumor island is further dissected, and the tumor removed.

Before submitting the tissue for pathologic examination, some surgeons will place orientation dyes in addition to the orientation suture.

Using an electrodessicator, or other electrosurgical/radiofrequency device, small bleeding points can be lightly cauterized (Figs. 23.27 and 23.28). Where a vessel is large enough to bleed in surges or spurts, it is grasped by mosquito forceps and clamped. When it is apparent that bleeding from the vessel has been controlled, the needle of the cautery electrode is

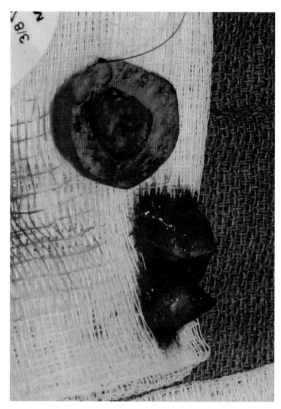

Fig. 23.26 An example of a suture used to mark orientation. (This tumor was shown in Fig. 23.17.)

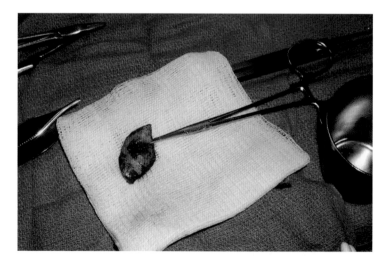

Fig. 23.25 A hemostat is placed for orientation.

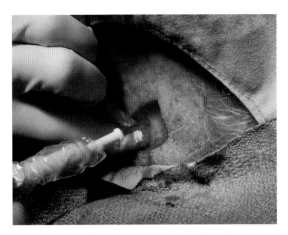

Fig. 23.27 Use of a Hyfrecator to control bleeding of small vessels.

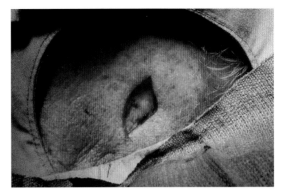

Fig. 23.28 A dry field after cautery, ready for closure.

pressed gently against the shaft of the forceps and the current activated with the foot pedal. Slight contraction of the tissue at the tip of the clamp should be noted. The clamp can then be released gently and the area observed to determine whether bleeding is controlled.

Occasionally a larger vessel may be cut. In these instances, the vessel is also clamped with mosquito forceps, and 5-0 absorbable suture such as Vicryl is used as a ligature. If the absorbable suture is swaged on a needle, it can be passed close under the tip of the clamp through the tissue adjacent to it. A triple knot in this case assures good control of the bleeding vessel.

After initial control of bleeding, preparation is made for closure of the defect. Ordinarily, most small lesions will be closed in a line by side-to-side approximation. In cases in which this is not feasible, a flap may be advanced or rotated into position or the defect closed by a free graft removed from another, "donor" site. Detailed discussions of surgical techniques are available in many excellent texts [7–12]. If a circle is to be made into a fusiform defect, it will be necessary to remove a standing cone, the location to be determined as previously mentioned by drawing the skin edges together (Figs. 23.18 through 23.21). The need for removal of standing cones may be assessed only after approximation of the defect's side walls. It will often be discovered that the standing cone removal is no longer required.

Small standing cones left behind will flatten over a few months on active or convex areas, leaving patients with smaller surgical scars—an option that may be worth discussing with the patient beforehand. Fig. 23.29 shows how standing cones do self-correct.

If the standing cones are removed, they may also be marked for pathologic evaluation to facilitate recognition of a subclinical neoplasm within them that may extend to an excision margin. The margins of this fusiform defect are then undermined, usually at the level of the base of the dermis or deeper, depending on the anatomic site. For the nose, undermining is accomplished below muscle, whereas for much of the midface, undermining may take place above the superficial muscular aponeurotic system. The more extensive the undermining, the less tension there is on the closure (Fig. 23.30). However, the more extensive the undermining, the greater the risk for postoperative bleeding and hematoma formation. Of note, excellent cosmetic results may be obtained with either no or minimal undermining.

Closure of the incision may then be done using dermal sutures in any one of several techniques, including mattress, running, and interrupted sutures. If buried absorbable sutures are used to close the defect (Figs. 23.31 to 23.33, 23.37), skin sutures that are used for precise apposition of skin edges are under no tension and can be removed and replaced by

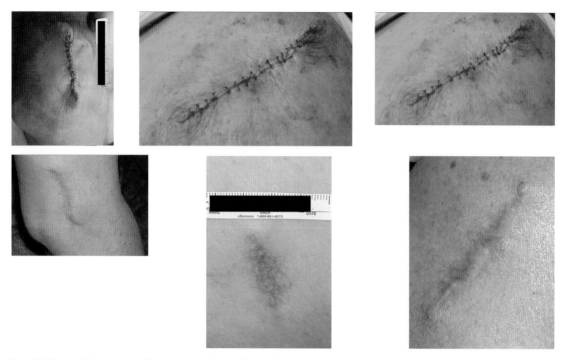

Fig. 23.29 Standing cones self-correcting. The top three photos demonstrate small standing cones left at the time of surgery from the arm, back, and shoulder. The bottom three photos of the scar line at 6 weeks postoperation demonstrate flattening of the standing cone from the arm, back, and shoulder.

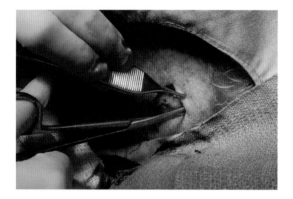

Fig. 23.30 Undermining of tissue margins.

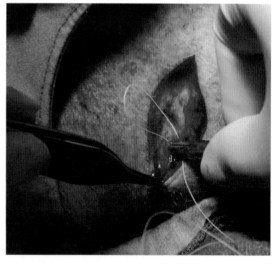

Fig. 23.31 Placing of the first subcuticular suture in a planned two-layer closure.

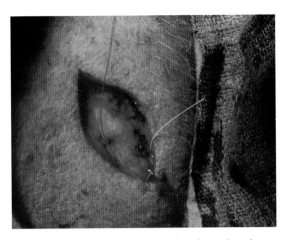

Fig. 23.32 The subcuticular suture is tightened, and wound edges begin to approximate each other.

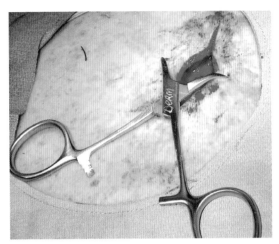

Fig. 23.34 A towel clamp bringing together tissue under tension.

tape closures in 6 or 7 days, reducing the chance of suture marks along the incision line. At times, a towel clamp may be used to stretch tissue and bring skin edges together to allow for easy placement of buried sutures (Figs. 23.34 to 23.36). When skin edges are under no tension, fast-absorbing gut sutures may be used for closure (Fig. 23.38). This allows the use of a waterproof, maintenance-free dressing as described later in the chapter.

Sometimes longer support is desired for active patients, such as children, or for mobile body parts, including the chest and back. In that case, a running intradermal suture may be employed, entering the skin at one end of the incision and exiting from the other, zigzagging from side to side horizontally in the dermis [12: fig. 16.13, p. 240]. It may then be

tied over a bolus of gauze, which also helps to stabilize the incision line. This type of suture may be left in for 2 weeks. Alternatively, if Prolene sutures are used, these may be left in for longer periods of time. Smooth monofilament synthetic material can easily be drawn out up to 2 inches. If a greater length than this is buried, it is well to bring a loop to the surface

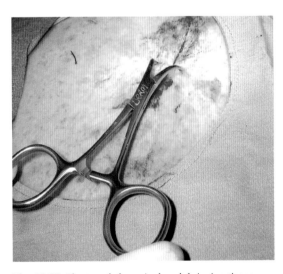

Fig. 23.35 The towel clamp is closed, bringing tissue together when a suture is placed and allowing for intraoperative tissue stretch.

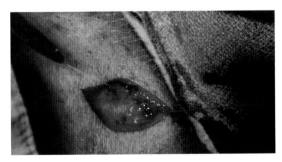

Fig. 23.33 Tying of the first subcuticular suture in a planned two-layer closure.

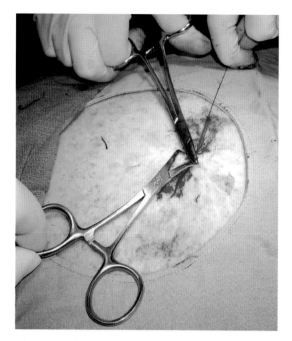

Fig. 23.36 The tissue is tied with the towel clamp in place.

at intervals along the incision to reduce the length of suture to be pulled out later. Incisions have very little strength in 5 to 7 days. When sutures are removed, especially where there may be either more than usual motion or pull on the closure, it is well to

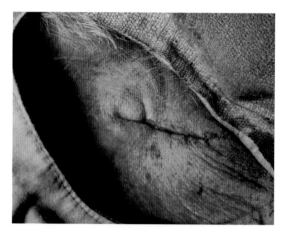

Fig. 23.37 All deep subcuticular sutures have been placed, and wound edge well approximated.

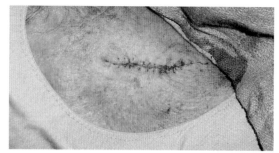

Fig. 23.38 In this case, running fast-absorbing gut sutures are used for fine cutaneous approximation.

reinforce thoroughly with tape closures, prolonged application of a "splint" of tape, or DuoDerm.

After the surgery is completed, it is of utmost importance to have an adequate and appropriate pressure dressing. This greatly reduces the chance of postoperative complications. The principles of a good dressing are simple. The wound must be kept clean and moist, and pressure should be applied for a minimum of 48 hours. To accomplish these goals, two techniques are outlined in Figs. 23.39 to 23.48.

Technique for a standard pressure dressing
(Figs. 23.39 to 23.43)

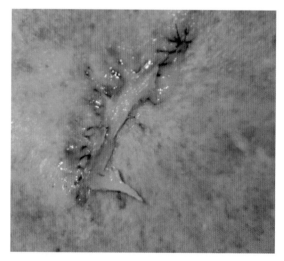

Fig. 23.39 The surgical margins are coated with emollient (Vaseline).

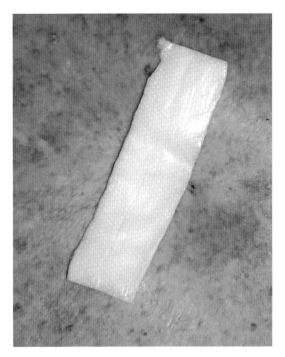

Fig. 23.40 A Telfa nonstick dressing is cut to size and applied.

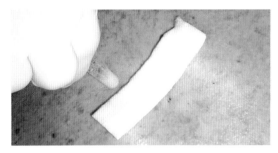

Fig. 23.41 Mastisol is used around the area to improve the adherence of the pressure dressing.

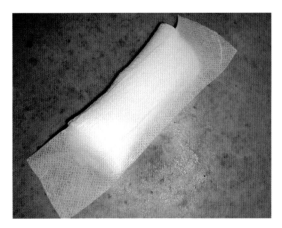

Fig. 23.42 Gauze is rolled or "fluffed" and held in place with a piece of Hypafix elastic tape.

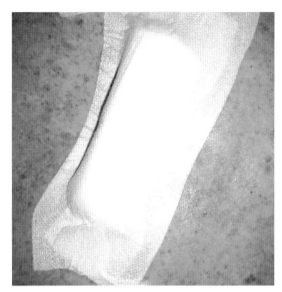

Fig. 23.43 Hypafix is placed over the bolster of gauze so that pressure is applied over the gauze but not on the skin edges.

Technique for a waterproof, maintenance-free dressing (used when wound is closed with 5-0 or 6-0 fast-absorbing gut suture)

(Figs. 23.44 to 23.48)

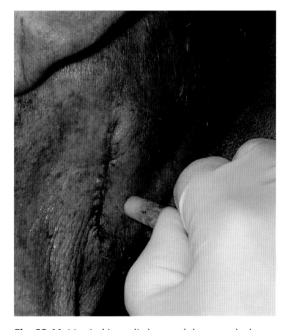

Fig. 23.44 Mastisol is applied around the wound edge.

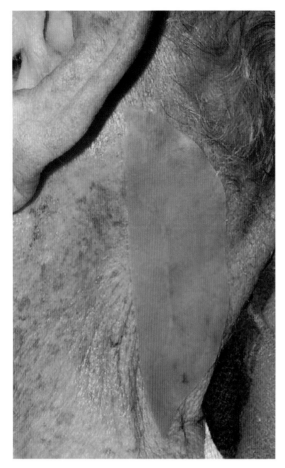

Fig. 23.45 A hydrocolloid dressing such as Duoderm or Restore is applied over the wound (note, no Vaseline is used).

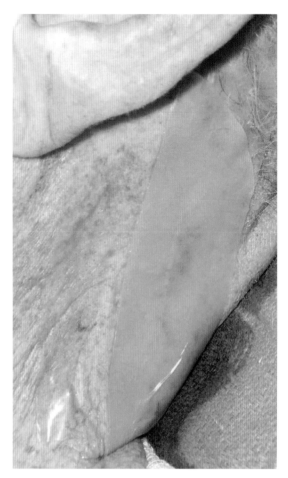

Fig. 23.46 Opsite or Tegaderm is applied over the hydrocolloid dressing. This dressing will be left in place for the next week and, if applied correctly, is watertight.

Complications

The principal complications of excision are:

1 Hemorrhage: This usually occurs in the first 24 hours. If a significant hematoma has formed, the incision should be reanesthetized and opened as needed, the clot removed, any bleeders controlled, and the defect reclosed. This will result in much faster healing and a better cosmetic result. At times, it may be possible to aspirate a hematoma with an 18-gauge needle after appropriate anesthesia. If this fails, one may always convert to opening part or all of the original defect.

2 Infection: Some ulcerated cancers are frankly infected. When infection is present, antibiotics should be started 2 to 3 days before surgery and continued until healing is well under way and the surgical site appears free of infection.

3 Dehiscence: Occasionally a wound will open even when sutures are removed 10 days to 2 weeks postsurgically. Either timely resuturing or allowing the defect to heal by secondary intention is an acceptable option, with the decision based on the cause of the dehiscence. Wounds dehisced under grossly contaminated circumstances are best left to heal by secondary intention.

4 Keloid/hypertrophic scar: The patient should be warned regarding this possibility. Injections of triamcinolone into the scar may arrest keloid

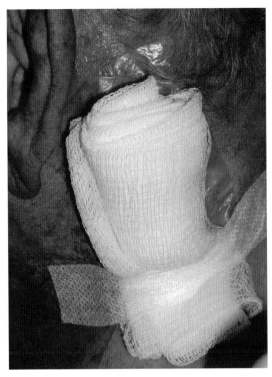

Fig. 23.47 A bolster of gauze is placed over the waterproof dressing and held in place with a strip of Hypafix.

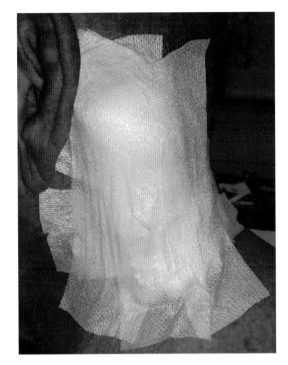

Fig. 23.48 Additional Hypafix is applied to create uniform pressure over the bolster with no pressure on the surrounding skin. This pressure dressing will be removed in 48 hours by the patient at home.

formation. Concentrations of 4 to 40 mg/mL may be appropriate, depending on the clinical context.

Pathology

If the physician decides to dye the specimen for orientation, blue dye (laundry bluing), black (India ink), red (Mercurochrome), or other tissue dyes are applied to the margins and base. This confirms that what appears as the margins on the slide, are in fact the surgical margins and not artifacts caused by fragmenting of the tissue in fixation or a bias cut of the tissue in the block. The excised specimen, marked with a suture and dye, is then sent to the lab with instructions for cutting and sectioning. It is essential to have a close working relationship with the technician who prepares the slides and the pathologist.

If malignant cells are found to extend to a margin, inking the pathologic specimen for orientation allows for timely clinical correlation to facilitate necessary re-excision. The second excision includes the former scar with additional tissue on the side where microscopic examination indicated failure. Alternatively, one may consider Mohs micrographic surgery for any residual tumor.

At times, a margin will appear clear but insufficiently wide. In such instances, it may be useful to remove additional tissue. Because there is always a chance of involved margins between cuts [1], especially in a diffuse lesion with relatively narrow margins, the patient is instructed to observe the area regularly throughout his or her life. As a routine, scars from surgical excisions should be examined as part of follow-up visits. Scars showing change in the opinion of the patient or on physical examination should be biopsied with a punch or excisional technique to identify recurrence.

In the majority of tumors, borders can be ascertained clinically with considerable accuracy, and there is sufficient adjacent healthy tissue to permit closure with adequate margins. In those cases, closure may be done immediately and the excised tissue submitted to the dermatopathologist for standard fixed sections. In cases in which microscopic evaluations of margins following simple excision are felt to be critical, as in the case of a difficulty in defining those margins, surgical repair may be delayed. This is particularly important in neoplasms in which repair requires a graft or flap.

Flap rotation particularly alters the anatomy, making localization of a positive margin a challenge. Frozen sections produced on modern equipment are good for evaluating borders when performed by a skilled technician or pathologist. The specimen is dyed in the usual way, frozen, sectioned, strained, and microscopically evaluated before closure is done. Mohs technique, which allows visualization of 100% of the surgical margin, is an ideal approach in cases in which margins are critical.

Conclusion

It cannot be emphasized enough that skin cancer is a progressive, serious problem and that the physician who first treats a malignancy should approach it aggressively and vigorously. The first physician to treat it has the best chance to cure it. Failure to do so may result in a tragic, disfiguring, and often miserable problem years later.

References

1 Abide JM, Nahai F, Bennett RG. The meaning of surgical margins. Plastic Reconstr Surg 1984;73:492–7.

2 Trizna Z, Wagner RF Jr. Surgical pearl: preventing self-inflicted injuries to the dermatologic surgeon. J Am Acad Dermatol 2001;44:520–2.

3 Siegel DM, Sun DK, Artman N. Surgical pearl: a novel cost-effective approach to wound closure and dressings. J Am Acad Dermatol 1996;34:673–5.

4 Wolf DJ, Zitelli JA. Surgical margins for basal cell carcinoma. Arch Dermatol 1987;123:340–4.

5 Brodland DG, Zitelli JA. Surgical margins for excision of primary cutaneous squamous cell carcinoma. J Am Acad Dermatol 1992;27:241.

6 Melman D, Siegel DM. Prefilled syringes: safe and effective. Dermatol Surg 1999;25:492–3.

7 Stegman SJ, Tromovitch TA, Glogau RG. Basics of dermatologic surgery. Chicago: Yearbook Medical Publishers; 1982.

8 Epstein E, Epstein E Jr. Skin surgery. 6th ed. Philadelphia: WB Saunders Co.; 1987.

9 Hill GJ. Outpatient surgery. 3rd ed. Philadelphia: WB Saunders Co; 1988.

10 Anderson R, Hoopes J. Symposium on malignancies of the head and neck. Vol. 11. St. Louis: CV Mosby; 1975.

11 Limberg AA. The planning of local plastic operations on the body surface: theory and practice. Translated by Wolfe SA. New York: Simon & Schuster; 1984.

12 Robinson JK, Hanke W, Sengelmann RD, Siegel DM. Surgery of the skin: textbook with DVD. Philadelphia: Elsevier; 2005.

CHAPTER 24

Local flap closure in the management of skin cancer

James W. Trimble and James R. Trimble

After surgical excision of skin cancer, it is routine to choose between wound closure by secondary intention, direct approximation, skin flaps, or skin grafts. Many variables that influence the restoration of cosmesis and function are weighed to achieve the "best" closure. There is not always an absolute best way to close a surgical wound. In fact, two different approaches can ultimately yield similarly good results. The choice of skin closure that is best suited for a particular situation rests on the experience and judgment of the surgeon and circumstances of the patient. Specific skin flap designs for each anatomic site and the surgical techniques for flap elevation and placement are beyond the scope of this chapter. Our remarks are limited to some fundamental considerations that go into local flap design for wound reconstruction after skin cancer removal (Table 24.1). For a more detailed discussion of surgical principles of specific flap techniques, the reader is referred to several texts and periodicals [1–16].

Importance of vascular supply

A skin flap is a tongue of skin and subcutaneous tissue that is severed from its bed but left attached to the surrounding skin at one selected point, called the flap base or pedicle. Rarely, a flap may be designed with two pedicles. The tissue layers included in a flap are skin, underlying superficial fascia, fat, and occasionally muscle. During flap closure, normal skin adjacent to a postoperative wound is mobilized and transferred into the defect resulting from cancer excision. Unlike the situation in skin graft-

ing, success of the transfer depends on maintenance of an adequate vascular system between the flap and the adjacent skin through the pedicle. Venous outflow and arterial supply are both very important [17]. Previously it was thought that pedicle flaps most often died in cyanosis from venous congestion rather than in pallor from ischemic arterial flow [2]. Other evidence has suggested that loss of arterial flow is probably the main cause of flap tip necrosis [18]. Reinisch [19] believed that arteriovenous shunting in the proximal flap was the specific cause of decreased arterial flow to the distal tip. Whatever the exact mechanism of necrosis, flaps depend on the maintenance of an intact flow system.

Local skin flaps can be subdivided into two categories based on their source of blood supply: axial flaps and random flaps. A flap that is designed around the blood supply of a specific anatomic arterial tree is called an axial flap. This type of flap has a single pedicle whose long axis parallels the vasculature of a recognized arterial system. Small cutaneous arteries that flow into the dermal–subdermal plexus may run for a significant distance in an axis parallel and just deep to the plane of the dermal–subdermal plexus [3]. Axial flaps have an increased chance of survival, which permits some easing of flap design restrictions such as length-to-base width ratio and amount of tension on a flap during closure. These flaps survive up to 50% greater lengths than flaps with a random blood supply [20,21]. Axial flaps are designed over arteriovenous systems such as the superficial temporal, supraorbital, supratrochlear, posterior auricular, labial, facial, and scalp arteries.

Table 24.1 Indications for skin flaps

When flap repair would offer the best cosmetic and functional result

When defect closure by direct approximation would lead to the sacrifice of extra normal tissue, an increase of resultant scar, or a distortion of natural boundaries

To "break up" the linear configuration of a long linear surgical scar

When characteristics of defect base preclude the use of a graft (i.e., exposed bone or cartilage)

Most local flaps used about the head and neck for surgical reconstruction are called random flaps because their design is not based on the circulation of a particular vessel. A random flap is nourished by the blood flow of the dermal–subdermal capillary network within the pedicle of the flap and small arterioles from musculocutaneous and cutaneous perforating vessels that may be included in the pedicle [20]. When a flap is raised and transferred to the recipient site, flap survival is dependent on adequate flow in and out through this system. Factors that would diminish blood flow through the flap must be considered during flap design and watched for in the postoperative period (Table 24.2). Efficiency of blood flow in the random flap differs from one location to another. The face and scalp have a richer circulation than do the trunk and extremities. Venous stasis and decreased peripheral flow are often present below the knees. Circulation in

Table 24.2 Clinical factors that influence blood flow efficiency in cutaneous flaps

Presence of peripheral vascular disease
   Hypertension
   Diabetes mellitus
   Atherosclerosis
Age of patient
Trimming of the flap at closure
Tension on the flap at closure
Kinking of vessels within the pedicle
Postoperative: edema, surgical trauma, infection
Hematoma or seroma

elderly adults may be diminished in comparison with young adults because of hypertension, diabetes, atherosclerosis, or other causes of peripheral vascular disease. Previous surgical scars may also alter blood flow.

Wound evaluation

Proper planning of a flap is essential to ensure the best possible outcome. Before the selection of a flap design, characteristics of the wound and properties of the surrounding skin should be evaluated. Particular attention is given to (1) the type of tissue missing; (2) the wound size, depth, and shape; (3) proximity to natural boundaries, free borders, and skin folds; (4) the elasticity and mobility of the wound edges and surrounding donor skin; and finally (5) the surface color, texture, and hair of surrounding skin. Local flaps are often favored for reconstruction because they most nearly match the missing skin in texture, color, thickness, and hair pattern.

The first question is what tissues need to be replaced to restore the best cosmesis and function. Tissues missing may include bone, cartilage, muscle, fat, and skin. Planning a flap should take into account the normal anatomy of the specific wound site so that during the reconstruction, by tissue replacement or realignment, the natural contours and muscle movement patterns are recreated. For example, specific realignment of the muscle layer by interrupted sutures is necessary during reconstruction in a wedge resection of the lower lip, and the addition of a Z-plasty below the vermilion may help elevate the vermilion border, which might otherwise become notched after primary closure and wound contracture. Similar principles of realigning the muscle layers apply when closing wounds involving eyelids.

The size and depth of the wound may preclude the use of certain local flaps. For example, on the forehead, where skin tends to be inelastic, single or even double advancement flaps may not be able to close a defect without undue tension. Instead, a rhomboid flap or double rotation flaps to either side of the defect may more easily close the wound. Depending on the situation, various combinations of closures might be appropriate, such as flap and free graft, flap partial closure and granulation, interpolation flaps, and so forth. Some defects may require a staged procedure, as in the forehead flap reconstruction of the nose or the Estlander flap for lip reconstruction [3]. The surgeon trying to achieve the best possible closure will rely on his or her experience, creativity, and attention to detail.

Proximity to natural boundaries and folds is important in two ways. First, the secondary scar at the donor site may often be hidden in a boundary or skin fold. Second, the unwanted distortion of a boundary or free border resulting from the forces of flap closure can be avoided (e.g., eyelids, eyebrow, vermilion border, ala nasi rim, nasolabial fold). The surgeon should carefully consider whether a specific flap design will cause the secondary movement of a natural boundary, particularly a free border. Forces of tension after closure should be directed so that distortion is minimal, to avoid problems such as ectropion and eclabium. Also, it is an unfortunate problem to get "webbing" across a concavity if an incision crosses an anatomic area that is naturally concave. When possible, it is better to skirt the edge of a natural concavity rather than transect it. Trapdoor deformities may be exaggerated when a flap crosses a concave area such as the inner canthus, ala nasi groove, or nasolabial fold. In concave areas, consider the possibility of a graft or granulation. Trapdoor deformities may also be more apparent when the edge of the flap does not incorporate a boundary or fold. These deformities are particularly noticeable in small-angle pedicle flaps such as the nasolabial pedicle flap to the lip or cheek pedicle flap to the nose. Wider undermining around the flap base may help lessen the trapdoor effect, but alternative closures can sometimes give superior results. For instance, a flap design using a rotation flap might hide the flap edges into the boundaries of the lip or nose better and avoid the trapdoor deformity altogether. Sometimes removal of the entire cosmetic unit before flap design might be preferred.

Elasticity and mobility of the skin near the wound are important to successful flap movement. When evaluating possible donor sites, look first to find the point of maximum redundancy and mobility. Try to determine the line of maximal extensibility (LME), which is perpendicular to relaxed skin tension lines. This line will be useful when designing and orienting a flap. Flap skin is most easily delivered to the recipient site when taken from the area of maximal extensibility along the LME. This brings us to flap motion. Skin flaps have three fundamental motions: advancement, rotation, and stretch. Advancement and rotation occur as the flap slides in a forward or diagonal direction into a recipient site. Skin mobility influences the degree to which flaps can be advanced or rotated. Stretch is a force that tries to enlarge the flap above its resting size, and skin elastic forces work in the opposite direction. A stretching force applied to a flap edge is one cause of tip necrosis, secondary to reduced perfusion in that area. Ischemia is manifested clinically by blanching of the flap as it is sutured into position. In general, flap design should ensure the necessary flap size and mobility so that during advancement and rotation into the recipient site, stretching forces are kept to a minimum.

Another important aspect of tissue movement during flap closure is secondary motion of the wound edges at the recipient site. This was emphasized by Stegman [22]. Secondary motion consists of movement of the skin around the wound in a direction opposite to the movement of the flap. This secondary motion helps close the surgical wound and may be enhanced by undermining the wound edges to which the flap will be attached. Secondary movement is also influenced by closure of the donor site and by closure of a Burow's triangle, which may have been added to equilibrate unequal wound edges. These result in partial closure of the wound before placement of the flap. An unwanted result of secondary motion may be distortion of a natural fold or boundary. As mentioned, this should be anticipated and avoided. Understanding the basic dynamics of skin movement before flap design will aid in the overall success and ease of transfer.

Finally, one should not neglect to evaluate the skin color, texture (including actinic damage and porosity), and hair pattern before flap design. Sometimes the quality of skin to be replaced is quite different from nearby potential donor sites, and this will be reflected in the final cosmetic result. For example, forehead or cheek skin on the nose may never gain the porous or oily texture that is often found on the nose.

Design

There are a myriad of names assigned to various flaps. The classification of flaps has been done using distance of movement, source of blood supply, pedicle characteristics, type of motion, and alphabetical design. Understanding the changes in geometry and the forces of skin tension during flap movement is the key to choosing the best repair design. It should be remembered that skin retracts after incision and swells during surgery from trauma and from injection of local anesthetics. This edema may obliterate natural skin folds and distort the flap. Important landmarks and flap design should be marked with gentian violet before surgery.

After tumor excision, elastic forces inherent in the wound edges will cause the defect to grow larger than expected. After flap mobilization, the skin flap will shrink in size. These changes should be anticipated. Flaps usually have to be planned slightly wider and longer than the defects they must fill. It is easier to trim excess tissue from a large flap than to try to compensate for a small flap with excess tension at closure, backcutting of the pedicle, or partial closure of the recipient site with Burow's triangle.

Selection of the most appropriate flap design is based on the skills and experience of the skin surgeon as he or she considers the multiple factors previously discussed. It is helpful sometimes to use a template cut out of gauze or Telfa to simulate closing the wound with a flap. The pattern should be cut in the shape of the planned flap and long enough and wide enough to cover the wound as the flap moves into place. The surgeon may reenact the flap movement with the template before incising the flap. Using a skin hook at the flap tip, the surgeon can test flap movement as surgery proceeds with undermining and continued incision. Three of the most commonly used types of flaps are the advancement, rotation, and transposition flaps.

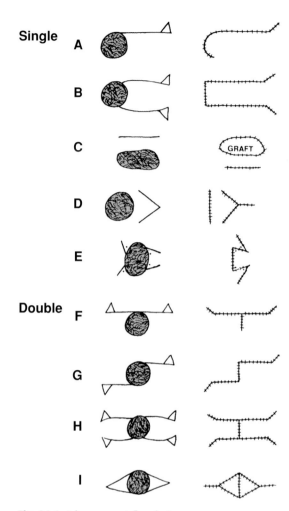

Fig. 24.1 Advancement flap designs.

Advancement flaps

Advancement flaps have a minimal rotational component. Closure is accomplished by linear movement of the flap to the defect and secondary movement of wound edges to the flap. Mobility that is produced by undermining both the wound edges around the defect and flap is helpful in minimizing stretch. Burow's triangles with a wide base may be added to enhance the advancement motion by creating an extra force that moves the flap in the direction of wound closure (Fig. 24.1).

The length of the flap in relation to its base width may vary slightly depending on the vascular supply of the flap and factors that influence blood supply. However, increasing the base width does not necessarily allow a longer flap length. Milton [23] showed that flaps with similar blood supplies will survive to the same length, irrespective of flap base width. To some extent, the maximum allowable length will also be influenced by the amount of stretching force that is placed on the flap at closure. Gibson and Kenedi [24] have shown that a very small stretching force on a flap will permit maximum expansion. Increasing the force of stretch to a higher level yields little increase in expansion and a great increase in risk to flap circulation, as evidenced by blanching. In his studies on flap length and base width in triangular flaps, Stell [25] found that flap viability is not directly governed by a length/width ratio or an area/width ratio. However, because he found a tendency to increasing surviving lengths with increasing pedicle width, some relation must exist. He concluded that the length to which a random flap (triangular or rectangular) will survive is determined primarily on the "pumping load" or circulation across the flap.

The classic single advancement flap (Fig. 24.1B) is limited in how much coverage it can give without pushing the limit of too much tension. This may result in flap tip necrosis, even in a very vascular area, such as the nasal bridge (in the repair of the nasal tip) or the helix of the ear. The movement of the flap is along only one directional vector and does not borrow from looser skin nearby as a transposition flap does. If it is possible to add a second flap to the closure (Fig. 24.1F–H), a greater area of coverage can be achieved.

The island pedicle flap (Fig. 24.1I) is one of the variations of an advancement flap that may be useful in reconstructing defects around the nose. It may be axial or random. Unlike other advancement flaps, the island pedicle flap is severed circumferentially from the surrounding dermis but remains attached by a subcutaneous pedicle. The flap is vascularized by perforating arterioles that rise up vertically from the underlying fascia or muscle through the subcutaneous pedicle to the subdermal plexus. The island of skin can be advanced directly from the skin contiguous to the edge of the defect or tunneled under intact skin to the recipient site. The

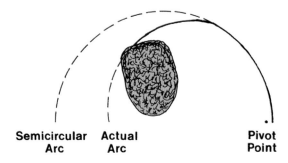

Fig. 24.2 Rotation flap. Rotation around a fixed pivot point causes the flap to "fall" short of a true semicircular arc.

island pedicle flap has advantages and disadvantages and is a more complicated advancement flap to mobilize and transfer. A thorough understanding of its limitations is necessary to successfully use this flap [12].

Rotation flaps

Rotation flaps pivot around a point of maximum tension (Fig. 24.2). It is important to accurately identify this point before incision. The pivot point tends to be relatively fixed, and a straight line drawn from this rotational point to the furthest extent of the defect will be the actual flap length required. Failure to properly identify the point will result in a flap too short for the defect. As the flap rotates into place, the arc "falls" short of a true semicircle because of limited rotation around the pivot point. This can be easily demonstrated by using a gauze template of the flap to simulate closing the defect.

Movement of the flap toward the defect and secondary motion of the wound edges to the flap are enhanced by undermining both the flap and the recipient site. A Burow's triangle placed at any point along the wound edge adjacent to the flap or the recipient wound edge accomplishes two objectives: (1) it creates a force that tends to close the wound (partial closure) and (2) it equalizes unequal lengths between the recipient wound edges and the edges of the flap. Backcutting the flap pedicle to increase mobility and dog ear repairs should be done with caution to avoid compromising blood supply. The flap donor site may be closed in a curvilinear line to

Single

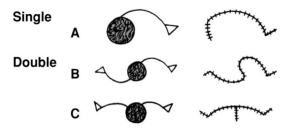

Double

Fig. 24.3 Rotation flap designs.

the trailing edge of the flap or with a graft or with a second flap. Dog ears that may form on either side of the pedicle will often flatten out in time, but a small Burow's triangle directed away from the flap can be used to flatten the redundant tissue. A rotation flap has some movement in a linear direction, like the advancement flap, but also captures some of the advantage of the looser skin nearby with rotation, like a transposition flap. Even with the extra direction of flap motion, it is sometimes humbling to find that the actual flap movement is far less than the expected movement, especially when the skin around the defect is inelastic as it is on the scalp and forehead. For this reason, a rotation is often designed much larger than the defect to be closed. Some have suggested that the length of the flap should be four times the width of the base of the defect [5]. Again, if the situation permits, adding a second rotation flap to the design can facilitate closure (Fig. 24.3B,C).

The O-to-T double rotation flap closure (Fig. 24.3C) is useful for defects adjacent to natural boundaries where the surgeon would like to direct tension of closure in a line parallel to the boundary rather than perpendicular to it. This helps avoid tension that would distort the natural line of the boundary. This design also allows the scar from the long arms of the flaps to fall into the boundary. These flaps may have components of advancement and rotation, depending on design. The specific repair situation will dictate which motion should predominate. Each flap has a wide base width to ensure survival. The O-to-S double rotation flap closure (Fig. 24.3B) may also be useful in situations in which closure tension should be directed away from

a boundary or in locations where skin is relatively inelastic.

Transposition flaps

Like rotation flaps, transposition flaps also rotate around a point of maximum tension, the pivot point. A transposition flap may be thought of as a narrow rotation flap with a small pedicle width that crosses (but does not span) an area of normal skin during transfer. Transposition flaps that span an area of normal skin are called interpolation flaps [7]. Interpolation flaps require a second stage to remove the pedicle that spans the intervening normal skin after the flap tip and edges have reestablished a new blood supply at the recipient site. Similar guidelines for planning the correct length and width for a rotation flap apply to a transposition flap except that the transposition flap has a much narrower pedicle (Fig 24.4). Therefore, the blood supply through the pedicle is more tenuous and likely to be adversely affected by too much stretching force, a pedicle that is too long, or vessel kinking within the pedicle. A length-to-width ratio of 3:1 has been suggested for a transposition flap that has a random blood supply, but sites that are not particularly vascular or under tension may not be able to sustain this ratio [6]. The choice of when to use a transposition or a rotation flap is based on the specific anatomic situation, the surgeon's understanding of the many different variations of local flaps, and his or her experience with flap movement.

The rhomboid flap [26] and its modification, the DuFourmentel flap [27], represent useful transposition flaps [26–30]. This flap has a rotational and a smaller advancement component to its motion. Like the rotation flap, the transposition flap will tend to fall short of that point on the recipient wound edge that is furthest from the pivot point at the pedicle base. However, secondary movement of the recipient wound edge to the flap will help make up for this shortfall. In theory, a properly designed rhomboid flap puts minimal closure tension across the wound recipient site and thus avoids distortion of a natural boundary to which the defect is adjacent. The flap is simple in design and based on an equilateral parallelogram of 60° and 120° angles (Fig. 24.5). The

Single

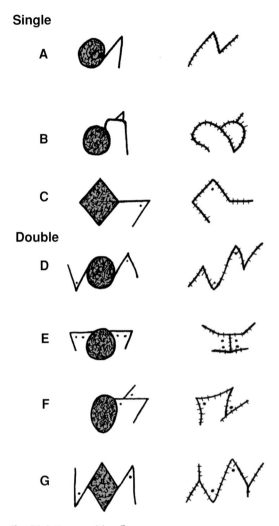

A

B

C

Double

D

E

F

G

Fig. 24.4 Transposition flap.

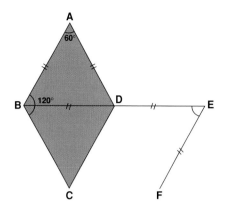

Fig. 24.5 Rhomboid flap. *ABCD* represents a surgical defect that is an equilateral parallelogram with angles of 60° and 120°. Line *BD* is extended to point *E*, a distance equal to *AD* with an incident angle of 60°. Line *EF* should then be parallel to *DC*. The diameter *DF* of the flap and the length *CE* of the flap will tend to shrink after incision.

shortest diameter of the rhombus is extended in a length equal to the length of one of the sides. From this extension arm, a new equilateral parallelogram is constructed abutting one side of the original parallelogram. The flap designed is a rhomboid with sides equal to the sides of the original rhombus. If possible, it is best to arrange for a line through *DF* (see Fig. 24.5) to fall along the direction of the LME. This insures easier flap transfer. If a natural skin fold is nearby, the flap can be designed so that one arm of

the resultant scar will fall into the fold. During flap movement, points *D* and *F* come together under moderate tension. It is paramount that this tension does not distort a natural boundary, such as a free border.

The DuFourmentel flap is a modification of the rhomboid flap and is not restricted to an equilateral parallelogram of angles 60° and 120° [31]. The rhomboid of the DuFourmentel design is composed of two equal isosceles triangles, with their bases superimposed to form the short diameter of the parallelogram (Fig. 24.6). The short diameter is extended, and one of the sides is extended to form an acute angle. This acute angle is then bisected by a line *JK*, which is equal in length to one of the sides of the original rhomboid. From point *K*, another line is constructed that is parallel to the longest diameter of the original rhomboid with a length equal to one of the sides.

Concentrating for a moment on the acute angle of the rhomboidal defect and the acute angle at the DuFourmentel flap tip, one can see that with a defect angle of less than 45°, the flap tip will be progressively larger than the defect it is to fill. Less advantage is gained with acute angles below 45°, and primary closure may be preferred. Defect angles above

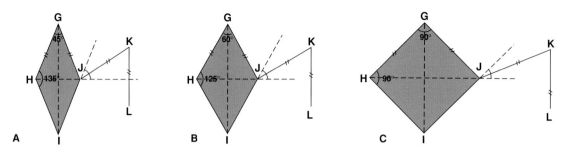

Fig. 24.6 DuFourmentel flap. *GHIJ* represents a rhomboidal defect. Lines *HJ* and *IJ* are extended, and the angle thus formed is bisected by a line *JK*, which is equal in length to line *HG*. Line *KL* is constructed from a point *K* so that line *KL* is parallel to line *GI* (the longest diameter of the defect) and equal in length to *GJ*.

90° have a progressively smaller flap tip size than defect to be filled and a much greater distance of flap movement during closure. As the defect angle exceeds 90°, too much force is necessary to

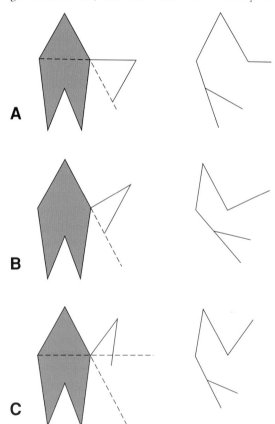

Fig. 24.7 *A*, Rhomboid flap with M-plasty. *B*, Webster [33] 30°-angle flap. *C*, Monheit [35] 30°-angle flap.

rotate and stretch the flap into position. In the middle range with defect angles between 45° and 90°, the DuFourmentel flap can be useful to know. In practice, the experienced skin surgeon designs a rhomboid flap to meet the specific requirements of the situation and may not exactly follow the textbook; however, a complete understanding of the geometry of rhomboid flaps and the forces at work during flap movement is a basic requirement for deviation from the standard design. There are a number of variations in rhomboid design [32–34]. Familiarity with these modifications will help the surgeon tailor his or her flap to achieve the best results.

Webster [33] has advocated the use of a 30° angle flap that is a variation of the 60° angle rhomboid flap (Fig. 24.7B). Loose or atrophic, thin skin may cause a permanent "dog ear" when a 60° angle is closed. This may happen in the rhomboid design at the flap base and the donor site. Closing a 30° angle eliminates this problem. In addition, tension at the closed donor site of a rhomboid flap is fairly great, whereas the tension at the closed donor site for a 30° angle flap is approximately half. These are the advantages of Webster's modification. The disadvantages are (1) a narrower flap tip with a decreased width-to-length ratio and (2) more stretch tension placed on the flap at closure because the flap was designed smaller than the original defect. However, in highly vascular areas around the face or when the flap is axial, the 30°-angle flap should be able to tolerate these design limitations (i.e., stretching force and small pedicle width) [33].

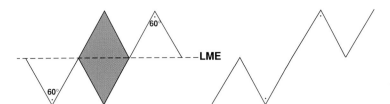

LME

Fig. 24.8 Double-Z rhomboid closure. Flap skin should be taken from skin along the LME.

In describing the 30°-angle flap, Monheit [35] slightly rotated the flap base axis away from the wound (Fig. 24.7C). This would lessen the total rotation necessary to secure closure and thereby reduce the chance of vessel kinking. In addition, vessels approaching the flap base would less likely be compromised. However, as the 30°-angle flap base is positioned more laterally, closure of the flap donor area produces more tension across the recipient site. Using any design, placement of a 30°-angle flap near a free border should be done with caution. In the 60°-rhomboid flap, maximal tension can be directed across the donor site and away from the free border more effectively. In a 30°-angle flap, tension across the donor site is reduced, which results in increased pull across the recipient wound site. This may be enough force to cause displacement of a free border.

Cuono [34] suggested employing the double Z-plasty repair of rhomboid defects. He used two 60°-angle flaps designed to either side of the rhomboid (Fig. 24.8). Each flap was constructed from an extension of one side of the rhomboid. The flaps were equilateral triangles whose bases were located in line with the short diameter of the rhomboid and with the flap tips pointing in opposite directions. Notice that each flap is actually part of a Z-plasty, so the Z-plasty flaps are then transposed. The key to proper design is to be sure the long axis of the rhomboidal defect is parallel to the relaxed skin tension line. This will ensure that 60°-angle Z-plasty flaps are taken from skin oriented along the LME [34]. In commenting on the use of the double Z-plasty repair of rhomboid defects, Roggendorf [36] emphasized that a large skin reserve from which to move the flaps is necessary. For a circular defect with a 5-cm radius, 11 cm of lax skin is needed in the direction of the LME to close the wound using the double-Z rhomboid technique [36].

Interpolation flaps are transposition flaps whose donor site is not contiguous with the defect to be closed. In elevating and transposing the interpolation flap, the pedicle must span an area of normal skin to reach the recipient site. Because the interpolation flap generally has a greater distance to travel to reach the defect, its pedicle may be long for the width of the base of the pedicle; that is, it may be greater than a 3:1 ratio. For this reason, the interpolation flap may need to be an axial flap or at very least have a rich vascular supply. The paramedian forehead flap and melolabial flap to the nose and the preauricular and postauricular interpolation flap to the ear are variations of the interpolation flap that may be very useful in reconstructing these areas [7].

The bilobed flap is also a variation of the transposition flap. The bilobed flap is useful to know when closing defects on the lower third of the nose at the nasal tip [10,13]. This flap is designed with two transposition flaps connected at the base by a single pedicle. The long axes of the two flaps are designed to be separated by a 90° angle. The defect is closed in the usual way by transposing the primary flap into the defect. The secondary flap is then transposed into the defect created at the donor site of the primary flap. Zitelli [13] suggested a modification by reducing the angle separating the primary and secondary flaps to 45°, which reduced the total rotation of the two flaps. This made transposition easier and helped reduce the dog ear distortion at the base of the pedicle.

Surgical technique

In closing, we would like to make some general comments on surgical technique. In the preoperative instructions, a patient should be advised not to take any aspirin or nonsteroidal anti-inflammatory–

containing products 7 days before surgery because diminution of the primary platelet-clotting mechanism will increase oozing during and after surgery. Niacin-containing vitamins should be avoided the day of surgery because this drug may cause flushing by peripheral vasodilation, which may also increase bleeding during surgery. If medically possible, consider stopping anticoagulants before flap or graft surgery. Also, patients should avoid smoking in the early postoperative period because of the vasoconstrictive effects of nicotine.

Of course, sterile technique is mandatory, and surgical preparation should include mechanical removal of oil, dirt, and superficial loose keratin with alcohol followed by a surgical scrub. An antimicrobial solution or scrub should be reapplied during surgery to maintain sterility within the surgical field. Using clippers to shave hair rather than a razor will also help minimize wound infections [37]. Fortunately, wound infections are uncommon, but attention to maintaining sterility until the wound is closed will go a long way to avoiding infection.

Hemostasis is a cardinal rule in cutaneous surgery to insure visibility during surgery and prevent hematoma after surgery. Use low concentrations of epinephrine with the local anesthetic whenever possible to aid with hemostasis. Suction and good lighting are very important tools for securing adequate visibility during surgery. Hemostasis by electrocautery, hot knife (Shaw scalpel), or suture is essential before closure. Suturing techniques such as the vertical mattress suture or the far-near-near-far suture, or bolsters may also be useful on large donor sites, but attention should be paid to how they influence blood supply to the flap.

As the flap is incised, try not to bevel the edges unless this is deliberately done in areas of hair-bearing skin. Facial folds may make a precise cut perpendicular to the skin surface difficult, but try to achieve this goal. As the flap is raised, use a skin hook rather than forceps to elevate the flap to reduce trauma on the flap. Directly observe the cutting and elevation of the undermined skin and secure pinpoint hemostasis with each step. Magnifying head loupes are very helpful.

Undermining should be at a level appropriate to preserve the blood supply that is intended to feed the flap and also fill the defect with adequate bulk. This is usually at a level of superficial fat or just below hair bulbs in the case of hair-bearing areas; however, in several areas of the face, facial muscles may be too close to lower dermis to permit undermining at this level. To preserve larger vessels, the depth may need to be full-thickness fat. In special areas, such as the scalp, undermining will be at a level just above periosteum but under galea. These variations of technique underscore the necessity of understanding the anatomy of the specific location involved.

If the flap tip blanches from pale pink to white during flap incision, elevation, or transfer, this indicates inadequate blood supply. The cause for blanching should be sought and corrected if possible. Causes include epinephrine effects, vessel kinking, inadequate blood supply for flap length, or too much tension at closure. In clinical practice, some flaps can withstand more tension than others, depending on flap design, local circulation, and host factors. Tension can be relieved somewhat by adding a Burow's triangle or partial closure to the recipient wound edge (preferably put in a facial fold or boundary). Infrequently, a second flap, graft, or granulation will be used in combination with the primary flap to relieve excess tension.

Potential spaces in the deep fatty layers should be closed with absorbable suture material to prevent seroma or hematoma. Skin edges should be approximated with deep dermal–buried absorbable suture at "key" points along the wound edges using the smallest-gauge suture possible. Surface sutures of a small gauge (preferably monofilament nylon) are placed to precisely close epithelial edges. One important point of surface suture placement is avoiding too much tension on each stitch. A continuous running epidermal or intradermal suture helps avoid excess tension as the wound swells postoperatively. The best closure technique will occur when the closure is all but perfect with buried suture alone and the epidermal sutures simply add to fine approximation of the edges. Constriction of tissue at the wound edges may cause tissue necrosis, which increases the resultant scar and ischemic entry points for bacteria.

Finally, a cool pack (not ice pack) applied over or around the flap for several hours after surgery may provide pressure over the area and help reduce postoperative edema. This will also insure that the patient is at rest and the surgical site is relatively immobile, which will minimize oozing under the flap resulting from a loss of epinephrine effect. Cool packs will greatly reduce eyelid edema and bruising, for which the patient will be grateful. The flap should be checked at 24 or 48 hours for any early sign of infection or hematoma. When in doubt about infection, do a culture and begin antibiotics. Early intervention could avoid a poor outcome. Wound edges should be gently cleaned each day with peroxide and covered with an antibiotic ointment to prevent air desiccation. Crusts that form around sutures act as a medium for bacterial growth around the foreign body. Crusts along the wound edge will contribute to a slight depression of the scar. Patients with very oily skin should avoid excessive ointment, especially around the nose, because a flare of rosacea or seborrhea could compromise wound healing. Also important in the postoperative period is the patient's understanding that wound healing is "teamwork" that requires his or her cooperation. Cooperation includes commonsense limitations on physical activity and refraining from all tobacco products during the initial 1- to 2-week postoperative healing phase. We are convinced that smoking is associated with an increase in postoperative flap and graft failure. The final result of surgery will depend on this teamwork and the patient's ability to heal the reconstructed wound.

In summary, local flap closure is an excellent alternative along with the choices of skin graft or granulation wound closure following surgical excision of skin cancer. Flaps are routinely done for immediate or delayed reconstruction. They often provide the best possible replacement for the tissue excised and can restore near-normal cosmesis and function. The foregoing has been a consideration of some basic concepts in local flap surgery. Their applicability and usefulness in reconstructive surgery are well accepted.

References

1 McGregor IA. Fundamental techniques of plastic surgery and their surgical applications. 7th ed. London: Churchill-Livingstone; 1980.
2 Converse JM. Plastic surgery and transplantation of skin. In: Epstein E, Epstein E Jr, editors. Skin surgery. 5th ed. Springfield, IL: Charles C Thomas; 1982. p. 245–77.
3 Grabb WC, Smith JW. Plastic surgery. 3rd ed. Boston: Little, Brown; 1980. p. 51–101, 451–554.
4 Rohrer TE, Bhatia A. Transposition flaps in cutaneous surgery. Dermatol Surg 2005;31:1014–23.
5 Tschoi M, Hoy EA, Granick MS. Skin flaps. Clin Plast Surg 2005;32:261–73.
6 Clark JM, Wang TD. Local flaps in scar revision. Facial Plast Surg 2001;17:295–308.
7 Mellette JR, Ho DQ. Interpolation flaps. Dermatol Clin 2005;23:87–112.
8 Pletcher SD, Kim DW. Current concepts in cheek reconstruction. Facial Plast Surg Clin North Am 2005; 13:267–81.
9 Murillo WL, Fernandez W, Caycedo DJ, Dupin CL, Black ES. Cheek and inferior eyelid reconstruction after skin cancer ablation. Clin Plast Surg 2004;31: 41–67.
10 Aasi SZ, Leffell DJ. Bilobed transposition flap. Dermatol Clin 2005;23:55–64.
11 Zavod MB, Zavod MB, Goldman GD. The dorsal nasal flap. Dermatol Clin 2005;23:73–85.
12 Kimyai-Asadi A, Goldberg LH. Island pedicle flap. Dermatol Clin 2005;23:113–27.
13 Zitelli JA. The bilobed flap for nasal reconstruction. Arch Dermatol 1989;125:957–9.
14 Chen EH, Johnson TM, Ratner D. Introduction to flap movement: reconstruction of five similar nasal defects using different flaps. Dermatol Surg 2005;31: 982–5.
15 Brodland DG. Paramedian forehead flap reconstruction for nasal defects. Dermatol Surg 2005;31: 1034–45.
16 Robinson JK, Hanke CW, Sengelmann RD, Siegel DM. Surgery of the skin, procedural dermatology. Philadelphia: Elsevier Mosby; 2005. p. 311–64.
17 Fontaine R, Pereira S. Obliterations etresections veineuses experimentales; contribution a l'etude de la circulation collaterale veineuse. Rev Chir 1937;75: 161.
18 Kerrigan CL. Skin flap failure: pathophysiology. Plast Reconstr Surg 1983;72:766–73.

19 Reinisch JF. Discussion: skin flap failure: pathophysiology. Plast Reconstr Surg 1983;72:775–7.

20 Daniel RK, Williams HB. Skin flaps: a reappraisal. I. The vascular supply to the skin. II. Experimental cutaneous arterial and island flaps. III. Experimental island flap transfer by microvascular anastomoses. Plast Reconstr Surg 1973;52:16–31.

21 Milton S. The effects of "delay" on the survival of experimental pedicled skin flaps. Plast Reconstr Surg 1969;22:244–52.

22 Stegman S. Design and movement of flaps. J Dermatol Surg Oncol 1980;6:182–6.

23 Milton SH. Pedicled skin flaps: the fallacy of the length:width ratio. Br J Surg 1970;57:502.

24 Gibson T, Kenedi RM. Biomechanical properties of skin. Surg Clin North Am 1967;47:279–94.

25 Stell PM. The viability of triangular skin flaps. Br J Plast Surg 1975;28:247–50.

26 Limberg AA. Design of local flaps. In: Gibson T, editor. Modern trends in plastic surgery. 2nd ed. London: Butterworths; 1966. p. 38–61.

27 DuFourmentel C. An L-shaped flap for lozenge shaped defects. In: Transactions of the Third International Congress of Plastic Surgery. Amsterdam: Excerpta Medical Foundation; 1963. p. 772.

28 Borges AF. Choosing the correct Limberg flap. Plast Reconstr Surg 1978;62:542–5.

29 Borges AF. The rhombic flap. Plast Reconstr Surg 1981;67:458–66.

30 Larrabee WF, Trachy R, Sutton D, Cox K. Rhomboid flap dynamics. Arch Otolaryngol 1981;107:755–7.

31 Lister GD, Gibson T. Closure of rhomboid skin defects: the flaps of Limberg and DuFourmentel. Br J Plast Surg 1972;25:300–14.

32 Becker H. The rhomboid-to-W technique for excision of some skin lesions and closure. Plast Reconstr Surg 1979;64:444–7.

33 Webster RC, Davidson TM, Smith RC. The 30% transposition flap. Laryngoscope 1978;88:85–94.

34 Cuono CB. Double Z-plasty repair of large and small rhombic defects: the double-Z rhomboid. Plast Reconstr Surg 1983;71:658–6.

35 Monheit GD. The rhomboid transposition flap reevaluated. J Dermatol Surg Oncol 1980;6:464–71.

36 Roggendorf E. Discussion: double Z-plasty repair of large and small rhombic defects: the double-Z rhomboid. Plast Reconstr Surg 1983;71:667.

37 Preoperative depilation [editorial]. Lancet 1983; 1:1311.

CHAPTER 25

The role of skin grafts in the management of skin malignancies

James R. Trimble and James W. Trimble

Dermatologic surgery has become simplified to such an extent that it is now routinely performed in an office or outpatient surgical facility. This includes skin flap and grafting procedures. Widespread acceptance of office-based skin surgery has resulted from the numerous medical advances in knowledge and techniques that have insured a low rate of complication. Good surgical technique, good wound care, and antibiotics have almost eliminated infection as a cause of graft failure. If we understand the various factors that influence graft survival and failure we can control them to a great extent.

Skin grafts are often useful in reconstruction of wounds resulting from surgical excision of cancer. This chapter focuses on the current role of skin grafting in the management of cutaneous malignancies. Skin grafting procedures are relatively uncomplicated, and the risk of failure is low. Any surgeon should be able to graft and should know the advantages of grafting. In general, skin grafting is easier than skin flap procedures. This is particularly true of complicated flaps such as interpolation, tubed flaps, and myocutaneous flaps. Numerous articles and books have been written describing proper skin grafting techniques [1–11]. These techniques are simple and if followed, will result in a successful outcome routinely.

When dealing with skin cancers, grafts are at times indispensable because of wound size or location. They give the surgeon confidence to close large surgical defects. This means that one can deal more radically with skin cancer if the need arises. Skin malignancies, particularly basal and squamous

cell carcinomas, recur more often because of an inadequate lateral margin than a deep margin. Wider margins reduce the chance of recurrence. Unlike flap closures, adjacent tissue is not rearranged with a graft closure. Grafting offers the practical advantage of not shifting undetected cancer cells. In the event of recurrence, theoretically, the tumor will recur focally at the positive margin. Recurrence under a flap or graft is problematic in either case.

Full-thickness grafts

The major goal of reconstructive dermatologic surgery is to achieve wound closure with the best cosmetic and functional result. The experience and skill of the surgeon should dictate whether a graft would be preferable to a flap or to granulation. There are a number of variables that need to be considered during graft selection. Skin grafts can be divided into several types: full-thickness, split-thickness, pinch, and composite skin grafts. By definition, the full-thickness graft contains the complete thickness of the epidermis and dermis. However, the thickness of the dermis varies with each individual and with different donor sites. Therefore, full-thickness grafts will vary in thickness depending on the donor site. In general, full-thickness grafts provide the best cosmetic and functional coverage. After the graft heals, it undergoes less contraction, withstands injury better, and retains its color better than other types. These advantages are attributable to the thick dermal layer that full-thickness grafts contain. Therefore, it is the graft of choice whenever possible, particularly on the face, where the cosmetic result is of paramount importance, and especially where the wound is adjacent to a free mobile border. Free borders are easily shifted by graft contraction.

It is important to select a donor site that will most closely match the host site. In general, the nearer the donor site is to the host site, the better the skin will match. A helpful method to select the best skin match is to cut a dime-sized hole in a strip of white 3×5 card. Hold this against the skin of the proposed donor site and compare it to the skin at the recipient site. There is no substitute for careful preoperative evaluation during graft site selection. Standard donor sites for facial grafts are preauricular, postauricular, infra-auricular, nasolabial fold, glabellar, cervical, supraclavicular, eyelid, and normal excess skin contiguous with the defect sacrificed during partial closure of the defect (i.e., Burow's graft). Although facial skin usually produces an excellent result, one disadvantage is the secondary scar resulting from closure of the donor site. For this reason, the surgeon should select an area where a donor site scar can be concealed by blepharoplasty, by facelift closure, behind the ear, within the supraclavicular sulcus, or in the nasolabial fold.

One of the most commonly used donor sites for facial grafts is skin from behind the ear and adjacent mastoid process. This retroauricular skin often matches facial skin very well, and moderate-sized full-thickness grafts may be harvested from this source. The donor site can be healed by primary closure, granulation, or split-thickness graft and is easily hidden behind the ear. Another good source for full-thickness facial grafts is supraclavicular skin and lower neck. This often matches the face quite well, and large grafts can be obtained from these areas. Again, whatever source is selected, it is important to carefully examine various donor sites to see how well they match the host site before a decision is made. Other donor sites for full-thickness facial skin grafts are less desirable than those already mentioned. For example, skin from the inner arm, anterior shoulder, or abdomen when placed on the face retains its pale color, it has few sebaceous glands and pores, and there is little actinic damage, features that accentuate the mismatch between donor and recipient sites.

In addition to its cosmetic advantage, the full-thickness graft is indicated in functionally important areas such as the eye. Full-thickness grafts undergo less postoperative contraction. Contraction may lead to serious distortion of the eyelid margin. The lip is another area on the face where contraction may lead to distortion of a free border. Although most defects in this location can be healed by an appropriate local skin flap, this area occasionally requires a graft. Postoperative wound contraction may also interfere with the extension or flexion of joints, particularly of the fingers, toes, wrists, knees, and elbows. At times, full-thickness grafts are indicated in these locations. One important point about wound edge distortion that needs special mention involves delayed grafts. Defects near free borders (eyelid, lip, ala nasi, and eyebrow) should be grafted soon after surgery, before contraction has time to begin. Once the myofibroblasts are in place and contraction begins, a skin graft will not prevent distortion of a free border. Finally, a full-thickness graft resists wear and tear better than other types. These grafts are indicated in areas such as the sole, palm, or near joints that are subject to repeated injury.

Wound depth is always a consideration when deciding on a flap or graft repair. Full-thickness skin grafts are limited in their thickness, and with deeper wounds, immediate grafting will result in a concavity. There may be exposed cartilage or bone. In these situations, a flap would be a better choice. Delayed grafting does offer another alternative in the situation in which wound edge contraction is not a problem. The wound may be allowed to granulate enough to fill the defect and cover cartilage or bone so that the skin graft can have a more successful outcome. Thin periosteum or perichondrium provides a risky recipient bed. Inattentive technique during surgery or the postoperative period (in the case of a delayed graft) that allows thin periosteum or perichondrium to dry out or be exposed to harsh or oxidizing chemicals, such as hydrogen peroxide, increases the risk of graft failure or slowed granulation time.

Split-thickness grafts

The split-thickness graft is a second type of graft that is useful in skin surgery. Split grafts are used less

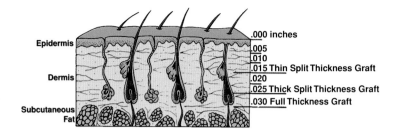

Fig. 25.1 Types of skin grafts. (Reprinted with modifications from Trimble [27] with permission of *Dermatologic Clinics*.)

frequently than full-thickness grafts. These grafts consist of the epidermis and a variable amount of dermis, depending on the depth of the excision (Fig. 25.1). They can be divided into thin grafts that are between 0.010 and 0.015 inches in depth, medium-thickness grafts between 0.015 and 0.022 inches, and thick grafts between 0.022 and 0.025 inches in depth. The cosmetic and functional properties are directly proportional to the thickness of the dermis. Thicker grafts always have better functional and cosmetic properties. Thick grafts undergo less postoperative contraction and withstand injury better than thin grafts. All split-thickness grafts undergo postoperative contraction. Thick grafts on a firm bed such as periosteum or perichondrium may contract 10% to 20%, whereas thin grafts on a soft bed such as the neck or eyelid may contract as much as 60%. To counter this predictable effect, split grafts should be greater than 0.022 inches in thickness, and graft size should be calculated based on a fully expanded recipient wound. It is wise to add slightly more skin than is actually necessary. It is much easier to trim away extra graft skin than to go back and add more skin.

The cosmetic properties of the split-thickness graft depend on the donor site. This fact severely limits its usefulness on the face. Because these grafts are usually large, they must be cut from a large flat surface. In addition, the donor site heals slowly and with a permanent scar. These considerations limit the choice of donor sites to places such as the lower abdomen, thighs, and buttocks, although almost any area of the body may be used. Unfortunately, the color match from these donor sites is poor when split grafts are applied to the face. They should only be used when the wound is so large that it is difficult to find a full-thickness donor site with enough skin or when a cosmetic reconstruction is being

delayed while the wound site is followed for tumor recurrence.

Other types of grafts that should be discussed are thin split-thickness grafts and pinch grafts (Figs. 25.1 and 25.2). Pinch grafts are obtained by elevating a small portion of skin on the tip of a

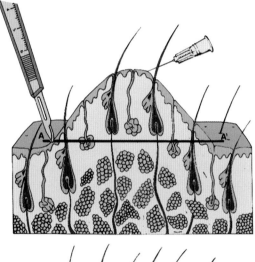

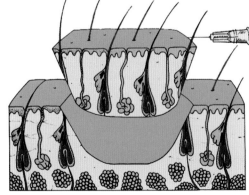

Fig. 25.2 Pinch grafts. (Reprinted with modifications from Trimble [27] with permission of *Dermatologic Clinics*.)

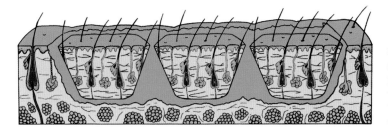

Fig. 25.3 Pinch grafts (small deep grafts). Host site: rows of pinch grafts placed on open wound. (Reprinted with modifications from Trimble [27] with permission of *Dermatologic Clinics*.)

needle and cutting the base. They should include the dermis but not subcutaneous fat. These small islands of epidermis and dermis are usually 4 to 6 mm in diameter. Pinch grafts are placed closely together on the wound in rows (Fig. 25.3). After the grafts take, the intervening spaces fill in with scar tissue. Pinch and thin split-thickness grafts have little place during reconstruction after most skin cancer surgery because their cosmetic appearance is so poor. Their only advantage over other grafts is that they can survive in situations in which a thick graft might fail. These situations include recipient sites with poor blood supply or poor granulations, such as wounds on the lower legs or foot, vascular ulcers, postradiation sites, chronic lymphedema, and sites with exposed perichondrium or periosteum. In general, the thinner the graft, the more likely it will survive. A final use of a thin graft might be to temporarily close a wound that is to be observed for tumor recurrence. Recurrence of skin cancer under a thin split-thickness graft can be identified earlier than if the wound is allowed to heal by granulation, a flap, or a thick graft.

Composite grafts

Certain specialized types of skin grafts are useful in the management of skin malignancies. One example is the composite graft. The composite graft contains more than one tissue, such as skin and fat or skin and cartilage. Most commonly, it is used to repair wounds around the nose, such as the rim of the ala nasi, nasal tip, or septum following the removal of tumor. For instance, a tumor is excised in a semicircular fashion from the nasal rim. A pattern of this defect is then traced on the rim of the ear above the lobe. This small portion of the helix

is excised. The excision is made completely through the ear so that the graft contains skin on both sides and cartilage or fat in the center. This piece of ear is trimmed and sutured to fit the defect on the nose. The donor site is closed as a "V" excision and closed in layers to prevent notching of the ear. A composite graft taken from posterior ear skin and conchal cartilage may be used to repair the ala, tip, or septum if structural support is necessary. This graft may have direct attachment between skin and cartilage, or separate pieces of cartilage in the form of round punches or strips may be placed under the graft skin [12,13].

Another form of composite graft is the hair transplant. The hair transplant graft involves moving strips, plugs, or single hairs of hair-bearing scalp and transplanting them to a location that needs hair. It can be used to camouflage scars and grafts of the eyebrows, eyelashes, or scalp [14–16].

Dermal overgraft

Another specialized graft that may be useful to the surgeon is the dermal overgraft [17–22]. It was originally described in 1958 by Webster [18], who used it to help prevent chronic leg ulcers from recurring. Webster removed the epidermis from a healed graft or healed ulcer scar and from a zone of surrounding normal skin. He then applied a skin graft to this dermal bed. The process was repeated at 3-month intervals until he built up a thick dermal layer over the ulcer. He discovered that this helped prevent a recurrence of the ulcer. Since his description, the dermal overgraft has been used for other purposes, such as improving the appearance of scars and grafts. It may be used to elevate depressed scars and grafts or to help camouflage the color of a scar or graft if it is too pale, red, or pigmented. In addition, the overgraft can improve the appearance of x-ray scars, even though these scars have a notoriously poor blood supply.

When to use a skin graft

The question of when the surgeon should close a wound with a skin graft following excision of a malignancy depends on whether or not use of a graft will restore cosmesis and function best. The surgeon must choose between the various alternative methods for healing wounds (direct approximation, graft, granulation, skin flap, and partial closure combined with granulation, flap, or graft) and use his or her experience to tailor the repair to fit the particular situation. All individuals heal slightly differently, and various sites on the same individual may heal differently. Therefore, unfortunately, one cannot exactly predict the result of any surgical procedure. The patient should be aware of this fact.

One variable that affects healing is the patient's age. Young adults may occasionally heal with pink hypertrophic scars. Also, young individuals have fewer creases and wrinkles on their face in which scars can be concealed. Their skin is not as loose as the skin in older patients, and a large flap may be necessary to close a small defect, whereas partial closure combined with a graft might produce less scarring. A graft can always be excised later in a second stage when the skin loosens. Flaps around the nose may be puffy or bulky and require subsequent procedures to correct problems such as ectropion, partial obstruction of an airway, webbing of the inner canthus, distortion of an ala nasi, or "pin cushioning." A graft may be a better choice. On the other hand, older patients have skin that is lax. They have wrinkles and lines of expression that run perpendicular to the underlying facial muscles. Their contour lines around the nose, hair line, eyebrows, and ears are more pronounced. The folds of dependency, such as sagging cheeks and chin, are more obvious. These features lend themselves to wound closure either by linear closure or by local skin flaps, because the scars can often be concealed in these lines and folds.

A second factor influencing healing is the wound location. Different sites of the body do not heal with the same good result. For example, skin flaps on the nasal tip or ala nasi may produce depressed incision lines with prominent suture marks, particularly in patients with thick sebaceous skin, or distortion of the ala rim. For this reason, a graft or granulation might be the preferable method of closing a wound on the ala and nasal tip. The skin of the cheeks and forehead lend themselves to closure by skin flaps. Areas around the eyelids and inner canthus heal extremely well with a graft. Skin wounds over the chest, neck, and shoulders occasionally heal with hypertrophic scars or keloids with any method of closure. Large full-thickness wounds on the trunk and extremities that are closed by direct approximation under great tension result in a stretched "fish mouth," pale, depressed scar that looks more artificial than a round scar with ill-defined edges resulting from healing by secondary intention. However, the healing time for a full-thickness wound left open to granulate may be very prolonged and in areas of poor circulation, may not heal at all. Although the healing time may be shorter with a graft, grafts to full-thickness wounds on the trunk and extremities are cosmetically poor because they look like a patch and may be depressed. If the wound is large, one must individualize the repair choice to what is best for the patient. An elderly patient may be unable to tolerate the delayed healing time and constant wound care of a granulating wound.

There are other individual variables that influence the ultimate cosmetic appearance of a healed graft, such as technique of the surgeon, postoperative complications, and compliance of the patient during healing. An experienced surgeon is able to control most of these factors, but after close inspection, a skin graft may end up looking like a patch, even with good technique. This is a result of several factors: (1) a color mismatch between graft and recipient skin, (2) a prominent scar at the junction between graft and recipient skin, (3) a contour defect with a depressed graft, and (4) a texture difference with a shiny, reflective surface quality. These problems can be minimized by careful selection of donor skin, meticulous operative technique, and attentiveness to wound healing in the early post-operative days.

A color mismatch may result even if the donor skin initially matches the host site. This is less common with full-thickness skin grafts. If hypopigmentation occurs, makeup can restore near-normal color or a very superficial dermabrasion around the graft may help blend the color transition. Hyperpigmentation may be cautiously treated with bleaching agents, cryosurgery, superficial laser, or dermabrasion. A small test area would be prudent. It is important to remember that wound healing is active for many months after surgery, and before secondary cosmetic procedures are attempted on a graft, one should try to wait 8 to 12 months before evaluating the cosmetic outcome.

A graft may look like a patch because of a prominent scar at the junction between graft and host site. This can be helped by placing the junction into wrinkle lines, folds, or cosmetic boundaries or replacing an entire cosmetic unit instead of just a part of the unit. Dermabrasion or superficial laser may help flatten an elevated scar ridge and blend color tones at the edge. Pressure therapy and intralesional steroids may help a hypertrophic scar line. The graft might not match the recipient site if the graft is depressed below the surrounding skin. If the surgeon notes a significant disparity between surgical wound depth and proposed donor site skin thickness before grafting, he or she may delay grafting until healing by granulation has "filled up" the wound base. Sometimes a horizontal excision of the wound edge and/or use of horizontal mattress sutures can lower the height of the wound edge or bring the base up to the level of the wound edge. The use of cartilage composite grafts and dermal overgrafts to elevate a depressed graft has been mentioned. Injectable materials such as collagen are available for elevating a graft [23]. Finally, a graft may be apparent because its surface texture is more shiny and reflective. This seems to happen more in grafts that peel or blister off their epidermis during the early postoperative period. The condition tends to improve with time, but a makeup with an oily base or powder can camouflage this defect.

Selected sites

The skin on the eyelids requires a certain laxity to function properly. Direct closure of large wounds on the lower eyelid may cause an ectropion. Similarly, a skin flap may result in ectropion by the effect of gravity or by the downward tension caused by closure of a flap donor site. Healing by secondary intention with wound contraction may cause the same problem. Thus, a graft is an excellent choice for healing wounds of the eyelid. The full-thickness graft does best because it contracts the least and retains its color the best. The donor site depends on the amount of skin needed. In order of preference, these are (1) upper eyelid skin, (2) posterior ear or retroauricular skin, and (3) supraclavicular skin. Graft size should be calculated with the wound maximally expanded. A split-thickness graft is a poor choice for closing eyelid wounds because this graft contracts to a greater degree.

Skin grafts are indicated on the ear. The skin on the surface of the auricle is attached firmly to the cartilage. This makes it difficult to close small wounds primarily or by the use of a flap. Healing by secondary intention is slow, requires twice-daily wound care, may be painful, and leaves the wound open to *Staphylococcus* or *Pseudomonas* infection, which is particularly worrisome in diabetics. The full-thickness graft or thick split graft is the preferred method of closure. Donor skin from the retroauricular area matches best, and the donor scar can be concealed behind the ear. It must be remembered that bare cartilage will not support a graft. If the graft cannot be placed on perichondrium, there are two alternatives. The cartilage may be removed entirely, and the graft may be placed on the exposed soft tissue of the skin on the back of the ear. However, this may result in a depressed graft or a change in normal contour. The alternative is to remove multiple 3- to 4-mm plugs of cartilage or 3- to 4-mm strips of cartilage using the "plow" technique with a dermal punch or curved iris scissor to expose the perichondrium and soft tissue of the back of the ear. The graft may be sutured to this base, or the wound may be allowed to granulate before grafting. Trying to granulate over solid cartilage (without perforations or complete removal) with only a thin perichondrium is much slower and will need to be followed closely for infection.

The nose has two distinct surgical zones. Skin on the upper two thirds of the nose is loosely attached to the bone and underlying cartilage. It also has contours and rhytids in which scars can be concealed. This is an ideal area for the use of local skin flaps. The skin on the lower third of the nose is firmly attached to the cartilage. Furthermore, the ala nasi and tip of the nose have few contours or wrinkles to hide the scars. Direct approximation can deform the ala nasi and tip, even with defects as small as 0.3 cm. Thus, it is obvious that if a cancer is going to be removed from this site with a margin of safety, it will be difficult to close primarily or with a flap. Of course, these wounds can be healed by secondary intention, but this may result in a pale, shiny, depressed scar on the tip or a notched ala rim. Full-thickness skin grafts are often the method of choice for wounds on the nasal tip or ala. Donor sites include the posterior ear, preauricular skin, nasolabial fold, and glabella. If it is necessary to remove much cartilage from the nasal tip or ala nasi, small portions of cartilage may be excised from the back of the ear with a 4-mm dermal punch or a #15 blade and placed under the graft to build it up to the proper level. Defects on the rim of the ala nasi or nasal septum may be repaired with a composite graft from the helix, as previously discussed. A through-and-through nasal defect above the ala nasi rim may be closed with a combination flap and graft or flap and composite graft.

Wounds elsewhere on the face, such as the forehead, cheeks, chin, or lips, are best repaired with methods other than a graft. With exception of the scalp, the skin in these locations is loose. There are numerous wrinkles, lines of dependency, and contours that make them ideal locations for closure with local skin flaps. Occasionally, a graft will be necessary with an unusually large wound and may be used in combination with a flap.

Grafts combined with partial closure are indicated in large wounds of the trunk and extremities. In these areas, there are few wrinkles or folds to hide a flap or a graft. There is little cosmetic advantage to flap closure because of the increased scar length. In addition, the reduced vascularity of the trunk and extremities raises the risk of flap failure, dehiscence, and stretch-back. The cosmetic result of both flaps and grafts in these areas is poor. However, partial closure and grafting may result in the smallest defect. As skin stretches over time, the graft may be eliminated in a second procedure.

Preparing the full-thickness skin graft

Once the donor site and graft size have been determined, removal of the graft skin is no more difficult than a simple excision. Using a skin hook so as not to crush or pinch the graft and a #15 scalpel blade or scissors, an attempt should be made to limit the amount of fat that is removed with the graft. The deeper one goes in removing the graft, the more the risk of injury to the normal anatomy below. This is particularly true when removing graft skin from the upper eyelid, where muscle approximates the deep dermis.

Trimming the fat from the graft should be done with good lighting and a magnification head loupe. With magnification, the surgeon can easily discriminate between fat, superficial fascia, and deep dermis. The yellow fat and transparent superficial fascia are carefully trimmed away, to leave a glistening white dermis. The connective tissue of the deep dermis appears more opaque, white, and firm than the transparent and mobile fascial tissue between fat and dermis. Tiny yellow nodules representing sebaceous glands may begin to appear if the surgeon continues to trim. Only experience can teach the proper depth for trimming. During the trimming procedure, great care should be taken not to allow air desiccation of the recipient wound or the graft. Both should be kept moist with sterile saline or lidocaine at all times. Care should be taken while trimming to prevent unnecessary manipulation of the graft and "button" holes.

An alternative method for elevating a full-thickness skin graft is faster and does not require defatting. Infiltrate with lidocaine at an intradermal level to expand the dermal thickness with the lidocaine. Using a template and a #15 scalpel blade, score the epidermis around the entire perimeter of the template about 2 mm deep. Turn the scalpel blade tangential to the skin surface. Using light pressure and a slicing motion along the length of the donor graft perimeter that was previously scored, elevate the graft with repeated slicing strokes. With practice, the graft can be cut as thick as a full-thickness skin graft or as thin as a thick split-thickness skin graft. The supraclavicular donor site is a good place to try this technique first. As the cutting proceeds, watch the angle of the blade. If the angle is too superficial, it will cause a "button hole." A deeper angle will yield a thicker graft. The partial-thickness donor wound left after the graft has been elevated may be excised further and closed [24–26].

Finally, the graft should be sutured into position with fine approximation of epidermal edges and occasional tacking sutures at the base to prevent lateral shift of the graft across its wound base and to eliminate dead space in which seromas and hematomas may develop. Hemostasis must be complete before applying the graft. Although every surgeon has his or her own preferred dressing, we advocate the tie-over bolster dressing using Telfa and a cotton ball wet with chlorhexidine gluconate 4% solution (Hibiclens). A tie-over dressing will give more uniform pressure over the graft to prevent hematoma and seroma and more protection from lateral shearing forces that could cause breaking of the fragile vascular connections between the graft and the bed. There may also be some advantage in counteracting the forces of contraction when the defect is near a free border by stretching the donor site. Dressings are not usually removed until 5 to 7 days on the face and 12 to 14 days on nonfacial areas unless signs of infection or hematoma are evident. A quick, easy method for the tie-over dressing is the "figure 8" method [24]. Using 5-0 or 6-0 monofilament nylon, enter the skin surface 2 to 3 mm beyond the grafted wound edge. Make a second pass (in the same direction) 180° across the graft at a point 2 to 3 mm beyond the edge of the grafted wound. Finally, place the piece of Telfa cut to size and the cotton ball over the graft and tie a square knot over the top of the cotton ball to hold it in place. If done properly, the knot and suture will form a figure 8. This tie-over suture may be done in multiple directions until the surgeon is satisfied with graft sta-

bility. The reader is referred to a more detailed description of the surgical technique for full-thickness grafting [1].

Preparing a split-thickness skin graft

After the donor site, size, and thickness of the split graft have been determined, the donor area is prepared with local anesthetic and sterile drape. Wheals resulting from the injection of anesthetic should be entirely flat before cutting the graft. We use the Brown dermatome for large grafts because it is easy to work with and is accessible in many hospital operating rooms. For small grafts, we use the Davol dermatome because it is easy to use, inexpensive, and battery operated and has disposable dermatome heads. On the Davol dermatome, the cutting thickness is preset to a medium thickness. The Brown requires the surgeon to set the thickness. The Brown dermatome blade should be properly set and locked into position before use. Using a magnifying head loupe, sight down the blade. When the dermatome is closed down completely, there should be a very thin rim of light passing through and along the entire blade edge. This lighted slit should be equal along the length of the blade. If the aperture is not equal along the entire blade, the dermatome may need calibration.

On the Brown dermatome, advance the dermatome thickness dials a little at a time (i.e., 0.005 inch), alternating sides. Turning one side too far without alternating sides may ruin the calibration. When the thickness setting is achieved, sight down the blade again to make certain that the lighted opening is equal along the blade edge. The standard #15 stainless steel blade is approximately 0.015 inches in thickness, so it may be used as a gross guide to double-check the aperture width.

The donor site and the bottom of the dermatome are lubricated with a thin film of chlorhexidine gluconate solution (Hibiclens). The dermatome is placed on the skin surface with a firm pressure that indents the skin surface 0.5 to 1.0 cm. If assistants are available, a moderate stretching of the skin at two equal points out in front of the advancing dermatome may help prevent "bunching" of the skin

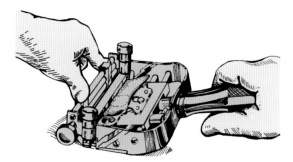

Fig. 25.4 Two-handed method of cutting a split-thickness graft with the Brown dermatome. The thumb and index finger of the left hand depress the dermatome into the skin. The right hand grasps the handle and advances the dermatome.

graft as the dermatome moves forward. The most important point to cutting a high-quality split graft is correct orientation to the skin surface. The plane of the bottom of the dermatome should be kept parallel to the skin surface at all times while the machine advances. The two-handed method of harvesting a split graft is illustrated in Fig. 25.4. The forward hand delivers moderate downward pressure. The back hand maintains a perfectly parallel orientation. Very little forward pressure is required if the skin is wet with chlorhexidine gluconate solution and the motor is kept at high speed. An assistant may use pickups or a hemostat to help brush graft skin away from the cutting edge as the graft is taken. At no time should the dermatome be allowed to angle upward during the advancement. This will result in a torn or shredded graft. When the graft has been cut, angle the blade upward to separate graft skin from donor site.

The split-thickness skin graft may be applied to the recipient site in the same manner as a full-thickness graft. The skin around the donor site may be cleaned with alcohol, dried, and painted with benzoin, which will facilitate the adherence of an Opsite dressing. Excess skin that was not used for reconstruction may be sutured back to the open donor site. If there is no history of allergy, a small amount of antibiotic ointment may be applied to the remaining uncovered donor wound before the application of the Opsite. The reader is referred to a more detailed description of the techniques of split-thickness grafting [1,27].

Summary

The dermatologic surgeon is commonly confronted with the four alternatives for wound closure after skin cancer excision: flap, graft, primary closure, and healing by granulation. Skin grafting is a technique that is indicated in certain situations during reconstruction and offers some advantages over alternative closures. Grafting has a relatively low risk of complication and a high degree of success when done properly in an outpatient surgery setting. The foregoing discussion is a short summary of the role of skin grafting in the management of skin malignancies.

References

1 Epstein E, Epstein E Jr. Skin surgery. 6th ed. Philadelphia: Saunders; 1987.
2 McGregor IA. Fundamental techniques of plastic surgery. 7th ed. Edinburgh and London: Churchill-Livingstone; 1980.
3 Converse JM, McCarthy JG, Litter JW. Reconstructive plastic surgery. 2nd ed. Philadelphia: WB Saunders; 1977.
4 Grabb WC, Smith JW. Plastic surgery. 3rd ed. Boston: Little, Brown; 1980.
5 Rudolph R, Fisher JC, Ninnemann JL. Skin grafting. Boston: Little, Brown; 1979.
6 Petruzzelli GJ, Johnson JT. Skin grafts. Otolaryngol Clin North Am 1994;27:25.
7 Cram AE, Chang P. Clinical applications of free skin grafts. In: Bardach J, editor. Local flaps and free skin grafts. St Louis: Mosby; 1992. p. 157–178.
8 Mailland GF, Clavel PR. Aesthetic units in skin grafting of the face. Ann Plast Surg 1991;26:347.
9 Adams DC, Ramsey ML. Grafts in dermatologic surgery: review and update on full- and split-thickness skin grafts, free cartilage grafts, and composite grafts. Dermatol Surg 2005;31(8 Pt 2):1055–67.
10 Gloster HM. The use of full-thickness skin grafts to repair nonperforating nasal defects. J Am Acad Dermatol 2000;42:1041–50.
11 Robinson JK, Hanke CW, Sengelmann RD, Siegel DM. Surgery of the skin, procedural dermatology. Philadelphia: Elsevier Mosby; 2005. p. 365–79.

12 Trimble JR. The use of multicartilage composite grafts to repair wounds of the lower third of the nose. Cutis 1976;17:777.

13 Adams C, Ratner D. Composite and free cartilage grafting. Dermatol Clin 2005;23:129–40.

14 Nordstrom RE. Punch hair grafting under split-skin grafts on scalps. Plast Reconstr Surg 1979;64:9–12.

15 Marritt E. Transplantation of single hairs from the scalp as eyelashes. J Dermatol Surg Oncol 1980;6:271–3.

16 Lewis LA, Resnik SS. Strip and punch grafting for alopecia of the eyebrow. J Dermatol Surg Oncol 1979;5:557–9.

17 Trimble JR. Dermal overgrafting in dermatology. J Dermatol Surg Oncol 1983;9:987–93.

18 Webster GV, Peterson RA, Stein HL. Dermal overgrafting of the leg. J Bone Joint Surg 1958;40A:796.

19 Hynes W. "Shaving" in plastic surgery with special reference to the treatment of chronic radiodermatitis. Br J Plast Surg 1959;12:43–54.

20 Rees ID, Casson PR. The indications for cutaneous dermal overgrafting. Plast Reconstr Surg 1966;38:522.

21 Hynes W. The treatment of pigmented moles by shaving and skin graft. Br J Plast Surg 1956;9: 47.

22 Hynes W. The treatment of scars by shaving and skin graft. Br J Plast Surg 1957;10:1.

23 Bailin P, Bailin M. Correction of depressed scars following Mohs surgery: the role of collagen implantation. J Dermatol Surg Oncol 1982;8:845–9.

24 Trimble JW. Full thickness grafts simplified. Presented during the scientific program at the second annual meeting of the Florida Society of Dermatologic Surgeons; 1983 May 22; Orlando, FL.

25 Cardon OP, Farhood VW. A freehand technique for harvesting dermal grafts. J Oral Maxillofac Surg 1990;48:1009–11.

26 Snow SN, Stiff M, Lambert D, Tsoi C, Mohs FE. Freehand technique to harvest partial-thickness skin to repair superficial facial defects. J Dermatol Surg Oncol 1995;21:153–7.

27 Trimble JR. Skin grafting as an office procedure in dermatology. Dermatol Clin 1984;2:251–70.

CHAPTER 26

Mohs micrographic surgery

David J. Goldberg and Eds Chua

Mohs micrographic surgery (MMS) is a procedure used to treat various forms of malignant skin neoplasms that leads to the highest success or cure rate with maximal tissue conservation [1–3].

The principle behind this technique is based on the idea of excision with minimal margins (sparing normal tissue) and immediate histologic examination through frozen sections while the patient waits [1–4]. The histopathologic examination is done by the Mohs surgeon, who plays a dual role as surgeon and pathologist.

Mohs surgery involves the use of a tangential excision, which permits the whole cutaneous tumor margin to be examined histologically. This then allows tracing or "graphically mapping" of the extent of the neoplasm until it is completely removed or cleared, as evaluated on histopathologic examination, thus sparing uninvolved normal tissue and facilitating easier reconstruction. Because it employs horizontal frozen sections of the excised neoplasm, Mohs surgery permits a more complete microscopic examination of the surgical margin compared with traditional surgical methods [1]. Furthermore, it allows complete removal of skin tumors while minimizing loss of normal tissue [2–4]. Because of its safety, success rate, and low recurrence rate, Mohs surgery has become the "gold standard" for the removal of many skin tumors [2,3] and has become the technique of choice for almost all recurrent skin tumors.

Historical insights

Mohs surgery, generally but not exclusively performed by specially trained dermatologists, was first developed by Dr. Frederic Mohs, a general surgeon,

in the 1930s [5–8]. His original method, named *chemosurgery*, involved the use of a 20% zinc chloride paste applied as fixative to skin cancers under occlusive dressing for 12 to 24 hours, followed by excision of a saucer-shaped tissue sample and histologic examination by frozen section. Precise mapping and examination of the tissue specimen, specifically the border, permitted greater assessment of the surgical margin [1–3]. Sectioning of the tissue was done horizontally so as to be able to simultaneously microscopically evaluate the epidermis and entire subcutaneous tissue. The fixation process was repeated if tumor remained at the excision margins. This technique allowed the surgeon to return to the exact location of the residual tumor. Once no more tumor was found on histology, the wound was allowed to heal by second intention [1].

This original technique offered several disadvantages. Although it was associated with a high success rate, this approach was time-consuming and uncomfortable for the patient because of the associated fixative-induced pain, and immediate wound reconstruction was not possible.

In 1953, Dr. Mohs made a modification of this technique that was simpler, effective, and less time-consuming. The new method, called *fresh tissue technique*, was initially employed for small tumors, especially those involving the eyelids, and used frozen tissue section processing. This also avoided irritation and pain caused by the zinc chloride fixative [5].

It was, however, Dr. Theodore Tromovitch in 1970 who initially described the now more popular use of the fresh tissue technique, but still using Mohs' original concept of tangential excision. This procedure offered a simpler technique, faster turnaround time, and less patient discomfort and allowed for most skin tumors to be removed in a single day, with same-day wound reconstruction [5]. Tromovitch's approach has been adopted as the standard of today's MMS [1,2,5].

Mohs micrographic surgery has developed into a special subspecialty field in dermatology and dermatologic surgery, with a universally recognized accredited training overseen by the American College of Mohs Micrographic Surgery and Cutaneous Oncology [1,5,7].

Today, the majority of Mohs micrographic surgeons exclusively use the fresh tissue section technique. The fixed tissue technique, however, is still occasionally employed in special situations, including cases of vascular tumors, tumors involving highly vascular areas, and tumors with bone invasion [1,7].

Indications

General indications
Recurrent tumors
In general, Mohs surgery is indicated especially for many recurrent skin tumors [1]. This technique offers three-dimensional mapping of the recurrent tumor, allowing for a more correct determination of tumor-free surgical margins and lower incidence of future recurrence. The overwhelming majority of trials show a lower recurrence rate for most recurrent cutaneous malignant neoplasms treated with Mohs surgery [9,10].

Indistinct clinical margins
Mohs surgery is indicated in untreated carcinoma with indistinct clinical margins [1–3]. These tumors have subclinical spread that may not be observed before traditional surgical excision—unless wide margins and generous amounts of normal tissue are excised. For these cases, Mohs surgery provides a greater chance of complete removal while sparing normal, uninvolved tissue [1].

High-risk locations
Tumors in specific anatomic areas are associated with greater unrecognized spread. These high-risk areas, which include the skin around the eyes, nose, ears, and lips, have a higher statistical frequency

of local recurrence and distant metastasis; hence a surgical technique that offers complete tumor excision and the lowest risk of recurrence is indicated. Skin overlying cartilage (i.e., pinna of the ear), skin overlying bony structures (i.e., scalp, temple, upper nose, nasal tip, forehead), and skin in embryonic fusion planes (preauricular area, retroauricular sulcus, nasolabial fold, inner canthus) are high-risk regions. Tumors involving the so-called H zone of the face, which includes the nasal ala, nasal septum, medial and lateral canthi, preauricular and postauricular areas, philtrum, and vermilion border of the lip—all of which involve cosmetically and functionally critical areas—should be managed by Mohs surgery [1,3]. The digits and genital areas are other areas that are high risk and should be managed by Mohs surgery [1,4,11].

Large tumors
Mohs surgery is indicated in any skin cancer with a diameter larger than 2 cm [3]. These tumors tend to have significant subclinical spread and have a higher incidence of recurrence when treated by traditional surgical excision compared with MMS [1].

Perineural, periappendageal, perivascular involvement
Mohs surgery offers the lowest risk of recurrence for tumors with perineural, periappendageal (e.g., nails), and perivascular involvement [1].

Failed traditional excision
When histopathologic examination of a routinely excised neoplasm reveals it to be incompletely removed, Mohs surgery is indicated [1–3].

Specific indications
Specific indications for Mohs surgery include the following [2,3]:

Basal cell carcinoma
Mohs surgery has become the treatment of choice for recurrent basal cell carcinomas (BCCs). In addition, Mohs surgery is ideal for aggressive subtypes of BCCs, which include the morpheaform, adenoidal, superficial, and infiltrating types. These

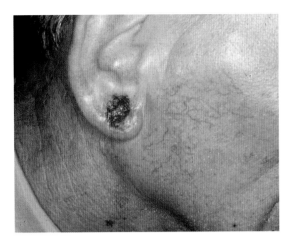

Fig. 26.1 Primary ulcerative BCC of the ear lobule. Mohs surgery preserved most of this patient's ear.

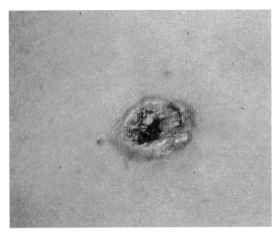

Fig. 26.3 Classic BCC with rolled pearly border and overlying telangiectases.

tumors have high rates of recurrence [1,2,3,11]. Overall, BCC is the most common indication and comprises the majority of Mohs surgery cases [1–3] (Figs. 26.1 to 26.6). Mohs surgery offers the best cure rate and lowest recurrence rate for both primary and recurrent BCCs. Studies have shown a 99% cure rate for these tumors, compared with 90% following traditional surgical excision [1]. For recurrent tumors, the cure rate using this procedure ranges between 90% and 95% compared with other modalities, which average around 77% to 80%

[2,3]. The 5-year recurrence rate for BCC ranges from 1.4% to 3.2% for primary BCC and 4% to 6.7% for recurrent BCC. [12,13].

Squamous cell carcinoma

Squamous cell carcinoma (SCC) is treated similarly as BCC. Indications for Mohs surgery are similar (Figs. 26.7 to 26.12). For SCC of the skin, reported cure rates are 96.9% compared with 92.1% for other modalities [2,3]. Recurrence rate after Mohs surgery is relatively low. The recurrence rate

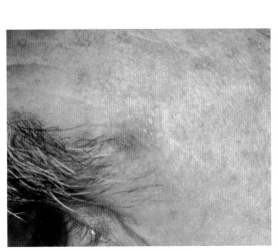

Fig. 26.2 Poorly defined BCC of the forehead that extended into the eyebrow during Mohs surgery.

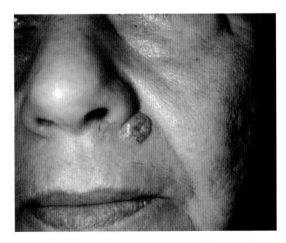

Fig. 26.4 Primary BCC of the nasolabial fold extending toward the nose. Mohs surgery is indicated here to provide a high cure rate and optimal cosmetic results.

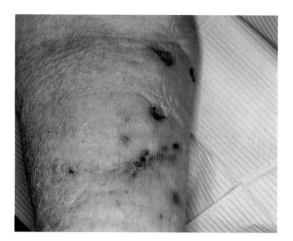

Fig. 26.5 Multiply recurrent BCC of the arm. This patient ultimately required amputation.

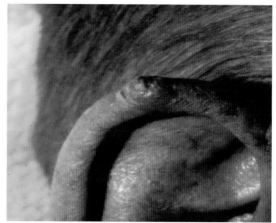

Fig. 26.7 Primary SCC of the ear.

is 2.6% for primary SCC and 5.9% for recurrent SCC [14].

Other indications

Other lesions that have been reported in the literature as having been treated using this method include the following:

1 SCC in situ [1,3]. Mohs surgery is particularly useful for extensive lesions with poorly defined margins.

2 Dermatofibrosarcoma protuberans. Various studies have shown excellent results in the treatment

of this tumor with Mohs surgery, resulting in low recurrences [1,15–17].

3 Verrucous carcinoma [1,18]. Mohs surgery offers advantages for this tumor because of its tissue-sparing ability, especially when the tumor involves the foot or penis [1].

4 Keratoacanthoma [1,3]. Mohs surgery is recommended especially for recurrent keratoacanthoma and keratoacanthoma in high-risk areas, given the similarity in clinical and histopathologic features between this tumor and SCC.

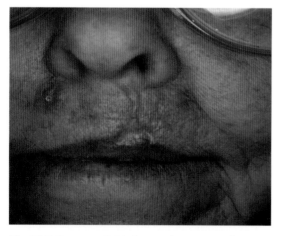

Fig. 26.6 Recurrent BCC after previous non-Mohs excision. Mohs surgery led to cure.

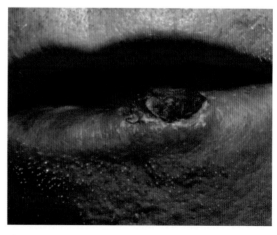

Fig. 26.8 Recurrent SCC of the lip, an ideal indication for Mohs surgery.

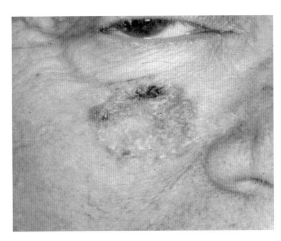

Fig. 26.9 Recurrent SCC of the cheek before Mohs surgery.

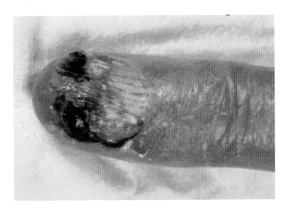

Fig. 26.10 Primary SCC of the finger and nail bed. Mohs surgery may lessen the likelihood of digital amputation.

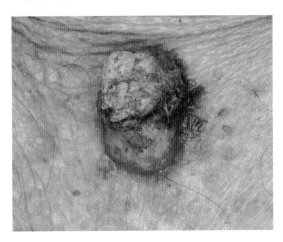

Fig. 26.11 Primary necrotic SCC of the skin.

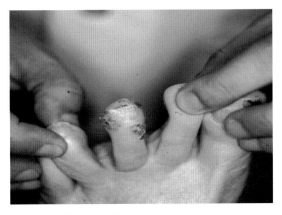

Fig. 26.12 Primary SCC of the toe. Mohs surgery may lessen the likelihood of digital amputation. Here, Mohs surgery led to cure and preservation of the toe.

5 Extramammary Paget's disease. Mohs surgery for this condition has resulted in lower recurrences compared with conventional excision and is specifically preferred when the anogenital region, the most commonly involved site, is affected, because of its tissue-sparing effect [1,19,20].
6 Sebaceous carcinoma (Fig. 26.13) [3]
7 Microcystic adnexal carcinoma [1,17,21]. Because of this tumor's high rate of recurrence and predisposition for deep tissue and neural invasion, Mohs surgery is an indicated treatment.
8 Merkel cell carcinoma [1,3,17]

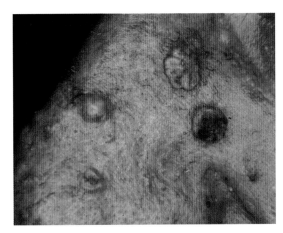

Fig. 26.13 A variety of sebaceous neoplasms, including a crusted lesion that proved to be sebaceous carcinoma.

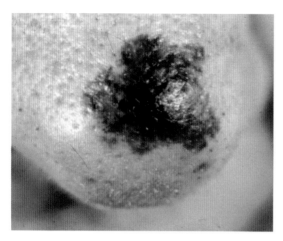

Fig. 26.14 Malignant melanoma of the nose. Mohs surgery may be tissue sparing in this case.

Treatment	BCC	SCC
Simple Surgical Excision	89.9	91.9
Radiotherapy	91.3	90.0
Cryotherapy	92.5	NA
ED&C	92.3	96.3
Mohs Surgery	99.0	96.9

Fig. 26.16 Cure rates for BCC and SCC with a variety of commonly used treatment modalities. Note the high cure rates after Mohs surgery. ED&C, electrodessication and curettage; NA, not applicable.

9 Primary cutaneous melanoma [22], including lentigo maligna and lentigo maligna melanoma (Figs. 26.14 and 26.15) [1,23]. Although there is still some debate as to the use of Mohs surgery for melanoma, data have shown outstanding results with this malignancy [1,23]. Mohs surgery has increasingly come to be an accepted therapeutic modality for lentigo maligna and lentigo maligna melanoma. Compared with standard excision, Mohs surgery offers better margin control and lower rates of recurrence (4% to 5% vs. 8% to 20% in one study) for this condition [22].

Most authors recommend that any skin tumor that has a contiguous and radial growth pattern and that may be examined on frozen section can be managed using Mohs surgery [2] (Fig. 26.16).

Preprocedural management

Mohs surgery is performed in an outpatient setting under local anesthesia. Proper preoperative evaluation is important and consists of a thorough history and physical examination. As in any other minor surgical procedure, preoperative evaluation of any concomitant comorbid illness that may affect outcome, especially wound healing, is important. Besides doing a comprehensive physical examination, especially of the skin and the lesion, it may also be helpful to take a photograph of the carcinoma preoperatively (Fig. 26.17). Although laboratory examinations may be ordered only as dictated by indications according to the patient's clinical history and evaluation, some authors encourage a chest radiograph for any patient with unusually aggressive or multiply recurrent SCC or BCC to rule out metastatic disease [3].

As is usually done in all procedures, patients should be made aware of the risks, benefits, and complications of the procedures, which should be thoroughly explained by the physician.

Alcohol intake and nonsteroidal anti-inflammatory drugs are usually avoided 1 week

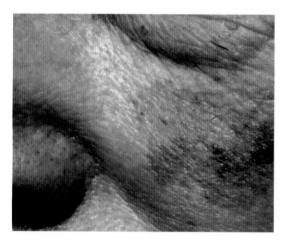

Fig. 26.15 Lentigo maligna melanoma of the cheek. Evidence suggests a high cure after Mohs surgery.

TUMOR IN THE SKIN

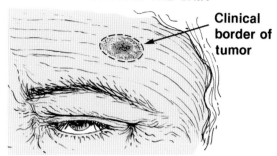

Clinical border of tumor

Fig. 26.17 Clinical evaluation of tumor prior to Mohs surgery.

CUT IN A THIN, FLAT SECTION
Establish orientation

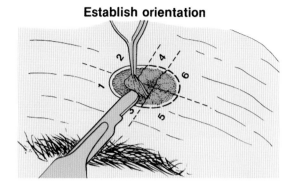

Fig. 26.18 Removal of tumor during Mohs surgery.

before the procedure. For patients who need to be on anticoagulants because of a medical indication, hemostasis may be achieved by electrocoagulation.

Mild sedation may be given on the morning of the procedure for anxious patients. As with any surgical procedure, informed consent must be provided.

Operating room setup

The surgical setup requires an appropriately equipped minor surgery procedure room, a well-trained staff, and a histopathologic laboratory and technician trained in tissue processing.

Proper instrumentation is mandatory. Necessary instruments include scalpel, curette, tissue forceps, needle holder, scissors, and electrocautery machine.

Preparation

After observing proper aseptic technique, the in-volved area is properly draped and the skin tumor is identified and infiltrated with local anesthesia. Some authors recommend application of ice to the involved area for 5 to 10 minutes, followed by slow injection of the local anesthesia (usually lidocaine 1% solution combined with epinephrine 1:100,000) using a 30-gauge needle [3].

Technique

The lesion is then debulked using a curette and scalpel to further delineate the size. This allows the

surgeon to "feel" for tumor extensions and take thinner samples during excision [1].

The planned excision is delineated on the skin 2 to 3 mm beyond the curetted margin. As a guide for orientation, identifying marks are made on the edge of the defect and the edges of the specimen using suture, staples, tattoos, or scalpel incisions [1]. This is followed by incision of the tissue by the scalpel blade held at a 45° angle to the skin surface. The tumor is excised 2 to 3 mm beyond the curetted margin. The excision continues entirely around the surface tumor and continues under the skin parallel to the surface (Fig. 26.18). The wound is bandaged and the tissue is processed while the patient waits.

The tissue is subdivided into smaller sections and numbered (Figs. 26.19 and 26.20). The tissue is cut

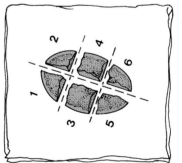

folded edge at top

Maintain orientation

Fig. 26.19 Coding of Mohs sections.

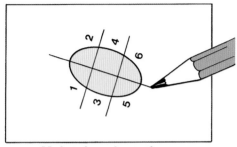

Maintain orientation

Fig. 26.20 Mapping of Mohs sections.

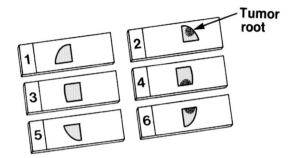

Fig. 26.22 Mohs sections placed on slides for evaluation.

into even smaller sections and surgical mapping is done using different colored dyes for orientation during histologic examination. The tissue is laid flat on a cryostat "chuck" so that the epidermis and the deepest margin are on a single plane. The tissue is frozen, sectioned horizontally, placed on a slide, and generally stained with hematoxylin and eosin (Figs. 26.21 and 26.22). Some physicians, as an alternative, prefer toluidine blue as the stain. The stained specimens are then examined by the Mohs surgeon (Fig. 26.23).

In a survey on different techniques used in different institutions by different Mohs surgeons, there was great variability in the mapping and processing techniques used in Mohs surgery. Most surgeons personally prepare the map of the tissue with a hand-drawn picture [24].

One of the advantages and a unique aspect of the Mohs procedure is that the operator/surgeon also serves a dual role as the pathologist, hence facilitating a good clinicopathologic correlation and an

increase in accuracy. The surgeon performs microscopic examination of the slides. Then if there are persistent malignant cells along the margin, the cells are properly marked. Then additional sections along the area of the persistent tumor are excised. This process is repeated until tumor-free margins are obtained.

It is important to control hemostasis, as the usual complications of this procedure commonly involve postoperative bleeding. Electrocoagulation is usually done for this purpose. Large blood vessels may be ligated with absorbable suture.

Wound reconstruction

Closure of the skin wound is done by side-to-side closures, flaps, or grafts, depending on the size of the

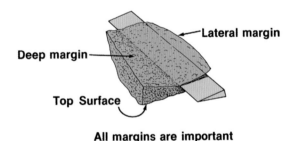

Fig. 26.21 Mohs section evaluation of all horizontal margins.

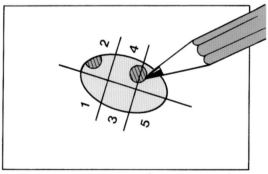

Return to areas of tumor and spare normal tissue

Fig. 26.23 Marked areas where there is persistence of tumor.

wound. Antibiotic ointment and occlusive dressings are generally left in place for at least 24 hours.

Postprocedural management

The patient is instructed to uncover the wounds after 24 hours, clean the sutures, and apply antibiotic ointment. For wounds that are closed by grafts, bolster dressings are applied and occasionally left in place for a week. Postprocedural pain, although minimal, may be managed by oral analgesics.

Success rate

As discussed above, overall, MMS has a high success rate, especially for BCCs, and the lowest recurrence rate among all treatment options for this condition [2,3,12]. Prognostic factors for recurrence include aggressive and infiltrating histopathologic subtype, more than four Mohs stages, size of defect, previous tumor recurrence, and long tumor duration [12–14].

Procedure safety

Asadi and colleagues [25] compared complication rates between office-based and hospital-based procedures in 3937 patients and showed no difference in complication rates, concluding that MMS can be safely done and is equally safe in either setting. Intraoperative adverse events are also rare, with minimal fluctuations in patients' vital signs [26].

Complications

Mohs surgery, like any surgical procedure, leads to some scarring. The degree of scarring is minimized by the minimal amounts of tissue removed. The extent of scar depends on wound size, depth, and location. Nerve damage may also complicate this procedure, leading to disruption of sensation, postoperative anesthesia, and paresthesia, but these usually resolve in a few months and are rarely long lasting. Immediate complications, such as bleeding and hematoma formation, are rare but may occur, as may secondary bacterial infection and dehiscence. In a comprehensive review of 1343 cases

of MMS, 1.6% developed complications, most commonly bleeding, postoperative hematomas, infection, and wound dehiscence [27].

New concepts and techniques

Mapping techniques and aids

Fluorescence imaging has been used for Mohs skin tumor demarcation. It appears to show a good correlation with standard Mohs histopathologic mapping [28]. The use of in vivo real-time confocal reflectance microscopy and ex vivo confocal scanning laser microscopy has also aided in the noninvasive optical imaging of skin sections, thus acting as a guide in Mohs surgery [28–31]. This approach may aid in confirmation of residual tumor [32].

Immunostaining

Immunohistochemical staining during Mohs surgery using MART-1 (melanoma antigen recognized by T cells) has proven to better visualize atypical melanocytes on frozen section, hence allowing for easier identification of lentigo maligna, facilitating complete removal of tumor [33], and improving the diagnostic accuracy of surgeons [34]. HMB-45 and Melan-A staining of tissue specimens also aids in the interpretation of frozen sections during MMS [35,36]. Immunoperoxidase techniques such as cytokeratin antibodies for SCCs, BCCs, and extramammary Paget's disease; CD34 for dermatofibrosarcoma protuberans; and S-100 staining for desmoplastic melanoma and lentigo maligna have also been useful in the removal of some high-risk carcinomas, sarcomas, and melanomas [37–39]. Mel-5 immunostaining has also yielded good results as an adjunct to the Mohs surgical treatment of lentigo maligna and lentigo maligna melanoma [40].

Unfortunately, although immunohistochemical techniques have proven to be helpful in the diagnostic interpretation of specimens, current practices of Mohs surgery laboratories rarely allow for the use of these immunostains because of the high cost of reagents, lack of reliable automated processes, additional expertise needed, and long times involved in doing such stains [41].

Photographic aids and telepathology

Recently, digital photography has been used for mapping Mohs tissue specimens, increasing the accuracy of depicting the excision defect [42]. With the widespread use of computers in all laboratories, this concept may soon become the norm in most Mohs laboratories.

Several investigators have reported on the utility of Internet transmission of digital images of the histopathology of tissue specimens (telepathology) during surgery for immediate opinion by a dermatopathologist at a remote site, hence facilitating more confident diagnosis of tissue samples [43–45].

The use of Polaroid photography for mapping sections has also been advocated, as it provides a less expensive alternative when compared with digital photography [46].

Adjuncts and adjuvant treatment

Light curettage done before Mohs surgery offers an increase in the ability to delineate subclinical extensions of the tumor margin [47].

The use of photodynamic therapy as adjuvant treatment for extensive carcinoma has been reported and advocated. Kuijpers and colleagues [48] reported on the usefulness of photodynamic therapy as treatment for the remaining superficial tumor remnants after MMS for advanced BCC. This was done to preserve normal tissue while adequately removing all tumor cells. This concept is especially useful for tumors in the face and for patients with a history of multiple BCCs.

Reported modifications of MMS also include the "peripheral in-continuity" tissue examination [49].

New applications and indications

Recent reports have described the use of Mohs surgery for the effective treatment of primary cutaneous mucinous carcinoma [32,50], atypical fibroxanthoma [51], myofibrosarcoma [52], syringocystadenocarcinoma papilliferum [53], superficial leiomyosarcoma [54], pilomatrix carcinoma [55], angiolymphoid hyperplasia with eosinophilia [56], and granular cell myoblastomas [57].

Reports on the success of Mohs surgery in the removal of rare skin neoplasms, such as atypical cellular neurothekeoma [58] and eccrine porocarcinoma [59,60], have also been described. In addition, its indication has expanded to include some benign tumors with aggressive growth characteristics, including cylindroma, desmoplastic trichoepithelioma, granular cell tumor, pilomatricoma, and proliferating trichilemmal tumor [61–63]. It has also been advocated as an alternative treatment for cutaneous mucormycosis [64]. Finally, a recent report has demonstrated the efficacy of Mohs surgery in the treatment of phaeohyphomycosis, with potential elimination of the need for antifungal treatment [65].

Conclusions

Mohs micrographic surgery as originally described was a time-consuming yet effective technique for the removal of various BCCs and SCCs. Today, Mohs surgery is a highly effective, fairly simple, and expedient technique used not only for a variety of BCCs and SCCs, but also for an increasing list of both malignant and benign cutaneous neoplasms.

References

1 Shriner DL, McCoy DK, Goldberg DJ, Wagner RF. Mohs micrographic surgery. J Am Acad Dermatol 1998;39:79–97.

2 Lee KK, Swanson NA. Mohs micrographic surgery. In: Freedberg I, Eisen A, Wolff K, Austen K, Goldsmith L, Katz S, editors. Fitzpatrick's dermatology in general medicine. New York: McGraw-Hill; 2003. p. 2581–5.

3 Finley E, Ratz JL. Mohs micrographic surgery. In: Ratz J, editor. Textbook of dermatologic surgery. Philadelphia: Lippincott-Raven; 1998:417–37.

4 Nouri K, Rivas MP. A primer of Mohs micrographic surgery: common indications. Skinmed 2004;3: 191–6.

5 Mohs FE. Mohs micrographic surgery: a historical perspective. Dermatol Clin 1989;7:609–11.

6 Brodland DG, Amonette R, Hanke CW, Robins P. The history and evolution of Mohs micrographic surgery. Dermatol Surg 2000;26:303–7.

7 Bennett RG. Current concepts in Mohs micrographic surgery. Dermatol Clin 1991;9:777–88.

8 Kimyai-Asadi A, Hale EK, Schmultz CA, Goldberg D, Hanke CW, Moy R. Mohs surgery revisited: 25 key articles. J Drugs Dermatol 2002;1:185–9.

9 Cohen PR, Schulze KE, Nelson BR. Basal cell carcinoma with mixed histology: a possible pathogenesis for recurrent skin cancer. Dermatol Surg 2006;32: 542–51.

10 Leibovitch I, Huilgol SC, Selva D, Richards S, Paver R. Basal cell carcinoma treated with Mohs surgery in Australia I: experience over 10 years. J Am Acad Dermatol. 2005;53:445–51.

11 Lang PG, Osguthorpe J. Indications and limitations of Mohs micrographic surgery. Dermatol Clin 1989;7:627–44.

12 Smeets NW, Kuijpers D, Nelemans P, et al. Mohs micrographic surgery for treatment of basal cell carcinoma of the face—results of a retrospective study and review of the literature. Br J Dermatol 2004;151:141–7.

13 Leibovitch I, Huilgol SC, Selva D, Richards S, Paver R. Basal cell carcinoma treated with Mohs surgery in Australia II: outcome at 5-year follow-up. J Am Acad Dermatol 2005;53:452–7.

14 Leibovitch I, Huilgol SC, Selva D, Richards S, Paver R. Cutaneous squamous cell carcinoma treated with Mohs micrographic surgery in Australia I: experience over 10 years. J Am Acad Dermatol 2005;53: 253–60.

15 Snow SN, Gordon EM, Larson PO, Bagheri MM, Bentz ML, Sable DB. Dermatofibrosarcoma protuberans: a report on 29 patients treated by Mohs micrographic surgery with long-term follow up and review of the literature. Cancer 2004;101:28–38.

16 DuBay D, Cimmino V, Lowe L, Johnson TM, Sondak VK. Low recurrence rate after surgery for dermatofibrosarcoma protuberans: a multidisciplinary approach from a single institution. Cancer 2004;100:1008–16.

17 Sei JF, Chaussade V, Zimmermann U, et al. Mohs micrographic surgery: history, principles, critical analysis of its efficacy and indications. Ann Dermatol Venereol 2004:131;173–82.

18 Alkalay R, Alcalay J, Shiri J. Plantar verrucous carcinoma treated with Mohs micrographic surgery: a case report and literature review. J Drugs Dermatol 2006;5:68–73.

19 O'Connor WJ, Lim KK, Zalla MJ, et al. Comparison of Mohs micrographic surgery and wide excision for extramammary Paget's disease. Dermatol Surg 2003;29:723–7.

20 Hendi A, Brodland DG, Zitelli JA. Extramammary Paget's disease: surgical treatment with Mohs micrographic surgery. J Am Acad Dermatol 2004;51:767–73.

21 Khachemoune A, Olbricht SM, Johnson DS. Microcystic adnexal carcinoma: report of four cases treated with Mohs micrographic surgical technique. Int J Dermatol 2005;44:507–12.

22 Bricca GM, Brodland D, Ren D, Zitelli J. Cutaneous head and neck melanoma treated with Mohs micrographic surgery. J Am Acad Dermatol 2005;52:92–100.

23 McKenna JK, Florell SR, Goldman GD, Bowen GM. Lentigo maligna/lentigo maligna melanoma: current state of diagnosis and treatment. Dermatol Surg 2006;32:493–504.

24 Silapunt S, Peterson SR, Alcalay J, Goldberg LH. Mohs tissue mapping and processing: a survey study. Dermatol Surg 2003;29:1109–12.

25 Kimyai-Asadi A, Goldberg LH, Peterson SR, Silapint S, Jih MH. The incidence of major complications from Mohs micrographic surgery performed in office-based and hospital-based settings. J Am Acad Dermatol 2005;53:628–34.

26 Larson MJ, Taylor RS. Monitoring vital signs during outpatient Mohs and post-Mohs reconstructive surgery performed under local anesthesia. Dermatol Surg 2004;30:777–83.

27 Cook JL, Perone JB. A prospective evaluation of the incidence of complications associated with Mohs micrographic surgery. Arch Dermatol 2003;139:143–52.

28 Stenquist B, Ericson MB, Strandeberg C, et al. Bispectral fluorescence imaging of aggressive basal cell carcinoma combined with histopathological mapping: a preliminary study indicating a possible adjunct to Mohs micrographic surgery. Br J Dermatol 2006;154:305–9.

29 Tannous Z, Torres A, González S. In vivo real-time confocal reflectance microscopy: a noninvasive guide for Mohs micrographic surgery facilitated by aluminum chloride, an excellent contrast enhancer. Dermatol Surg 2003;29:839–46.

30 Chung VQ, Dwyer PJ, Nehal KS, et al. Use of ex-vivo confocal scanning laser microscopy during Mohs surgery for nonmelanoma skin cancers. Dermatol Surg 2004;30:1470–8.

31 Curiel-Lewandrowski C, Williams CM, Swindells KJ, et al. Use of in vivo confocal microscopy in malignant melanoma: an aid in diagnosis and assessment of

surgical and nonsurgical therapeutic approaches. Arch Dermatol 2004;140:1127–32.

32 Marra DE, Torres A, Schanbacher CF, Gonzalez S. Detection of residual basal cell carcinoma by in vivo confocal microscopy. Dermatol Surg 2005;31:538–41.

33 Kelley LC, Starkus L. Immunohistochemical staining of lentigo maligna during Mohs micrographic surgery using MART-1. J Am Acad Dermatol 2002;46:78–84.

34 Albertini JG, Elston DM, Libow LF, Smith SB, Farley MF. Mohs micrographic surgery for melanoma: a case series, a comparative study of immunostains, an informative case report, and a unique mapping technique. Dermatol Surg 2002;28:656–65.

35 Zalla MJ, Lim KK, DiCaudo DJ, Gagnot MM. Mohs micrographic excision of melanoma using immunostains. Dermatol Surg 2000;26:771–84.

36 Menaker GH, Chiang JK, Tabila B, Moy RL. Rapid HMB-45 staining in Mohs micrographic surgery for melanoma in situ and invasive melanoma. J Am Acad Dermatol 2001;44:833–6.

37 Mondragon RM, Barrett TL. Current concepts: the use of immunoperoxidase techniques in Mohs micrographic surgery. J Am Acad Dermatol 2000;43:66–71.

38 Smeets NW, Stavast-Kooy AJ, Krekels GA, Daemen MJ, Neumann HA. Adjuvant cytokeratin staining in Mohs micrographic surgery for basal cell carcinoma. Dermatol Surg 2003;29:375–7.

39 Smith SB, Farley MF, Albertini JG, Elston DM. Mohs micrographic surgery for granular cell tumor using S-100 immunostain. Dermatol Surg 2002;28:1076–8.

40 Bhardwaj SS, Tope WD, Lee PK. Mohs micrographic surgery for lentigo maligna and lentigo maligna melanoma using Mel-5 immunostaining: University of Minnesota experience. Dermatol Surg 2006;32:690–6.

41 Robinson JK. Current histologic preparation methods for Mohs micrographic surgery. Dermatol Surg 2001;27:555–60.

42 Lin BB, Taylor RS. Digital photography for mapping Mohs micrographic surgery sections. Dermatol Surg 2001;27:411–4.

43 Chandra S, Elliott T, Vinciullo C. Telepathology as an aid in Mohs micrographic surgery. Dermatol Surg 2004;30:945–7.

44 Nehal LS, Busam LK, Halpern AC. Use of dynamic telepathology in Mohs surgery: a feasibility study. Dermatol Surg 2002;28:422–6.

45 Sukal SA, Busam KJ, Nehal KS. Clinical application of dynamic telepathology in Mohs surgery. Dermatol Surg 2005;31:1700–3.

46 Jih MH, Goldberg LH, Friedman PM, Kimyai-Asadi A. Surgical pearl: the use of Polaroid photography for mapping Mohs micrographic surgery sections. J Am Acad Dermatol 2005;52:511–3.

47 Chung VQ, Bernardo L, Jiang SB. Presurgical curettage appropriately reduces the number of Mohs stages by better delineating the subclinical extensions of tumor margins. Dermatol Surg 2005;31:1094–9.

48 Kuijpers DI, Smeets NW, Krekels GA, Thissen MR. Photodynamic therapy as adjuvant treatment of extensive basal cell carcinoma treated with Mohs micrographic surgery. Dermatol Surg 2004;30:794–8.

49 Strong JW, Worsham GF, Hagerty RC. Peripheral in-continuity tissue examination: a modification of Mohs micrographic surgery. Clin Plast Surg 2004;31: 1–4.

50 Cecchi R, Rapicano V. Primary cutaneous mucinous carcinoma: report of two cases treated with Mohs micrographic surgery. Australas J Dermatol 2006;47: 192–4.

51 Seavolt M, McCall M. Atypical fibroxanthoma: review of literature and summary of 13 patients treated with Mohs micrographic surgery. Dermatol Surg 2006;32:435–41.

52 Chiller K, Parker D, Washington C. Myofibrosarcoma treated with Mohs micrographic surgery. Dermatol Surg 2004;30:1565–67.

53 Chi CC, Tsai RY, Wang SH. Syringocystadenocarcinoma papilliferum: successfully treated with Mohs micrographic surgery. Dermatol Surg 2004;30:468–71.

54 Humphreys TR, Finkelstein DH, Lee JB. Superficial leiomyosarcoma treated with Mohs micrographic surgery. Dermatol Surg 2004;30:108–12.

55 Sable D, Snow SN. Pilomatrix carcinoma of the back treated by Mohs micrographic surgery. Dermatol Surg 2004;30:1174–6.

56 Miller CJ, Ioffreda MD, Ammirati CT. Mohs micrographic surgery for angiolymphoid hyperplasia with eosinophilia. Dermatol Surg 2004;30:1169–73.

57 Chilukuri S, Peterson SR, Goldberg LH. Granular cell tumor of the heel treated with Mohs technique. Dermatol Surg 2004;30:1046–9.

58 Benbenisty KM, Andea A, Metcalf J, Cook J. Atypical cellular neurothekeoma with Mohs micrographic surgery. Dermatol Surg 2006;32:582–7.

59 Cowden A, Dans M, Militello G, Junkins-Hopkins J, Van Voorhees AS. Eccrine porocarcinoma arising in two African American patients: distinct presentations both treated with Mohs micrographic surgery. Int J Dermatol 2006;45:146–50.

60 D'Ambrosia RA, Ward H, Parry E. Eccrine porocarcinoma of the eyelid treated with Mohs micrographic surgery. Dermatol Surg 2004;30:570–71.

61 Behroozan DS, Goldberg LH, Glaich AS, Kaplan B, Kaye VN. Mohs micrographic surgery for deeply penetrating, expanding benign cutaneous neoplasms. Dermatol Surg 2006;32:958–65.

62 Schweiger E, Spann CT, Weinberg JM, Ross B. A case of desmoplastic trichilemmoma of the lip treated with Mohs surgery. Dermatol Surg 2004;30:1062–4.

63 Tierney E, Ochoa MT, Rudkin G, Soriano TT. Mohs micrographic surgery of a proliferating trichilemmal tumor in a young black man. Dermatol Surg 2005; 31:359–63.

64 Clark FL, Batra RS, Gladstone HB. Mohs micrographic surgery as an alternative treatment method for cutaneous mucormycosis. Dermatol Surg 2003;29: 882–5.

65 Bogle MA, Rabkin MS, Joseph AK. Mohs micrographic surgery for the eradication of phaeohyphomycosis of the hand. Dermatol Surg 2004;30:231–3.

CHAPTER 27

Photodynamic therapy

David J. Goldberg and Eds Chua

Photodynamic therapy (PDT) is a noninvasive technique used in the treatment of various skin disorders. Used primarily for cutaneous tumors, its objective is to cause selective destruction of the desired target tissue without inducing damage to other normal surrounding structures. In dermatology, its application includes precancerous lesions such as actinic keratosis (AK) and Bowen's disease, malignant conditions including basal cell carcinoma (BCC) and squamous cell carcinoma (SCC), and benign inflammatory processes such as psoriasis and acne vulgaris. PDT has become an increasingly safe and effective treatment modality [1].

Historical insights

Photodynamic therapy was first introduced in the early 1900s as an experimental treatment that consisted of oxygen, light, and a photosensitizing agent to cause tumor cell destruction [2,3]. Systemic photosensitizing drugs were used because these agents accumulated selectively in tumor cells, and therefore led to selective cell destruction. PDT was first used for the treatment of internal malignancies such as tumors of the bladder and esophagus as well as some skin conditions [2,3]. The drawback to these early treatments was the prolonged cutaneous photosensitivity of the systemic agents used. It was not until 1990, when Kennedy and Pottier [4] introduced the use of 5-aminolevulinic acid (ALA) that PDT as we know it today dramatically changed. ALA became a potent topical photosensitizing agent that could be used for PDT without significant phototoxicity. This agent was approved by the US Food and Drug Administration (FDA) in 1999 in combination with light for the treatment of AK. Since then, the

field of PDT has generated vast interest in terms of research and clinical application. In Europe, PDT is being used for AK and BCC. Off-label uses, in both the United States and Europe, include Bowen's disease, cutaneous T-cell lymphoma, psoriasis, acne, and most recently, photorejuvenation and hair removal [5,6].

Mechanism of action

Photodynamic therapy is a form of photochemotherapy [7]. It uses a photosensitizer, light, and molecular oxygen to selectively kill cells. The photosensitizer is activated by light with specific light wavelengths. When localized to the tissue concerned, PDT produces oxygen intermediates that cause destruction of abnormal target cells [7–12]. Neither drug nor light alone is effective as a therapeutic agent; as such, PDT should be regarded as a combined drug and light device therapy [7].

Because of the easy access of the skin to light-based therapy, PDT has been used by dermatologists in treating a variety of skin conditions. It has been most successful in the treatment of AK, Bowen's disease, and superficial BCC [8,12,13].

The first and now most widely used photosensitizing agent, ALA, is a prodrug that is metabolized inside the cell to form protoporphyrin IX (PpIX), a photosensitizing molecule. Once activated by light, a photodynamic reaction is triggered, and PpIX generates cytotoxic reactive oxygen species and free radicals, which cause destruction of malignant and nonmalignant hyperproliferative tissues, decreasing their size and eventually eliminating them [3,10,13]. With a sufficient dose of light,

ALA-induced PpIX is completely photobleached within the treatment field, thus leading to no further significant phototoxic effects [3].

The introduction of topical ALA has significantly reduced the morbidity associated with earlier systemic photosensitizing agents because it does not make patients susceptible to significant phototoxicity. The most common adverse side effects seen with today's PDT are transient erythema or irritation and pain [14]. For optimal effect, the drug must be released at an appropriate rate from the preparation and penetrate the skin, ideally to reach the target tissue at sufficiently high concentrations [15].

Photosensitizing drugs

Currently, there are two topical agents that are widely used as photosensitizing drugs for PDT: ALA and methyl aminolevulinic acid (MAL). These agents stimulate the production of porphyrins, which act as powerful photosensitizers.

Aminolevulinic acid

5-Aminolevulinic acid is an endogenous sensitizer and a metabolite of heme biosynthesis. It is the first approved photosensitizing agent and the most commonly used drug for PDT. Various clinical trials have proven its benefit as a photosensitizer in the photodynamic therapy of AK, BCC, and Bowen's disease [16–22]. Its main limitation is its poor penetration into the skin because of its hydrophilic and charge characteristics [23]. The use of different enhancers of PpIX production, as well as the development of new drug delivery systems and the modification of its molecule, have improved its penetration.

The use of dimethyl sulfoxide (DMSO) as a vehicle improves skin penetration of ALA and leads to higher porphyrin accumulation in tumor tissue [24–27]. Addition of topical glycolic acid also has been shown to enhance ALA's penetration in tissue [28]. One study evaluated the effectiveness of the use of a water-soluble adhesive patch for drug delivery [29], whereas another concluded that elevating the skin temperature during topical ALA application can induce greater penetration, thus improving treatment results [30]. A recently proposed

concept to enhance the efficacy of PDT, especially in the treatment of thicker lesions, is through the use of intralesional ALA [31].

Methyl aminolevulinic acid

Methyl 5-aminolevulinate is an ester derivative of ALA. It is more lipophilic when compared with ALA and has been approved by the US FDA solely for the management of AK. MAL has been registered in Europe, Australia, and New Zealand for the treatment of AK and superficial and nodular BCC [11]. MAL leads to high penetration in tumor cells (high ratio of porphyrin fluorescence depth to tumor depth) with less fluorescence in adjacent normal tissues [32] and acceptable cosmetic results [33]. Clinical trials have proven its efficacy for both AK and BCC [34–38].

In a study done by Kuijpers and colleagues [39], there was no difference in short-term efficacy and side effects between ALA and MAL. Both can be equally recommended as topical photosensitizers in PDT. Kasche and colleagues [40], however, demonstrated in a trial in 69 patients with AK, that PDT with MAL induced less pain than ALA and was better tolerated.

The absorption spectra of these current sensitizing agents are in the range of 600 to 700 nm, which limits their use to superficial tumors because light penetration at these wavelengths is only up to 3 mm [2].

Other photosensitizing agents

Initial studies utilizing mono-L-aspartyl chlorine e6 (NPe6) as a photosensitizer for PDT in the treatment of BCC showed good efficacy and patient tolerance with minimal side effects [41,42].

The systemic photosensitizing agent metatetrahydroxyphenylchlorin (temoporfin) has been the subject of several studies demonstrating its effectiveness as an initial treatment for several cutaneous tumors, including vulvar intraepithelial neoplasia [43] and oral SCC [44]. Studies have revealed a good cosmetic outcome, selective effect, and conservation of function. Another systemic photosensitizer, verteporfin, showed good tumor response and excellent cosmetic results for nonmelanoma skin cancers [45].

Another novel photosensitizer, ATX-S10(Na), has also been studied for PDT of SCC and was shown to be effective in an early pilot study [46]. Further clinical trials are required.

Light sources

Several light sources are available for PDT. Human tissue has the highest absorption for ALA in a spectral range of 600 to 800 nm [47]. However, numerous other wavelengths have been successfully used. Nevertheless, it would appear that the ideal wavelength that matches the absorption spectra of photosensitizers is 630 nm [2]. At spectra of 630 to 700 nm, malignant tumor cells of BCC and SCC have been demonstrated to have a higher intensity of PpIX fluorescence compared with normal tissue [3]. Initially, large complex lasers were used for PDT because these have a wavelength of 630 nm. Presently, however, these are being replaced by smaller laser diodes and nonlaser light sources such as noncoherent filtered lamps and sources containing light-emitting diodes [10].

There are, at this time, no established guidelines for standard optimal irradiance, wavelength, and total dose characteristics for PDT. Light dosimetry also depends on the disease being treated [2,48].

Commercially available light sources have appropriate red or blue light emission designed for treatment of large areas. For dermatologic purposes, either incoherent lamps or light-emitting diode arrays may be used. The effects of either cytotoxic destruction of tumor cells or immunomodulatory effects on inflammatory conditions depend on the applied light dose and concentration of the photosensitizer [12].

Red

Most studies that have employed ALA for PDT have used red light. Red light is capable of deep skin penetration [10,49] and can activate porphyrins produced by ALA and MAL. The Aktilite lamp (Photocure ASA), designed for use with MAL, has an emission spectrum that closely matches the red light absorption profile of PpIX [10].

Radakovic-Fijan [50] compared the efficacy and tolerability of three different doses of red light for ALA-PDT for AK and found that a red light dose of 70 J/cm^2 was sufficient for effective treatment of AK on the face and scalp [50].

Green

In a study done by Morton and colleagues [49], green light was shown to be less effective than red light in the treatment of Bowen's disease by topical ALA-PDT.

Blue

Blue light is commonly used for the successful treatment of non-hyperkeratotic AK of the face and scalp [13,20,51]. Some reports have also demonstrated a good response with its use for the treatment of superficial and nodular BCC [52].

Violet

Violet light provides maximal overlap with excitation spectrum of PpIX and uses less light energy to induce phototoxic reaction. Hence, it is well tolerated and serves as an effective alternative light source in the treatment of premalignant and malignant skin disorders, especially for multiple and large lesions [53].

Lasers

Lasers have been employed in PDT for the curative treatment of AK, superficial BCC, and Bowen's disease, and even as palliative treatment for cutaneous metastases in some patients [54]. Kaviani and his colleagues [55] used laser light in the PDT of different kinds of BCC and obtained excellent response rates, except for the pigmented type.

Pulsed dye laser

Britton and associates [56] investigated the use of pulsed dye laser as the light source for PDT in Bowen's disease. In this study, PDT was shown to be an effective treatment. Treatment was well tolerated in spite of significant discomfort and some posttreatment crusting [57].

Erbium:yttrium-aluminum-garnet laser

Animal studies have shown an effect of the erbium:yttrium-aluminum-garnet laser in increasing the amount of PpIX in tumors, thereby enhancing the efficacy of ALA-PDT [58,59].

Ultraviolet A light

Ultraviolet A (UV-A) ALA-PDT is a potentially interesting new approach. This approach has been shown to be more potent than green light in human skin fibroblasts, although no clinical trials have been conducted [60]. Fink-Puches and colleagues [61] found no difference in the outcome between PDT using UV-A and PDT using visible light in the treatment of superficial BCC.

In an in vitro and in vivo study comparing two light sources, Babilas and colleagues [19] found no difference in cytotoxicity, efficacy, remission rates, side effects, patient satisfaction, and cosmetic outcome between light-emitting diodes and incoherent lamp in patients with AK. Likewise, Clark and associates [16] found similar efficacy between broadband and laser light sources. However, their study demonstrated a higher frequency of pain in PDT using broadband and laser sources compared with a low-output xenon source.

Ericson and coworkers [62] demonstrated that both the photobleaching rate and the primary treatment outcome were dependent on fluence rate and that a low fluence rate (30 mW/cm^2) was preferable for PDT of AK, resulting in a better treatment outcome.

Indications/applications

Basal cell carcinoma

Photodynamic therapy has been shown to be highly effective for the treatment of superficial BCC [11,13,14,18,48,55,63]. A large number of clinical trials and observational studies using ALA-PDT [16,21,22,61,64–68] have demonstrated its superior effect as treatment for superficial BCC, with lesser recurrence rates for the treatment of this form of BCC when compared with other forms of BCC (Figs. 27.1 and 27.2). Studies on nodular BCC showed varying results, with response rates ranging from as low as 50% to as high as 83% to 91% [33,53,55,69]. In Kaviani's study [55], he concluded

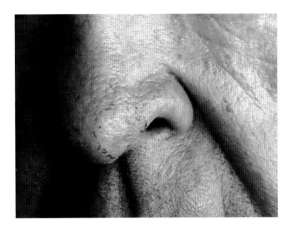

Fig. 27.1 Irregularly defined, superficial, previously untreated BCC of the nose in a patient seeking a nonsurgical, cosmetically elegant form of treatment.

that PDT is not recommended for pigmented BCC.

Actinic Keratosis

Photodynamic therapy is a well-established therapeutic modality for AK [20,36–38,48,51,70–72]. Both ALA and MAL are effective in the PDT for AK and have been approved by the US FDA. Trials comparing PDT with other modalities of AK treatments have proved that PDT is a safe and effective treatment and that it offers excellent cosmetic outcome (Figs. 27.3 to 27.6).

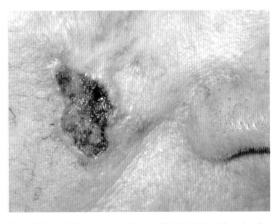

Fig. 27.2 Well-demarcated superficial BCC of the cheek amenable to PDT.

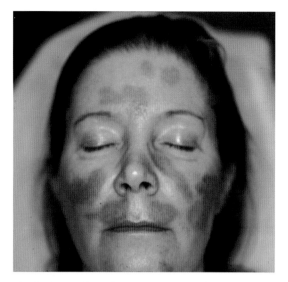

Fig. 27.3 Two days after PDT treatment of AKs. Note PDT-induced photoactivation of lesions.

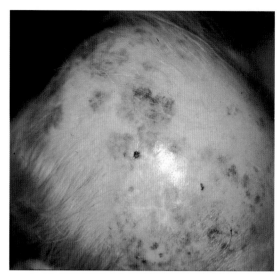

Fig. 27.5 Myriad AKs of the scalp before PDT treatment.

Squamous cell carcinoma in situ/Bowen's disease

5-Aminolevulinic acid PDT is now considered one of the first-line options for Bowen's disease [18,73], especially for large and multiple areas [63,74]. Large lesions, however, often require multiple treatments.

Previous studies have shown excellent response rates [16,73]. Its use in subungual Bowen's disease has also proved to be effective [75].

A recent randomized trial in 225 patients that compared MAL-PDT and cryotherapy for the treatment of Bowen's disease showed that PDT was

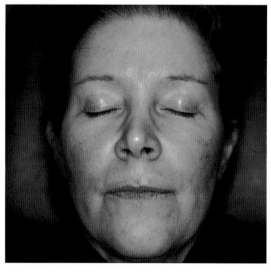

Fig. 27.4 Clearance of AKs 2 weeks after PDT. Note the excellent cosmetic result.

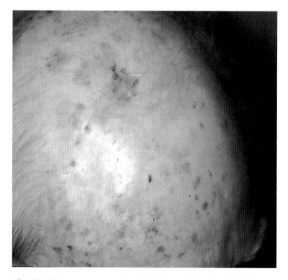

Fig. 27.6 Improvement in AKs 1 month after PDT. A second treatment is required.

superior to cryotherapy, with excellent cosmetic results [76].

Others

Several authors have described the effect of PDT as a useful adjuvant treatment modality for patients with cutaneous T-cell lymphoma resistant to conventional therapy [77–79]. PDT may also be used for cutaneous anaplastic large cell lymphoma [80], achieving complete remission in some reported cases.

There are data suggesting benefit of ALA-PDT in acne vulgaris, verrucae, psoriasis, and human papillomavirus infection [12,13]. These studies demonstrate a good clinical response and objective histologic effects.

Studies have also shown a good clinical response, with less scarring and recurrence rates comparable with those of standard therapies, in patients with extramammary Paget's disease [81].

In a study done by Gold and Goldman [82], PDT was also found to be effective for photorejuvenation. Potential future use includes its effect on melanocytic activation for skin disorders characterized by hypopigmentation [83].

Photodynamic therapy is not indicated for primary malignant melanoma and invasive SCC [54]. Pigmented BCC, as described above, also shows a poor response to this modality [55].

Protocol/guidelines

Although PDT is a relatively simple technique, there are multiple variables in drug formulation, delivery, and duration of application, and different light-specific parameters, which ultimately affect its efficacy [48].

Optimal irradiance, wavelength, and total dose characteristics vary for specific diseases. Furthermore, PDT success rates are also compounded by difficulties comparing different light sources [48].

5-Aminolevulinic acid is applied topically using a 20% solution. Light is then applied, generally 3 to 6 hours later, using red light, typically in the intensity range of 100 to 150 mW/cm^2 with a fluence of 100 to 150 J/cm^2. Treated tumor thickness should not exceed 2 to 3 mm. Although single treatments

may be effective, repeated treatments are recommended for thicker or nonresponding lesions [84] and have been shown to enhance efficacy [64,65]. The literature cites an optimal interval of 3.5 to 5 hours between ALA application and irradiation for BCC and AK [85].

The MAL regimen, as used in clinical trials, is 160 mg/g applied for 3 hours, followed by illumination with red light (570 to 670 nm) at a total light dose of 75 J/cm^2 [86].

Success and recurrence rates

Clinical trials using ALA-PDT [16,18,21,22,33,48, 53,61,63–69,72,75] have reported clearance rates ranging from 89% to 99% for AK, 80% to 98% for Bowen's disease, 86% to 97% for superficial BCC, and 50% to 92% for nodular BCC. Overall, PDT is an effective treatment with an excellent cosmetic outcome.

Reported recurrence rates ranged from 16% to 31% for AK, 0% to 52% for Bowen's disease, 0% to 31% for superficial BCC, 44% for nodular BCC, and 82% for invasive SCC [3]. Superficial BCC has the lowest recurrence rates after PDT, whereas invasive SCC has the highest. Success and recurrence depend largely on the size, localization, and histologic type of the lesion; the chemical structure of the chosen photosensitizer; and the light source used as well as its dosimetry.

Data from several clinical trials proved that PDT is as efficacious as surgery and cryotherapy, and superior to 5-fluorouracil, for the treatment of AK. In addition, PDT is superior to cryotherapy, 5-fluorouracil, and excisional surgery in terms of cosmetic outcome and patient satisfaction [21,33,36,38,73,76].

Complications/adverse events

The most common side effects are mild, tolerable pain and a burning or stinging sensation [14]. Severe pain has been noted more when high-output broadband and laser sources have been used than with low-output xenon arc sources [16].

Pigmentary change and minor scarring may occur in a minority of cases [16]. A case of photocontact urticaria after PDT has also been reported [87]. The carcinogenic risk of ALA-PDT is clearly very low, if present at all [48].

Advantages/disadvantages

Photodynamic therapy is noninvasive. It involves a targeted therapy approach, affecting only the tumor tissue, with relative sparing of normal tissue. Therefore, PDT is associated with excellent cosmetic results because the healing process results in little or no scarring [54]. It is associated with minimal discomfort and can be performed easily on any part of the body. Furthermore, repeated doses, without limitations of dose, can be given [44]. PDT is also very convenient for large and multiple lesions [44]. It has been proven advantageous for lesions in which the size, site, or number of lesions limits the efficacy and acceptability of conventional treatment [48] and may be the only choice for patients with contraindications to surgery or radiotherapy.

Disadvantages include the lack of histologic control, limited depth of tissue penetration [54], and the high recurrence rate in some series.

Combination with other treatment

The use of PDT as an adjuvant treatment with Mohs micrographic surgery has resulted in the clearing of any remaining lesions in patients with extensive superficial BCC, potentially leading to complete cure of the tumor with maximal skin conservation and excellent cosmetic outcome [88].

Efficacy and usefulness in immunocompromised patients

Photodynamic therapy has an overall reduced efficacy in immunosuppressed patients compared with immunocompetent patients. Immunosuppressed patients, such as transplant recipients, require more aggressive optimization of cytotoxic pathways [89]. Nevertheless, several trials have shown the promising efficacy of PDT treatment of skin tumors in organ-transplanted patients [90,91]. Yet, its role as a preventive treatment for new skin lesions in trans-

plant patients, although promising, is still controversial and has had conflicting results [92,93]. Paech and colleagues [94] described good response to PDT for the treatment of mycosis fungoides in a patient with advanced HIV infection. Animal studies showed a prophylactic effect in delaying the appearance of UV-induced skin tumors [95].

Conclusions

Photodynamic therapy continues to flourish as one of the primary therapeutic modalities for selected skin cancers, offering advantages of excellent cosmetic outcome and outstanding results. New indications will continue to emerge as research and clinical trials continue to offer new techniques and concepts to improve the efficacy of this treatment option.

References

1 Nestor MS, Gold MH, Kauvar AN, et al. The use of photodynamic therapy in dermatology: results of a consensus conference. J Drugs Dermatol 2006;5:140–54.

2 Honigsmann H, Szeimies RM, Knobler R, Fitzpatrick TR, Pathak MA, Wolff K. Photochemotherapy and photodynamic therapy. In: Freedberg IM, Eisen AZ, Wolff K, Austen KF, Goldsmith LA, Katz SI, editors. Fitzpatrick's dermatology in general medicine. 6th ed. Vol. 2. New York: McGraw-Hill; 2003. p. 2477–93.

3 Marmur ES, Schmults CD, Goldberg DJ. A review of laser and photodynamic therapy for the treatment of nonmelanoma skin cancer. Dermatol Surg 2004;30:264–71.

4 Kennedy JC, Pottier RH. Endogenous protoporphyrin IX, a clinically useful photosensitizer for photodynamic therapy. J Photochem Photobiol B Biol 1992;14:275–92.

5 Garcia-Zuazaga J, Cooper KD, Baron ED. Photodynamic therapy in dermatology: current concepts in the treatment of skin cancer. Expert Rev Anticancer Ther 2005;5:791–800.

6 Touma DJ, Gilchrest BA. Topical photodynamic therapy: a new tool in cosmetic dermatology. Semin Cutan Med Surg 2003;22:124–30.

7 Marcus SL, McIntyre WR. Photodynamic therapy systems and applications. Expert Opin Emerg Drugs 2002;7:321–34.

8 Taub AF. Photodynamic therapy in dermatology: history and horizons. J Drugs Dermatol 2004;3(1 Suppl):S8–25.

9 Zeitouni NC, Oseroff AR, Shieh S. Photodynamic therapy for nonmelanoma skin cancers. Current review and update. Mol Immunol 2003;39:1133–36.

10 Brown SB. The role of light in the treatment of non-melanoma skin cancer using methyl aminolevulinate. J Dermatolog Treat 2003;14 Suppl 3:11–14.

11 Szeimies RM, Morton CA, Sidoroff A, Braathen LR. Photodynamic therapy for non-melanoma skin cancer. Acta Derm Venereol 2005;85:483–90.

12 Babilas P, Karrer S, Sidoroff A, Landthaler M, Szeimies RM. Photodynamic therapy in dermatology—an update. Photodermatol Photoimmunol Photomed 2005;21:142–9.

13 Gupta AK, Ryder JE. Photodynamic therapy and topical aminolevulinic acid: an overview. Am J Clin Dermatol 2003;4:699–708.

14 Morton CA. Methyl aminolevulinate (Metvix) photodynamic therapy—practical pearls. J Dermatolog Treat 2003;14 Suppl 3:23–26.

15 Lopez RF, Lange N, Guy R, Bentley MV. Photodynamic therapy of skin cancer: controlled drug delivery of 5-ALA and its esters. Adv Drug Deliv Rev 2004;56:77–94.

16 Clark C, Bryden A, Dawe R, Moseley H, Ferguson J, Ibbotson SH. Topical 5-aminolaevulinic acid photodynamic therapy for cutaneous lesions: outcome and comparison of light sources. Photodermatol Photoimmunol Photomed 2003;19:134–41.

17 Baptista J, Martinez C, Leite L, Cochito M. Our PDT experience in the treatment of non-melanoma skin cancer over the last 7 years. J Eur Acad Dermatol Venereol 2006;20:693–7.

18 Clayton TH, Tait J, Whitehurst C, Yates VM. Photodynamic therapy for superficial basal cell carcinoma and Bowen's disease. Eur J Dermatol 2006;16:39–41.

19 Babilas P, Kohl E, Maisch T, et al. In vitro and in vivo comparison of two different light sources for topical photodynamic therapy. Br J Dermatol 2006;154:712–8.

20 Jeffes EW, McCullough JL, Weinstein GD, Kaplan R, Glazer SD, Taylor JR. Photodynamic therapy of actinic keratoses with topical aminolevulinic acid hydrochloride and fluorescent blue light. J Am Acad Dermatol 2001;45:96–104.

21 Wang I, Bendsoe N, Klinteberg CA, et al. Photodynamic therapy vs. cryosurgery of basal cell carcinomas: results of a phase III clinical trial. Br J Dermatol 2001;144:832–40.

22 Thissen MR, Schroeter CA, Neumann HA. Photodynamic therapy with delta-aminolaevulinic acid for nodular basal cell carcinomas using a prior debulking technique. Br J Dermatol 2000;142:338–9.

23 De Rosa FS, Bentley MV. Photodynamic therapy of skin cancers: sensitizers, clinical studies and future directives. Pharm Res 2000;17:1447–55.

24 De Rosa FS, Marchetti JM, Thomazini JA, Tedesco AC, Bentley MV. A vehicle for photodynamic therapy of skin cancer: influence of dimethylsulphoxide on 5-aminolevulinic acid in vitro cutaneous permeation and in vivo protoporphyrin IX accumulation determined by confocal microscopy. J Control Release 2000;65:359–66.

25 Casas A, Fukuda H, Di Venosa G, Batlle AM. The influence of the vehicle on the synthesis of porphyrins after topical application of 5-aminolaevulinic acid. Implications in cutaneous photodynamic sensitization. Br J Dermatol 2000;143:564–72.

26 Harth Y, Hirshowitz B, Kaplan B. Modified topical photodynamic therapy of superficial skin tumors, utilizing aminolevulinic acid, penetration enhancers, red light, and hyperthermia. Dermatol Surg 1998;24:723–6.

27 Casas A, Perotti C, Fukuda H, Rogers L, Butler AR, Batlle A. ALA and ALA hexyl ester-induced porphyrin synthesis in chemically induced skin tumours: the role of different vehicles on improving photosensitization. Br J Cancer 2001;85:1794–800.

28 Ziolkowski P, Osiecka BJ, Oremek G, et al. Enhancement of photodynamic therapy by use of aminolevulinic acid/glycolic acid drug mixture. J Exp Ther Oncol 2004;4:121–9.

29 McCarron PA, Donnelly RF, Zawislak A, Woolfson AD. Design and evaluation of a water-soluble bioadhesive patch formulation for cutaneous delivery of 5-aminolevulinic acid to superficial neoplastic lesions. Eur J Pharm Sci 2006;27:268–79.

30 van den Akker JT, Boot K, Vernon DI, et al. Effect of elevating the skin temperature during topical ALA application on in vitro ALA penetration through mouse skin and in vivo PpIX production in human skin. Photochem Photobiol Sci 2004;3:263–7.

31 Cappugi P, Mavilia L, Campolmi P, Reali EF, Mori M, Rossi R. New proposal for the treatment of nodular basal cell carcinoma with intralesional 5-aminolevulinic acid. J Chemother 2004;16:491–3.

32 Peng Q, Soler AM, Warloe T, Nesland JM, Giercksky KE. Selective distribution of porphyrins in skin thick basal cell carcinoma after topical application of methyl 5-aminolevulinate. J Photochem Photobiol B 2001;62:140–5.

33 Rhodes LE, de Rie M, Enstrom Y, et al. Photodynamic therapy using topical methyl aminolevulinate vs surgery for nodular basal cell carcinoma: results of a multicenter randomized prospective trial. Arch Dermatol 2004;140:17–23.

34 Angell-Petersen E, Sorensen R, Warloe T, et al. Porphyrin formation in actinic keratosis and basal cell carcinoma after topical application of methyl 5-aminolevulinate. J Invest Dermatol 2006;126:265–71.

35 Vinciullo C, Elliott T, Francis D, et al. Photodynamic therapy with topical methyl aminolaevulinate for 'difficult-to-treat' basal cell carcinoma. Br J Dermatol 2005;152:765–72.

36 Freeman M, Vinciullo C, Francis D, et al. A comparison of photodynamic therapy using topical methyl aminolevulinate (Metvix) with single cycle cryotherapy in patients with actinic keratosis: a prospective, randomized study. J Dermatolog Treat 2003;14:99–106.

37 Pariser DM, Lowe NJ, Stewart DM, et al. Photodynamic therapy with topical methyl aminolevulinate for actinic keratosis: results of a prospective randomized multicenter trial. J Am Acad Dermatol 2003;48:227–32.

38 Szeimies RM, Karrer S, Radakovic-Fijan S, et al. Photodynamic therapy using topical methyl 5-aminolevulinate compared with cryotherapy for actinic keratosis: a prospective, randomized study. J Am Acad Dermatol 2002;47:258–62.

39 Kuijpers DI, Thissen MR, Thissen CA, Neumann MH. Similar effectiveness of methyl aminolevulinate and 5-aminolevulinate in topical photodynamic therapy for nodular basal cell carcinoma. J Drugs Dermatol 2006;5:642–5.

40 Kasche A, Luderschmidt S, Ring J, Hein R. Photodynamic therapy induces less pain in patients treated with methyl aminolevulinate compared to aminolevulinic acid. J Drugs Dermatol 2006;5:353–6.

41 Chan AL, Juarez M, Allen R, Volz W, Albertson T. Pharmacokinetics and clinical effects of mono-L-aspartyl chlorin e6 (NPe6) photodynamic therapy in adult patients with primary or secondary cancer of the skin and mucosal surfaces. Photodermatol Photoimmunol Photomed 2005;21:72–8.

42 Wong TW, Aizawa K, Sheyhedin I, Wushur C, Kato H. Pilot study of topical delivery of mono-L-aspartyl chlorin e6 (NPe6): implication of topical NPe6-photodynamic therapy. J Pharmacol Sci 2003;93:136–42.

43 Campbell SM, Gould DJ, Salter L, Clifford T, Curnow A. Photodynamic therapy using meta-tetrahydroxyphenylchlorin (Foscan) for the treatment of vulval intraepithelial neoplasia. Br J Dermatol. 2004;151:1076–80.

44 Hopper C, Kubler A, Lewis H, Tan IB, Putnam G. mTHPC-mediated photodynamic therapy for early oral squamous cell carcinoma. Int J Cancer. 2004;111:138–46.

45 Lui H, Hobbs L, Tope WD, et al. Photodynamic therapy of multiple nonmelanoma skin cancers with verteporfin and red light-emitting diodes: two-year results evaluating tumor response and cosmetic outcomes. Arch Dermatol 2004;140:26–32.

46 Takahashi H, Itoh Y, Nakajima S, Sakata I, Iizuka H. A novel ATX-S10(Na) photodynamic therapy for human skin tumors and benign hyperproliferative skin. Photodermatol Photoimmunol Photomed 2004;20:257–65.

47 Silva JN, Filipe P, Morliere P, et al. Photodynamic therapies: principles and present medical applications. Biomed Mater Eng 2006;16(4 Suppl):S147–54.

48 Morton CA, Brown SB, Collins S, et al. Guidelines for topical photodynamic therapy: report of a workshop of the British Photodermatology Group. Br J Dermatol 2002;146:552–67.

49 Morton CA, Whitehurst C, Moore JV, MacKie RM. Comparison of red and green light in the treatment of Bowen's disease by photodynamic therapy. Br J Dermatol 2000;143:767–72.

50 Radakovic-Fijan S, Blecha-Thalhammer U, Kittler H, Honigsmann H, Tanew A. Efficacy of 3 different light doses in the treatment of actinic keratosis with 5-aminolevulinic acid photodynamic therapy: a randomized, observer-blinded, intrapatient, comparison study. J Am Acad Dermatol 2005;53:823–7.

51 Piacquadio DJ, Chen DM, Farber HF, et al. Photodynamic therapy with aminolevulinic acid topical solution and visible blue light in the treatment of multiple actinic keratoses of the face and scalp: investigator-blinded, phase 3, multicenter trials. Arch Dermatol 2004;140:41–6.

52 Itkin A, Gilchrest BA. Delta-aminolevulinic acid and blue light photodynamic therapy for treatment of multiple basal cell carcinomas in two patients with nevoid basal cell carcinoma syndrome. Dermatol Surg 2004;30:1054–61.

53 Dijkstra AT, Majoie IM, van Dongen JW, van Weelden H, van Vloten WA. Photodynamic therapy with violet light and topical 6-aminolaevulinic acid in the treatment of actinic keratosis, Bowen's disease and basal cell carcinoma. J Eur Acad Dermatol Venereol 2001;15:550–4.

54 Karrer S, Szeimies RM, Hohenleutner U, Landthaler M. Role of lasers and photodynamic therapy in the treatment of cutaneous malignancy. Am J Clin Dermatol 2001;2:229–37.

55 Kaviani A, Ataie-Fashtami L, Fateh M, et al. Photodynamic therapy of head and neck basal cell carcinoma according to different clinicopathologic features. Lasers Surg Med 2005;36:377–82.

56 Britton JE, Goulden V, Stables G, Stringer M, Sheehan-Dare R. Investigation of the use of the pulsed dye laser in the treatment of Bowen's disease using 5-aminolaevulinic acid phototherapy. Br J Dermatol 2005;153:780–4.

57 Karrer S, Baumler W, Abels C, Hohenleutner U, Landthaler M, Szeimies RM. Long-pulse dye laser for photodynamic therapy: investigations in vitro and in vivo. Lasers Surg Med 1999;25:51–9.

58 Shen SC, Lee WR, Fang YP, Hu CH, Fang JY. In vitro percutaneous absorption and in vivo protoporphyrin IX accumulation in skin and tumors after topical 5-aminolevulinic acid application with enhancement using an erbium:YAG laser. J Pharm Sci 2006;95:929–38.

59 Fang JY, Lee WR, Shen SC, Fang YP, Hu CH. Enhancement of topical 5-aminolaevulinic acid delivery by erbium:YAG laser and microdermabrasion: a comparison with iontophoresis and electroporation. Br J Dermatol 2004;151:132–40.

60 Buchczyk DP, Klotz LO, Lang K, Fritsch C, Sies H. High efficiency of 5-aminolaevulinate-photodynamic treatment using UVA irradiation. Carcinogenesis. 2001;22:879–83.

61 Fink-Puches R, Soyer HP, Hofer A, Kerl H, Wolf P. Long-term follow-up and histological changes of superficial nonmelanoma skin cancers treated with topical delta-aminolevulinic acid photodynamic therapy. Arch Dermatol 1998;134:821–6.

62 Ericson MB, Sandberg C, Stenquist B, et al. Photodynamic therapy of actinic keratosis at varying fluence rates: assessment of photobleaching, pain and primary clinical outcome. Br J Dermatol 2004;151:1204–12.

63 Morton CA, Whitehurst C, McColl JH, Moore JV, MacKie RM. Photodynamic therapy for large or multiple patches of Bowen disease and basal cell carcinoma. Arch Dermatol 2001;137:319–24.

64 Calzavara-Pinton PG. Repetitive photodynamic therapy with topical delta-aminolevulinic acid as an appropriate approach to the routine treatment of superficial non-melanoma skin tumours. J Photochem Photobiol B 1995;29:53–7.

65 Haller JC, Cairnduff F, Slack G, et al. Routine double treatments of superficial basal cell carcinomas using aminolaevulinic acid-based photodynamic therapy. Br J Dermatol 2000;143:1270–5.

66 Soler AM, Angell-Petersen E, Warloe T, et al. Photodynamic therapy of superficial basal cell carcinoma with 5-aminolevulinic acid with dimethylsulfoxide and ethylendiaminetetraacetic acid: a comparison of two light sources. Photochem Photobiol 2000;71:724–9.

67 Svanberg K, Andersson T, Killander D, et al. Photodynamic therapy of non-melanoma malignant tumours of the skin using topical delta-amino levulinic acid sensitization and laser irradiation. Br J Dermatol 1994;130:743–51.

68 Varma S, Wilson H, Kurwa HA, et al. Bowen's disease, solar keratoses and superficial basal cell carcinomas treated by photodynamic therapy using a large-field incoherent light source. Br J Dermatol 2001;144:567–74.

69 Horn M, Wolf P, Wulf HC. Topical methyl aminolaevulinate photodynamic therapy in patients with basal cell carcinoma prone to complications and poor cosmetic outcome with conventional treatment. Br J Dermatol 2003;149:1242–9.

70 Jeffes EW, McCullough JL, Weinstein GD, et al. Photodynamic therapy of actinic keratosis with topical 5-aminolevulinic acid. A pilot dose-ranging study. Arch Dermatol 1997;133:727–32.

71 Kurwa HA, Yong-Gee SA, Seed PT, et al. A randomized paired comparison of photodynamic therapy and topical 5-fluorouracil in the treatment of actinic keratoses. J Am Acad Dermatol 1999;41:258–62.

72 Goldman M, Atkin D. ALA/PDT in the treatment of actinic keratosis: spot versus confluent therapy. J Cosmet Laser Ther 2003;5:107–10.

73 Salim A, Leman JA, McColl JH, Chapman R, Morton CA. Randomized comparison of photodynamic therapy with topical 5-fluorouracil in Bowen's disease. Br J Dermatol 2003;148:539–43.

74 Stables GI, Stringer MR, Robinson DJ, Ash DV. Large patches of Bowen's disease treated by topical aminolaevulinic acid photodynamic therapy. Br J Dermatol 1997;136:957–60.

75 Tan B, Sinclair R, Foley P. Photodynamic therapy for subungual Bowen's disease. Australas J Dermatol 2004;45:172–4.

76 Morton C, Horn M, Leman J, et al. Comparison of topical methyl aminolevulinate photodynamic therapy with cryotherapy or fluorouracil for treatment of squamous cell carcinoma in situ: results of a multicenter randomized trial. Arch Dermatol 2006;142:729–35.

77 Coors EA, von den Driesch P. Topical photodynamic therapy for patients with therapy-resistant lesions of cutaneous T-cell lymphoma. J Am Acad Dermatol 2004;50:363–7.

78 Leman JA, Dick DC, Morton CA. Topical 5-ALA photodynamic therapy for the treatment of cutaneous T-cell lymphoma. Clin Exp Dermatol 2002;27:516–8.

79 Edstrom DW, Porwit A, Ros AM. Photodynamic therapy with topical 5-aminolevulinic acid for mycosis fungoides: clinical and histological response. Acta Derm Venereol 2001;81:184–8.

80 Umegaki N, Moritsugu R, Katoh S, et al. Photodynamic therapy may be useful in debulking cutaneous lymphoma prior to radiotherapy. Clin Exp Dermatol 2004;29:42–5.

81 Shieh S, Dee AS, Cheney RT, Frawley NP, Zeitouni NC, Oseroff AR. Photodynamic therapy for the treatment of extramammary Paget's disease. Br J Dermatol 2002;146:1000–5.

82 Gold MH, Goldman MP. 5-aminolevulinic acid photodynamic therapy: where we have been and where we are going. Dermatol Surg 2004;30:1077–83.

83 Monfrecola G, Procaccini EM, D'Onofrio D, et al. Hyperpigmentation induced by topical 5-aminolaevulinic acid plus visible light. J Photochem Photobiol B 2002;68:147–55.

84 Tarstedt M, Rosdahl I, Berne B, Svanberg K, Wennberg AM. A randomized multicenter study to compare two treatment regimens of topical methyl aminolevulinate (Metvix)-PDT in actinic keratosis of the face and scalp. Acta Derm Venereol 2005;85:424–8.

85 Stefanidou M, Tosca A, Themelis G, Vazgiouraki E, Balas C. In vivo fluorescence kinetics and photodynamic therapy efficacy of delta-aminolevulinic acid-induced porphyrins in basal cell carcinomas and actinic keratoses; implications for optimization of photodynamic therapy. Eur J Dermatol 2000;10:351–6.

86 Siddiqui MA, Perry CM, Scott LJ. Topical methyl aminolevulinate. Am J Clin Dermatol 2004;5:127–37.

87 Yokoyama S, Nakano H, Nishizawa A, Kaneko T, Harada K, Hanada K. A case of photocontact urticaria induced by photodynamic therapy with topical 5-aminolaevulinic acid. J Dermatol 2005;32:843–7.

88 Kuijpers DI, Smeets NW, Krekels GA, Thissen MR. Photodynamic therapy as adjuvant treatment of extensive basal cell carcinoma treated with Mohs micrographic surgery. Dermatol Surg 2004;30:794–8.

89 Oseroff A. PDT as a cytotoxic agent and biological response modifier: Implications for cancer prevention and treatment in immunosuppressed and immunocompetent patients. J Invest Dermatol 2006;126:542–4.

90 Schleier P, Hyckel P, Berndt A, et al. Photodynamic therapy of virus-associated epithelial tumours of the face in organ transplant recipients. J Cancer Res Clin Oncol 2004;130:279–84.

91 Dragieva G, Hafner J, Dummer R, et al. Topical photodynamic therapy in the treatment of actinic keratoses and Bowen's disease in transplant recipients. Transplantation 2004;15:115–21.

92 Wulf HC, Pavel S, Stender I, Bakker-Wensveen CA. Topical photodynamic therapy for prevention of new skin lesions in renal transplant recipients. Acta Derm Venereol 2006;86:25–8.

93 de Graaf YG, Kennedy C, Wolterbeek R, Collen AF, Willemze R, Bouwes Bavinck JN. Photodynamic therapy does not prevent cutaneous squamous cell carcinoma in organ-transplant recipients: results of a randomized-controlled trial. J Invest Dermatol 2006;126:569–74.

94 Paech V, Lorenzen T, Stoehr A, et al. Remission of a cutaneous mycosis fungoides after topical 5-ALA sensitisation and photodynamic therapy in a patient with advanced HIV-infection. Eur J Med Res 2002;7:477–9.

95 Sharfaei S, Juzenas P, Moan J, Bissonnette R. Weekly topical application of methyl aminolevulinate followed by light exposure delays the appearance of UV-induced skin tumours in mice. Arch Dermatol Res 2002;294:237–42.

CHAPTER 28

Cutaneous cancer and radiotherapy

Thomas N. Helm, Klaus Helm, Kyu H. Shin, and Robert A. Schwartz

Radiation therapy uses high-energy rays to stop cancer cells from growing and multiplying. If radiation is given when a cell is reproducing, it prevents the cell from dividing and kills it. Because cancer cells grow rapidly, a larger proportion of tumor cells are in the process of mitosis as compared with normal cells and therefore are more sensitive to radiation.

Modern radiotherapy is highly effective in treating basal cell carcinomas (BCCs), squamous cell carcinomas (SCCs), keratoacanthomas, classic Kaposi's sarcoma, and cutaneous lymphomas. Although all cancer cells can be destroyed by radiation if a high enough dose is given, the x-ray dose is limited because of damage to adjacent normal tissue.

Unfortunately, radiation therapy in recent years has fallen in popularity, and only a few dermatologists consider x-ray therapy as an integral part of their therapeutic armamentarium. Much of the damage done in the past by x-rays could have been avoided by the suitable use of proper technique. Radiation treatment should be given by a person who knows the natural biologic behavior of the different types of skin cancer and is well trained in the selection and application of the particular radiation. Although each skin cancer needs an individualized assessment, some well-established techniques and dose schemes have evolved that allow the treatment of almost any superficial cancer by x-rays with relative ease. Improvements in computerization have allowed variables such as tumor metabolism, surrounding normal tissue, and organ movement to be considered in addition to setup problems and other difficulties [1]. New techniques such as intensity-modulated radiotherapy (IMRT); three-dimensional radiotherapy that is guided by computed tomography (CT) and takes into account unusual contours, such as those found on the neck; and computer models that offer adjustments to daily variations in target motion and tumor volume offer improvements in therapy that hold great promise for improving outcomes. Radiation therapy given at the time of surgery is now used in the treatment of breast cancer and may be applicable to the management of skin cancer, employing equipment such as the Intrabeam, made by Zeiss Surgical, Oberkochen, Germany, for intraoperative radiotherapy.

Advantages

Radiation therapy has particular merits for older patients and for those in poor health. It is bloodless, painless, and associated with little or no emotional or physical stress. As it preserves the normal anatomic contours, it frequently does not require hospitalization or reconstructive therapy. This is especially important for neoplasms of the eyelids, canthi, nose, ears, and lips, where it is frequently the preferred treatment, as surgical removal may result in objectionable cosmetic deformities. Carcinomas of the nasolabial fold and preauricular area show a tendency to spread along embryonal fusion planes and therefore are well treated by radiation. X-rays may be given in patients with hemorrhagic diathesis, those on anticoagulants, and patients prone to keloid formation. Use of radiation may allow larger treatment fields, thereby permitting a greater safety margin and increased cure rate without causing disfigurement.

Disadvantages

All forms of ionizing radiation are cumulative. There is no safe minimum dose. The accumulative threshold dose leading to chronic radiodermatitis appears to be greater than 1000 rads. The potential risk of cataracts, leukemogenesis, carcinogenesis (thyroid cancer, etc.), and genetic effects can be greatly reduced by proper shielding and adherence to proper dose limits. X-ray therapy requires expensive equipment, and the patient must make many return visits for the fractionated dose schedule, which gives better cosmetic results than a single dose or a few large doses. Some degree of chronic radiodermatitis with scarring, telangiectasia, and pigment changes is to be expected; worsening of the scars may be seen as time passes owing to additional actinic damage. Poor tolerance to radiation and unsatisfactory cosmetic results are found in areas where the amount of subcutaneous tissue is thin and the skin overlies cartilage and bone. The cosmetic results of radiation on extremities and trunk may be unsatisfactory, and therefore radiation treatment in these areas is usually avoided.

Common skin cancers such as BCCs and SCCs measuring 0.5 to 4.0 cm in diameter can be easily treated by soft x-ray, which produces radiation of a certain quality, measured in terms of the half-value layer (HVL) of 0.7 to 1.4 mm of aluminum. (HVL equals the thickness of any specific material, usually aluminum, that reduces the intensity of the incident beam to one half its original value.) Small lesions can often be removed more effectively by surgical excision or electrodesiccation and curettage. X-ray therapy can be successfully used for BCC induced by radiotherapy 20 to 50 years earlier [2].

Nevertheless, the risk of side effects due to ionizing radiation must be considered in weighing benefit versus risk for starting any patient on radiation therapy. The biologic characteristic of the carcinoma and of the surrounding tissue has to be taken into account. Techniques such as IMRT, quantification of volumetric and geometric changes, low-dose megavoltage cone-beam CT, and others now widely employed for prostate and head and neck tumors promise to minimize disadvantages to radiotherapy [3–7].

Table 28.1 Comparison of different x-ray qualities

	Wavelength		
	kV	A	HVL, mm Al
Grenz ray	5–20	130–2	0.02–0.04
Soft x-ray (beryllium window)	10–50	2–0.4	0.06–1.5
Contact x-ray	4–50	0.8	3 (at 60 kVp)
Low-voltage superficial x-ray	60–100	0.5	0.25–3
Deep x-ray	200–250	0.14	
Super-voltage x-ray	700–1000	0.03	

Al, aluminum; kVp, kilovolt peak.

Types of dermatologic x-ray therapy

A comparison of different x-rays is given in Table 28.1.

The *superficial x-ray technique* (Grenz rays) used to be the most widely used by practicing dermatologists.

Modern soft x-ray units have a beryllium window that is less filtering and therefore are gradually replacing superficial x-ray machines, because they allow a greater versatility by producing softer x-rays (i.e., less-penetrating wavelengths). The Dermopan by Siemens permits a wide range of half-value layers. An automatic filter safety device gives radiation only with the filter intended for the desired voltage. However, high cost limits its widespread use.

Contact therapy, produced by Chaoul tubes, is x-ray therapy given with a small target skin distance (TSD). These machines yield a high dose rate (roentgen per minute [R/min]) and a steep fall of dose, so the underlying tissue is not greatly affected. A disadvantage of this method is the limited field size. With the wide acceptance of soft x-ray therapy, contact x-ray machines are mostly replaced by more modern units.

Electron-beam therapy uses high-energy electrons that are presently available at many radiation centers and offer an almost ideal form of ionizing radiation [8–13]. The action of these electrons is similar to that of roentgen rays but permits

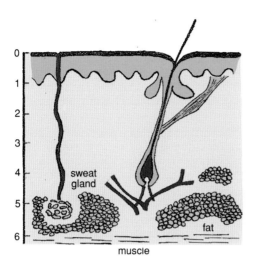
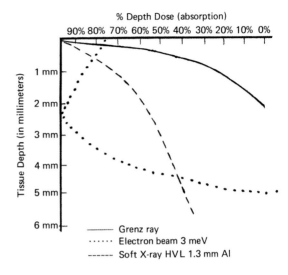

Fig. 28.1 Absorption curves, schematic, in millimeters.

optimal dose distribution throughout the treatment field. Conventional x-ray treatment of skin lesions is associated with unavoidable amounts of radiation reaching the underlying tissues. In contrast, the electron beam reaches maximum dose under the skin surface, which is especially beneficial in the treatment of cutaneous lymphomas; it also spares the mucous membranes and the bone marrow. By controlling the voltage, the depth of penetration can be adjusted with some precision, and beyond this the dose rapidly decreases to zero, which explains the better cosmetic results. For the electron beam, the inverse square law does not apply; therefore, this therapy is advantageous in cases in which the tumor is not located on an even plane (see Fig. 28.1). Electron-beam therapy is ideal for the treatment of radiosensitive widespread neoplastic lesions, in which damage to underlying structures such as bone marrow has to be avoided. Generalized lymphoma (particularly T-cell lymphomas and Hodgkin's disease), Kaposi's sarcoma, extensive skin metastases, and more circumscribed malignancies near bone and cartilage (e.g., ear) respond well to electron-beam therapy. Electron-beam therapy may be given with other therapies such as psoralen plus ultraviolet A (PUVA) to further enhance results.

The main consideration in treating cancer is its cure. A dose of x-rays big enough to destroy the cancer but not so large as to seriously damage the surrounding normal tissue is desirable.

Selection of treatment factors

The selection of appropriate radiation factors will depend on the size, location, thickness, invasiveness, type of cancer, and body response to radiation. Experience shows that when the size of the irradiated area is between 3 cm^2 and 20 cm^2, a *total surface dose* of 3500 to 6000 R is usually sufficient to eradicate skin cancers. *Fractionation* means subdividing the total dose into increments, a technique that increases the tissue tolerance and gives overall better cosmetic results, as normal cells recover more rapidly than do tumor cells after each dose. Dividing the total amount of radiation is especially important in large tumors and those in certain locations, as on the ears above cartilage. Biologic effects are also influenced by the dose rate (R/min). *Time–dose relationship* is the overall time in which the fractionated radiation is given and the total dose has to be considered. If a change in the overall treatment time occurs, the whole dose has to be increased.

The quality of radiation is selected for the estimated thickness of the tumor and depends on the proportion of different wavelengths. The shorter the wavelength, the "harder" its penetrating power. To define the quality of a given radiation, the term *half-value layer* is used. One millimeter of aluminum will absorb about the same amount of radiation as 15 mm of tissue. Instead of the term *HVL*, the term *half-value depth* (HVD, or D$\frac{1}{2}$) is gaining acceptance, because it is more meaningful. D$\frac{1}{2}$ indicates the tissue depth in millimeters, at which depth the absorbed dose is 50% of the surface dose.

The HVL is influenced by properties of the x-ray tube, kilovoltage, and filter. The selection of the appropriate HVL will depend on the depth of the lesion. As a rule of thumb, the base of the cancer should receive half the surface dose of x-rays. The depth of the lesion is estimated by visual inspection and also by histologic examination, which is not always reliable because the depth of the tumor may vary in different sections (Fig. 28.1). As most cancers have a depth less than 5 mm, it is apparent that in most instances radiation with HVL of less than 1 mm of aluminum should be sufficient to treat the majority of skin cancers.

The formula

$$I = \frac{mA \times kV^2 \times t}{D^2}$$

shows the relationships of *I* (intensity of radiation) to mA (milliampere), kV (kilovoltage), *t* (time), and *D* (distance). An increase in peak kilovoltage will increase the energy of the x-rays, with a greater proportion of shorter wavelengths. An increase in milliamperes leads to a greater number of x-rays, with no change in the quality of the x-ray beam. The intensity of radiation is inversely proportional to its distance squared. This law (the inverse square law) does not strictly apply to very soft radiation, which is partially absorbed by air, or to electron-beam therapy.

To deliver a uniform dose throughout the field, the *target skin distance* (distance between the metal of the x-ray tube on which the electrons impinge and the tumor) should be approximately twice the diameter of the radiated area.

Filters, mostly made from aluminum, are used to get a more homogeneous beam. They diminish the quantity of the radiation, mainly by filtering the softer radiation.

The *size of a radiated area* also has a distinctive influence on the biologic effects of radiation. For areas smaller than 2 cm^2, a greater radiation dose is required. Cones and lead shields are used for delineating the field and for radiation protection. Small cones (< 10 mm in diameter) reduce the x-ray dose, whereas apertures exceeding 5 cm increase the dose appreciably. The tumor is outlined and the field size is marked with a marker. In well-defined smaller lesions, a 5- to 10-mm margin is sufficient. In ill-defined lesions (e.g., morphea-like BCCs or recurrent cancer), a margin of a least 10 mm is given.

Practical approach to treatment of skin cancer

Planning for radiotherapy can begin as soon as the clinical diagnosis is verified by histologic examination. A shave biopsy may be preferable to a punch, which may leave a depressed scar in the radiation field. Radiotherapy should be started after the biopsy site has healed. The patient is provided with an instruction sheet. We begin a radiotherapy record form (as shown on the next page).

Radiation protection

Select the amount and quality of radiation properly suited for the type and depth of the pathologic process. Radiosensitive tissues, such as the lenses, thyroid gland, gonads, breasts, and blood-forming organs, have to be protected by proper lead shields: ordinarily a thickness of 0.15 mm is satisfactory. The lead is available in sheets and is cut according to the size and shape of the lesion to be treated. Lead shielding is also present under the x-ray table, and a lead apron is placed over the patient's body.

When *tumors in the orbital area* are treated, the lens must be shielded with eyecups, which consist of a lead core, electroplated with copper and covered with cadmium. In addition, the eye shields are sometimes coated with a layer of paraffin. If eyecups have to be put directly on the eyes, a local anesthetic (e.g., 0.5% pantocaine) is used.

For *cancers of the nose*, in addition to eye shielding, lead strips are inserted into the nose to reduce the exit dose and thus protect the nasal septum. When

INSTRUCTION SHEET FOR PATIENT UNDERGOING RADIATION THERAPY

You are about to undergo a course of radiation therapy. You will be treated every day except Thursday, Sunday, Holidays, and on occasion, other days. You will be treated over one or possibly several areas each day. The length of each treatment may vary during your course of therapy due to a change of dosage.

The areas to be treated may be marked on your skin with a marking fluid. These marks serve as a guide for further treatments, so please do not try to remove them. Ordinary washing with soap and water will not remove them, unless you try to scrub them off.

> DO NOT APPLY ANY MEDICINE, LOTIONS, OR SALVES (this includes cosmetics, deodorants, and antiperspirants) to the areas of the skin being treated except those recommended by me.
>
> Extreme caution should be exercised so that no other form of light treatment (UV), or overexposure to the sun is given.
>
> Should you have any questions concerning your treatments or need any advice, do not hesitate to contact me.
>
> After completion of your course of radiation therapy you will receive a return appointment. As is customary for most treatment centers, you will be followed the first year in three month intervals, the second year, bi-yearly, and from then on yearly.
>
> At that point, you will have completed your course of radiation therapy and are given a return appointment card for a check-up.

Following radiation treatment the skin often becomes red with itching and burning sensations. These reactions are unavoidable in order to obtain a beneficial result. If this has already occurred, you have been instructed in its proper care. If it has not occurred, in most cases it will within a short time after completion of your x-ray treatments, and the proper care of this mild stage is to use cold cream or preferably Polysporin ointment on the areas. If the reaction becomes more intense (with cracking, blisters, etc.), a 1% water solution of Gentian Violet may be painted on the skin with a cotton swab twice a day for a few days. Should open sores or thick crusts develop, they may be bathed with a solution of normal saline (three level teaspoonfuls of salt mixed in a quart of water) — such wet dressings often help in cleaning up infections. If the reaction does not improve within a few days, consult me.

If you have any further questions concerning your condition or your treatment, be sure to consult or call me.

a *cancer of the lips* has to be treated by radiation, lead shields properly cut and covered with tape are inserted behind the lips.

Radiation sequelae

Using x-ray increments of 400 R (HVL = 1.2 mm aluminum), erythema usually appears after the sixth to eighth treatment and increases in intensity for up to 6 to 10 days even after treatment has already been completed. Oozing, crusting, and ulceration may follow, especially in large tumors. Healing may take several weeks. In treatment of cancer with underlying mucosa, mucositis and erosion may develop on the surface underneath the irradiated area. The patient should be forewarned of this possibility. Painful ulcerations may appear immediately at the end of the irradiation, and healing may be prolonged. A few months after treatment, the cosmetic result, with exception of occasional hyperpigmentation, is mostly excellent; the skin appears completely normal. Unfortunately, later signs of chronic radiodermatitis usually develop.

Occasionally, it may take up to 5 months for complete disappearance of the neoplasm (delayed tumor regression). If the tumor does not involute, the neoplasm is considered radioresistant and is treated

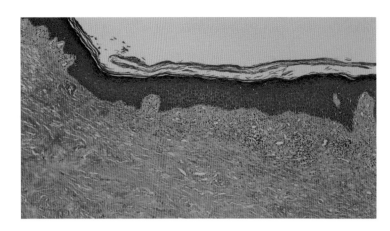

Fig. 28.2 Radiation dermatitis revealing thickened collagen bundles (hematoxylin-eosin [H&E] 10×).

by a different modality. Rarely, one sees the appearance of a growth at the previous tumor site, which on histologic examination does not reveal cancer but granulation tissue. This lesion is called pseudo-recidive and may be clinically worrisome. Years after successful treatment, a necrosis in the radiation field may develop. The differential diagnosis between recurrent tumor versus radiation necrosis may be difficult. Close observation and skin biopsies at times are necessary to establish the definitive diagnosis. Such radiation ulcers unfortunately heal very slowly, and grafting in such damaged skin is difficult. Postradiation leukoplakia on palpebral conjunctiva and epiphora after treatment of eyelid epithelioma is fortunately rare, but it is an unpleasant occurrence. The development of comedones at the periphery of the radiation field is not infrequently seen, especially on the face. These blackheads may persist for many months. Chronic radiation dermatitis may occur after many years and is characterized by fibrosis and atypical fibroblasts (Figs. 28.2 and 28.3).

Recurrences

Recurrences after radiation are mostly the result of inadequate depth, too small a field, or inadequate total dose. The cure rate is approximately 95% and compares well with other treatment modalities, except the Mohs technique, which has an even higher cure rate. However, the choice of treatment methods cannot be based by cure rates alone; other factors, such as cosmetic consideration, general health, age of the patient, and so forth, have to be evaluated.

Specific x-ray therapy

Basal cell carcinoma and squamous cell carcinoma

Nonmelanoma skin cancers (BCCs, SCCs, keratoacanthomas) are all treated in a similar way: HVL = 0.2 to 1.2 mm aluminum, depending on the tumor depth; TSD = 15 cm; 400 R (350 rads) × 13, total dose 5200 R (4550 rads) given in the course of 3 weeks, 5 days a week. The main exception is a low-grade type of SCC, the verrucous carcinoma, for which radiotherapy is controversial and probably contraindicated because of the risk of its transformation into an aggressive SCC [14–16]. If it is difficult for the patient to come for several treatments, less fractionation—for instance, 700 rads × 5—may be given in a 2- to 3-week time period. To use a massive single tumor dose is not advisable but may be given under certain circumstances when the tumor is less than 1 cm in diameter. This single dose of 2500 R obviously is lower than a total dose after fractionation during a 3-week course. Late complications of radiation therapy increase with the dose given per fraction of radiation. In the past, doctors and patients wanted to reduce the number of treatments given so that treatment was most practical. Unfortunately, the incidence of late complications of this strategy was fairly high. The role of radiation therapy for BCCs, SCCs,

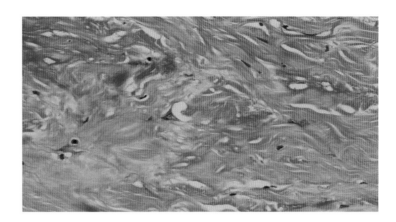

Fig. 28.3 Radiation dermatitis showing prominent fibroblasts (H&E 20×).

and keratoacanthomas has been revised [17–21]. Over the last decade, delivery of a large number of smaller doses has been used to take advantage of a differential sparing of the tissues responsible for the acute effects of radiation. Hyperfractionation or altered fractionation may improve local control and minimize side effects. Excellent cosmetic results can be achieved (Figs. 28.4 to 28.9). Skin cancers larger than 10 cm in diameter are usually unsuitable for radiotherapy, with the exception of superficial, so-called multicentric basal cell epitheliomas, which may be treated by Grenz rays (radiation of low energy, HVL = 0.02 to 0.05 mm aluminum) of 4 × 2000 R. Above bone and cartilage, soft radiation qualities and more frequent increments are used. Radiation on the trunk and extremities shows more radiation sequelae than on the face.

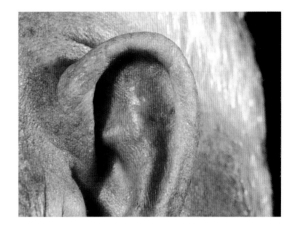

Fig. 28.5 Patient in Fig. 28.4 after radiation therapy.

Soft x-ray therapy for Bowen's disease and erythroplasia of Queyrat has achieved excellent results [22].

Radiotherapy may also be employed after surgical excision. Patients who have a cutaneous SCC with perineural invasion may benefit from postoperative radiation therapy to minimize the risk of recurrence [23]. Magnetic resonance imaging can detect and define the extent of perineural invasion; CT can document regional lymph node metastases. Those with apparently resectable SCCs or BCCs undergo surgery usually followed by postoperative radiotherapy [24]. Patients with incompletely resectable cancers get definitive radiotherapy. The 5-year local control, cause-specific survival, and overall survival rates were approximately 87%, 65%, and 50%,

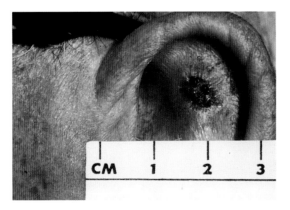

Fig. 28.4 Basal cell carcinoma on the ear.

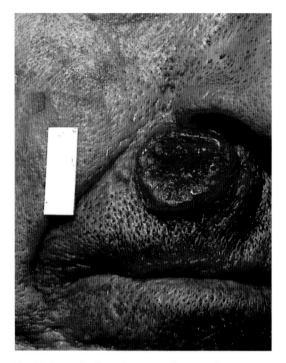

Fig. 28.6 Basal cell carcinoma on the upper lip.

respectively, for patients with incidental perineural invasion compared with 55%, 59%, and 55%, respectively, for those with clinical perineural invasion.

Melanomas

Superficial spreading melanomas are not usually treated with radiotherapy. Desmoplastic melanoma

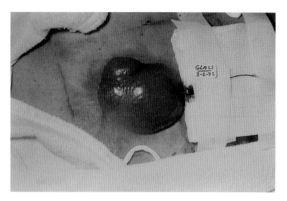

Fig. 28.8 Metastatic breast cancer.

and lentigo maligna are exceptions [25–30]. Total doses of up to 10,000 to 20,000 R are required, which cause necrosis. Fractionated radiation therapy is associated with results that are comparable to conventional surgical excision. Margin control remains the most important factor in the successful treatment of desmoplastic melanoma. Surgical treatment without adjuvant radiation but with careful margin control gave better results than historical results for conventional surgery and additional radiation therapy. Radiation therapy may have a wider role in the management of melanoma than previously assumed. It is covered in detail in the chapter on treatment of melanoma.

Kaposi's sarcoma

The treatment of Kaposi's sarcoma has evolved over the past few years [31–34]. Both protease

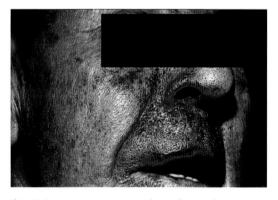

Fig. 28.7 Patient in Fig. 28.6 after radiation therapy.

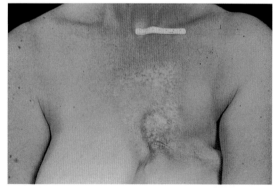

Fig. 28.9 Patient in Fig. 28.8 after radiation therapy and hyperthermia.

inhibitor–based and non-nucleoside reverse transcription inhibitor–based regimens reduce the incidence of AIDS-Kaposi's sarcoma. Topical alitretinoin gel may be a useful agent. Systemic chemotherapy with doxorubicin, bleomycin, or vincristine may be of value. Kaposi's sarcoma arising in the setting of HIV infection is also responsive to radiation therapy. It is best to begin with doses of 150 to 300 R once weekly or biweekly up to 2000 to 3000 R, total dose. Because of the development of new lesions, the long-term prognosis is guarded. The quality of radiation (HVL) will depend on the depth and age of the lesion. Radiotherapy may be palliative for AIDS-associated Kaposi's sarcoma. The higher dose of 40 Gy given over 20 fractions is associated with higher complete response and less residual purple pigmentation than lower dosages. Complete response of lesions to 20 Gy given in 10 fractions or 40 Gy in 20 fractions may be slightly superior to lesions treated with 8 Gy as a single fraction. Radiation therapy for Kaposi's sarcoma in the setting of HIV-1 infection has its greatest use in resource-poor settings or for palliation. Treatment of oral lesions with radiotherapy should be avoided because of the predictable development of severe radiation mucositis.

B-cell lymphoma

Cutaneous B-cell lymphoma usually responds well initially to radiation therapy [35,36]. The thickness of the lesions will determine what kind of HVL to choose. A single dose of 200 R four to five times in weekly intervals to a total dose of 1000 R is given. Radiotherapy is useful in primary cutaneous large cell lymphomas of follicular center cell origin. In fact, we have found it valuable in patients with lymphoma cutis in general. Follicular center cell lymphomas have a rather indolent clinical course and may be treated with localized radiotherapy alone, compared with diffuse large B-cell lymphoma, which warrants more aggressive therapy. Unlike diffuse large B-cell lymphoma presenting in nodal or noncutaneous sites, primary large B-cell lymphoma has an indolent course and may be treated with local radiotherapy alone [36].

T-cell lymphoma

Mycosis fungoides (a cutaneous T-cell lymphoma) is usually very sensitive to ionizing radiation and is treated with the minimal effective dose (low-dose regimen), local field radiation, and total skin electron-beam radiation [37–39]. Total-body electron-beam irradiation may be combined with chemotherapy, such as doxorubicin and cyclophosphamide, with good results. A consensus report outlines a useful protocol for total electron-beam therapy. The treatment is effective and may be coupled with PUVA or extracorporeal phototherapy.

Cutaneous metastatic disease

As with solitary cutaneous lymphomas, cutaneous metastases may respond to palliative radiotherapy. We have found radiation therapy to be beneficial in selected patients (Figs 28.8 and 28.9). X-ray therapy should be considered for metastases, including chondrosarcoma cutaneous metastases[40] and melanoma [41]. Radiotherapy has been used for metastatic sweat gland carcinoma [42].

Merkel cell carcinoma

Merkel cell carcinoma is also sensitive to radiation therapy. Adjuvant local irradiation is extremely useful in enhancing results [43]. Patients who receive postoperative radiation in the tumor bed appear to have a lower number of recurrences. Radiation therapy with a mean dose of 50 to 60 Gy to the primary tumor and 45 to 50 Gy to the regional lymphatics is typically employed. Merkel cell carcinoma is the subject of a separate chapter, which details radiotherapy for this rare but important entity.

Curious phenomena associated with cutaneous radiotherapy

Radiotherapy may induce or exacerbate underlying disease expression like bullae formation in bullous pemphigoid [44] or cutaneous metastases in areas of radiation dermatitis [45]. Certain chemotherapeutic agents may severely damage tissues that have been previously irradiated [46–48]. Such "radiation recall" reactions may occur concurrent with, or even after, administration of chemotherapy and present as intense erythema, which sometimes progresses to cutaneous necrosis. The most frequent offenders are doxorubicin, 5-fluorouracil, and actinomycin D. It occurred in about 9% of patients in one series, usually within 6 weeks after the completion of radiotherapy, and varied in intensity from mild to severe exfoliative dermatitis [49]. Similar reactions also arise after electron-beam therapy and to a lesser extent with ultraviolet light. In addition, we have noted a variety of cutaneous vascular reaction patterns, such as urticaria, erythema multiforme, and leukocytoclastic vasculitis, after radiotherapy [50]. Tumor antigen released or altered by radiotherapy may induce such cutaneous reactions. Paradoxically, radiated skin sites may be spared generalized skin eruptions [51].

Consequences of long-term radiotherapy

Ionizing radiation may produce serious effects in the skin. It has been emphasized that chronic radiation skin damage is a sign of possible cancer not only of the skin but of underlying structures, including thyroid, breasts, and vascular and appendageal structures [52]. Benign neurilemmomas and salivary gland tumors of the head and neck may follow childhood irradiation [53,54]. Sebaceous carcinomas, angiosarcomas, eccrine porocarcinoma, and malignant fibrous histiocytomas may also occur [55–58]. Unusual vascular neoplasms may arise after radiation therapy. These vascular neoplasms may be difficult to classify but should be excised in their entirety [56]. Because the carcinogenic lag is up to 50 years, it is very important to examine patients critically for evidence of previous irradiation and to watch for the development of neoplasms. BCCs in childhood may result from ionizing radiation, especially in the setting of basal cell nevus syndrome, albinism, or xeroderma pigmentosum [59]. Therapeutic radiation therapy is much more closely associated with the development of BCCs than with that of SCCs [60].

Clearly, even low-energy "soft" or Grenz rays are carcinogenic in a few patients who received large doses, as a study of 14,140 patients treated with Grenz rays indicates [61]. But the risk-to-benefit ratio of dermatologic x-ray therapy in the treatment of cutaneous neoplasms is still accept-

able, when properly trained dermatologists use this modality.

Nonionizing radiotherapeutic options

Psoralens and ultraviolet light

Ultraviolet light in the long-wave "A" range (UV-A) together with psoralens (PUVA) has been used predominately to treat patients with benign inflammatory disorders. However, this modality has also been employed in patients with chronic cutaneous T-cell lymphomas, Sézary syndrome, and lymphomatoid papulosis. At times, UV-A therapy is combined with oral retinoids or other chemotherapy. However, enthusiasm for the use of PUVA together with oral retinoids in cancer has waned. The development of primary skin cancers in patients receiving PUVA therapy must be kept in mind. Extracorporeal photochemotherapy for cutaneous T-cell lymphomas may be a promising modality.

Other photochemotherapies

Hematoporphyrin derivatives and cationic dyes have been used to preferentially destroy skin cancer cells [62,63]. The latter, relatively new technique, also called "selective carcinoma cell photolysis," has a higher degree of localization to tumor cells. Hematoporphyrin phototherapy has been employed for many years for human skin cancers. Photodynamic therapy has been an exciting area of study. Excellent response rates have been reported for SCCs of the head and neck [64].

Hyperthermia

Like hematoporphyrin phototherapy, hyperthermia employing microwaves by itself or in combination with other modalities, such as conventional x-rays or chemotherapy, has been used for superficial cutaneous skin cancer with enthusiasm by a small number of physicians [65].

Conclusion

The risk of side effects due to ionizing radiation must be considered in weighing benefits versus risks for starting any patient on radiation therapy. The biologic characteristics of the neoplasm and of its surrounding tissue have to be taken into account. Radiation therapy remains a very useful tool in the treatment of skin cancer and lymphomas. Because of improved techniques and better radiation sources, past mistakes can be avoided, and radiation treatment should regain some popularity in the future. When accurately administered under proper indications, it has a good safety record and yields excellent results. The dosage of radiotherapy should be kept to a minimum, and the underlying and surrounding tissues should be protected. Particular attention should be paid to the protection of eyes, thyroid, and genitalia.

References

1 Bucci MK, Bevan A, Roach M 3rd. Advances in radiation therapy: conventional to 3D, to IMRT, to 4D, and beyond. CA Cancer J Clin 2005;55:117–34.

2 Short KA, Calman FM, Ross DA, et al. Can radiotherapy cure radiation-induced skin cancer? Clin Exp Dermatol 2007;32:109–11.

3 Intensity Modulated Radiation Therapy Collaborative Working Group. Intensity-modulated radiotherapy: current status and issues of interest. Int J Radiat Oncol Biol Phys 2001;51:880–914.

4 Barker JL Jr, Garden AS, Ang KK, et al. Quantification of volumetric and geometric changes occurring during fractionated radiotherapy for head-and-neck cancer using an integrated CT/linear accelerator system. Int J Radiat Oncol Biol Phys 2004;59:960–70.

5 Hansen EK, Bucci MK, Quivey JM, et al. Repeat CT imaging and replanning during the course of IMRT for head-and-neck cancer. Int J Radiat Oncol Biol Phys 2006;64:355–62.

6 Welsh JS, Patel RR, Ritter MA, et al. Helical tomotherapy: an innovative technology and approach to radiation therapy. Technol Cancer Res Treat 2002;1:311–6.

7 Pouliot J, Bani-Hashemi A, Chen J, et al. Low-dose megavoltage cone-beam CT for radiation therapy. Int J Radiat Oncol Biol Phys 2005;61:552–60.

8 Diamandidou E, Cohen PR, Kurzrock R. Mycosis fungoides and Sezary syndrome. Blood 1996;88:2385–409.

9 Jones GW, Hoppe RT, Glatstein E. Electron beam treatment for cutaneous T-cell lymphoma. Hematol Oncol Clin North Am 1995;9:1057–76.

10 Jones GW, Tadros A, Hodson DI, et al. Prognosis with newly diagnosed mycosis fungoides after total skin electron radiation of 30 or 35 Gy. Int J Radiat Oncol Biol Phys 1994;28:839–45.

11 Jones G, Wilson LD, Fox-Goguen L. Total skin electron beam radiotherapy for patients who have mycosis fungoides. Hematol Oncol Clin North Am 2003;17:1421–34.

12 Parida DK, Verma KK, Chander S, et al. Total skin electron irradiation therapy in mycosis fungoides using high-dose rate mode: a preliminary experience. Int J Dermatol 2005;44:828–30.

13 Friedman M, Pearce JI. Electron beam therapy. In: Helm F, editor. Cancer dermatology. Philadelphia: Lea & Febiger; 1979. p. 353–62.

14 Schwartz RA. Verrucous carcinoma of the skin and mucosa. J Am Acad Dermatol 1995;32:1–21; quiz 22–4.

15 Rush B. Radiotherapy for verrucous carcinoma of the oral cavity. J Surg Oncol 2006;94:639; author reply 640–1.

16 Micali G, Nasca MR, Innocenzi D, et al. Penile cancer. J Am Acad Dermatol 2006;54:369–91; quiz 391–4.

17 Wilder RB, Shimm DS, Kittelson JM, et al. Recurrent basal cell carcinoma treated with radiation therapy. Arch Dermatol 1991;127:1668–72.

18 Sherr DL. Therapeutic options for superficial basal cell carcinoma: the role of radiation therapy. Arch Dermatol 1998;134:752.

19 Schulte KW, Lippold A, Auras C, et al. Soft x-ray therapy for cutaneous basal cell and squamous cell carcinomas. J Am Acad Dermatol 2005;53:993–1001.

20 Pipitone MA, Gloster HM. Superficial squamous cell carcinomas and extensive actinic keratoses of the scalp treated with radiation therapy. Dermatol Surg 2006;32:756–9.

21 Mendenhall WM, Amdur RJ, Siemann DW, et al. Altered fractionation in definitive irradiation of squamous cell carcinoma of the head and neck. Curr Opin Oncol 2000;12:207–14.

22 Blank AA, Schnyder UW. Soft-X-ray therapy in Bowen's disease and erythroplasia of Queyrat. Dermatologica 1985;171:89–94.

23 Han A, Ratner D. What is the role of adjuvant radiotherapy in the treatment of cutaneous squamous cell carcinoma with perineural invasion? Cancer 2007;109:1053–9.

24 Mendenhall WM, Amdur RJ, Hinerman RW, et al. Skin cancer of the head and neck with perineural invasion. Am J Clin Oncol 2007;30:93–6.

25 Ballo MT, Ang KK. Radiation therapy for malignant melanoma. Surg Clin North Am 2003;83:323–42.

26 Schmid-Wendtner MH, Brunner B, Konz B, et al. Fractionated radiotherapy of lentigo maligna and lentigo maligna melanoma in 64 patients. J Am Acad Dermatol 2000;43:477–82.

27 Salmi R, Holsti P. Effects of roentgen irradiation on human melanoma metastases in the skin. Acta Oncol 1987;26:37–40.

28 Arora A, Lowe L, Su L, et al. Wide excision without radiation for desmoplastic melanoma. Cancer 2005;104:1462–7.

29 Stevens G, Hong A. Radiation therapy in the management of cutaneous melanoma. Surg Oncol Clin N Am 2006;15:353–71.

30 Stevens G, McKay MJ. Dispelling the myths surrounding radiotherapy for treatment of cutaneous melanoma. Lancet Oncol 2006;7:575–83.

31 Dedicoat M, Vaithilingum M, Newton R. Treatment of Kaposi's sarcoma in HIV-1 infected individuals with emphasis on resource poor settings. Cochrane Database Syst Rev 2003:CD003256.

32 el-Akkad S, Bull CA, el-Senoussi MA, et al. Kaposi's sarcoma and its management by radiotherapy. Arch Dermatol 1986;122:1396–9.

33 Stelzer KJ, Griffin TW. A randomized prospective trial of radiation therapy for AIDS-associated Kaposi's sarcoma. Int J Radiat Oncol Biol Phys 1993;27:1057–61.

34 Huang KM, Hsu CH, Cheng JC, et al. Radiotherapy of classic Kaposi's sarcoma in Taiwan, an area where classic Kaposi's sarcoma is not prevalent. Anticancer Res 2006;26:4659–63.

35 Ulutin HC, Ozturk B, Onguru O, et al. Treatment of primary cutaneous B-cell lymphoma with radiotherapy. Radiat Med 2005;23:292–5.

36 Smith BD, Glusac EJ, McNiff JM, et al. Primary cutaneous B-cell lymphoma treated with radiotherapy: a comparison of the European Organization for Research and Treatment of Cancer and the WHO classification systems. J Clin Oncol 2004;22:634–9.

37 Wilson LD, Jones GW, Kim D, et al. Experience with total skin electron beam therapy in combination with extracorporeal photopheresis in the management of patients with erythrodermic (T4) mycosis fungoides. J Am Acad Dermatol 2000;43:54–60.

38 Maingon P, Truc G, Dalac S, et al. Radiotherapy of advanced mycosis fungoides: indications and results of total skin electron beam and photon beam irradiation. Radiother Oncol 2000;54:73–8.

39 van Vloten WA, de Vroome H, Noordijk EM. Total skin electron beam irradiation for cutaneous T-cell lymphoma (mycosis fungoides). Br J Dermatol 1985;112:697–702.

40 Sherr DL, Fountain KS, Kalb RE. Cutaneous metastases from chondrosarcoma. J Dermatol Surg Oncol 1986;12:146–9.

41 Trefzer U, Sterry W. Topical immunotherapy with diphenylcyclopropenone in combination with DTIC and radiation for cutaneous metastases of melanoma. Dermatology 2005;211:370–1.

42 Voutsadakis IA, Bruckner HW. Eccrine sweat gland carcinoma: a case report and review of diagnosis and treatment. Conn Med 2000;64:263–6.

43 Lewis KG, Weinstock MA, Weaver AL, et al. Adjuvant local irradiation for Merkel cell carcinoma. Arch Dermatol 2006;142:693–700.

44 Mul VE, Verschueren TA, van Geest AJ, et al. Bullous pemphigoid (BP) induced by radiotherapy. Radiother Oncol 2007;82:105.

45 Marley NF, Marley WM. Skin metastases in an area of radiation dermatitis. Arch Dermatol 1982;118:129–31.

46 Dunagin WG. Clinical toxicity of chemotherapeutic agents: dermatologic toxicity. Semin Oncol 1982;9:14–22.

47 Kundranda MN, Daw HA. Tamoxifen-induced radiation recall dermatitis. Am J Clin Oncol 2006;29:637–8.

48 Deland MM, Weiss RA, McDaniel DH, et al. Treatment of radiation-induced dermatitis with light-emitting diode (LED) photomodulation. Lasers Surg Med 2007;39:164–8.

49 Kodym E, Kalinska R, Ehringfeld C, et al. Frequency of radiation recall dermatitis in adult cancer patients. Onkologie 2005;28:18–21.

50 Yoshitake T, Nakamura K, Shioyama Y, et al. Erythema multiforme and Stevens–Johnson syndrome following radiotherapy. Radiat Med 2007;25:27–30.

51 Cochran RJ, Wilkin JK. Failure of drug rash to appear in a previously irradiated site. Arch Dermatol 1981;117:810–1.

52 Schwartz RA, Burgess GH, Milgrom H. Breast carcinoma and basal cell epithelioma after x-ray therapy for hirsutism. Cancer 1979;44:1601–5.

53 Whatley WS, Thompson JW, Rao B. Salivary gland tumors in survivors of childhood cancer. Otolaryngol Head Neck Surg 2006;134:385–8.

54 Preston DL, Ron E, Yonehara S, et al. Tumors of the nervous system and pituitary gland associated with atomic bomb radiation exposure. J Natl Cancer Inst 2002;94:1555–63.

55 Clarke LE, Julian KG, Clarke JT, et al. Reactive angioendotheliomatosis in association with a

well-differentiated angiosarcoma. Am J Dermatopathol 2005;27:422–7.

56 Brenn T, Fletcher CD. Radiation-associated cutaneous atypical vascular lesions and angiosarcoma: clinicopathologic analysis of 42 cases. Am J Surg Pathol 2005;29:983–96.

57 Rao J, Dekoven JG, Beatty JD, et al. Cutaneous angiosarcoma as a delayed complication of radiation therapy for carcinoma of the breast. J Am Acad Dermatol 2003;49:532–8.

58 Kose R, Coban YK, Ciralik H. Eccrine porocarcinoma arising from preexisting eccrine poroma of the scalp after radiotherapy for cervical cancer. Dermatol Online J 2006;12:18.

59 Marin-Gutzke M, Sanchez-Olaso A, Berenguer B, et al. Basal cell carcinoma in childhood after radiation therapy: case report and review. Ann Plast Surg 2004;53:593–5.

60 Karagas MR, McDonald JA, Greenberg ER, et al. Risk of basal cell and squamous cell skin cancers after ionizing radiation therapy. For The Skin Cancer Prevention Study Group. J Natl Cancer Inst 1996;88: 1848–53.

61 Lindelof B, Eklund G. Incidence of malignant skin tumors in 14,140 patients after Grenz-ray treatment for benign skin disorders. Arch Dermatol 1986;122: 1391–5.

62 Blume JE, Oseroff AR. Aminolevulinic acid photodynamic therapy for skin cancers. Dermatol Clin 2007;25:5–14.

63 Oseroff AR, Shieh S, Frawley NP, et al. Treatment of diffuse basal cell carcinomas and basaloid follicular hamartomas in nevoid basal cell carcinoma syndrome by wide-area 5-aminolevulinic acid photodynamic therapy. Arch Dermatol 2005;141:60–7.

64 Biel MA. Photodynamic therapy and the treatment of head and neck neoplasia. Laryngoscope 1998;108:1259–68.

65 El-Tonsy MH, El-Domyati MM, El-Sawy AE, et al. Continuous-wave Nd:YAG laser hyperthermia: a successful modality in treatment of basal cell carcinoma. Dermatol Online J 2004;10:3.

CHAPTER 29

Local chemotherapy

Ulrich R. Hengge

Several forms of local chemotherapy are being used in the treatment of skin cancers (Table 29.1). They are particularly valuable for diffuse actinic damage on large skin surfaces, possibly to avoid field cancerization. Thus, topical chemotherapies are particularly appealing.

Topical 5-fluorouracil

Topical 5-fluorouracil (5-FU) has represented the mainstay of treatment for actinic keratoses (AKs) since it was pioneered by Klein [1–4] in the 1960s (Fig. 29.1). 5-FU is a chemotherapeutic agent that blocks DNA synthesis by ribosylation and phosphorylation. Specifically, 5-FU inhibits thymidylate synthetase, the enzyme responsible for converting deoxyoridine-5 to thymidine-5-monophosphate. The depletion of thymidine leads to reduced DNA synthesis. As a consequence, the effect on DNA synthesis is more pronounced in rapidly proliferating malignant cells in comparison with normal cells. Thus, it causes cell death in AKs, but not in normal skin.

Topical 5-FU has been approved by the Food and Drug Administration (FDA) for the treatment of AKs. Treatment regimens include once- or twice-daily application for 2 to 6 weeks (Table 29.2). However, there are no well-designed large studies demonstrating the actual effectiveness of 5-FU cream because its approval was granted decades before the actual rigorous FDA standards for proving the effectiveness of new medications were implemented.

To resolve the question of whether treatment of AKs with intermittent doses of topical 5-FU is effective, 85 AKs in 53 patients were treated with 5-FU

in decreasing intensity [5]. The initial treatment frequency was four applications per week in week 1, followed by a reduction to two times per week if significant irritation occurred. Complete clearance occurred in 88.6% of treated AKs. For individuals who continued the four applications–per-week schedule, time to complete response was 7.4 weeks as opposed to 10.2 weeks when therapy was reduced to two times per week.

5-Fluorouracil is available as a 0.5%, 1%, or 5% cream as well as a 1% or 2.5% topical solution. A recent study of 177 patients examined the efficacy of 0.5% 5-FU in a randomized, double-blind, vehicle-controlled design [6]. Treatment duration consisted of 1, 2, or 4 weeks, with a percentage reduction in the number of AKs from baseline of 78.5%, 83.6%, and 88.7%, respectively ($P < 0.001$). Mild to moderate facial irritation with dryness and erythema was noted in up to 73% of treated individuals. Total clearance occurred in 26.3%, 19.5%, 47.5%, and 3.4% of patients in the 1-, 2-, and 4-week fluorouracil and vehicle groups, respectively. A study conducted by Gupta [7] suggested that the topical 0.5% 5-FU cream is more cost-effective than the higher concentrations (1% and 5%), most likely because of the once-daily regimen.

Another study also concluded that 5-FU 5% cream twice daily for 3 weeks is more effective than two applications once weekly [8]. Moreover, topical 5-FU 0.5% applied once daily for 7 days followed by cryosurgery of any residual AKs at the 4-week follow-up visit was compared with cryotherapy alone of AKs in a randomized, vehicle-controlled trial with 144 patients [9]. At the 6-month outcome, 30% and 8% had achieved complete clinical clearance in the 5-FU plus cryotherapy

Table 29.1 Local chemotherapeutic agents/procedures

Photodynamic therapy using 5-aminolevulinic acid (ALA)
  or methyl aminolevulinate (MAL)
Topical 5-fluorouracil (5-FU)
Diclofenac
Colchicine
Retinoids
Chemical peels (e.g., Jessner's solution, trichloroacetic acid)

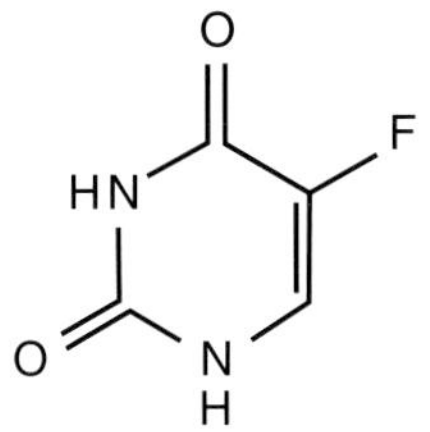

Fig. 29.1 Chemical structure of 5-FU.

Table 29.2 Instructions for the use of 5-FU for treatment
of actinic keratoses and other precancerous lesions

1 Apply 5-FU cream or lotion with fingertips twice daily
   (morning and evening) to those areas of your skin
   that are affected with "rough spots," called actinic
   keratosis. The medication should be given to the
   entire general area involved with keratoses, including
   normal-looking skin between them. Special attention,
   however, should be given to the sites of the keratoses.
2 Do not use other cosmetics or creams on the treated
   area, unless otherwise instructed.
3 During the course of treatment, avoid excessive
   exposure to the sun.
4 Do not be surprised if at the end of the second week
   or early in the third week, your skin looks worse than
   before treatment. You can expect some redness,
   dryness, and possibly even oozing and discomfort
   similar to that in a severe sunburn. These are signs of
   a normal process in the treatment. It is essential for
   you to follow these instructions and to continue to
   use the 5-FU cream for a prescribed length of time
   (usually 4 weeks).
5 5-FU is very effective for actinic keratoses, but after
   completion of one course of treatment, your skin
   should be checked by a dermatologist, who will
   determine whether all keratoses are removed. 5-FU,
   however, does not prevent the development of new
   keratoses in the future. Therefore, regular follow-up
   visits are essential.
6 In case of severe irritation or any other problems,
   please contact our clinic.

group and the vehicle and cryotherapy group,
respectively.

Among the different 5-FU–containing preparations, a 0.5% 5-FU cream was compared with 5%
5-FU cream applied to each side of the face in patients with AKs in a randomized study [10]. In this
trial, the 0.5% 5-FU cream achieved a significantly
greater reduction of AKs than the 5% cream, yielding a reduction from 11.3 to 2.5 lesions as compared
with 10.3 to 4.2, respectively. There was no difference between the two treatments in the percentage
of total clearance or the percent reduction in AKs
from baseline or in investigator-rated local irritation.

5-Fluorouracil has also been used in patients
with xeroderma pigmentosum, arsenical and radiation keratoses, and basal cell nevus syndrome
and in transplantation recipients. In contrast to immunomodulatory treatments, 5-FU has no effect on
immune defense. Therefore, it seems well suited for
the treatment of nonmelanoma skin cancer in this
patient population [11]. In a case series, five renal
transplant recipients with in situ squamous cell carcinoma receiving chronic immunosuppressive therapy were treated with 5-FU and imiquimod cream.
All five patients achieved a complete clearance.

In addition, 5-FU has been used successfully either topically or intralesionally to treat keratoacanthoma since pioneered by Klein [1] in 1962 [12–15].
The treatment of actinic cheilitis with topical 5-FU
has been performed but is no longer recommended
because of significant edema and discomfort [16]. It
may also be used for superficial basal cell carcinomas
(BCCs) [2].

Diclofenac

Diclofenac, a nonsteroidal anti-inflammatory drug,
has also been evaluated for the treatment of
AKs. The effect occurs through inhibition of

the cyclooxygenase enzymes, which decrease the metabolic products of the arachidonic acid metabolism. Some of these by-products are involved in immunosurveillance, inhibition of apoptosis, and angiogenesis [17,18]. In the pivotal study by Wolf and colleagues [19], the efficacy and safety of 3% diclofenac in 2.5% hyaluronan gel was documented in 120 subjects. The gel was applied twice daily for 3 months. At the 1-month follow-up evaluation, 50% of treated patients and 20% of placebo patients experienced a total clearance of target AKs. Generally, the preparation was well tolerated. Side effects from using diclofenac include pruritus, application site reactions, dry skin, and erythema.

In a second study including 195 patients, both 30- and 60-day application periods of 3% diclofenac in 2.5% hyaluronan gel and placebo were conducted [20]. Significant improvement was reported only with the 60-day regimen, with 33% of treated patients experiencing clearance of their initial AKs. In contrast, McEwan and Smith [21] evaluated 130 patients employing 3% diclofenac applied twice daily for 180 days. This study showed no significant benefit of diclofenac for the treatment of AKs.

Colchicine

Colchicine is known for the treatment of gout. It inhibits the formation of the mitotic spindle by disrupting the polymerization of tubulin and is therefore useful for inhibiting cellular migration of inflammatory cells and proliferation of tumor cells [22]. This was first recognized by Marshall [23]. Two recent studies addressed colchicine's therapeutic efficacy on AKs. In one study, 20 patients were treated with topical application of 1% colchicine twice daily for 10 days [24]. At day 10, a significant inflammatory response appeared at the treated AKs, which patients described as a sunburn-like feeling, which was followed by the development of a pustular reaction in most cases. In seven of 10 treated patients, complete clearance was reported at day 16. Another randomized trial using 16 patients compared 0.5% and 1% colchicine cream applied twice daily [25]. Clearance of target AKs occurred in seven of eight

patients in the 0.5% group and in six of eight patients in the 1% group.

Retinoids

Retinoids have potent antiproliferative and differentiation-inducing effects known to improve the manifestations of skin photodamage. This effect was analyzed by Kligman and Thorne [26], who performed a multicenter, double-blind study on 1265 patients with histologically confirmed AKs randomly assigned to receive either 0.05% tretinoin, 0.1% tretinoin, or vehicle twice daily for up to 15 months. The most effective treatment was 0.1% tretinoin applied twice daily, which led to an excellent response in 73% of patients compared with 40% of those in the vehicle-treated group ($P < 0.001$). In a similar study, topical 0.05% tretinoin cream applied once or twice daily was shown to decrease the number and size of facial AKs by 50% after 6 to 15 months [27]. Another trial with 100 patients reported similar reduction rates for facial AKs treated with topical 0.1% isotretinoin cream twice daily for 24 weeks, whereas no benefit was observed for AKs of the scalp or upper extremities [28].

Retinoids were also described to enhance the effectiveness of 5-FU in a randomized, double-blind controlled study with 19 patients. In this study, 5-FU cream was administered to AKs on one arm, followed by nightly application of 0.05% tretinoin cream to the same arm and a control cream to the other arm, until significant discomfort precluded further application [29]. At 3 months, the tretinoin-treated arms had 3.4 ± 2.6 AKs versus 15.7 ± 6.1 AKs before treatment. The control arm had 4.2 ± 2.5 lesions after treatment as compared with 15.3 ± 6.9 before treatment. Similar results were reported for the treatment of disseminated AKs on photodamaged skin with a combination of oral low-dose isotretinoin (20 mg daily) and topical 5-FU [30].

Tazarotene

Tazarotene is the first topical receptor-selective retinoid approved for the treatment of plaque psoriasis. Tazarotene 0.1% gel has also been used for the treatment of nonmelanoma skin cancer. It was applied daily for 24 weeks to patients with a total of 154 small superficial and nodular BCCs [31]. At 24 weeks of therapy, 70.8% of BCCs showed greater than 50% clinical and dermatoscopic regression, whereas 30.5% achieved a complete response. This outcome was associated with reduced proliferation and increased apoptosis, as demonstrated by Ki-67 and TdT-mediated dUTP-biotin-nick-end labeling [32]. It was also linked to enhanced retinoid acid receptor-α and bax expression, providing evidence that tazarotene induces BCC regression by synergistic retinoid acid receptor–dependent antiproliferative and proapoptotic pathways.

Alitretinoin

Some years ago, topical 0.1% alitretinoin was licensed for the treatment of Kaposi's sarcoma [33]. In a phase III vehicle-controlled, randomized trial, 134 patients with Kaposi's sarcoma were included. The overall patient response rate (complete plus partial response) was 37% (23 of 62) for the alitretinoin-treated patients and 7% (5 of 72) for the vehicle-treated patients. Generally, treatment with alitretinoin gel was well tolerated. However, several other treatment modalities exist for the therapy of a limited number of disseminated mucocutaneous Kaposi's sarcoma lesions [34].

Nitrogen mustard

Nitrogen mustard (mechlorethamine; HN2) is a cytotoxic compound that acts via intramolecular cyclization to form a cyclic onium cation (ethylenimonium). The onium cations are highly reactive and can alkylate carboxyl and amino groups of proteins (Fig. 29.2). On a cellular level, multiple chromosome breaks, cross-links, and translocations as well as nuclear fragmentation occur.

Clinically, topical nitrogen mustard has been used for more than 50 years in the treatment of mycosis fungoides, especially for plaque stage mycosis fungoides. Nitrogen mustard can be administered in an aqueous solution (10 mg/d in 50 mL of water) or in an ointment base. The ointment is

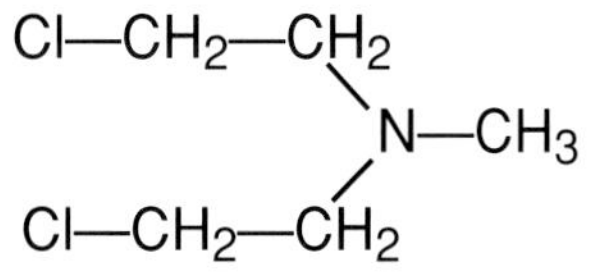

Fig. 29.2 Chemical structure of mechlorethamine (nitrogen mustard).

prepared by dissolving 10 mg of mechlorethamine in 5 mL water and then mixing it into white petrolatum (Aquaphor). Ointment-based nitrogen mustard shows increased stability and fewer hypersensitivity reactions. In addition, it does not dry the skin. Complete blood cell counts should be performed to detect possible pancytopenia. In addition, skin cancer was increased in patients treated with topical nitrogen mustard [35–37]. However, it was often impossible to differentiate whether the increased rate of skin cancer was the result of topical nitrogen mustard therapy or of other well-known risk factors. Pruritus and temporary hyperpigmentation are also occasionally observed.

It is important to treat the entire body surface. The maximum daily dose is 10 mg of mechlorethamine. Particular care has to be taken to avoid contact with mucous membranes such as eyelids, lips, and genitals. Typically, some clinical improvement is observed following 2 to 3 weeks of daily therapy. After 2 to 3 months of therapy, maintenance treatment should be performed; this treatment consists of 3-week–long intermittent courses administered every 3 months in the first year and every 4 months in the following years.

Carmustine (BCNU)

The nitrosourea carmustine, also known as BCNU, is another alkylating agent in the treatment of cutaneous T-cell lymphoma. It acts mainly by inhibiting DNA repair [38]. A 0.2% stock solution is prepared by dissolving carmustine in 95% ethanol. For total body applications, 10 mL of the 0.2% stock solution (20 mg) is added to 60 mL of water. This aqueous solution is applied daily for 6 to 8 weeks, by which time clinical response should have occurred. BCNU is absorbed through the skin and may cause myelosuppression in up to 10% of patients. Frequently, patients will develop mild to moderate erythema after 4 weeks of treatment and occasionally some erosions as well as tenderness.

Chemical peels

Various peeling agents have been used to treat patients with disseminated AKs of the scalp. The most superficial peeling agent is glycolic acid, for which a double-blind, vehicle-controlled study showed statistically significant improvement with the application of 50% glycolic acid in 41 patients [39]. Treatment was performed by topical application for 5 minutes once weekly for 4 weeks. Chemical peeling using Jessner's solution and 35% trichloroacetic acid on one side of the face has been compared with twice-daily application of 5% 5-FU cream for 3 weeks [40]. Both treatments reduced the number of visible AKs by 75% and showed equivalent histologic reduction of keratinocyte atypia. The long-term efficacy of both regimens was comparable at 32 months [41]. The Jessner's solution and 35% trichloroacetic acid was the preferred treatment in terms of patient satisfaction [40].

References

1 Klein E, Helm F, Milgrom H, et al. Tumors of the skin. II. Keratoacanthoma; local effect of 5-fluorouracil. Skin (Los Angeles) 1962;1:153–6.

2 Klein E, Stoll HL Jr, Milgrom H, et al. Tumors of the skin. V. Local administration of anti-tumor agents to multiple superficial basal cell carcinomas. J Invest Dermatol 1965;45:489–95.

3 Klein E. Tumors of skin. IX. Local cytostatic therapy of cutaneous and mucosal premalignant and malignant lesions. N Y State J Med 1968;68:886–9.

4 Klein E, Stoll HL Jr, Milgrom H, et al. Tumors of the skin. XII. Topical 5-fluorouracil for epidermal neoplasms. J Surg Oncol 1971;3:331–49.

5 Labandeira J, Pereiro M Jr, Valdes F, et al. Intermittent topical 5-fluorouracil is effective without significant irritation in the treatment of actinic keratoses but prolongs treatment duration. Dermatol Surg 2004;30:517–20.

6 Weiss J, Menter A, Hevia O, et al. Effective treatment of actinic keratosis with 0.5% fluorouracil cream for 1, 2, or 4 weeks. Cutis 2002;70:22–9.

7 Gupta AK. The management of actinic keratoses in the United States with topical fluorouracil: a pharmacoeconomic evaluation. Cutis 2002;70:30–6.

8 Jury CS, Ramraka-Jones VS, Gudi V, et al. A randomized trial of topical 5% 5-fluorouracil (Efudix cream) in the treatment of actinic keratoses comparing daily with weekly treatment. Br J Dermatol 2005;153:808–10.

9 Jorizzo J, Weiss J, Furst K, et al. Effect of a 1-week treatment with 0.5% topical fluorouracil on occurrence of actinic keratosis after cryosurgery: a randomized, vehicle-controlled clinical trial. Arch Dermatol 2004;140:813–6.

10 Loven K, Stein L, Furst K, et al. Evaluation of the efficacy and tolerability of 0.5% fluorouracil cream and 5% fluorouracil cream applied to each side of the face in patients with actinic keratosis. Clin Ther 2002;24:990–1000.

11 Smith KJ, Germain M, Skelton H. Squamous cell carcinoma in situ (Bowen's disease) in renal transplant patients treated with 5% imiquimod and 5% 5-fluorouracil therapy. Dermatol Surg 2001;27:561–4.

12 Goette DK, Odom RB, Arrott JW, et al. Treatment of keratoacanthoma with topical application of fluorouracil. Arch Dermatol 1982;118:309–11.

13 Morse LG, Kendrick C, Hooper D, et al. Treatment of squamous cell carcinoma with intralesional 5-fluorouracil. Dermatol Surg 2003;29:1150–3; discussion 1153.

14 Leonard AL, Hanke CW. Treatment of giant keratoacanthoma with intralesional 5-fluorouracil. J Drugs Dermatol 2006;5:454–6.

15 Yuge S, Godoy DA, Melo MC, et al. Keratoacanthoma centrifugum marginatum: response to topical 5-fluorouracil. J Am Acad Dermatol 2006;54:S218–9.

16 Epstein E. Treatment of lip keratoses (actinic cheilitis) with topical fluorouracil. Arch Dermatol 1977;113:906–8.

17 Marnett LJ. Generation of mutagens during arachidonic acid metabolism. Cancer Metastasis Rev 1994;13:303–8.

18 Masferrer JL, Leahy KM, Koki AT, et al. Antiangiogenic and antitumor activities of cyclooxygenase-2 inhibitors. Cancer Res 2000;60:1306–11.

19 Wolf JE Jr, Taylor JR, Tschen E, et al. Topical 3.0% diclofenac in 2.5% hyaluronan gel in the treatment of actinic keratoses. Int J Dermatol 2001;40:709–13.

20 Rivers JK, Arlette J, Shear N, et al. Topical treatment of actinic keratoses with 3.0% diclofenac in 2.5% hyaluronan gel. Br J Dermatol 2002;146:94–100.

21 McEwan LE, Smith JG. Topical diclofenac/hyaluronic acid gel in the treatment of solar keratoses. Australas J Dermatol 1997;38:187–9.

22 Ben-Chetrit E, Levy M. Colchicine: 1998 update. Semin Arthritis Rheum 1998;28:48–59.

23 Marshall J. Treatment of solar keratoses with topically-applied cytostatic agents. Br J Dermatol 1968;80:540–2.

24 Grimaitre M, Etienne A, Fathi M, et al. Topical colchicine therapy for actinic keratoses. Dermatology 2000;200:346–8.

25 Akar A, Bulent Tastan H, Erbil H, et al. Efficacy and safety assessment of 0.5% and 1% colchicine cream in the treatment of actinic keratoses. J Dermatolog Treat 2001;12:199–203.

26 Kligman AL, Thorne EG. Topical therapy of actinic keratoses with tretinoin. In: Marks R, editor. Retinoids in cutaneous malignancy. Oxford: Blackwell Scientific; 1991. p. 66–73.

27 Thorne EG. Long-term clinical experience with a topical retinoid. Br J Dermatol 1992;127 Suppl 41: 31–6.

28 Alirezai M, Dupuy P, Amblard P, et al. Clinical evaluation of topical isotretinoin in the treatment of actinic keratoses. J Am Acad Dermatol 1994;30:447–51.

29 Bercovitch L. Topical chemotherapy of actinic keratoses of the upper extremity with tretinoin and 5-fluorouracil: a double-blind controlled study. Br J Dermatol 1987;116:549–52.

30 Sander CA, Pfeiffer C, Kligman AM, et al. Chemotherapy for disseminated actinic keratoses with 5-fluorouracil and isotretinoin. J Am Acad Dermatol 1997;36:236–8.

31 Bianchi L, Orlandi A, Campione E, et al. Topical treatment of basal cell carcinoma with tazarotene: a clinicopathological study on a large series of cases. Br J Dermatol 2004;151:148–56.

32 Orlandi A, Bianchi L, Costanzo A, et al. Evidence of increased apoptosis and reduced proliferation in basal cell carcinomas treated with tazarotene. J Invest Dermatol 2004;122:1037–41.

33 Bodsworth NJ, Bloch M, Bower M, et al. Phase III vehicle-controlled, multi-centered study of topical alitretinoin gel 0.1% in cutaneous AIDS-related Kaposi's sarcoma. Am J Clin Dermatol 2001;2:77–87.

34 Hengge UR, Ruzicka T, Tyring SK, et al. Update on Kaposi's sarcoma and other HHV8 associated diseases. Part 1: epidemiology, environmental predispositions, clinical manifestations, and therapy. Lancet Infect Dis 2002;2:281–92.

35 Du Vivier A, Vonderheid EC, Van Scott EJ, et al. Mycosis fungoides, nitrogen mustard and skin cancer. Br J Dermatol 1978;99:61–3.

36 Kravitz PH, McDonald CJ. Topical nitrogen mustard induced carcinogenesis. Acta Derm Venereol 1978;58:421–5.

37 Abel EA, Sendagorta E, Hoppe RT. Cutaneous malignancies and metastatic squamous cell carcinoma following topical therapies for mycosis fungoides. J Am Acad Dermatol 1986;14:1029–38.

38 Zackheim HS, Epstein EH Jr, McNutt NS, et al. Topical carmustine (BCNU) for mycosis fungoides and related disorders: a 10-year experience. J Am Acad Dermatol 1983;9:363–74.

39 Newman N, Newman A, Moy LS, et al. Clinical improvement of photoaged skin with 50% glycolic acid. A double-blind vehicle-controlled study. Dermatol Surg 1996;22:455–60.

40 Lawrence N, Cox SE, Cockerell CJ, et al. A comparison of the efficacy and safety of Jessner's solution and 35% trichloroacetic acid vs 5% fluorouracil in the treatment of widespread facial actinic keratoses. Arch Dermatol 1995;131:176–81.

41 Witheiler DD, Lawrence N, Cox SE, et al. Long-term efficacy and safety of Jessner's solution and 35% trichloroacetic acid vs 5% fluorouracil in the treatment of widespread facial actinic keratoses. Dermatol Surg 1997;23:191–6.

CHAPTER 30
Topical immunotherapy

Ulrich R. Hengge

Assessment of immunocompetence

The mammalian immune system has most likely developed to fight infectious agents such as viruses. The immunologic defense against tumors follows the same basic principles, with innate and adaptive immunity playing a major role. Whereas the innate immunity is triggered mainly by toll-like receptors (TLRs) that serve as evolutionary conserved pattern recognition receptors stimulated by bacterial glycoproteins, lipoproteins, or viral or bacterial RNA and DNA—and is therefore readily available but at a low degree of specificity—the adaptive immunity takes some weeks to develop but is highly specific.

To assess the immunocompetence of individuals who may be subjected to topical immunotherapy, the skin-derived immune system as well as systemic immunity can be checked for their reactivity. Therefore, recall that an antigen such as tuberculin or tetanus toxoid may be applied to the skin and the delayed-type hypersensitivity (type IV reaction according to Coombs and Gell) can be assessed in sensitized individuals.

Systemic immunity can be examined by immunophenotyping lymphocytic cells in the blood. Importantly, the number of CD4$^+$ helper T (T$_H$) cells (CD4$^+$ lymphocytes) and the cytotoxic or effector T cells (CD8$^+$) can be assessed by fluorescence-activated cell sorting (FACS). In addition, the produced cytokines can be measured by intracytoplasmic staining of T$_H$1 (interleukin [IL]-2, IL-12, interferon-γ)- and T$_H$2 (IL-4, IL-10)-type cytokines.

In general, topical immunotherapies are less effective in patients with iatrogenic or acquired immunodeficiency such as HIV, in transplant patients, and in those receiving immunosuppressive therapy.

Topical immunomodulators

Topical immunomodulators (TIMs) include both immunostimulatory and immunosuppressive agents. If successful, topical immunotherapy may represent an important improvement in the therapy of inflammatory dermatoses, viral infections, and skin cancers. Immune enhancers lead to increased innate and adaptive immunity, whereas immunosuppressors decrease the activity of the cellular immune system and its associated cytokines. In the following review, topical immune enhancement is discussed (Table 30.1).

Contact sensitizers

Immunotherapy of cutaneous neoplasms, pioneered by Edmund Klein more than 40 years ago, is a concept also applied in patients with alopecia areata and for warts to clear them in previously sensitized individuals [1–7]. Contact sensitization has been used since for topical immunotherapy using dinitrochlorobenzene (DNCB), diphencyprone, and squaric acid dibutyl ester against alopecia areata [2,3], viral warts [1,4,5], basal cell (BCC) and squamous cell carcinomas (SCC) [6,7], and malignant melanoma [8].

Mechanisms of action

Contact immunotherapy is believed to work by the induction of type IV hypersensitivity. This cell-mediated response presumably acts against a complex of the contact sensitizer, serving as hapten

Table 30.1 Topical immune enhancers

Microbial agents (bacillus Calmette-Guérin, thymic
  peptides)

Obligate contact allergens
  Dinitrochlorobenzene (DNCB)
  Diphencyprone
  Squaric acid dibutyl ester

Immune response modifiers
  Interferon
  Imiquimod
  Resiquimod

bound to viral or cancerous antigens, and elicits antigen presentation through epidermal antigen-presenting Langerhans cells. The exact mechanisms of action remain to be elucidated. Various theories have been propounded, such as alterations of cytokine levels and nonspecific inflammation with predominance of CD8 T cells.

Nonmelanoma skin cancer

Topical immunotherapy of superficial cutaneous neoplasms has been performed since the late 1960s using DNCB and 2,3,5-triethylene-imino-benzoquinone (TEIB), leading to a greater than 80% regression of BCCs, SCCs, and actinic keratoses (AKs) from a total of 2000 lesions [6] and yielding a 32% complete responses in another trial evaluating 113 tumors [9]. Interestingly, the surrounding normal skin remains unaffected, pointing to involvement of certain tumor/viral antigens in the generation of an inflammatory response.

Cutaneous melanoma metastases

Contact sensitization also has been used to treat primary melanoma metastases [10]. Forty-six of 50 patients with primary melanoma responded to topical 1-chloro, 2,4-dinitrobenzene (DNCB) [10]. The 5-year survival rate for primary tumors was in excess of 87% in this cohort. Similarly, patients with cutaneous melanoma recurrences or melanoma metastases have also shown benefit from topical DNCB treatment combined with systemic dacarbazine (DTIC) [11]. Fifteen of 59 patients (25%)

attained a complete response with a median duration of 10 months (range: 3 to 210 months). Seven patients (12%) achieved a partial response, with no response being detectable in 37 patients (63%). Interestingly, the severity of the local reaction to DNCB was associated with the clinical response. These findings have been confirmed by another independent study using topical DNCB and systemic DTIC for cutaneous melanoma metastases [12], in which seven complete remissions and three partial remissions were achieved in a cohort of 15 treated patients.

BCG vaccination

Historically, intralesional application of the BCG (bacille Calmette-Guérin) vaccine has been used to treat cutaneous melanoma metastases [13,14]. Collectively, these early studies showed regression of small cutaneous metastases in up to 80% of patients. The response to BCG was characterized by flu-like reactions with nausea, vomiting, muscular pain, and joint pain [14]. It is generally accepted that BCG causes a nonspecific immune stimulation with activation of innate and adaptive immunity.

Imidazoquinolines

Imiquimod (1-(2-methylpropyl)-1H-imidazo[4,5-c]-quinolin-4-amin) and resiquimod (R-848; 4-amino-α,α-dimethyl-2-ethoxymethyl-1H-imidazo[4,5-c]-quinoline-1-ethanol) belong to the recently discovered family of imidazoquinolines that have proven antiviral and antitumor properties in animal models, although they do not display direct antiviral or antiproliferative actions. Their immune effects appear to be mediated, at least in part, through stimulation of innate immunity.

Mechanisms of action

Topical imidazoquinolines bind to TLR-7 and -8 and seem to stimulate several arms of acquired immunity, resulting in the production of monocyte-macrophage–derived cytokines, such as interferon-α (IFN-α), tumor necrosis factor-α (TNF-α), IL-1α, IL-12, and interferon-γ (IFN-γ), producing a T_H1-dominant response (Fig. 30.1)[15–18].

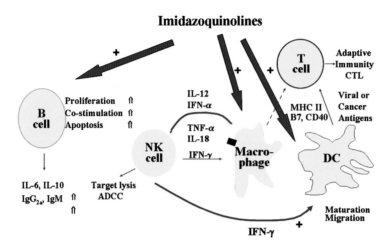

Imidazoquinolines

Fig. 30.1 Mechanism of action of TLRs and CpG. Direct and indirect effects with regard to cells of the innate and adaptive immune system are outlined. ADCC, antibody-dependent cellular cytotoxicity; CTL, cytotoxic T lymphocytes; DC, dendritic cell; IFN, interferon; Ig, immunoglobulin; IL, interleukin; MHC, major immunohistocompatibility complex; NK, natural killer.

Following topical application to the skin, IL-6, IL-8, and IFN-α synthesis by keratinocytes has also been shown [19–21]. IFN-α's antiviral activity is mediated in part by a number of proteins, including the 2′-5′-oligoadenylatsynthetase (2′-5′-AS) and the MxA protein[22,23]. Imiquimod and resiquimod have also been shown to enhance antigen presentation and maturation of Langerhans cells via TNF-α and IFN-γ as well as their migration to regional lymph nodes[6,16,24,25]. TLR signaling also seems to induce maturation of dendritic cells and may lead to the activation of the adaptive immune system [26,27]. The ability of imiquimod and resiquimod to induce antigen-specific proliferation of B lymphocytes and the expression of differentiation markers such as MHC class-II and B7.2 has recently been discovered [28,29]. Furthermore, resiquimod but not imiquimod was effective at inducing immunoglobulin (Ig)M synthesis and aided class switching from IgE to IgG$_{2a}$ in the presence of IFN-γ[30]. The results on B cell activation and differentiation suggest the potential activity of resiquimod and other imidazoquinolines to act as adjuvant and to boost antigen-specific immune responses. Indeed, resiquimod was capable of enhancing ovalbumin-specific IgG$_{2a}$ levels

and suppressed IgE when given along with the antigen [31].

Thus, the ability to enhance cutaneous adaptive responses and innate immunologic responses seems a key feature of imidazoquinolines. Meanwhile, the exact receptors and intracellular pathways have been discovered [18]. Innate immune cells recognize certain molecular structures that are present in pathogens in a simple yet elegant manner by using "pattern recognition receptors" (PRRs) that are expressed on certain innate immune cells, such as dendritic cell subsets, macrophages, monocytes, and neutrophils [32]. Imiquimod and resiquimod exert their effects upon binding to intracellular endosomal TLR-7 and -8 [33]. The best-characterized family of PRRs are the TLRs, of which 10 members have been identified in humans [32]. Signaling occurs through the TLR-MyD88 pathway [18].

Besides the immunomodulatory activity in increasing T$_H$1-type cytokines, including IFN-α and TNF-α through binding of TLR-7 and TLR-8 [34], the proinflammatory milieu was found to initiate a profound tumor-directed cellular immune response. In addition, imiquimod exhibits considerable direct proapoptotic activity [35,36]. This effect was independent of membrane-bound death

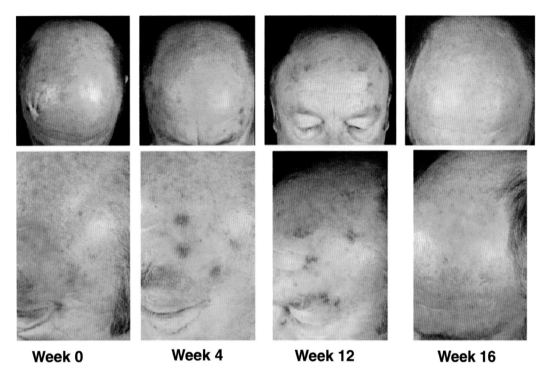

Week 0   **Week 4**   **Week 12**   **Week 16**

Fig. 30.2 Several AKs on the forehead were treated with imiquimod. A close-up of the left temple with one clinically identifiable AK next to the eyebrow is depicted in the *lower panel*. At week 4, some lesions had become erythematous (*second column from the left*). Interestingly, imiquimod treatment highlighted (demarcated) additional AKs that were not clinically identified. At week 12, multiple ones were present with erythema and excoriations (*third column from the left*). At week 16 (4 weeks after termination of treatment), no evidence of AKs was present on the forehead and the left temple (*fourth column from the left*). (Reprinted from Eklind et al. [39], with permission.)

receptors (e.g., CD95, TNF, and TRAIL receptor) but involved caspase activation. This direct apoptosis seemed to be mediated through Bcl-2–dependent release of mitochondrial cytochrome-c and the subsequent activation of caspase-9.

Actinic keratosis

As more than 1 million cases of nonmelanoma skin cancer are reported annually in the United States, topical immunomodulatory treatments are particularly attractive as they permit patient-friendly application and good cosmesis. Given the high prevalence of ultraviolet light–induced transformation, the prevalence of AKs and in situ SCC and the incidence of skin cancers are increasing [37]. Current treatment modalities include cryotherapy, laser, excision, Mohs surgery, chemical peeling, photody-namic therapy, and 5-fluorouracil, which are locally destructive and cause substantial patient discomfort. Especially in patients with preexisting medical conditions or in a particular localization, topical, easy-to-use therapy may be desirable.

Imiquimod has been licensed for the treatment of BCC and AKs (Fig. 30.2). Two phase III, randomized, vehicle-controlled trials investigated imiquimod 5% cream for multiple actinic keratoses applied two times per week over 16 weeks [38]. Complete clearance at 8 weeks posttreatment was observed in 97 of 215 patients (45%) receiving imiquimod compared with 7 of 221 patients (3%) treated with vehicle ($P < 0.001$). Partial clearance was observed in 59% of 215 patients treated with imiquimod and in 12% of 221 patients receiving vehicle.

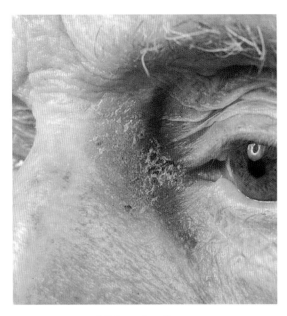
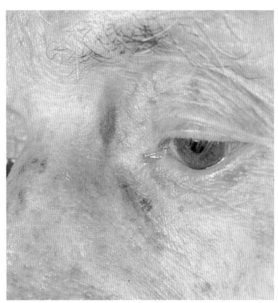

Week 0   Week 17

Fig. 30.3 An 87-year-old patient with severe cardiac arrhythmia and SCC in situ (Bowen's disease). Imiquimod treatment given intermittently for 17 weeks resulted in complete clinical and histologic clearance.

Squamous cell cancer in situ (Bowen's disease)

After initial reports [17,39–41], a phase II open-label study in 16 patients was performed to treat Bowen's disease with imiquimod applied daily for 16 weeks [42]. In this trial, 14 of 15 patients (93%) cleared histologically at 6 weeks posttreatment. However, local skin reactions were severe and prompted six patients to stop treatment between weeks 4 and 8. In addition, a randomized, double-blind, placebo-controlled trial used imiquimod 5% cream monotherapy for Bowen's disease[43]. In this trial, 31 patients with biopsy-proven cutaneous SCC in situ were randomly assigned to placebo or imiquimod cream once daily for 16 weeks. Eleven of 15 patients (73%) in the imiquimod group achieved complete clearance of Bowen's disease, with no relapse during the 9-month follow-up period, as opposed to none in the placebo group ($P < 0.001$). We successfully treated an 87-year-old patient with severe arrhythmia for hypertrophic AK and Bowen's disease (Fig. 30.3). In addition, we have treated two patients with invasive SCC under special circumstances, leading to complete clearance during 18 months of follow-up [39]. Moreover, topical imiquimod has been evaluated in four cases with grade 3 vulvar intraepithelial neoplasia, with good results [42].

Invasive squamous cell carcinoma

A small case series has reported the treatment of seven invasive SCC lesions, with clearance in five of seven cases (71.4%) after 16 weeks of treatment [44]. In addition, previously we suggested that transplant recipients can also be effectively treated for SCC despite the systemic immunosuppression [39].

Basal cell carcinoma

Several trials have evaluated imiquimod for the treatment of superficial BCC [45,46]. A randomized, double-blind, vehicle-controlled, dose-response study was performed in 128 patients with small superficial BCCs [47]. In this dose-finding trial, complete responses occurred between 52% and 100%. Two pivotal trials were performed according to an identical randomized, vehicle-controlled, phase III design with 724 patients receiving imiquimod 5% cream applied five or seven times per week for 6 weeks [48]. Clinical and histologic clearance was observed in 75% of 185 patients treated with imiquimod five times per week 12 weeks posttreatment. Interestingly, the high (93%) negative predictive value (probability that a tumor clinically assessed by a physician as negative will be confirmed histologically as negative) observed in the study suggested that most clinicians will be able to accurately determine the appropriate response of the BCC to imiquimod treatment. Application-site reactions were also dose dependent, occurring in 28% of imiquimod-treated patients, and included erythema, erosion, and crusting.

The response of nodular BCC to imiquimod 5% treatment was also investigated in two phase II trials: a 6-week randomized, open-label study including 99 patients and a 12-week randomized, vehicle-controlled study including 92 patients [49,50]. In the imiquimod three-times-per-week group, 60% of complete responses were achieved, compared with 70% in the five-times-per-week group and 76% in the seven-times-per-week group [49].

Transplant recipients

Moreover, the safety and efficacy of 5% imiquimod cream have been demonstrated for cutaneous dysplasia (viral warts and hyperkeratotic AKs) in renal transplant patients who were treated in a randomized, double-blind, placebo-controlled trial [51]. Seven of 14 patients receiving imiquimod developed fewer AKs and viral warts. Renal function was not affected adversely. It was concluded that topical 5% imiquimod cream was safe on skin areas up to 60 cm^2 in renal transplant recipients.

The successful treatment of AKs in organ transplant recipients has been documented in additional small surveys [52]. The AKs cleared with organ transplant recipients experiencing no adverse events. Interestingly, human papillomavirus was identified in transplant-associated porokeratoses of

Mibelli that cleared upon treatment with 5% imiquimod cream [53]. Moreover, a randomized, double-blind, placebo-controlled trial in high-risk renal transplantation patients was performed using 5% imiquimod for the treatment of actinically damaged skin [51]. In all seven patients assigned to imiquimod, skin atypia and viral warts were significantly reduced as opposed to the placebo group. Interestingly, in the subsequent year, fewer cutaneous SCCs arose in imiquimod-treated skin than in control areas.

Lentigo maligna

Lentigo maligna is associated with chronically exposed and sun-damaged skin. In an open-label trial in 30 patients with lentigo maligna 2 cm or more in diameter, imiquimod 5% cream once daily for 12 weeks led to histologically confirmed complete clearance in 26 of 28 patients (93%)[54]. No recurrence was reported for 80% of the cohort that was followed for at least 12 months.

A recent meta-analysis on the treatment of lentigo maligna with imiquimod has been performed [55,56]. The authors identified 11 case reports and four open-label studies, comprising a total of 67 patients who completed treatment for lentigo maligna. Despite variability in treatment schedules and regimens, 59 patients responded to therapy with clinical and/or histologic clearance. Eight patients failed to respond, with lentigo maligna melanoma developing in two individuals within a short follow-up period of less than 1 year. In successfully treated patients, a CD68$^+$ macrophage-rich infiltrate and T cells of the CD8$^+$ phenotype were observed, accompanied by depletion of epidermal and dermal CD1a$^+$ dendritic cells [57]. In addition, granzyme B and TIA-1 were expressed in the epidermis and the dermoepidermal junction, suggesting a cytotoxic T cell–mediated immune response to malignant melanocytes.

Treatment of metastases

The local treatment of cutaneous melanoma metastases has been performed using diphenylcyclopropenone in combination with DTIC and radiation [58] and with a combination of topical imiquimod, pegylated IFN-α-2b and IL-2 [59]. In the latter, a macrophage (MAC387[+] and CD68[+])-rich infiltrate together with CD4[+] and CD25[+] lymphocytes was found. Cytotoxic T lymphocytes were sparse as shown by TIA-1 and granzyme B staining. The gene regulation upon treatment of cutaneous melanoma metastases with topical imiquimod has been analyzed in more detail [60]. By real-time polymerase chain reaction, matrix metalloproteinase (MMP)-1 and tissue inhibitor of metalloproteinase (TIMP)-1 and KiSS-1 were significantly up-regulated, with MMP-9 expression being substantially reduced. Imiquimod seems to down-regulate metastatic invasion and angiogenesis as the result of slightly increased expression of angiogenesis inhibitors. Nevertheless, further studies need to confirm these initial findings before the mode of action in treating cutaneous melanoma metastases with imiquimod can be generalized.

Cutaneous metastases of different types of cancers, such as breast cancer (erysipelas carcinomatosum and Paget's disease), have also been successfully treated using topical imiquimod [61,62]. Alternatively, miltefosine was used to treat cutaneous metastases of a cutaneous SCC in a small trial [63].

Other potential indications

A small number of patients with erythroplasia of Queyrat have been treated with imiquimod 5% cream [64,65]. In addition, successful management of chronic radiation dermatitis has been described in a few people using topical imiquimod [66,67]. Our group has analyzed the gene expression profile in AKs before and during therapy with imiquimod [68], describing a significant up-regulation of IFN, IL-6, IL-10 receptor, and TLR-7 and a significant down-regulation in antiapoptotic genes such as hurpin and *HAX-1*.

References

1 Lewis HM. Topical immunotherapy of refractory warts. Cutis 1973;12:863–7.

2 Happle R, Echternacht K. Induction of hair growth in alopecia areata with D.N.C.B. Lancet 1977;2:100–23.

3 Happle R. Antigenic competition as a therapeutic concept for alopecia areata. Arch Dermatol Res 1980;267:109–14.

4 Naylor MF, Neldner KH, Yarbrough GK, et al. Contact immunotherapy of resistant warts. J Am Acad Dermatol 1988;19:679–83.

5 Rampen FH, Steijlen PM. Diphencyprone in the management of refractory palmoplantar and periungual warts: an open study. Dermatology 1996;193:236–8.

6 Williams AC, Klein E. Experiences with local chemotherapy and immunotherapy in premalignant and malignant skin lesions. Cancer 1970;25:450–62.

7 Schwartz RA. Edmund Klein (1921–1999). J Am Acad Dermatol 2001;44:716–8.

8 Harland CC, Saihan EM. Regression of cutaneous metastatic malignant melanoma with topical diphencyprone and oral cimetidine. Lancet 1989;2:445.

9 Levis WR, Kraemer KH, Klingler WG, et al. Topical immunotherapy of basal cell carcinomas with dinitrochlorobenzene. Cancer Res 1973;33:3036–42.

10 Illig L, Paul E, Bodeker RH. Epifocal dinitrochlorobenzene therapy in malignant melanoma (experience during the last eight years). Anticancer Res 1984;4:293–8.

11 Strobbe LJ, Hart AA, Rumke P, et al. Topical dinitrochlorobenzene combined with systemic dacarbazine in the treatment of recurrent melanoma. Melanoma Res 1997;7:507–12.

12 Trcka J, Kampgen E, Becker JC, et al. [Immunochemotherapy of malignant melanoma. Epifocal administration of dinitrochlorobenzene (DNCB) combined with systemic chemotherapy with dacarbazine (DTIC)]. Hautarzt 1998;49:17–22.

13 Holmes EC, Eilber FR, Morton DL. Immunotherapy of malignancy in humans. Current status. JAMA 1975;232:1052–5.

14 Sopkova B, Kolar V. Intralesional BCG application in malignant melanoma. Neoplasma 1976;23:421–6.

15 Imbertson LM, Beaurline JM, Couture AM, et al. Cytokine induction in hairless mouse and rat skin after topical application of the immune response modifiers imiquimod and S-28463. J Invest Dermatol 1998;110:734–9.

16 Wagner TL, Ahonen CL, Couture AM, et al. Modulation of TH1 and TH2 cytokine production with the immune response modifiers, R-848 and imiquimod. Cell Immunol 1999;191:10–9.

17 Hengge UR, Stark R. Topical imiquimod to treat intraepidermal carcinoma. Arch Dermatol 2001;137:709–11.

18 Hemmi H, Kaisho T, Takeuchi O, et al. Small antiviral compounds activate immune cells via the TLR7 MyD88-dependent signaling pathway. Nat Immunol 2002;3:196–200.

19 Kono T, Kondo S, Pastore S, et al. Effects of a novel topical immunomodulator, imiquimod, on keratinocyte cytokine gene expression. Lymphokine Cytokine Res 1994;13:71–6.

20 Slade HB, Owens ML, Tomai MA, et al. Imiquimod 5% cream (Aldara). Expert Opin Investig Drugs 1998;7:437–49.

21 Arany I, Tyring SK, Stanley MA, et al. Enhancement of the innate and cellular immune response in patients with genital warts treated with topical imiquimod cream 5%. Antiviral Res 1999;43:55–63.

22 Testerman TL, Gerster JF, Imbertson LM, et al. Cytokine induction by the immunomodulators imiquimod and S-27609. J Leukoc Biol 1995;58:365–72.

23 Tomai MA, Gibson SJ, Imbertson LM, et al. Immunomodulating and antiviral activities of the imidazoquinoline S-28463. Antiviral Res 1995;28:253–64.

24 Baca LM, Genis P, Kalvakolanu D, et al. Regulation of interferon-alpha-inducible cellular genes in human immunodeficiency virus-infected monocytes. J Leukoc Biol 1994;55:299–309.

25 Burns RP Jr, Ferbel B, Tomai M, et al. The imidazoquinolines, imiquimod and R-848, induce functional, but not phenotypic, maturation of human epidermal Langerhans' cells. Clin Immunol 2000;94:13–23.

26 Takeda K, Akira S. Roles of toll-like receptors in innate immune responses. Genes Cells 2001;6:733–42.

27 Vasselon T, Detmers PA. Toll receptors: a central element in innate immune responses. Infect Immun 2002;70:1033–41.

28 Suzuki H, Wang B, Shivji GM, et al. Imiquimod, a topical immune response modifier, induces migration of Langerhans cells. J Invest Dermatol 2000;114:135–41.

29 Tomai MA, Imbertson LM, Stanczak TL, et al. The immune response modifiers imiquimod and R-848 are potent activators of B lymphocytes. Cell Immunol 2000;203:55–65.

30 Frotscher B, Anton K, Worm M. Inhibition of IgE production by the imidazoquinoline resiquimod in nonallergic and allergic donors. J Invest Dermatol 2002;119:1059–64.

31 Vasilakos JP, Smith RM, Gibson SJ, et al. Adjuvant activities of immune response modifier R-848: comparison with CpG ODN. Cell Immunol 2000;204:64–74.

32 Uhlmann E, Vollmer J. Recent advances in the development of immunostimulatory oligonucleotides. Curr Opin Drug Discov Devel 2003;6:204–17.

33 Edwards AD, Diebold SS, Slack EM, et al. Toll-like receptor expression in murine DC subsets: lack of TLR7 expression by CD8 alpha+ DC correlates with unresponsiveness to imidazoquinolines. Eur J Immunol 2003;33:827–33.

34 Hengge UR, Benninghoff B, Ruzicka T, et al. Topical immunomodulators—progress towards treating inflammation, infection, and cancer. Lancet Infect Dis 2001;1:189–98.

35 Schon MP, Schon M. Immune modulation and apoptosis induction: two sides of the antitumoral activity of imiquimod. Apoptosis 2004;9:291–8.

36 Schon M, Bong AB, Drewniok C, et al. Tumor-selective induction of apoptosis and the small-molecule immune response modifier imiquimod. J Natl Cancer Inst 2003;95:1138–49.

37 Marks R, Rennie G, Selwood TS. Malignant transformation of solar keratoses to squamous cell carcinoma. Lancet 1988;1:795–7.

38 Lebwohl M, Dinehart S, Whiting D, et al. Imiquimod 5% cream for the treatment of actinic keratosis: results from two phase III, randomized, double-blind, parallel group, vehicle-controlled trials. J Am Acad Dermatol 2004;50:714–21.

39 Eklind J, Tartler U, Maschke J, et al. Imiquimod to treat different cancers of the epidermis. Dermatol Surg 2003;29:890–6; discussion 896.

40 Hengge UR, Schaller J. Successful treatment of invasive squamous cell carcinoma using topical imiquimod. Arch Dermatol 2004;140:404–6.

41 Hengge UR, Schaller J. Imiquimod and squamous cell cancer. Arch Dermatol 2005;141:787–8.

42 Mackenzie-Wood A, Kossard S, de Launey J, et al. Imiquimod 5% cream in the treatment of Bowen's disease. J Am Acad Dermatol 2001;44:462–70.

43 Patel GK, Goodwin R, Chawla M, et al. Imiquimod 5% cream monotherapy for cutaneous squamous cell carcinoma in situ (Bowen's disease): a randomized, double-blind, placebo-controlled trial. J Am Acad Dermatol 2006;54:1025–32.

44 Peris K, Micantonio T, Fargnoli MC, et al. Imiquimod 5% cream in the treatment of Bowen's disease and invasive squamous cell carcinoma. J Am Acad Dermatol 2006;55:324–7.

45 Beutner KR, Geisse JK, Helman D, et al. Therapeutic response of basal cell carcinoma to the immune response modifier imiquimod 5% cream. J Am Acad Dermatol 1999;41:1002–7.

46 Marks R, Gebauer K, Shumack S, et al. Imiquimod 5% cream in the treatment of superficial basal cell carcinoma: results of a multicenter 6-week dose-response trial. J Am Acad Dermatol 2001;44:807–13.

47 Geisse JK, Rich P, Pandya A, et al. Imiquimod 5% cream for the treatment of superficial basal cell

carcinoma: a double-blind, randomized, vehicle-controlled study. J Am Acad Dermatol 2002;47:390–8.

48 Geisse J, Caro I, Lindholm J, et al. Imiquimod 5% cream for the treatment of superficial basal cell carcinoma: results from two phase III, randomized, vehicle-controlled studies. J Am Acad Dermatol 2004;50:722–33.

49 Shumack S, Robinson J, Kossard S, et al. Efficacy of topical 5% imiquimod cream for the treatment of nodular basal cell carcinoma: comparison of dosing regimens. Arch Dermatol 2002;138:1165–71.

50 Sterry W, Ruzicka T, Herrera E, et al. Imiquimod 5% cream for the treatment of superficial and nodular basal cell carcinoma: randomized studies comparing low-frequency dosing with and without occlusion. Br J Dermatol 2002;147:1227–36.

51 Brown VL, Atkins CL, Ghali L, et al. Safety and efficacy of 5% imiquimod cream for the treatment of skin dysplasia in high-risk renal transplant recipients: randomized, double-blind, placebo-controlled trial. Arch Dermatol 2005;141:985–93.

52 Ulrich C, Busch JO, Meyer T, et al. Successful treatment of multiple actinic keratoses in organ transplant patients with topical 5% imiquimod: a report of six cases. Br J Dermatol 2006;155:451–4.

53 Esser AC, Pittelkow MR, Randle HW. Human papillomavirus isolated from transplant-associated porokeratoses of Mibelli responsive to topical 5% imiquimod cream. Dermatol Surg 2006;32:858–61.

54 Naylor MF, Crowson N, Kuwahara R, et al. Treatment of lentigo maligna with topical imiquimod. Br J Dermatol 2003;149 Suppl 66:66–70.

55 Wolf IH, Smolle J, Binder B, et al. Topical imiquimod in the treatment of metastatic melanoma to skin. Arch Dermatol 2003;139:273–6.

56 Rajpar SF, Marsden JR. Imiquimod in the treatment of lentigo maligna. Br J Dermatol 2006;155:653–6.

57 Michalopoulos P, Yawalkar N, Bronnimann M, et al. Characterization of the cellular infiltrate during successful topical treatment of lentigo maligna with imiquimod. Br J Dermatol 2004;151:903–6.

58 Trefzer U, Sterry W. Topical immunotherapy with diphenylcyclopropenone in combination with DTIC and radiation for cutaneous metastases of melanoma. Dermatology 2005;211:370–1.

59 Loquai C, Nashan D, Metze D, et al. [Imiquimod, pegylated interferon-alpha-2b and interleukin-2 in the treatment of cutaneous melanoma metastases]. Hautarzt 2004;55:176–81.

60 Hesling C, D'Incan M, Mansard S, et al. In vivo and in situ modulation of the expression of genes involved in metastasis and angiogenesis in a patient treated with topical imiquimod for melanoma skin metastases. Br J Dermatol 2004;150:761–7.

61 Qian Z, Zeitoun NC, Shieh S, et al. Successful treatment of extramammary Paget's disease with imiquimod. J Drugs Dermatol 2003;2:73–6.

62 Hengge UR, Roth S, Tannapfel A. Topical imiquimod to treat recurrent breast cancer. Breast Cancer Res Treat 2005;94:93–4.

63 Mahieu-Renard L, Richard MA, Dales JP, et al. [Treatment of cutaneous metastases of a squamous cell carcinoma of the leg with topical miltefosine]. Ann Dermatol Venereol 2005;132:346–8.

64 Kaspari M, Gutzmer R, Kiehl P, et al. Imiquimod 5% cream in the treatment of human papillomavirus-16-positive erythroplasia of Queyrat. Dermatology 2002;205:67–9.

65 Micali G, Nasca MR, De Pasquale R. Erythroplasia of Queyrat treated with imiquimod 5% cream. J Am Acad Dermatol 2006;55:901–3.

66 Beyeler M, Urosevic M, Pestalozzi B, et al. Successful imiquimod treatment of multiple basal cell carcinomas after radiation therapy for Hodgkin's disease. Eur J Dermatol 2005;15:52–5.

67 Sachse MM, Zimmermann J, Bahmer FA. Efficiency of topical imiquimod 5% cream in the management of chronic radiation dermatitis with multiple neoplasias. Eur J Dermatol 2006;16:56–8.

68 Lysa B, Tartler U, Wolf R, et al. Gene expression in actinic keratoses: pharmacological modulation by imiquimod. Br J Dermatol 2004;151:1150–9.

CHAPTER 31

Treatment of melanoma

Maja A. Hofmann, Wolfram Sterry, and Robert A. Schwartz

Melanoma is a deadly and all-too-frequent cancer that is rising in incidence [1–3]. It has been estimated that there will be 59,940 new cases of melanoma in the United States in 2007 [3]. This incidence represents 5% of new cancers (excluding cutaneous basal cell carcinomas [BCCs] and squamous cell carcinomas [SCCs]) in men and 4% in women. New cases of in situ melanoma were projected to be 48,290 for 2007. Although the total number of melanoma cases is much less than the more than 1 million new cases of basal cell and squamous cell skin cancer projected for 2007, 8110 people in the United States alone are likely to die from melanoma in 2007. Nearly three fourths of all deaths from skin cancer are the result of melanoma (Table 31.1). In parts of Europe, too, there seems to be an increasing incidence, with the mean annual age-standardized incidence of invasive cutaneous melanoma in Styria, a region of Austria, recently calculated to have risen to 24.5 per 100,000, representing a lifetime risk of one in 52 [4].

The reasons for this rise in incidence of melanoma have been debated [5–7]. Because preventive measures have thus far been unable to reduce the increasing incidence, melanoma is likely to remain a significant problem. Early diagnosis facilitates therapy and improves prognosis. Importantly, the outcome of treatment from melanoma is not as easily predicted as in many other malignancies; late treatment failures are commonplace, even after a decade in remission. This pernicious virulent malignancy has a serious financial and emotional impact on patients, many of whom are in their active, productive years of life, as well as on their families. The success or failure of treatment depends almost entirely on surgery. In contrast to many types of cancer, other treatment modalities, such as radiation therapy and chemotherapy, have not played a curative role, and are mainly used for palliation.

Therapeutic data need to be analyzed using the relatively new American Joint Committee on Cancer (AJCC) staging criteria. It is uniform with the International Union Against Cancer as of January 1, 2003. They reflect the prognostic value of histologic tumor ulceration, the number of positive lymph nodes as a better prognostic indicator than the size of nodal metastasis, and similar prognostic value provided by nodal, in-transit, and local recurrences. They also consider pathologic information about staging provided by lymphatic mapping and sentinel lymphadenectomy, with adjustments for updating in light of more recent data and modifications [8].

In this chapter, the major treatment methods for melanoma are discussed. Emphasis is placed on surgery, because that is the major curative modality. Various forms of systemic therapy are outlined, including chemotherapy and biologic response modifiers. The present role of radiation therapy is described.

Surgery

The role of surgery in the treatment of melanoma includes a broad spectrum of procedures. The indications for surgery in melanoma can be grouped into eight major categories, as shown in Table 31.2.

Suspicious lesions

Suspicious lesions should prompt histologic examination. Ten years or more of experience in dermatology was linked with a clinical diagnostic

Table 31.1 Estimated new American cancer cases and deaths for 2007

Primary Site	Estimated New Cases			Estimated Deaths		
	Total	Males	Females	Total	Males	Females
Skin (excl. basal & squamous)	65,050	37,070	27,980	10,850	7140	3710
Melanoma of the skin	59,940	33,910	26,030	8110	5220	2890
Other nonepithelial skin	5110	3160	1950	2740	1920	820

Source: National Cancer Institute. Surveillance epidemiology and end results [online]. Available from: http://seer.cancer.gov.

accuracy rate for melanoma of only 80% on the basis of naked eye examination and clinical history [9]. With this potentially fatal malignancy, it is desirable to overdiagnose rather than underdiagnose, creating a proportion of false positives. The essential steps in the preoperative workup of a suspected melanoma appear in Table 31.3.

Table 31.2 Role of surgery in melanoma

Diagnosis	Incisional or excisional biopsy, needle or punch biopsy (in selected cases); excision of metastatic lesion
Staging	Sentinel lymph node biopsy, regional node dissection; needle biopsy of metastatic lesions; staging laparotomy
Cure	Wide local excision, regional node dissection; excision of solitary metastasis
Adjuvant	Combined with other methods as regional node dissection
Palliation	When local control is achieved, even though distant metastases develop When surgery is done for control of pain, bleeding, obstruction due to metastases
Prevention	Removal of nevi and moles that are traumatized regularly, or atypical acral lentiginous nevi, or dysplastic nevi
Research	Removal of metastatic lesions for study, as in tumor antigen presentations; may or may not be potentially beneficial to patient
Rehabilitation	Reconstruction of defect with skin flap or skin graft

Judgment must be exercised regarding the need to biopsy. After all, most pigmented nodules are not melanomas. Nonpigmented ones may be amelanotic melanomas, or other skin cancers, including cutaneous metastases from visceral cancers. It is often best to biopsy anything suspicious or when concern is expressed by the patient, family member, friend, or other health professional, simply because there may have been a subtle change that heralds malignancy. If there are numerous lesions of concern, a good approach is to start with two or three that are potentially the most serious, given size, location, or symptoms (e.g., pain, pruritus, bleeding). In general, melanomas are uncommon under the age of 17, and almost all primary cutaneous melanomas are at least 0.6 cm in greatest diameter at the time of diagnosis. Fulguration (electrocoagulation) and laser surgery of a mole are to be avoided; histologic examination is essential for every melanocytic nevus that is removed.

Table 31.3 Sagacious steps before biopsy of a suspected melanoma

1 Examine under good light (natural sunlight if possible) with magnifying lens
2 Perform dermoscopy
3 Photograph the lesion
4 Measure the lesion with a millimeter ruler, in two planes. In horizontal plane, measure the greatest two dimensions at right angles; measure height of elevation and depth of ulcer.
5 Describe the lesion (ABCDE rule): asymmetry, border, color, diameter, elevation
6 Examine the regional lymph nodes *before* biopsy

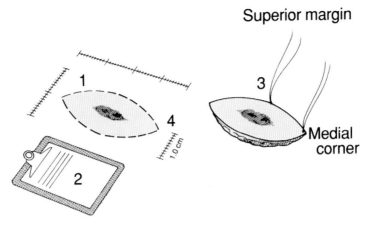

Fig. 31.1 Excisional biopsy: 1. Incision in skin lines; 2. Record size of incision and margins; 3. Orient specimen with sutures; 4. If preoperative diagnosis is melanoma, use apt biopsy margin.

A complete pertinent history and physical examination should be obtained in every patient with melanoma. Details of the history and physical examination before biopsy of a suspicious lesion vary among reported cases. Dermoscopy has been established in the last two decades as a noninvasive method for improving the diagnostic accuracy of malignant melanoma, and is the subject of Chapter 12. In the hands of experienced users, dermoscopy improves the diagnostic accuracy of pigmented skin lesions [10–13]. It would be ideal to have each suspicious nodule photographed before it is biopsied.

Biopsy

There had been considerable concern that an incisional biopsy into a melanoma could disrupt melanoma cells that would then metastasize. In 1985, Lederman and Sober [14] demonstrated no adverse effect on prognosis from performing a partial biopsy of cutaneous melanoma (incisional or punch biopsy vs. excisional biopsy) after correcting for thickness. Further efforts have substantiated this theory [15,16].

A well-planned and carefully performed excisional biopsy is essential in the diagnosis of melanoma (Fig. 31.1). Whenever possible, the neoplasm should be excised for diagnostic purposes. An excisional margin of 2 to 3 mm should be consid-

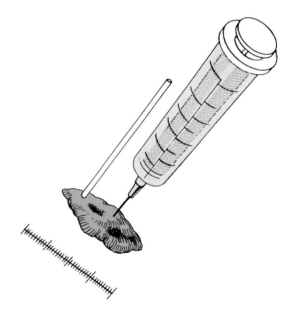

Fig. 31.2 Punch and needle biopsies.

ered when a suspect lesion is excised. For benign melanocytic nevi and dysplastic nevi, the procedure is therapeutic. If a neoplasm is larger than 5 to 6 cm and located on the face or distal extremity, a punch biopsy (Fig. 31.2) or incisional biopsy (Fig. 31.3) may be the best way to establish the diagnosis and start treatment planning. Additionally, a preoperative diagnosis of melanoma may not have

Step 1

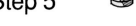

Step 2,3

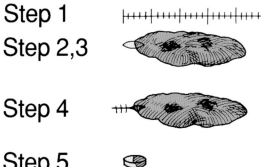

Step 4

Step 5

Fig. 31.3 Incisional biopsy: 1. Record biopsy size; 2. Include normal skin; 3. Biopsy to full length of neoplasm; 4. Suture normal skin; control bleeding with pressure; 5. Orient specimen for pathology.

been rendered, resulting in the margin of incision being very close to the melanoma. In every case, the pathologist should have the opportunity to examine the melanoma for deepest level of penetration. This usually requires step sections. Incisional biopsy specimens should include a portion of normal skin, as well as the neoplasm's thickest-appearing part. Among other things, the pathologist's ability to distinguish between a primary melanoma and a metastasis from an unknown primary site often depends on the examination of its margins. The biopsy specimen should be measured, oriented with sutures to mark anterior–posterior, right and left sides, and laid out flat for the pathologist. If the lesion is large, and a punch biopsy is done for diagnosis, the clinician must not rely on the biopsy for information regarding the depth of penetration, because the pathologist receives only a small sample of the tumor in such cases.

Clinicians planning treatment should personally examine the slides together with a pathologist/dermatopathologist. The greatest depth of penetration is a major determinant in prognosis, and a major guide to future therapy. The point is probably moot if the melanoma extends into fat (making it level V) or is greater than 4 mm in thickness, as these cases have a high likelihood of distant metastases. Further consultation is often desirable after the diagnosis of melanoma is confirmed histologically.

Staging of melanoma

A completely revised staging system for cutaneous melanoma, implemented in 2003, was validated with prognostic factor analysis involving 17,600 melanoma patients from prospective databases [17] (Tables 11.13 and 11.14 in Chapter 11). Thus, we now have what Balch and associates [17] have described as evidence-based staging. Major changes from previous staging included melanoma thickness and histologic ulceration as the dominant predictors of survival in patients with localized stage I or II melanoma and deeper level of invasion (stage IV and V) independently associated with reduced survival only in patients with thin melanomas 1 mm or less in thickness. Histologic ulceration occurs when the melanoma invades through the overlying epidermis rather than pushing it upward to produce an absent epidermis overlying the major portion of the melanoma. In addition, the number of metastatic lymph nodes and the tumor burden were the most dominant predictors of survival in patients with stage III melanoma; patients with metastatic nodes detected by palpation had a shorter survival compared with patients whose nodal metastases were first detected by sentinel node excision of clinically occult or "microscopic" metastases. The site of distant metastases (nonvisceral vs. lung vs. all other visceral metastatic sites) and the presence of elevated serum lactate dehydrogenase (LDH) were dominant predictors of outcome in patients with stage IV distant metastatic disease. Other important changes were that an upstaging should be implemented for all patients with stage I, II, and III disease when a primary melanoma is ulcerated by histopathologic criteria. Satellite and in-transit metastases are cutaneous metastases to skin situated around the site of a primary melanoma or between the primary melanoma and the regional lymph nodes. Satellite metastases are tumor cell aggregates located in the dermis and/or subcutis within radices of 2 to 5 cm of the primary melanoma [18]. This distinction from in-transit metastases, which are considered to be located somewhere between 5 cm from the primary melanoma and the regional lymph nodes, has become less important, as satellite metastases around a primary melanoma and in-transit metastases were merged into a single staging entity that is grouped into stage III disease. The designation *B* applies when there is ulceration, *A* if there is none. Stage T1 is a cutaneous melanoma equal to or less than 1.0 mm in thickness; T2 is 1.01 to 2.0 mm; T3 is 2.01 to 4.0 mm; T4 is more than 4.0 mm (see full staging in Chapter 11). In stage 0 (in situ) melanoma and stage IA (low-risk melanoma), no further staging examinations are necessary.

Treatment planning and assessment of prognosis are important considerations early in the management of patients with newly diagnosed melanoma. Melanoma stage correlates to prognosis, albeit imperfectly. The current staging system uses the histologic examination of the primary melanoma, ulceration of the primary melanoma, the presence or absence of satellites, the regional nodes (micro/macrometastases), and involvement of distant sites as factors assessed. Accurate melanoma staging is essential, because inadequate staging may lead to incorrect treatment and poor outcome. Surgical methods play a vital role in staging, because there is no perfect indirect, noninvasive method to evaluate regional lymph nodes. A surgical sentinel lymph node biopsy (SLNB) is employed to evaluate the presence or absence of nodal metastases; the metastatic status of the sentinel lymph node (SLN) should predict the status of an involved nodal region. However, if there are multiple large and/or matted lymph nodes, particularly if several nodal areas are involved, confirmation of nodal metastases may be accomplished with needle aspiration, if necessary. Patients with lymph node metastasis confirmed by fine-needle aspiration (FNA) should have a prompt regional lymphadenectomy, assuming there are no distant metastases [19–21].

Baseline staging therefore includes a careful history and physical examination, and searching for signs and symptoms of regional and distant metastases. In concordance with the guidelines of the National Cancer Comprehensive Network (NCCN) and the American Academy of Dermatology, the baseline evaluation of a primary cutaneous melanoma depends on the stage of the melanoma. Chest radiography is recommended mainly in intermediate and thick melanomas (stage IB, level II melanoma). Body computed tomography

(CT) scans to detect occult metastases in patients with primary melanoma greater than stage II are not warranted [19,22]. However, further imaging (CT scan, magnetic resonance imaging [MRI], positron emission tomography [PET]) should be performed if clinically indicated for stage IIB and IIC melanoma. Fluorodeoxyglucose (FDG) PET/CT has a high degree of accuracy for the diagnosis of both regional and distant melanoma in patients with cutaneous melanoma and was found to alter management in about 25% with stage II to IV disease [23]. In stage III melanoma, chest radiograph, serum LDH, and further imaging (CT scan, MRI, PET) should be performed if clinically indicated [20,21,24]. An FNA should be considered in patients with clinically positive lymph nodes. In patients first seen with likely stage IV distant metastatic disease, the suspicion of metastatic disease should be confirmed with either FNA (preferred) or with open biopsy of a metastasis. LDH level plus chest radiography and/or chest CT are recommended. Abdominal/pelvic CT, with or without PET, and/or head MRI should be performed; other imaging studies are appropriate if clinically indicated [20,21]. Radioisotope studies of lymph nodes, gallium scan, and lymphangiography are not recommended [22]. The use of PET/CT in patients undergoing SLNB for melanoma is not recommended, as SLNB appears to be a more sensitive staging modality in the detection of lymphatic metastasis [25].

Cure

Surgery is virtually the only treatment modality for melanoma that is curative, assuming it is detected early enough [26]. The word *cure*, however, must be defined to understand the role of surgery in treatment. Because relapse may occur with melanoma after years of complete remission, the word *cure* must be used advisedly. Benchmarks for success include "free of disease at 5 years" and "survival curve parallel to the normal population." Perhaps the only true proof of cure is the patient who dies of other causes, many years after apparent successful treatment for melanoma, and is found to be free of melanoma at autopsy. That degree of scrutiny provides little satisfaction for the patient. Therefore, the conventional, but admittedly imprecise, use of the

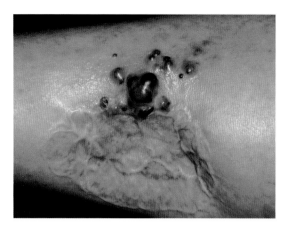

Fig. 31.4 Locally recurrent melanoma, occurring as cutaneous and subcutaneous reddish or black nodules adjacent to the skin graft site from a prior wide excision. (Courtesy of Eric D. Whitman, MD, FACS, Medical Director, Mountainside Hospital Cancer Center; Director, Melanoma Center, Montclair, NJ.)

word *cure* usually uses the 5-year NED (no evidence of disease) rate.

Surgical treatment for cure uses two major principles:

1 Wide local excision (WLE) of the primary tumor
2 SLNB and regional lymph node dissection (LND) to remove positive nodes before further spread occurs

However, in-transit metastasis may be an important morbidity factor after SLNB. In one study, the 5-year probability of developing in-transit metastases as a first recurrence was found to be 11.2%; after negative and positive SLNB, the probabilities were 6.3% and 24%, respectively [27]. If satellite metastases were identified and excised concurrently with the primary melanoma, there was a probability of recurrence with in-transit metastases of 41%. Long-term complete remission and apparent "cures" after resection of isolated metastases or resection of satellites and in-transit metastases [28] do occasionally occur (Fig. 31.4).

Width

A 1-cm margin for a local melanoma excision may in some cases be sufficiently wide to produce a cure. This has been the case for many melanomas of the face, and probably for some small melanomas elsewhere on the body. However, for many years, conventional teaching in the United States and elsewhere mandated a measured margin of 3 to 5 cm, a margin large enough that closure could not be accomplished without a skin graft [29]. In comparing outcomes, a 2-cm margin is as satisfactory as a 5-cm margin for local control and long-term remission. However, excessively narrow margins during standard surgery result in a higher rate of local recurrence.

Current recommendations are based on the results of prospective randomized clinical trials. A World Health Organization (WHO) trial for melanomas less than 2 mm in thickness was performed in 612 patients comparing 1-cm versus 3-cm margins. Overall survival rates were similar in both groups [30,31]. In a separate study, intermediate-thickness (1- to 4-mm) melanoma patients randomly received a 2-cm or a 4-cm margin. The rate of local recurrences was higher in the 4-cm margin group (1.7%) versus the 2-cm margin group (0.8%), a difference with no statistical significance [32]. A third randomized clinical trial was performed by the Swedish Melanoma Study Group comparing 2-cm versus 5-cm margins in primary melanoma 0.8 to 2.0 mm in thickness. With a median follow-up time of 5.8 years, no significant differences regarding local recurrences and survival times were observed [33]. In a British collaborative trial with about 900 patients, 1-cm and 3-cm excision margins were compared in high-risk melanomas (≥2 mm). A 1-cm margin for melanomas thicker than 2 mm was associated with a slightly greater risk of local recurrence than was a 3-cm margin, but no significant difference in overall survival was noted [34]. A prospectively collected series of 535 patients with 553 primary cutaneous melanomas proposed surgical margins for excision of melanoma or melanoma in situ by standard surgical techniques to include 1 cm of normal-appearing skin for melanomas on the trunk and proximal extremities that are smaller than 2 cm in diameter, or a 1.5-cm margin for tumors larger than 2 cm in diameter. For melanomas on the head, neck, hands, and feet, a minimum surgical margin of 1.5 cm was recommended, or a margin of 2.5 cm for melanomas

Table 31.4 Recommendations for excision margins based on tumor thickness and histologic confirmation that margins are tumor-free

Tumor Thickness	Excision Margin
In situ	0.5 cm
<2 mm	1 cm
≥ 2mm	2 cm

Source: Sober et al. [21].

larger than 3 cm in diameter [35]. Narrower margins are possible with Mohs surgery [36].

Thus, some uncertainty remains about optimal excision margins. The latest NCCN recommendation was that margins for invasive melanoma depend on the tumor thickness [20]. For in situ melanoma, a wide excision of 0.5 cm around the visible lesion should be considered with confirmation of histologically negative peripheral margins. Patients with stage IA melanoma should have a wide excision with a 1.0 cm margin, whereas those with melanomas measuring 1.01 to 2.0 mm in thickness should receive a wide excision with a 1- to 2-cm margin. A wide excision with 2.0 cm margins is advised for melanomas measuring more than 2.0 mm in thickness. The American Academy of Dermatology guidelines for primary cutaneous melanoma proposed an excision margin of 1 cm for melanomas less than 2 mm in thickness, and an excision margin of 2 cm for melanomas 2 mm or greater in thickness [21] (Table 31.4).

Micrographic surgery for melanoma has been most commonly reported in the management of lentigo maligna melanoma (LMM). Mohs surgery is of particular value in lentigo maligna (LM) and LMM in which characteristically unpredictable subclinical peripheral and periadnexal atypical junctional melanocytic hyperplasia may extend several centimeters beyond the visible clinical margins. Wide excision margins, especially of LMMs involving the face, would result in large defects. Different approaches, such as wide surgical excision with meticulous margin control, and Mohs surgery with and without immunoperoxidase staining with HMB-45, have demonstrated high local control rates [36–39]. Mohs surgery allows an incorrect tumor margin to be rapidly corrected after frozen section evaluation. Accordingly, the margin can be more narrowly constructed, as small as 6 mm, without increasing metastatic risk [36].

Depth

Depth of excision has been less controversial than margin width, although guidelines regarding the depth of the primary melanoma excision have never been outlined definitively. Until the present decade, many surgeons made a vertical excision down to the deep fascia underlying the subcutaneous fat, and then excised a portion of the deep fascia under the putative melanoma [29]. The resulting defect was then covered with a split-thickness skin graft. No undermining of the lateral edges was allowed, lest malignant cells be inadvertently deposited deep to the skin flaps, to grow unnoticed. As time has passed, this method (WLE with split-thickness graft) has gradually been abandoned by many surgeons. Newer methods include the depth of the excision as being down to the underlying muscular fascia. With the advent of decreased excision margins, primary closure using local anesthesia can now be accomplished and larger defects can be closed by rotating flaps or with a split-thickness skin graft. Some prefer the latter approach, because examination for local recurrence seems to be facilitated by the presence of a split-thickness graft rather than a full-thickness closure or rotated flap. No significant statistical difference in recurrence has been apparent between flap closure and skin grafting [40,41].

Subungual and acral lentiginous melanomas

Subungual, palmar, and plantar melanomas require a different approach that cannot be categorized in the same way regarding width and depth of excision [42]. At diagnosis, these acral melanomas are often at an advanced stage, at high risk for distant metastases, so local control may be more palliative than curative. In general, amputation of the terminal one and one-half phalanges is sufficient for subungual finger melanomas [43]. Subungual toe

Table 31.5 Prognosis of patients with lymph node metastases, cumulative 5- and 10-year survival employing the new AJCC staging system

Pathologic Stage	TNM	Thickness	Ulceration +	Nodes, no.	Nodal size	Patients, no.	5-Yr Survival, %	10-Yr Survival, %
IIIa	N1a	Any	No	1	Micro	252	70	63
	N2a	Any	No	2–3	Micro	130	63	57
IIIb	N1a	Any	Yes	1	Micro	217	53	38
	N2a	Any	Yes	2–3	Micro	111	50	36
	N1b	Any	No	1	Macro	122	59	48
	N2b	Any	No	2–3	Macro	93	46	39
IIIc	N1b	Any	Yes	1	Macro	98	29	24
	N2b	Any	Yes	2–3	Macro	109	24	15
	N3	Any	Any	4	Micro/Macro	396	27	18

Macro, macrometastasis; Micro, micrometastasis; TNM, tumor, node(s), metastasis.
Source: Balch et al. [17].

melanomas are best treated with a ray amputation, a minor amputation in which a toe and part of the corresponding metatarsal bone are removed, for the small four toes and a metatarsal–phalangeal disarticulation for melanoma of the great toe. Melanoma of the palm, which is rare, is probably best managed by a WLE, 1 to 2 cm in most cases. Melanoma of the sole of the foot, the most common anatomic location of foot melanomas, unfortunately is often advanced when it is first diagnosed [44]. Adequate excision produces a defect that is not amenable to primary closure. Secondary wound healing techniques with delayed split-thickness skin grafting are preferred [45].

Lymph node biopsy and node dissection

Excision of regional lymph nodes containing metastases may be of therapeutic benefit as well as being important in assessing prognosis (i.e., staging). Patients with lymph node metastases have a significantly decreased 5-year survival compared with those without lymph node involvement [46]. Furthermore, patients with clinically negative nodes that are found to contain cancer on microscopic examination (so-called clinically negative, histologically positive micrometastases) have a better prognosis than patients whose nodes are clinically positive and also histologically

positive (macrometastases) (Table 31.5). Until the early 1990s, elective lymphadenectomy was recommended in patients with high-risk melanomas. Several retrospective reports have demonstrated a survival benefit for patients who underwent elective LND (ELND) [47–50], but in prospective, randomized trials, no survival benefit from ELND instead of observation after wide excision could be demonstrated [51–53]. In addition, the morbidity that sometimes follows these procedures has to be considered, which may include trapezius muscle paralysis due to spinal accessory nerve damage from a modified radical neck dissection, pectoralis muscle atrophy after axillary node dissection, or lymphedema following inguinal node dissection.

In 1992, Morton and colleagues [54] introduced lymphatic mapping and SLNB as a method to identify regional nodal metastases for melanoma. They found that the sentinel node histology reflects the tumor status of the entire nodal basin [55]. The SLN is the first draining node between the primary tumor and the regional nodal basin. The SLN localization technique was initially performed using a vital blue dye injected intradermally at the primary site, a safe technique rarely eliciting a hypersensitivity reaction [56]. The first node(s) in the regional nodal basin could visually be identified and excised. SLN identification preoperatively was soon enhanced by the addition of radiolabeled sulfur colloid at the primary melanoma site with preoperative lymphoscintigraphy [57]. More valuable information was provided with the intraoperative use of the handheld gamma probe [58]. Lymphatic mapping and sentinel lymphadenectomy could be successfully learned and applied in a standardized fashion with high accuracy, producing a sentinel node identification rate of 97% [59]. SLNB is a minimally invasive procedure for identifying the nodal status in patients with clinically negative nodes. In several prospective studies, the prognostic value of the SLN status has been described [58,60,61]. In 1999, the WHO declared intraoperative lymphatic mapping with SLNB to be standard of care for melanoma [62].

However, a good case has been made for further research being necessary before SLNB should be considered the standard of care [63]. Three points should be emphasized [64]: (1) Rather than orderly melanoma dissemination with lymph nodes acting as barriers, melanoma cell spread may be organ specific, mediated by surface proteins [65]. (2) The significance of microscopic lymph node melanoma and the effect of selective lymphadenectomy are unclear, with thin melanomas commonly having positive nodes detectable with polymerase chain reaction analysis. Yet clinical disease and distant metastases are rare, and prognosis is excellent [66]. (3) The validity of a survival benefit from SLNB may need further analysis and clarification.

Multiple trials have been designed to address various questions that concern the application of SLNB [67–69]. The Multicenter Selective Lymphadenectomy Trial (MSLT) is a prospective randomized effort that will address whether the routine SLNB provides a survival benefit for patients with cutaneous melanoma thickness of 1 mm or greater, Clark level III or greater of any thickness, and Clark level IV or greater. First results showed the SLNB to be a safe and accurate method of identifying patients with lymph node metastases from a primary cutaneous melanoma [70]. Further results demonstrated that, in patients with intermediate-thickness melanoma (1.2 to 3.5 mm), the SLNB is an important prognostic factor. A survival benefit was achieved in patients with a tumor-positive sentinel node undergoing immediate lymphadenectomy [71]. The final results on the overall therapeutic outcome will be available after a longer follow-up period [70]. The Sunbelt Melanoma Trial (SBMT) will examine the role of molecular staging in patients who undergo SLNB [69]. In another arm of the study, the role of adjuvant interferon-α (IFN-α) versus observation will be analyzed. The Florida Melanoma Trial (FMT) will determine whether all patients with a positive SLN will benefit from a complete LND of the involved basin [69].

An SLNB is particularly recommended for the patient with an intermediate- or high-risk primary melanoma (stage IB to IIC) [20]. In patients with a tumor-positive sentinel node, a regional lymphadenectomy is suggested [72]. Furthermore, patients should receive adjuvant therapy.

Radical LND requires a thorough dissection of the relevant or involved nodal basin. In general, removal and examination of 10 nodes in the groin, 15 nodes in the axilla (levels I to III as clinically indicated), and 15 lymph nodes in the neck (levels I to V as clinically indicated) should be performed by an experienced team [20]. Unusual or rare LNDs including the posterior neck, epitrochlear area, and popliteal fossa should be individualized.

A well-performed regional lymphadenectomy provides useful quantitative information on the number of nodes examined and the ratio of positive to negative nodes, if positive nodes are present. Removal of only a few nodes does not provide information that is nearly as useful. An incomplete regional lymphadenectomy may be falsely interpreted as negative as a result of sampling error, and is not likely to be therapeutic if there are nodes present that contain melanoma.

In the majority of melanoma patients, mostly the SLNs are infiltrated by tumor cells whereas the draining nodes are not. Thus, it is unclear if therapeutic LNDs are warranted for a better prognosis. Some recommend that until further data are available, melanoma patients with a positive SLNB by routine histologic analysis should have a complete LND [73]. *However, the therapeutic effect of lymphadenectomy following positive sentinel node biopsy, especially with regard to patient survival, has yet to be determined accurately.*

Palliation

Palliation is achieved if the primary melanoma is controlled by WLE, with or without regional lymphadenectomy, even if distant metastases develop later. Local control is a goal that is well worth achieving, because the alternative may be dreadful. Extensive local melanoma regrowth may be painful and unsightly, and frequently becomes contaminated with foul-smelling clostridia and other anaerobes.

The traditional uses of surgery for palliation of cancer are relief of pain, bleeding, obstruction, and perforation. All of these indications exist in melanoma. Obstruction, bleeding, and perforation of hollow viscera are not uncommon events, because melanoma frequently metastasizes to gastrointestinal tract mucosa [74]. Craniotomy, laminectomy, and thoracotomy are occasionally indicated for progression of metastatic melanoma, if the patient is otherwise doing well. A large progressing necrotic cutaneous metastasis should be resected before it becomes too large to remove, if it is not responding to treatment with radiation therapy, chemotherapy, or biologic response modifiers [75].

Prevention

The removal of pigmented melanocytic nevi that are subject to repeated trauma has been a standard surgical recommendation. Admittedly, it cannot be proved that the development of melanoma is prevented by this procedure. Other lesions to consider for removal are pigmented nevi of the ear, the external genitalia, the hair-bearing scalp, and the palms and soles. All these sites are associated with a poor prognosis if melanocytic nevi develop into melanoma. In addition, enlarging Hutchinson's freckles (LM) should be excised, or the most active areas biopsied. A low overall rate of LMM in LM has been estimated, the lifetime risk of developing LMM from LM being less than 5%; the rate is highest in LMs that are undergoing obvious change [76]. Giant congenital melanocytic nevi (bathing suit nevi) should be considered for excision and grafting, because the risk of malignant degeneration has been estimated to be between 4% and 10% [77,78]. The risk of developing melanoma in small and medium-sized congenital melanocytic nevi

remains controversial [79]; we have no recommendation for these at this time, although we in general encourage excision of medium-sized ones.

The dysplastic nevus syndrome requires close attention and judicious use of biopsies for diagnosis and/or prevention [80,81]. Its incidence is about 7% of the general population. It is usually familial, characterized by multiple melanocytic nevi, some of which are unusually large (>1 cm in diameter), irregular in size and shape, variegated in color, and often noticeably changing. Up to 50% of melanomas are believed to occur within dysplastic nevi. Excisional biopsies are often indicated for diagnosis as well as prevention of melanoma in these patients [82]. Targeting of dysplastic nevi for melanoma chemoprevention with prolonged treatment with imiquimod or the use of other immune response modifiers has been suggested [81].

Rehabilitation

Plastic and orthopedic surgery techniques are often used to reconstruct the best appearance while preserving function following curative or palliative surgery for melanoma. External and implanted prostheses are often used, as in the replacement of the external ear or ocular globe. Health professionals should be aware of the new developments in reconstructive surgery and physical medicine and rehabilitation, and be sensitive to their patients' needs and desires. Because melanoma is largely a surface disease, disfigurement and disability are common following surgery and should be minimized whenever possible without compromising the best chance for cure.

Follow-up

Lifetime follow-up is needed after treatment for melanoma. Follow-up includes patient education, skin and lymph node self-examination, interval examinations by physicians, and laboratory and/or radiologic examination. Local recurrence should be detected and treated immediately. The regional lymph nodes should be examined, even if they were previously resected. The other major groups of lymph nodes should be examined at regular intervals, because metastases occasionally spread to several groups of nodes while initially sparing the deep viscera. Isolated metastases may be resected or, if a resection is not possible, radiated for palliation. Early treatment is preferable to late discovery and/or late treatment. The follow-up interval may be individualized depending on the prognosis. The type of follow-up depends on the location of the melanoma. Guidelines are available [20,21]. In general, the follow-up plan must balance the benefit from the timely detection of recurrence and the cost of the follow-up examination and tests. More follow-up visits are recommended for melanoma of a higher stage. This is based on the higher risk of recurrence when compared with less-advanced melanomas. A reduction in visits over time tends to follow [83]. There is no follow-up schedule with international consensus; different schedules have been reported [84]. Recently, a recommended follow-up schedule was published based on the new AJCC staging system. Following are the recommended intervals: stage I, annually; stage II, every 6 months for years 1 and 2 and annually thereafter; stage III, every 3 months for year 1, every 4 months for the next 2 years, and every 6 months for years 3 through 5; at year 6 and beyond, all patients should have surveillance annually because of the risk of late recurrence and metachronous multiple primaries [85]. NCCN guidelines recommend the following: stage 0 (in situ), annual skin examination for life, patient education, and monthly skin self-examination; stage IA, interval history and physical examination every 3 to 12 months as clinically indicated; stage IB to III, interval history and physical examination every 3 to 6 months for 3 years, every 4 to 12 months for the next 2 years, then annually as clinically indicated. Chest radiography, LDH levels, complete blood count, and liver function tests may be done every 3 to 12 months (optional). CT scans should be performed when clinically indicated [20].

Adjuvant treatment of melanoma

To improve surgical outcomes for high-risk, resectable melanoma, systemic therapy has been added. The concept of adjuvant therapy for melanoma is derived from the hypothesis that these therapies may target micrometastatic disease.

Different approaches have been studied, including the administration of postoperative chemotherapy, immunotherapy, vaccines, or combinations of these. Prospective randomized, controlled clinical trials are desirable when evaluating the efficacy of adjuvant therapy. It is not unusual to find that a reportedly effective treatment modality when compared with historical controls is not as promising when tested in a prospective, controlled manner. The results of adjuvant therapy for melanoma have been disappointing [86–89]. *In an adjuvant setting, only IFN-α has been shown to have a potential survival benefit for intermediate- and high-risk melanoma.*

Adjuvant chemotherapy

Dacarbazine (DTIC), the most active single agent used in advanced melanoma, is employed as monotherapy or in the adjuvant setting with other chemotherapeutic or immunotherapeutic agents [90,91]. In a meta-analysis including 10 adjuvant randomized studies, no statistical survival benefit was demonstrated when comparing chemotherapy with control [86].

As there are no regimens for advanced disease shown to demonstrate a high response rate, the ineffectiveness of adjuvant chemotherapy in early disease is not surprising.

Adjuvant immunotherapy: interferon

The most accepted adjuvant therapy for high-risk melanoma currently is IFN-α [92]. The family of interferons represents a broad spectrum of potent antiviral, antiproliferative, apoptosis-inducing, antiangiogenic, and immunomodulatory compounds. Their antitumor properties appear to be the result of a combination of direct antiproliferative as well as indirect immune-mediated effects [93,94]. IFN-α possesses pleiotropic and potentially antagonistic activity in immune cells and tumors. There are two types of IFN-α, 2a and 2b, which differ slightly in their chemical structure but have similar efficacy [86]. In several prospective randomized studies, a prolongation of disease-free survival was reported with different treatment regimens [92,95–101] (Table 31.6). However, only high-dose IFN-α showed significant improvement in overall survival in two prospective randomized trials

Table 31.6 Randomized, prospective trials comparing interferon-α versus observation (vs. others as indicated) in the adjuvant therapy of melanoma

Reference	Stage of Melanoma	Treatment Schedule	Patients, no.	Relapse-free Survival	Overall Survival (UICC 1992)
Creagan 1995 [98]	IIB–IIIB	20 MU/m^2 IV 3×/wk × 12 wk	262	NS	NS
Kirkwood 1996 (ECOG 1684) [96]	IIB–IIIB	20 MU/m^2 IV 5×/wk × 4 wk, then 10 MU/m^2 SC 3×/wk × 11 mo	287	$P = 0.0023$	$P = 0.00237$
Kirkwood 2000 (ECOG 1690) [97]	IIB–IIIB	20 MU/m^2 IV 5×/wk × 4 wk, then 10 MU/m^2 SC 3×/wk × 11 mo vs. 3 MU SC 3×/wk × 24 mo	608	$P = 0.003$	NS
Kirkwood 2001 (ECOG 1694) [95]	IIB–IIIB	20 MU/m^2 IV 5×/wk × 4 wk, then 10 MU/m^2 SC 3×/wk × 11 mo vs. ganglioside vaccine	880	$P = 0.0015$	$P = 0.009$
Grob 1998 [92]	IIA, IIB	3 MU SC 3×/wk × 18 mo	499	$P = 0.035$	$P = 0.059$
Pehamberger 1998 [99]	IIA, IIB	3 MU SC 3×/wk × 12 mo	311	$P = 0.02$	NS
Cascinelli 2001 [100]	IIIb	3 MU SC 3×/wk × 36 mo	427	NS	NS
Cameron 2001 [101]	IIB–IIIB	3 MU SC 3×/wk × 6 mo	96	NS	NS
Eggermont 2005 [102] (EORTC 18952)	IIB–IIIB	10 MU SC 5×/wk × 4 wk, then either 10 MU SC 3×/wk × 11 mo or 5 MU SC 3×/wk × 23 mo	1388	NS	NS

IV, intravenously; NS, not significant; SC, subcutaneously; UICC, International Union Against Cancer.

[95,96]. Low-dose IFN has been extensively tested in Europe and did not demonstrate the same survival benefit [92,99–102].

In 1995, the US Food and Drug Administration (FDA) approved the use of high-dose IFN-α-2b as adjuvant treatment in patients with high-risk melanoma (melanoma with tumor thickness $\geq$4 mm and/or positive nodes) on the basis of the results of the Eastern Cooperative Oncology Group (ECOG) 1684 trial [96]. This study randomized 287 patients to either observation or high-dose IFN-α-2b (20 MU/m^2/d intravenously for 1 month and 10 MU/m^2 three times per week subcutaneously for 48 weeks). After a median follow-up time of 6.9 years (range, 0.6 to 9.6 years), a significant impact on relapse-free survival ($P = 0.0023$) and overall survival ($P = 0.0237$) was demonstrated [103]. This and other studies before 2002 were often done before the prognostic value of nodal, in-transit, and local recurrences became evident [104]. Another trial, ECOG 1690, was initiated to confirm the results of ECOG 1684. High-dose IFN-α-2b and low-dose IFN-α-2b (3 × 10 MU/week) independently were compared with observation alone. No survival benefit was observed among the three arms after a median follow-up time of 4.3 years. The relapse-free survival was favorable for high-dose IFN compared with low-dose IFN or observation alone [97]. The third ECOG trial (1694), including 880 patients, compared a ganglioside vaccine with a high-dose IFN arm. In an interim analysis, a significant relapse-free and overall survival benefit was noted for the high-dose IFN arm [95]. In a pooled analysis of the ECOG and intergroup trials, a significant impact on relapse-free survival, but not on overall survival, was detected in patients with stage IIB and III melanoma receiving high-dose IFN [103]. A meta-analysis of the three ECOG trials yielded a reduction in 2-year mortality and an improvement in relapse-free survival [86].

It is evident that some patients have a clear survival benefit from interferon therapy whereas others do not. A recent study showed that patients with autoimmune phenomena (autoantibodies or clinical manifestations of autoimmunity) using IFN therapy have a favorable relapse-free and overall survival [105]. Nevertheless, the systemic toxicity of high-dose IFN, including flu-like symptoms, neurologic manifestations (especially depression), myelosuppression, and hepatotoxicity, is often dose limiting and may become life threatening [93,106].

Recombinant human pegylated (PEG) IFN-α-2a and -2b are both modified forms of IFN-α-2a/2b with a longer half-life, allowing a more convenient once-weekly dosing regimen and improved tolerability. Studies in melanoma patients with chronic hepatitis found that PEG-IFN-α-2a has superior efficacy to nonpegylated IFN-α [107,108]. Melanoma patients had safety and tolerability results demonstrating efficacy similar to that seen with standard IFN-α [109].

Other adjuvant immunotherapy

Based on the fact that melanoma cells are weakly antigenic and that melanoma patients appear to have some degree of immune dysfunction, nonspecific immunotherapy with bacille Calmette-Guérin (BCG) and *Cryptosporidium parvum* and specific immunotherapy with melanoma cell substances have been tested. The vast majority of prospective randomized, controlled trials in the adjuvant setting have shown no benefit [110–114]. Results of a phase III randomized trial showed no survival benefit in melanoma stages I to III regarding a 30-year survival analysis comparing BCG versus observation and BCG plus dacarbazine versus BCG alone [115]. Another nonspecific immunotherapeutic agent, the mistletoe preparation Iscador (Weleda), did not show any survival benefit in high-risk melanoma patients in adjuvant therapy [116]. However, a cohort study of 542 melanoma patients in six European countries and Israel showed that vaccination with vaccinia in early life significantly prolongs the survival of patients with a melanoma after initial surgical management [117]. BCG vaccination had a similar, although weaker, effect.

Attempts to use specific immunotherapy have included the use of viral lysates of melanoma cells [118]. In adjuvant randomized trials, different vaccine strategies, including vaccinia melanoma cell lysates [119], GM-2 ganglioside vaccine [95], autologous hapten-modified melanoma vaccine [120], vaccinia viral lysates of melanoma [121], and allogenic melanoma vaccine (Melacine, Corixa Corp.) [122] have been employed. However, none of these trials has reported a survival benefit in the vaccination arm [86]. The vaccine development is an active area of research [123].

A potentially less toxic approach is the use of gene therapy [124]. One idea is to use melanoma differentiation–associated gene-7/interleukin-24 (*mda-7/IL-24*) to get tumor cells to lose growth potential irreversibly and terminally differentiate [125]. Other gene therapy concepts for melanoma abound [126–130].

Adjuvant radiation therapy

For radiotherapy to be effective as an adjuvant treatment modality in increasing survival, it must be assumed that all melanoma cells are confined within the area to be radiated. However, this confinement is unlikely. One trial used this approach, with negative results [131]. The role of adjuvant irradiation after surgery of nodal metastases remains controversial. Postoperative adjuvant irradiation should be considered for stage III patients with extracapsular soft tissue extension and multi–lymph node involvement or incomplete dissection, especially in the head and neck region [20]. Furthermore, radiotherapy should be considered in patients with recurrence after previous LND without previous radiotherapy. Concerning adjuvant radiotherapy to a nodal field, prospective randomized trials are lacking; small retrospective observations are available [132,133].

Adjuvant isolation-perfusion

In many types of cancer, the role of surgery is diminishing as noninvasive alternatives such as radiation therapy and chemotherapy now exist. In melanoma, however, radiation and chemotherapy are of little benefit except in palliation. There is, on the other hand, another aspect of adjuvant therapy whose value remains controversial: adjuvant isolated limb perfusion (ILP).

Isolated limb perfusion has many advantages. In the hands of an experienced team, morbidity is low and operative mortality is almost nonexistent [134].

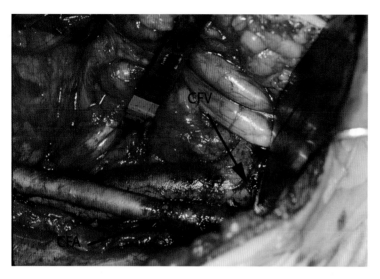

Fig. 31.5 Isolated hyperthermic limb perfusion of the right leg following removal of cannulae from the common femoral artery (CFA) and common femoral vein (CFV) and primary suture repair of the vessels. (Courtesy of Eric D. Whitman, MD, FACS, Medical Director, Mountainside Hospital Cancer Center; Director, Melanoma Center, Montclair, NJ.)

Improved cure rates were reported when the procedure was used as an adjunct to primary resection [135]. An ELND is usually performed, and the vessels exposed during the dissection are cannulated for perfusion. The limb volume has to be calculated before surgery [136]. A proximal tourniquet is applied to concentrate the drug to the extremity. The usual technique uses a moderate degree of hyperthermia (39°C to 41°C) and a chemotherapeutic agent such as melphalan, with dosages for ILPs between 10 mg/L for the lower limb and 13 mg/L for the upper limb of perfused tissue (Figs. 31.5 and 31.6). Furthermore, promising results were reported using ILP in combination with tumor necrosis factor-α (TNF-α) with or without interferon-γ [137–140].

Adjuvant isolated hyperthermic limb perfusion with high-dose melphalan was reported to improve the results of excision of melanomas of the extremities with thickness greater than 1.5 mm in unrandomized retrospective trials [135,141–143]. Another study was performed from a single university hospital of 85 patients with primary,

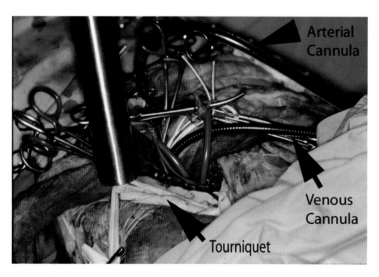

Fig. 31.6 Isolated hyperthermic limb perfusion of the right leg. Arterial and venous cannulae are in place and perfusing the right common femoral artery and vein, respectively. A tourniquet, secured to a pin in the right iliac crest and braced by the large metallic post, prevents leakage of chemotherapy via peripheral vessels. (Courtesy of Eric D. Whitman, MD, FACS, Medical Director, Mountainside Hospital Cancer Center; Director, Melanoma Center, Montclair, NJ.)

Table 31.7 Prognosis of patients with distant metastases, cumulative 1-, 2-, and 5-year survival regarding the new AJCC staging system

Pathologic Stage	TNM	Distant Metastasis	Patients, no.	1-Yr Survival, %	2-Yr Survival, %	5-Yr Survival, %
IV	M1a	Skin, SQ	179	59	37	19
	M1b	Lung	186	57	23	7
	M2b	Other visceral	793	41	24	9

SQ, subcutaneous.
Source: Balch et al. [32].

non-ulcerated limb melanoma who had undergone adjuvant ILP over 10 years (1986 to 1995). The observed and expected survival rates in patients receiving adjuvant ILP at the end of 3 and 5 years were comparable. The value of adjuvant ILP was judged unclear [144]. In a prospective multicenter trial, prophylactic limb perfusion for melanoma with a depth of 1.5 mm or greater after wide excision surgery showed a trend for a longer relapse-free interval, but no impact on survival was noted [145]. This study included a total of 832 patients; the median follow-up time was 6.4 years. The decision to perform elective LND was optional. A significant impact on relapse-free survival was noted in patients who received ELND. As would be anticipated, side effects were more severe after ILP, with two amputations being required. At present, on the basis of this prospective randomized trial, adjuvant ILP cannot be recommended in patients with high-risk melanomas following surgery of the primary melanoma.

To summarize, at the present time, only systemic therapy with IFN-α can be recommended to improve the results obtained by surgery in an adjuvant setting. Furthermore, the morbidity induced by the treatment itself has to be considered. All efforts must be made to enter patients at risk into prospective randomized trials.

Treatment of metastatic melanoma

Metastatic melanoma is uniformly fatal, but its behavior may vary significantly from patient to patient. Prolonged survival is exceptional (Table 31.7). Currently available therapy is palliative at best. Although long-term complete remissions are rare, a few cases are described after chemotherapy. Even the rare patients who experience a dramatic response will almost always eventually progress and die of melanoma [146].

Treatment causes morbidity, ranging from mild to life-threatening. The potential risks and benefits must be carefully balanced. Management of patients with disseminated melanoma may call for the use of one or more of the following modalities, simultaneously or sequentially: symptomatic treatment only, chemotherapy, regional or systemic immunotherapy, radiation, hyperthermia, and surgery. *Because existing therapeutic options are so poor, every effort should be made to enter patients on clinical trials to hasten progress in treatment research.*

Symptomatic treatment for metastatic melanoma

In some circumstances, it may be appropriate not to use any antineoplastic treatment. Other measures may be necessary to provide symptomatic relief, such as analgesia and nutritional support.

Chemotherapy for metastatic melanoma
Systemic monotherapy for metastatic melanoma

Dacarbazine is the single most commonly employed agent in melanoma therapy and has become the standard against which other drugs and regimens are compared. The objective response rate is about 10% to 25%, with a median survival of 6 to 9 months [147]. Complete responses (CRs) occur, at best, in about 4% of patients. It has been noted that subcutaneous disease and lymphadenopathy respond better than visceral disease [146]. A dose–response relationship has been suggested [148]. During the past two decades, more than 30 randomized trials were performed in which newer agents or combinations were compared with DTIC solo treatment. Nevertheless, no survival improvements have been noted.

Recently, the results of a multicenter trial comparing DTIC with and without bcl-2 antisense (oblimersen sodium) were published [149]. The overexpression of bcl-2 as an antiapoptotic regulatory protein confers resistance to a broad spectrum of antineoplastic agents [150]. This study, which included 771 patients, found an overall response rate of 13.5% for patients treated with oblimersen-DTIC and 7.5% for patients who received DTIC. Interestingly, a favorable overall survival in patients without an elevated baseline serum LDH was found in the oblimersen-DTIC group [149]. Temozolomide (TMZ), a prodrug given orally and metabolized to an alkylating agent, has advantageous pharmacokinetics as compared with DTIC. Recently, temozolomide was tested in clinical studies for patients with melanoma [151]. When temozolomide was compared with DTIC in previously untreated stage IV melanoma, the response rates and survival were found to be equivalent, but a lower incidence of subsequent brain metastases was obvious in the temozolomide group [152,153].

Nitrosoureas have modest activity, comparable with that of DTIC alone. The use of fotemustine in 153 stage IV melanoma patients showed three CRs and 34 partial responses, leading to an objective response rate of 24.2%. Furthermore, activity against cerebral metastases was noted in 25.0% [154]. In a prospective multicenter trial, patients receiving fotemustine as a first-line treatment of disseminated melanoma had a higher overall response rate but no significant impact on survival when compared with the DTIC arm [155]. As a chemotherapeutic agent with CNS activity, the alkylating agent temozolomide or the nitrosourea fotemustine may be used in patients with brain involvement [154,156]. Temozolomide in combination with thalidomide or in combination with radiotherapy has also been shown to be of some use, with acceptable toxicities, in this patient group [157,158]. Alkylating agents and vinca alkaloids have modest activity.

Other drugs with some activity include the platin analogues carboplatin and cisplatin [159]. However, the dose-limiting toxicity of cisplatin is its nephrotoxicity, ototoxicity, and gastrointestinal toxicity [160,161]. Carboplatin, a cisplatin analogue [162], has been described in combination with cisplatin as an active and safe second-line therapy [163]. Pegylated liposomal doxorubicin was well tolerated using a 2-week schedule but failed to show any activity in chemotherapy-naive patients with advanced malignant melanoma in another phase II effort [164].

Combination chemotherapy for metastatic melanoma

To improve the chemotherapeutic response rates, numerous clinical trials have been performed using combination chemotherapy. These regimens have produced good response rates and a trend to prolongation of median survival but have failed to demonstrate superiority to DTIC monotherapy [165]. Furthermore, DTIC monotherapy, like temozolomide and fotemustine monotherapy, is characterized by its simplicity of administration and its low toxicity. A recent randomized trial analyzed the combination of dacarbazine, vincristine, and carmustine in two different dosing schedules and two other regimens that included vindesine, bleomycin, cisplatin, and carmustine plus procarbazine, with no impact on survival [166].

In early studies, the addition of the antiestrogen tamoxifen to chemotherapy showed some beneficial therapeutic efficacy [167]. Subsequently, randomized trials addressed whether the addition of tamoxifen to systemic chemotherapy increases response or prolongs survival. In a small phase III trial that compared DTIC alone with DTIC plus tamoxifen, a significant impact on response rates and overall survival was observed [168]. This beneficial effect could not be confirmed investigating different monotherapy or polychemotherapy schedules with or without tamoxifen [169–172]. In a recent multicenter study [173] comparing DTIC and tamoxifen versus vindesine and tamoxifen, neither response nor survival correlated with gender [168]. The Dartmouth regimen including DTIC, cisplatin, carmustine, and tamoxifen with

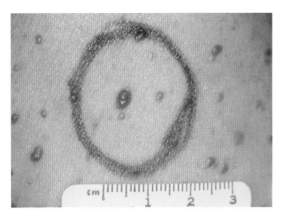

Fig. 31.7 Disseminated cutaneous metastatic melanoma, a model for modern immunotherapy.

a 55% response rate was first described in 1984 [174]. A variety of single-institution trials confirmed relatively high response rates of 40% to 50% [175–177]. In a multicenter phase III randomized trial that compared the Dartmouth regimen to single-agent DTIC, no difference in survival time was seen [178]. Therefore, tamoxifen, in addition to monochemotherapy or polychemotherapies, does not have a survival benefit in patients with metastatic melanoma.

Immunotherapy and biologic response modifiers for metastatic melanoma

As a rule, responses seen with immunotherapy are less common but are suspected to be more durable than those seen with chemotherapy. Several different approaches to modify the immune environment have been tried, including nonspecific stimulation of the immune system using BCG or methanol-extracted residue of BCG (MER), vaccination with tumor extracts, injection of visible lesions with BCG or MER for local control, monoclonal antibodies, and interleukin-2 (IL-2) with or without lymphokine-activated killer cells [179]. Disseminated metastatic cutaneous melanoma can serve as a model directly evaluating immunotherapy and other modalities (Fig. 31.7).

Interleukin-2 is a cytokine with pleiotropic immunostimulatory effects that has shown in vitro and in vivo activity against melanoma cells. IL-2,

with or without lymphokine-activated killer (LAK) cells, has resulted in some responses in patients with disseminated melanoma [180,181]. Based on the first encouraging results, immunotherapy using high-dose recombinant interleukin-2 (rIL-2) as a single agent has produced responses in up to 20% of melanoma patients in multiple randomized trials [182–184]. In some cases, durable CRs were achieved [184]. The clinical effect of adding LAK cells to high-dose IL-2 therapy has been discussed as controversial. In different trials, the clinical impact fell short [185,186]. Based on these data, the US FDA has approved the use of high-dose bolus administration of rIL-2 for the treatment of metastatic melanoma. IL-2 600,000 to 720,000 IU/kg is given by 15-minute intravenous infusion every 8 hours for up to 14 consecutive doses over 5 days as clinically tolerated. A second treatment cycle is repeated after 6 to 9 days of rest. Besides the positive clinical effects, various and severe toxicities, such as fever, chills, anemia, thrombocytopenia, renal toxicity, hypotension, cutaneous drug reactions, respiratory distress, and fluid retention, may occur [187,188]. Maximum support, including pressors, may be necessary. IL-2 used together with imiquimod was found to be effective in controlling mixed cutaneous and subcutaneous metastatic melanoma, and was well tolerated. Imiquimod alone often elicited a response in purely cutaneous metastases [18,189]. Imiquimod 5% cream may be applied three times weekly to cutaneous metastases with a 1-cm surrounding margin and washed off in the morning [18]. The addition of intralesional IL-2 increased the response rates in subcutaneous metastatic melanomas and in otherwise refractory cutaneous ones [189].

Interferon-α is widely used as an adjuvant therapeutic agent (see above). In metastatic melanoma, IFN-α as a single agent has only marginal activity, but the combination of IFN-α and IL-2 has shown response rates of up to 40% [190–192]. Trials with IFN were the subject of different reviews [193,194]. Many studies have used IFNs combined with DTIC. A meta-analysis of 3273 patients from 20 randomized trials suggests that the IFN-α plus DTIC combination produces a 53% greater response rate than DTIC alone [193]. Falkson and colleagues [195] reported that the combination of IFN-α and DTIC had significant impact on overall survival ($P < 0.01$). Other studies could not confirm these encouraging results [196–198].

Biochemotherapy for metastatic melanoma

When combining IFN-α with cytotoxic drugs, response rates of up to 50% have been observed [193]. The same was found when IL-2 was added to chemotherapy, with even durable CRs reported [199–205]. Legha and associates [206,207] compared an alternating biochemotherapy regimen and a sequential biochemotherapy using cisplatin, vinblastine, DTIC, IL-2 and IFN-α. The sequential biochemotherapy regimen produced an overall response rate of 60%, with 14 CRs out of 62 treated patients. Similar response rates have been reported using a concurrent biochemotherapy in a single-center trial [208]. However, in a phase III trial comparing this biochemotherapy with chemotherapy, the high number of CRs could not be confirmed. The biochemotherapy was significantly more toxic, but the median survival for biochemotherapy was 11.9 months, as compared with 9.2 months for chemotherapy [209]. Several cytotoxic drugs have now been investigated in combination with IFN-α with or without IL-2 in randomized prospective trials [210–215]. Favorable response rates were reported without significant impact on overall survival. Besides, polychemoimmunotherapies are invariably accompanied by increased and potentially hazardous toxicity. Therefore, to date, biochemotherapy cannot be recommended as standard first-line therapy for metastatic melanoma. DTIC monotherapy is well tolerated and appears to deliver clinical improvements similar to those of the biochemotherapies.

Therapeutic approaches with less toxicity and regimens with a benefit on overall survival are desired in the treatment of advanced malignant melanoma. There are many options. For example, a phase II study evaluated the combination of semaxanib, a small-molecule tyrosine kinase inhibitor of vascular endothelial growth factor (VEGF) receptor-2, and thalidomide in 12 patients with metastatic melanoma who failed to benefit from previous

therapy [216]. One patient had a complete remission lasting 20 months, and another had a partial remission, with four stabilized for up to 10 months. *No chemotherapeutic regimen has demonstrated clear-cut advantages over DTIC used alone for metastatic melanoma.*

Regional chemotherapy for metastatic melanoma

When metastatic disease occurs predominantly in a limb, good results may be achieved with isolation perfusion employing chemotherapeutic agents. High-dose melphalan as well as other drugs have been employed (see above). Recent reports have described the results of ILP using hyperthermia, TNF-α, and melphalan, with CR rates of up to 76% in patients with regionally advanced melanoma [138,217–219]. TNF-α was observed to increase response rates for in-transit melanoma when coadministered with melphalan [220]. ILP is generally applied with curative intent in patients without evidence of distant metastases. In melanoma stage IV patients, the decision for palliative ILP should be individualized. In a small study group, ILP appeared to be an effective palliative treatment option in 75% of stage IV melanoma patients with symptomatic advanced limb disease [221].

Immunotherapy has been used for the local control of melanoma since Edmund Klein pioneered the concept in the 1960s [222,223]. Two thirds of melanomas injected with BCG responded [224]. Noninjected melanomas situated in the vicinity of those injected may occasionally regress as well [225]. Other chemical substances, such as dinitrochlorobenzene, or cytokines such as IL-2 have yielded similar results [226,227].

Antibody treatments and vaccine approaches for metastatic melanoma

Monoclonal antibodies are used in the diagnosis and treatment of malignant melanoma, but their precise value still needs to be defined. Cutaneous melanoma may regress when injected with monoclonal antibodies. Melanoma antibody treatment has focused for decades on ganglioside antigens, as gangliosides are highly expressed on melanoma cells. Using EMD 273063, a humanized anti-GD2 monoclonal antibody linked to IL-2, in 33 metastatic melanoma patients, eight (24%) had disease stabilization [228]. In another trial, 17 melanoma patients were given KM 871, a chimeric monoclonal antibody against the ganglioside antigen GD3. Two patients had disease stabilization and one a partial response with inflammatory reactions at the tumor site [229]. Further phase II trials are under way.

The optimal methodology for vaccine therapy in metastatic melanoma has not been established. Encouraging results using the allogenic vaccine Canvaxin (CancerVax Corp.) were reported in metastatic melanoma patients [54]. Canvaxin is composed of cells from three melanoma cell lines mixed with BCG as an adjuvant. In 263 patients with complete resection of stage IV melanoma, post-operative adjuvant vaccine therapy was compared with observation. Five-year overall survival rates were significantly different, with 39% for vaccinated and 19% for nonvaccinated patients [230]. Multicenter phase III trials in stage III and IV melanoma were started, but both trials were halted because of lack of efficacy.

An autologous, hapten-modified melanoma vaccine showed two complete, four partial, and five mixed responses with a significant survival benefit for patients with tumor regression (median survival times for responders, 21.4 months; nonresponders, 8.7 months) in 79 metastatic melanoma patients [231]. Another vaccine consisting of autologous, tumor-derived heat-shock protein (gp96-peptide) complexes was given to 28 patients with metastatic melanoma; two had a CR and three had stable disease [232].

In using multipeptide vaccines with or without additive cytokines in metastatic melanoma, only few objective responses were noted. But immune responses could be detected [233–235]. In dendritic cell vaccines, the melanoma antigens are presented with the aid of dendritic cells. Different approaches were reported with occasionally impressive clinical responses in patient subgroups. Nevertheless, it has not been possible to identify these potential subgroups with immunologic methods so far [236,237]. DNA vaccines are generated by inserting the complementary DNA encoding the melanoma antigens of interest into bacterial expression plasmids with a constitutively active promoter, such as the cytomegalovirus promoter. Murine models are available [238]; clinical trials are under way.

Surgery for metastatic melanoma

Surgery is seldom used for metastatic melanoma involving multiple organs. However, complete metastasectomy in patients with stage IV melanoma may be considered [75]. It may be beneficial to remove a solitary metastatic nodule and a few isolated subcutaneous nodules, as there have been patients who have had a long disease-free survival following surgery for metastatic melanoma [239,240]. Surgery should be contemplated only if it would leave the patient free of clinically evident disease. On occasion, it may become necessary for palliation of a life-threatening complication in patients with advanced disease. Up to 75% of patients with metastatic melanoma suffer from cerebral metastases [241]. Therapeutic options often require individualized management with regard to age, the number of brain metastases, and performance status. In patients with a limited number of brain metastases, neurosurgical excision should be considered, as overall survival is improved in these patients [242]. In patients with pulmonary metastatic melanoma, improved survival was found after an analysis of 1720 patients with pulmonary metastasectomy [243]. It was associated with a survival advantage of 12 months for patients with a disease-free interval longer than 5 years (19 vs. 7 months) and of 10 months for patients without extrathoracic metastasis (18 vs. 8 months). *Given these results, resection of melanoma metastases in a selected group of patients may be beneficial* [244,245].

New prospects and research in systemic treatment of metastatic melanoma

A number of additional innovative approaches are being tried. One is the application of blocking cytotoxic T-lymphocyte antigen 4 (CTLA-4) antibodies in melanoma patients, resulting in an activation of T cells. Phase I and II studies were conducted, with response rates of 15% to 20% [246]. Limiting side effects included dermatitis, enterocolitis, hepatitis, and hypophysitis. Other possible molecular therapies target the melanoma-induced angiogenesis, the

Ras-MAPK and PI3K/AKT signal transduction pathways, and the proteasome and histone deacetylases. The Raf inhibitor sorafenib (BAY 43-9006) has little activity on its own in advanced melanoma patients [247], but in combination with the cytotoxic agents carboplatin and paclitaxel, encouraging results were reported [248]. Phase I or II studies are available for the proteasome inhibitor bortezomib [249], inhibitors of the PI3K/AKT pathway [250], antiangiogenic therapies [157], and histone-deacetylase inhibitors [251].

Clearly, there is a great need for more effective treatment for metastatic malignant melanoma.

Radiation therapy

Despite old in vitro and in vivo data suggesting that melanomas are radioresistant, current findings show a wide range of sensitivities, with some melanomas being highly sensitive; the findings also show that regimens with a high dose per fraction are more effective than those with a low dose per fraction [252]. *LM and LMM, particularly those on the face of an elderly person, can be effectively treated with conventional fractionated radiotherapy* [253]. *Local tumor control rates have been reported to be between 90% and 100%* [254,255].

Currently, there is no standard treatment schedule concerning radiotherapy of metastatic melanoma. A randomized trial compared melanoma patients treated with 4×8.0 Gy in 21 days once weekly to 20×2.5 Gy in 26 to 28 days, 5 days a week. No difference between conventional and hypofractionated schedules was detected [256]. Radiotherapy may be combined with other modalities, such as topical immunotherapy with diphenylcyclopropenone and DTIC for cutaneous metastases of melanoma [257].

Radiotherapy is generally reserved for metastases that may become life threatening because of growth in a strategic location. For instance, brain metastases or spinal cord compression are best palliated with external-beam radiation. Melanoma can be effectively controlled with modern radiation equipment and techniques. Brain metastases are common in melanoma patients. In patients with a limited number of small brain metastases, surgical excision or stereotactic radiosurgery (SRS) are possible treatment options. The combination of surgery or SRS with subsequent whole-brain radiotherapy (WBRT) is still a matter of debate [258]. *In patients with disseminated brain metastases, WBRT with or without chemotherapy is recommended* [259].

Overview

Curable if caught and excised early, a virtual death sentence if diagnosis is delayed, cutaneous melanoma represents an increasing challenge. Chemotherapy and radiotherapy have not provided substantial benefit. Immunotherapy, as pioneered by Edmund Klein, the Father of Modern Immunotherapy [260], remains an active dream that someday may awaken into reality.

References

1 Jemal A, Siegel R, Ward E, et al. Cancer statistics, 2006. CA Cancer J Clin 2006;56:106–30.

2 Crocetti E, Carli P, Miccinesi G. Melanoma incidence in central Italy will go on increasing also in the near future: a registry-based, age-period-cohort analysis. Eur J Cancer Prev 2007;16:50–4.

3 Jemal A, Siegel R, Ward E, et al. Cancer statistics, 2007. CA Cancer J Clin 2007;57:43–66.

4 Richtig E, Berghold A, Schwantzer G, et al. Clinical epidemiology of invasive cutaneous malignant melanoma in the Austrian province Styria in the years 2001–2003 and its relationship with local geographical, meteorological and economic data. Dermatology 2007;214:246–52.

5 Kraemer KH, Lee MM, Andrews AD, et al. The role of sunlight and DNA repair in melanoma and nonmelanoma skin cancer. The xeroderma pigmentosum paradigm. Arch Dermatol 1994;130:1018–21.

6 Bulliard JL, De Weck D, Fisch T, et al. Detailed site distribution of melanoma and sunlight exposure: aetiological patterns from a Swiss series. Ann Oncol 2007;18:789–94.

7 Richtig E, Gerger A, Berghold A, et al. Natural history of invasive cutaneous melanoma in Styria, Austria 2001–2003. J Dtsch Dermatol Ges 2007;5:293–9.

8 Ross MI. New American Joint Commission on Cancer staging system for melanoma: prognostic impact and future directions. Surg Oncol Clin N Am 2006;15:341–52.

9 Morton CA, Mackie RM. Clinical accuracy of the diagnosis of cutaneous malignant melanoma. Br J Dermatol 1998;138:283–7.

10 Pizzichetta MA, Stanganelli I, Bono R, et al. Dermoscopic features of difficult melanoma. Dermatol Surg 2007;33:91–9.

11 Henning JS, Dusza SW, Wang SQ, et al. The CASH (color, architecture, symmetry, and homogeneity) algorithm for dermoscopy. J Am Acad Dermatol 2007;56:45–52.

12 Bowling J, Argenziano G, Azenha A, et al. Dermoscopy key points: recommendations from the international dermoscopy society. Dermatology 2007;214:3–5.

13 Braun RP, Rabinovitz HS, Oliviero M, et al. Dermoscopy of pigmented skin lesions. J Am Acad Dermatol 2005;52:109–21.

14 Lederman JS, Sober AJ. Does wide excision as the initial diagnostic procedure improve prognosis in patients with cutaneous melanoma? J Dermatol Surg Oncol 1986;12:697–9.

15 Stell VH, Norton HJ, Smith KS, et al. Method of biopsy and incidence of positive margins in primary melanoma. Ann Surg Oncol 2007;14:893–8.

16 Sober AJ, Balch CM. Method of biopsy and incidence of positive margins in primary melanoma. Ann Surg Oncol 2007;14:274–5.

17 Balch CM, Soong SJ, Atkins MB, et al. An evidence-based staging system for cutaneous melanoma. CA Cancer J Clin 2004;54:131–49; quiz 82-4.

18 Wolf IH, Richtig E, Kopera D, et al. Locoregional cutaneous metastases of malignant melanoma and their management. Dermatol Surg 2004;30:244–7.

19 Hafner J, Schmid MH, Kempf W, et al. Baseline staging in cutaneous malignant melanoma. Br J Dermatol 2004;150:677–86.

20 National Comprehensive Cancer Network Clinical Practice Guidelines in Oncology™v.2.2006 melanoma. Available from: http://www.nccn.org/professionals/physician_gls/ PDF/melanoma.pdf.

21 Sober AJ, Chuang TY, Duvic M, et al. Guidelines of care for primary cutaneous melanoma. J Am Acad Dermatol 2001;45:579–86.

22 Buzaid AC, Sandler AB, Mani S, et al. Role of computed tomography in the staging of primary melanoma. J Clin Oncol 1993;11:638–43.

23 Falk MS, Truitt AK, Coakley FV, et al. Interpretation, accuracy and management implications of FDG PET/CT in cutaneous malignant melanoma. Nucl Med Commun 2007;28:273–80.

24 Wang TS, Johnson TM, Cascade PN, et al. Evaluation of staging chest radiographs and serum lactate dehydrogenase for localized melanoma. J Am Acad Dermatol 2004;51:399–405.

25 Kell MR, Ridge JA, Joseph N, et al. PET CT imaging in patients undergoing sentinel node biopsy for melanoma [published online ahead of print on January 3, 2007]. Eur J Surg Oncol. PMID: 17207956.

26 Young SE, Martinez SR, Faries MB, et al. Can surgical therapy alone achieve long-term cure of melanoma metastatic to regional nodes? Cancer J 2006;12:207–11.

27 Kretschmer L, Beckmann I, Thoms KM, et al. Factors predicting the risk of in-transit recurrence after sentinel lymphonodectomy in patients with cutaneous malignant melanoma. Ann Surg Oncol 2006;13:1105–12.

28 de Wilt JH, Farmer SE, Scolyer RA, et al. Isolated melanoma in the lung where there is no known primary site: metastatic disease or primary lung tumour? Melanoma Res 2005;15:531–7.

29 Goldman LI. The surgical therapy of malignant melanomas. Semin Oncol 1975;2:175–8.

30 Veronesi U, Cascinelli N, Adamus J, et al. Thin stage I primary cutaneous malignant melanoma. Comparison of excision with margins of 1 or 3 cm. N Engl J Med 1988;318:1159–62.

31 Veronesi U, Cascinelli N. Narrow excision (1-cm margin). A safe procedure for thin cutaneous melanoma. Arch Surg 1991;126:438–41.

32 Balch CM, Urist MM, Karakousis CP, et al. Efficacy of 2-cm surgical margins for intermediate-thickness melanomas (1 to 4 mm). Results of a multi-institutional randomized surgical trial. Ann Surg 1993;218:262–7; discussion 267–9.

33 Cohn-Cedermark G, Rutqvist LE, Andersson R, et al. Long term results of a randomized study by the Swedish Melanoma Study Group on 2-cm versus 5-cm resection margins for patients with cutaneous melanoma with a tumor thickness of 0.8–2.0 mm. Cancer 2000;89:1495–501.

34 Thomas JM, Newton-Bishop J, A'Hern R, et al. Excision margins in high-risk malignant melanoma. N Engl J Med 2004;350:757–66.

35 Zitelli JA, Brown CD, Hanusa BH. Surgical margins for excision of primary cutaneous melanoma. J Am Acad Dermatol 1997;37:422–9.

36 Zitelli JA, Brown C, Hanusa BH. Mohs micrographic surgery for the treatment of primary cutaneous melanoma. J Am Acad Dermatol 1997;37:236–45.

37 Johnson TM, Headington JT, Baker SR, et al. Useful-ness of the staged excision for lentigo maligna and lentigo maligna melanoma: the "square" procedure. J Am Acad Dermatol 1997;37:758–64.

38 Cohen LM, McCall MW, Hodge SJ, et al. Success-ful treatment of lentigo maligna and lentigo maligna melanoma with Mohs' micrographic surgery aided by rush permanent sections. Cancer 1994;73:2964–70.

39 Stonecipher MR, Leshin B, Patrick J, et al. Man-agement of lentigo maligna and lentigo maligna melanoma with paraffin-embedded tangential sec-tions: utility of immunoperoxidase staining and sup-plemental vertical sections. J Am Acad Dermatol 1993;29:589–94.

40 Cuono CB, Ariyan S. Versatility and safety of flap coverage for wide excision of cutaneous melanomas. Plast Reconstr Surg 1985;76:281–5.

41 Lent WM, Ariyan S. Flap reconstruction following wide local excision for primary malignant melanoma of the head and neck region. Ann Plast Surg 1994;33:23–7.

42 Yang CH, Yeh JT, Shen SC, et al. Regressed subun-gual melanoma simulating cellular blue nevus: man-aged with sentinel lymph node biopsy. Dermatol Surg 2006;32:577–80; discussion 580–1.

43 Furukawa H, Tsutsumida A, Yamamoto Y, et al. Melanoma of thumb: retrospective study for amputa-tion levels, surgical margin and reconstruction. J Plast Reconstr Aesthet Surg 2007;60:24–31.

44 Fortin PT, Freiberg AA, Rees R, et al. Malignant melanoma of the foot and ankle. J Bone Joint Surg Am 1995;77:1396–403.

45 Cowles RA, Johnson TM, Chang AE. Useful tech-niques for the resection of foot melanomas. J Surg Oncol 1999;70:255–9; discussion 259–60.

46 Balch CM, Buzaid AC, Soong SJ, et al. Final version of the American Joint Committee on Cancer stag-ing system for cutaneous melanoma. J Clin Oncol 2001;19:3635–48.

47 Balch CM, Soong SJ, Milton GW, et al. A compari-son of prognostic factors and surgical results in 1786 patients with localized (stage I) melanoma treated in Alabama, USA, and New South Wales, Australia. Ann Surg 1982;196:677–84.

48 Rompel R, Garbe C, Buttner P, et al. Elective lymph node dissection in primary malignant melanoma: a matched-pair analysis. Melanoma Res 1995;5:189–94.

49 Drepper H, Kohler CO, Bastian B, et al. Benefit of elective lymph node dissection in subgroups of

melanoma patients. Results of a multicenter study of 3616 patients. Cancer 1993;72:741–9.

50 McCarthy WH, Shaw HM, Milton GW. Efficacy of elective lymph node dissection in 2347 patients with clinical stage I malignant melanoma. Surg Gynecol Obstet 1985;161:575–80.

51 Sim FH, Taylor WF, Pritchard DJ, et al. Lymphadenec-tomy in the management of stage I malignant melanoma: a prospective randomized study. Mayo Clin Proc 1986;61:697–705.

52 Veronesi U, Adamus J, Bandiera DC, et al. Inefficacy of immediate node dissection in stage 1 melanoma of the limbs. N Engl J Med 1977;297:627–30.

53 Balch CM, Soong SJ, Bartolucci AA, et al. Efficacy of an elective regional lymph node dissection of 1 to 4 mm thick melanomas for patients 60 years of age and younger. Ann Surg 1996;224:255–63; discussion 263–6.

54 Morton DL, Wen DR, Wong JH, et al. Technical details of intraoperative lymphatic mapping for early stage melanoma. Arch Surg 1992;127:392–9.

55 Morton DL, Wen DR, Foshag LJ, et al. Intraopera-tive lymphatic mapping and selective cervical lym-phadenectomy for early-stage melanomas of the head and neck. J Clin Oncol 1993;11:1751–6.

56 Keller B, Yawalkar N, Pichler C, et al. Hypersensitivity reaction against patent blue during sentinel lymph node removal in three melanoma patients. Am J Surg 2007;193:122–4.

57 Uren RF, Howman-Giles R, Thompson JF, et al. Lym-phoscintigraphy to identify sentinel lymph nodes in patients with melanoma. Melanoma Res 1994;4:395–9.

58 Gershenwald JE, Colome MI, Lee JE, et al. Patterns of recurrence following a negative sentinel lymph node biopsy in 243 patients with stage I or II melanoma. J Clin Oncol 1998;16:2253–60.

59 Morton DL, Thompson JF, Essner R, et al. Vali-dation of the accuracy of intraoperative lymphatic mapping and sentinel lymphadenectomy for early-stage melanoma: a multicenter trial. Multicenter Se-lective Lymphadenectomy Trial Group. Ann Surg 1999;230:453–63; discussion 463–5.

60 Statius Muller MG, van Leeuwen PA, de Lange-De Klerk ES, et al. The sentinel lymph node status is an important factor for predicting clinical outcome in pa-tients with stage I or II cutaneous melanoma. Cancer 2001;91:2401–8.

61 Essner R, Conforti A, Kelley MC, et al. Efficacy of lymphatic mapping, sentinel lymphadenectomy, and selective complete lymph node dissection as a

therapeutic procedure for early-stage melanoma. Ann Surg Oncol 1999;6:442–9.

62 Thompson JF, Uren RF. Lymphatic mapping in management of patients with primary cutaneous melanoma. Lancet Oncol 2005;6:877–85.

63 Johnson TM, Sondak VK, Bichakjian CK, et al. The role of sentinel lymph node biopsy for melanoma: evidence assessment. J Am Acad Dermatol 2006;54:19–27.

64 Garcia C, Poletti E. Sentinel lymph node biopsy for melanoma is still controversial. J Am Acad Dermatol 2007;56:347–8.

65 Pacifico MD, Grover R, Richman PI, et al. Development of a tissue array for primary melanoma with long-term follow-up: discovering melanoma cell adhesion molecule as an important prognostic marker. Plast Reconstr Surg 2005;115:367–75.

66 Li W, Stall A, Shivers SC, et al. Clinical relevance of molecular staging for melanoma: comparison of RT-PCR and immunohistochemistry staining in sentinel lymph nodes of patients with melanoma. Ann Surg 2000;231:795–803.

67 Twomey P. Sentinel Node Biopsy for Early-Stage Melanoma: Accuracy and Morbidity in MSLT-1, an International Multicenter Trial. Ann Surg 2007;245:156–7.

68 Tsutsumida A, Furukawa H, Hata S, et al. Prediction of metastases in melanoma patients with positive sentinel node: histological and molecular approach. J Dermatol 2007;34:31–6.

69 Reintgen D, Pendas S, Jakub J, et al. National trials involving lymphatic mapping for melanoma: the Multicenter Selective Lymphadenectomy Trial, the Sunbelt Melanoma Trial, and the Florida Melanoma Trial. Semin Oncol 2004;31:363–73.

70 Morton DL, Cochran AJ, Thompson JF, et al. Sentinel node biopsy for early-stage melanoma: accuracy and morbidity in MSLT-I, an international multicenter trial. Ann Surg 2005;242:302–11; discussion 311–3.

71 Morton DL, Thompson JF, Cochran AJ, et al. Sentinel-node biopsy or nodal observation in melanoma. N Engl J Med 2006;355:1307–17.

72 Thompson JF, Scolyer RA, Kefford RF. Cutaneous melanoma. Lancet 2005;365:687–701.

73 Jakub JW, Reintgen DS, Shivers S, et al. Regional node dissection for melanoma: techniques and indication. Surg Oncol Clin N Am 2007;16:247–61.

74 Liang KV, Sanderson SO, Nowakowski GS, et al. Metastatic malignant melanoma of the gastrointestinal tract. Mayo Clin Proc 2006;81:511–6.

75 Ollila DW. Complete metastasectomy in patients with stage IV metastatic melanoma. Lancet Oncol 2006;7:919–24.

76 Weinstock MA, Sober AJ. The risk of progression of lentigo maligna to lentigo maligna melanoma. Br J Dermatol 1987;116:303–10.

77 Cruz MA, Cho ES, Schwartz RA, et al. Congenital neurocutaneous melanosis. Cutis 1997;60:178–81.

78 Marghoob AA, Agero AL, Benvenuto-Andrade C, et al. Large congenital melanocytic nevi, risk of cutaneous melanoma, and prophylactic surgery. J Am Acad Dermatol 2006;54:868–70; discussion 871–3.

79 Ingordo V, Gentile C, Iannazzone SS, et al. Congenital melanocytic nevus: an epidemiologic study in Italy. Dermatology 2007;214:227–30.

80 Kraemer KH, Tucker M, Tarone R, et al. Risk of cutaneous melanoma in dysplastic nevus syndrome types A and B. N Engl J Med 1986;315:1615–6.

81 Dusza SW, Delgado R, Busam KJ, et al. Treatment of dysplastic nevi with 5% imiquimod cream, a pilot study. J Drugs Dermatol 2006;5:56–62.

82 Armour K, Mann S, Lee S. Dysplastic naevi: to shave, or not to shave? A retrospective study of the use of the shave biopsy technique in the initial management of dysplastic naevi. Australas J Dermatol 2005;46:70–5.

83 Francken AB, Bastiaannet E, Hoekstra HJ. Follow-up in patients with localised primary cutaneous melanoma. Lancet Oncol 2005;6:608–21.

84 Garbe C, Paul A, Kohler-Spath H, et al. Prospective evaluation of a follow-up schedule in cutaneous melanoma patients: recommendations for an effective follow-up strategy. J Clin Oncol 2003;21:520–9.

85 Poo-Hwu WJ, Ariyan S, Lamb L, et al. Follow-up recommendations for patients with American Joint Committee on Cancer stages I–III malignant melanoma. Cancer 1999;86:2252–8.

86 Verma S, Quirt I, McCready D, et al. Systematic review of systemic adjuvant therapy for patients at high risk for recurrent melanoma. Cancer 2006;106:1431–42.

87 Lens MB, Dawes M. Interferon alfa therapy for malignant melanoma: a systematic review of randomized controlled trials. J Clin Oncol 2002;20:1818–25.

88 Wheatley K, Ives N, Hancock B, et al. Does adjuvant interferon-alpha for high-risk melanoma provide a worthwhile benefit? A meta-analysis of the randomised trials. Cancer Treat Rev 2003;29:241–52.

89 Hersey P. Adjuvant therapy for high-risk primary and resected metastatic melanoma. Intern Med J 2003;33:33–43.

90 Balch CM, Murray D, Presant C, et al. Ineffectiveness of adjuvant chemotherapy using DTIC and cyclophosphamide in patients with resectable metastatic melanoma. Surgery 1984;95:454–9.

91 Tranum BL, Dixon D, Quagliana J, et al. Lack of benefit of adjunctive chemotherapy in stage I malignant melanoma: a Southwest Oncology Group Study. Cancer Treat Rep 1987;71:643–4.

92 Grob JJ, Dreno B, de la Salmoniere P, et al. Randomised trial of interferon alpha-2a as adjuvant therapy in resected primary melanoma thicker than 1.5 mm without clinically detectable node metastases. French Cooperative Group on Melanoma. Lancet 1998;351:1905–10.

93 Jonasch E, Haluska FG. Interferon in oncological practice: review of interferon biology, clinical applications, and toxicities. Oncologist 2001;6:34–55.

94 Pestka S, Krause CD, Walter MR. Interferons, interferon-like cytokines, and their receptors. Immunol Rev 2004;202:8–32.

95 Kirkwood JM, Ibrahim JG, Sosman JA, et al. High-dose interferon alfa-2b significantly prolongs relapse-free and overall survival compared with the GM2-KLH/QS-21 vaccine in patients with resected stage IIB-III melanoma: results of intergroup trial E1694/S9512/C509801. J Clin Oncol 2001;19:2370–80.

96 Kirkwood JM, Strawderman MH, Ernstoff MS, et al. Interferon alfa-2b adjuvant therapy of high-risk resected cutaneous melanoma: the Eastern Cooperative Oncology Group Trial EST 1684. J Clin Oncol 1996;14:7–17.

97 Kirkwood JM, Ibrahim JG, Sondak VK, et al. High- and low-dose interferon alfa-2b in high-risk melanoma: first analysis of intergroup trial E1690/S9111/C9190. J Clin Oncol 2000;18:2444–58.

98 Creagan ET, Dalton RJ, Ahmann DL, et al. Randomized, surgical adjuvant clinical trial of recombinant interferon alfa-2a in selected patients with malignant melanoma. J Clin Oncol 1995;13:2776–83.

99 Pehamberger H, Soyer HP, Steiner A, et al. Adjuvant interferon alfa-2a treatment in resected primary stage II cutaneous melanoma. Austrian Malignant Melanoma Cooperative Group. J Clin Oncol 1998;16:1425–9.

100 Cascinelli N, Belli F, MacKie RM, et al. Effect of long-term adjuvant therapy with interferon alpha-2a in patients with regional node metastases from cutaneous melanoma: a randomised trial. Lancet 2001;358:866–9.

101 Cameron DA, Cornbleet MC, Mackie RM, et al. Adjuvant interferon alpha 2b in high risk melanoma—the Scottish study. Br J Cancer 2001;84:1146–9.

102 Eggermont AM, Suciu S, MacKie R, et al. Post-surgery adjuvant therapy with intermediate doses of interferon alfa 2b versus observation in patients with stage IIb/III melanoma (EORTC 18952): randomised controlled trial. Lancet 2005;366:1189–96.

103 Kirkwood JM, Manola J, Ibrahim J, et al. A pooled analysis of Eastern Cooperative Oncology Group and intergroup trials of adjuvant high-dose interferon for melanoma. Clin Cancer Res 2004;10:1670–7.

104 Kirkwood JM, Tarhini AA. Adjuvant high-dose interferon-alpha therapy for high-risk melanoma. Forum (Genova) 2003;13:127–40; quiz 87–8.

105 Gogas H, Ioannovich J, Dafni U, et al. Prognostic significance of autoimmunity during treatment of melanoma with interferon. N Engl J Med 2006;354:709–18.

106 Agarwala SS, Kirkwood JM. Interferons in melanoma. Curr Opin Oncol 1996;8:167–74.

107 Zeuzem S, Feinman SV, Rasenack J, et al. Peginterferon alfa-2a in patients with chronic hepatitis C. N Engl J Med 2000;343:1666–72.

108 Heathcote EJ, Shiffman ML, Cooksley WG, et al. Peginterferon alfa-2a in patients with chronic hepatitis C and cirrhosis. N Engl J Med 2000;343:1673–80.

109 Dummer R, Garbe C, Thompson JA, et al. Randomized dose-escalation study evaluating peginterferon alfa-2a in patients with metastatic malignant melanoma. J Clin Oncol 2006;24:1188–94.

110 Kaiser LR, Burk MW, Morton DL. Adjuvant therapy for malignant melanoma. Surg Clin North Am 1981;61:1249–57.

111 Ariyan S, Kirkwood JM, Mitchell MS, et al. Intralymphatic and regional surgical adjuvant immunotherapy in high-risk melanoma of the extremities. Surgery 1982;92:459–63.

112 Brocker EB, Suter L, Czarnetzki BM, et al. BCG immunotherapy in stage I melanoma patients. Does it influence prognosis determined by HLA-DR expression in high-risk primary tumors? Cancer Immunol Immunother 1986;23:155–7.

113 Veronesi U, Adamus J, Aubert C, et al. A randomized trial of adjuvant chemotherapy and immunotherapy in cutaneous melanoma. N Engl J Med 1982;307:913–6.

114 Czarnetzki BM, Macher E, Suciu S, et al. Long-term adjuvant immunotherapy in stage I high risk malignant melanoma, comparing two BCG preparations versus non-treatment in a randomised

multicentre study (EORTC Protocol 18781). Eur J Cancer 1993;29A:1237–42.

115 Agarwala SS, Neuberg D, Park Y, et al. Mature results of a phase III randomized trial of bacillus Calmette-Guerin (BCG) versus observation and BCG plus dacarbazine versus BCG in the adjuvant therapy of American Joint Committee on Cancer stage I–III melanoma (E1673): a trial of the Eastern Oncology Group. Cancer 2004;100:1692–8.

116 Kleeberg UR, Suciu S, Brocker EB, et al. Final results of the EORTC 18871/DKG 80-1 randomised phase III trial. rIFN-alpha2b versus rIFN-gamma versus ISCADOR M versus observation after surgery in melanoma patients with either high-risk primary (thickness >3 mm) or regional lymph node metastasis. Eur J Cancer 2004;40:390–402.

117 Kolmel KF, Grange JM, Krone B, et al. Prior immunisation of patients with malignant melanoma with vaccinia or BCG is associated with better survival. A European Organization for Research and Treatment of Cancer cohort study on 542 patients. Eur J Cancer 2005;41:118–25.

118 Spagnoli GC, Adamina M, Bolli M, et al. Active antigen-specific immunotherapy of melanoma: from basic science to clinical investigation. World J Surg 2005;29:692–9.

119 Wallack MK, Sivanandham M, Balch CM, et al. Surgical adjuvant active specific immunotherapy for patients with stage III melanoma: the final analysis of data from a phase III, randomized, double-blind, multicenter vaccinia melanoma oncolysate trial. J Am Coll Surg 1998;187:69–77; discussion 79.

120 Berd D, Maguire HC Jr, Schuchter LM, et al. Autologous hapten-modified melanoma vaccine as postsurgical adjuvant treatment after resection of nodal metastases. J Clin Oncol 1997;15:2359–70.

121 Hersey P, Coates AS, McCarthy WH, et al. Adjuvant immunotherapy of patients with high-risk melanoma using vaccinia viral lysates of melanoma: results of a randomized trial. J Clin Oncol 2002;20:4181–90.

122 Sosman JA, Unger JM, Liu PY, et al. Adjuvant immunotherapy of resected, intermediate-thickness, node-negative melanoma with an allogeneic tumor vaccine: impact of HLA class I antigen expression on outcome. J Clin Oncol 2002;20:2067–75.

123 Hamid O, Solomon JC, Scotland R, et al. Alum with interleukin-12 augments immunity to a melanoma peptide vaccine: correlation with time to relapse in patients with resected high-risk disease. Clin Cancer Res 2007;13:215–22.

124 Lu B, Makhija SK, Nettelbeck DM, et al. Evaluation of tumor-specific promoter activities in melanoma. Gene Ther 2005;12:330–8.

125 Fisher PB, Sarkar D, Lebedeva IV, et al. Melanoma differentiation associated gene-7/interleukin-24 (mda-7/IL-24): novel gene therapeutic for metastatic melanoma. Toxicol Appl Pharmacol 2007;7:577–86.

126 Wu XZ, Wei HM, Zheng XD, et al. [Induction and mechanism study of anti-melanoma immune response by M. tuberculosis Ag85B]. Xi Bao Yu Fen Zi Mian Yi Xue Za Zhi 2007;23:36–8.

127 Mitrus I, Delic K, Wrobel N, et al. Combination of IL-12 gene therapy and CTX chemotherapy inhibits growth of primary B16(F10) melanoma tumors in mice. Acta Biochim Pol 2006;53:357–60.

128 Jazowiecka-Rakus J, Jarosz M, Szala S. Combination of vasostatin gene therapy with cyclophosphamide inhibits growth of B16(F10) melanoma tumours. Acta Biochim Pol 2006;53:199–202.

129 Geng H, Zhang GM, Xiao H, et al. HSP70 vaccine in combination with gene therapy with plasmid DNA encoding sPD-1 overcomes immune resistance and suppresses the progression of pulmonary metastatic melanoma. Int J Cancer 2006;118:2657–64.

130 Morita N, Hiratsuka J, Kondoh H, et al. Improvement of the tumor-suppressive effect of boron neutron capture therapy for amelanotic melanoma by intratumoral injection of the tyrosinase gene. Cancer Res 2006;66:3747–53.

131 Creagan ET, Cupps RE, Ivins JC, et al. Adjuvant radiation therapy for regional nodal metastases from malignant melanoma: a randomized, prospective study. Cancer 1978;42:2206–10.

132 Ballo MT, Bonnen MD, Garden AS, et al. Adjuvant irradiation for cervical lymph node metastases from melanoma. Cancer 2003;97:1789–96.

133 Ballo MT, Zagars GK, Gershenwald JE, et al. A critical assessment of adjuvant radiotherapy for inguinal lymph node metastases from melanoma. Ann Surg Oncol 2004;11:1079–84.

134 Fletcher JR, White CR Jr, Fletcher WS. Improved survival rates of patients with acral lentiginous melanoma treated with hyperthermic isolation perfusion, wide excision, and regional lymphadenectomy. Am J Surg 1986;151:593–8.

135 Ghussen F, Nagel K, Groth W, et al. A prospective randomized study of regional extremity perfusion in patients with malignant melanoma. Ann Surg 1984;200:764–8.

136 Wieberdink J, Benckhuysen C, Braat RP, et al. Dosimetry in isolation perfusion of the limbs by

assessment of perfused tissue volume and grading of toxic tissue reactions. Eur J Cancer Clin Oncol 1982;18:905–10.

137 Hayes AJ, Neuhaus SJ, Clark MA, et al. Isolated limb perfusion with melphalan and tumor necrosis factor alpha for advanced melanoma and soft-tissue sarcoma. Ann Surg Oncol 2007;14:230–8.

138 Lienard D, Eggermont AM, Schraffordt Koops H, et al. Isolated perfusion of the limb with high-dose tumour necrosis factor-alpha (TNF-alpha), interferon-gamma (IFN-gamma) and melphalan for melanoma stage III. Results of a multi-centre pilot study. Melanoma Res 1994;4 Suppl 1:21–6.

139 Lienard D, Eggermont AM, Koops HS, et al. Isolated limb perfusion with tumour necrosis factor-alpha and melphalan with or without interferon-gamma for the treatment of in-transit melanoma metastases: a multicentre randomized phase II study. Melanoma Res 1999;9:491–502.

140 Cornett WR, McCall LM, Petersen RP, et al. Randomized multicenter trial of hyperthermic isolated limb perfusion with melphalan alone compared with melphalan plus tumor necrosis factor: American College of Surgeons Oncology Group Trial Z0020. J Clin Oncol 2006;24:4196–201.

141 Franklin HR, Schraffordt Koops H, Oldhoff J, et al. To perfuse or not to perfuse? A retrospective comparative study to evaluate the effect of adjuvant isolated regional perfusion in patients with stage I extremity melanoma with a thickness of 1.5 mm or greater. J Clin Oncol 1988;6:701–8.

142 Schraffordt Koops H, Kroon BB, Oldhoff J, et al. Controversies concerning adjuvant regional isolated perfusion for stage I melanoma of the extremities. World J Surg 1992;16:241–5.

143 Rege VB, Leone LA, Soderberg CH Jr, et al. Hyperthermic adjuvant perfusion chemotherapy for stage I malignant melanoma of the extremity with literature review. Cancer 1983;52:2033–9.

144 Nagabhushan JS, Murphy K, Angerson W, et al. Prognostic scoring in patients with melanoma after adjuvant isolated limb perfusion. J Surg Res 2007;138:22–4.

145 Koops HS, Vaglini M, Suciu S, et al. Prophylactic isolated limb perfusion for localized, high-risk limb melanoma: results of a multicenter randomized phase III trial. European Organization for Research and Treatment of Cancer Malignant Melanoma Cooperative Group Protocol 18832, the World Health Organization Melanoma Program Trial 15, and the North American Perfusion Group Southwest

Oncology Group-8593. J Clin Oncol 1998;16:2906–12.

146 Hill GJ 2nd, Krementz ET, Hill HZ. Dimethyl triazeno imidazole carboxamide and combination therapy for melanoma. IV. Late results after complete response to chemotherapy (Central Oncology Group protocols 7130, 7131, and 7131A). Cancer 1984;53:1299–305.

147 Eggermont AM, Kirkwood JM. Re-evaluating the role of dacarbazine in metastatic melanoma: what have we learned in 30 years? Eur J Cancer 2004;40:1825–36.

148 Hoelzer KL, Harrison BR, Luedke DW, et al. Dose-response relationship to dacarbazine demonstrated in a patient with malignant melanoma. Cancer Treat Rep 1986;70:1211–2.

149 Bedikian AY, Millward M, Pehamberger H, et al. Bcl-2 antisense (oblimersen sodium) plus dacarbazine in patients with advanced melanoma: the Oblimersen Melanoma Study Group. J Clin Oncol 2006;24:4738–45.

150 Soengas MS, Lowe SW. Apoptosis and melanoma chemoresistance. Oncogene 2003;22:3138–51.

151 Kaufmann R, Spieth K, Leiter U, et al. Temozolomide in combination with interferon-alfa versus temozolomide alone in patients with advanced metastatic melanoma: a randomized, phase III, multicenter study from the Dermatologic Cooperative Oncology Group. J Clin Oncol 2005;23:9001–7.

152 Middleton MR, Grob JJ, Aaronson N, et al. Randomized phase III study of temozolomide versus dacarbazine in the treatment of patients with advanced metastatic malignant melanoma. J Clin Oncol 2000;18:158–66.

153 Bleehen NM, Newlands ES, Lee SM, et al. Cancer Research Campaign phase II trial of temozolomide in metastatic melanoma. J Clin Oncol 1995;13:910–3.

154 Jacquillat C, Khayat D, Banzet P, et al. Final report of the French multicenter phase II study of the nitrosourea fotemustine in 153 evaluable patients with disseminated malignant melanoma including patients with cerebral metastases. Cancer 1990;66:1873–8.

155 Avril MF, Aamdal S, Grob JJ, et al. Fotemustine compared with dacarbazine in patients with disseminated malignant melanoma: a phase III study. J Clin Oncol 2004;22:1118–25.

156 Mornex F, Thomas L, Mohr P, et al. [Randomised phase III trial of fotemustine versus fotemustine plus whole brain irradiation in cerebral metastases of melanoma]. Cancer Radiother 2003;7:1–8.

157 Hwu WJ, Lis E, Menell JH, et al. Temozolomide plus thalidomide in patients with brain metastases from melanoma: a phase II study. Cancer 2005;103:2590–7.

158 Hofmann M, Kiecker F, Wurm R, et al. Temozolomide with or without radiotherapy in melanoma with unresectable brain metastases. J Neurooncol 2006;76:59–64.

159 Glover D, Glick JH, Weiler C, et al. WR-2721 and high-dose cisplatin: an active combination in the treatment of metastatic melanoma. J Clin Oncol 1987;5:574–8.

160 Creagan ET, Ahmann DL, Schutt AJ, et al. Phase II study of the combination of vinblastine plus cisplatin administered by continuous 120-hour infusion for patients with advanced malignant melanoma. Cancer Treat Rep 1987;71:769–70.

161 Oratz R, Speyer JL, Green M, et al. Treatment of metastatic malignant melanoma with dacarbazine and cisplatin. Cancer Treat Rep 1987;71:877–8.

162 Evans LM, Casper ES, Rosenbluth R. Phase II trial of carboplatin in advanced malignant melanoma. Cancer Treat Rep 1987;71:171–2.

163 Guven K, Kittler H, Wolff K, et al. Cisplatin and carboplatin combination as second-line chemotherapy in dacarbazine-resistant melanoma patients. Melanoma Res 2001;11:411–5.

164 Smylie MG, Wong R, Mihalcioiu C, et al. A phase II, open label, monotherapy study of liposomal doxorubicin in patients with metastatic malignant melanoma. Invest New Drugs 2007;25:155–9.

165 Eigentler TK, Caroli UM, Radny P, et al. Palliative therapy of disseminated malignant melanoma: a systematic review of 41 randomised clinical trials. Lancet Oncol 2003;4:748–59.

166 Jelic S, Babovic N, Kovcin V, et al. Comparison of the efficacy of two different dosage dacarbazine-based regimens and two regimens without dacarbazine in metastatic melanoma: a single-centre randomized four-arm study. Melanoma Res 2002;12:91–8.

167 McClay EF, Mastrangelo MJ, Bellet RE, et al. Combination chemotherapy and hormonal therapy in the treatment of malignant melanoma. Cancer Treat Rep 1987;71:465–9.

168 Cocconi G, Bella M, Calabresi F, et al. Treatment of metastatic malignant melanoma with dacarbazine plus tamoxifen. N Engl J Med 1992;327:516–23.

169 Rusthoven JJ, Quirt IC, Iscoe NA, et al. Randomized, double-blind, placebo-controlled trial comparing the response rates of carmustine, dacarbazine, and cisplatin with and without tamoxifen in patients with metastatic melanoma. National Cancer Institute of Canada Clinical Trials Group. J Clin Oncol 1996;14:2083–90.

170 Creagan ET, Suman VJ, Dalton RJ, et al. Phase III clinical trial of the combination of cisplatin, dacarbazine, and carmustine with or without tamoxifen in patients with advanced malignant melanoma. J Clin Oncol 1999;17:1884–90.

171 Falkson CI, Ibrahim J, Kirkwood JM, et al. Phase III trial of dacarbazine versus dacarbazine with interferon alpha-2b versus dacarbazine with tamoxifen versus dacarbazine with interferon alpha-2b and tamoxifen in patients with metastatic malignant melanoma: an Eastern Cooperative Oncology Group study. J Clin Oncol 1998;16:1743–51.

172 Agarwala SS, Ferri W, Gooding W, et al. A phase III randomized trial of dacarbazine and carboplatin with and without tamoxifen in the treatment of patients with metastatic melanoma. Cancer 1999;85:1979–84.

173 Cocconi G, Passalacqua R, Foladore S, et al. Treatment of metastatic malignant melanoma with dacarbazine plus tamoxifen, or vindesine plus tamoxifen: a prospective randomized study. Melanoma Res 2003;13:73–9.

174 Del Prete SA, Maurer LH, O'Donnell J, et al. Combination chemotherapy with cisplatin, carmustine, dacarbazine, and tamoxifen in metastatic melanoma. Cancer Treat Rep 1984;68:1403–5.

175 Saba HI, Cruse CW, Wells KE, et al. Treatment of stage IV malignant melanoma with dacarbazine, carmustine, cisplatin, and tamoxifen regimens: a University of South Florida and H. Lee Moffitt Melanoma Center Study. Ann Plast Surg 1992;28:65–9.

176 Lattanzi SC, Tosteson T, Chertoff J, et al. Dacarbazine, cisplatin and carmustine, with or without tamoxifen, for metastatic melanoma: 5-year follow-up. Melanoma Res 1995;5:365–9.

177 Richards JM, Gilewski TA, Ramming K, et al. Effective chemotherapy for melanoma after treatment with interleukin-2. Cancer 1992;69:427–9.

178 Chapman PB, Einhorn LH, Meyers ML, et al. Phase III multicenter randomized trial of the Dartmouth regimen versus dacarbazine in patients with metastatic melanoma. J Clin Oncol 1999;17:2745–51.

179 Kasper B, D'Hondt V, Vereecken P, et al. Novel treatment strategies for malignant melanoma: a new beginning? Crit Rev Oncol Hematol 2007;62:16–22.

180 Rosenberg SA, Lotze MT, Muul LM, et al. Observations on the systemic administration of autologous lymphokine-activated killer cells and recombinant

interleukin-2 to patients with metastatic cancer. N Engl J Med 1985;313:1485–92.

181 Lotze MT, Chang AE, Seipp CA, et al. High-dose recombinant interleukin 2 in the treatment of patients with disseminated cancer. Responses, treatment-related morbidity, and histologic findings. JAMA 1986;256:3117–24.

182 Thatcher N, Dazzi H, Johnson RJ, et al. Recombinant interleukin-2 (rIL-2) given intrasplenically and intra-venously for advanced malignant melanoma. A phase I and II study. Br J Cancer 1989;60:770–4.

183 Parkinson DR, Abrams JS, Wiernik PH, et al. Interleukin-2 therapy in patients with metastatic malignant melanoma: a phase II study. J Clin Oncol 1990;8:1650–6.

184 Atkins MB, Lotze MT, Dutcher JP, et al. High-dose recombinant interleukin 2 therapy for patients with metastatic melanoma: analysis of 270 patients treated between 1985 and 1993. J Clin Oncol 1999;17:2105–16.

185 Rosenberg SA, Lotze MT, Yang JC, et al. Prospective randomized trial of high-dose interleukin-2 alone or in conjunction with lymphokine-activated killer cells for the treatment of patients with advanced cancer. J Natl Cancer Inst 1993;85:622–32.

186 Weiss GR, Margolin KA, Aronson FR, et al. A randomized phase II trial of continuous infusion interleukin-2 or bolus injection interleukin-2 plus lymphokine-activated killer cells for advanced renal cell carcinoma. J Clin Oncol 1992;10:275–81.

187 Trefzer U, Hofmann M, Sterry W, et al. Cytokine and anticytokine therapy in dermatology. Expert Opin Biol Ther 2003;3:733–43.

188 Hofmann M, Audring H, Sterry W, et al. Interleukin-2-associated bullous drug dermatosis. Dermatology 2005;210:74–5.

189 Green DS, Bodman-Smith MD, Dalgleish AG, et al. Phase I/II study of topical imiquimod and intralesional interleukin-2 in the treatment of accessible metastases in malignant melanoma. Br J Dermatol 2007;156:337–45.

190 Rosenberg SA, Lotze MT, Yang JC, et al. Combination therapy with interleukin-2 and alpha-interferon for the treatment of patients with advanced cancer. J Clin Oncol 1989;7:1863–74.

191 Keilholz U, Scheibenbogen C, Tilgen W, et al. Interferon-alpha and interleukin-2 in the treatment of metastatic melanoma. Comparison of two phase II trials. Cancer 1993;72:607–14.

192 Sparano JA, Fisher RI, Sunderland M, et al. Randomized phase III trial of treatment with high-dose interleukin-2 either alone or in combination with interferon alfa-2a in patients with advanced melanoma. J Clin Oncol 1993;11:1969–77.

193 Huncharek M, Caubet JF, McGarry R. Single-agent DTIC versus combination chemotherapy with or without immunotherapy in metastatic melanoma: a meta-analysis of 3273 patients from 20 randomized trials. Melanoma Res 2001;11:75–81.

194 Bezwoda WR. The treatment of disseminated malignant melanoma with special reference to the role of interferons, vinca alkaloids and tamoxifen. Cancer Treat Rev 1997;23:17–34.

195 Falkson CI, Falkson G, Falkson HC. Improved results with the addition of interferon alfa-2b to dacarbazine in the treatment of patients with metastatic malignant melanoma. J Clin Oncol 1991;9:1403–8.

196 Thomson DB, Adena M, McLeod GR, et al. Interferon-alpha 2a does not improve response or survival when combined with dacarbazine in metastatic malignant melanoma: results of a multi-institutional Australian randomized trial. Melanoma Res 1993;3:133–8.

197 Bajetta E, Di Leo A, Zampino MG, et al. Multi-center randomized trial of dacarbazine alone or in combination with two different doses and schedules of interferon alfa-2a in the treatment of advanced melanoma. J Clin Oncol 1994;12:806–11.

198 Young AM, Marsden J, Goodman A, et al. Prospective randomized comparison of dacarbazine (DTIC) versus DTIC plus interferon-alpha (IFN-alpha) in metastatic melanoma. Clin Oncol (R Coll Radiol) 2001;13:458–65.

199 Richards JM, Mehta N, Ramming K, et al. Sequential chemoimmunotherapy in the treatment of metastatic melanoma. J Clin Oncol 1992;10:1338–43.

200 Legha SS, Buzaid AC. Role of recombinant interleukin-2 in combination with interferon-alfa and chemotherapy in the treatment of advanced melanoma. Semin Oncol 1993;20:27–32.

201 Atkins MB, O'Boyle KR, Sosman JA, et al. Multi-institutional phase II trial of intensive combination chemoimmunotherapy for metastatic melanoma. J Clin Oncol 1994;12:1553–60.

202 Khayat D, Borel C, Tourani JM, et al. Sequential chemoimmunotherapy with cisplatin, interleukin-2, and interferon alfa-2a for metastatic melanoma. J Clin Oncol 1993;11:2173–80.

203 Legha SS. Durable complete responses in metastatic melanoma treated with interleukin-2 in combination with interferon alpha and chemotherapy. Semin Oncol 1997;24:S39–43.

204 Proebstle TM, Fuchs T, Scheibenbogen C, et al. Long-term outcome of treatment with dacarbazine, cisplatin, interferon-alpha and intravenous high dose interleukin-2 in poor risk melanoma patients. Melanoma Res 1998;8:557–63.

205 Ridolfi R, Chiarion-Sileni V, Guida M, et al. Cisplatin, dacarbazine with or without subcutaneous interleukin-2, and interferon alpha-2b in advanced melanoma outpatients: results from an Italian multicenter phase III randomized clinical trial. J Clin Oncol 2002;20:1600–7.

206 Legha SS, Ring S, Bedikian A, et al. Treatment of metastatic melanoma with combined chemotherapy containing cisplatin, vinblastine and dacarbazine (CVD) and biotherapy using interleukin-2 and interferon-alpha. Ann Oncol 1996;7:827–35.

207 Legha SS, Ring S, Eton O, et al. Development of a biochemotherapy regimen with concurrent administration of cisplatin, vinblastine, dacarbazine, interferon alfa, and interleukin-2 for patients with metastatic melanoma. J Clin Oncol 1998;16:1752–9.

208 Eton O, Legha SS, Bedikian AY, et al. Sequential biochemotherapy versus chemotherapy for metastatic melanoma: results from a phase III randomized trial. J Clin Oncol 2002;20:2045–52.

209 Rosenberg SA, Yang JC, Schwartzentruber DJ, et al. Prospective randomized trial of the treatment of patients with metastatic melanoma using chemotherapy with cisplatin, dacarbazine, and tamoxifen alone or in combination with interleukin-2 and interferon alfa-2b. J Clin Oncol 1999;17:968–75.

210 Bajetta E, Del Vecchio M, Nova P, et al. Multicenter phase III randomized trial of polychemotherapy (CVD regimen) versus the same chemotherapy (CT) plus subcutaneous interleukin-2 and interferon-alpha2b in metastatic melanoma. Ann Oncol 2006;17:571–7.

211 Sertoli MR, Queirolo P, Bajetta E, et al. Multi-institutional phase II randomized trial of integrated therapy with cisplatin, dacarbazine, vindesine, subcutaneous interleukin-2, interferon alpha2a and tamoxifen in metastatic melanoma. BREMIM (Biological Response Modifiers in Melanoma). Melanoma Res 1999;9:503–9.

212 Johnston SR, Constenla DO, Moore J, et al. Randomized phase II trial of BCDT [carmustine (BCNU), cisplatin, dacarbazine (DTIC) and tamoxifen] with or without interferon alpha (IFN-alpha) and interleukin (IL-2) in patients with metastatic melanoma. Br J Cancer 1998;77:1280–6.

213 Atzpodien J, Neuber K, Kamanabrou D, et al. Combination chemotherapy with or without s.c. IL-2 and IFN-alpha: results of a prospectively randomized trial of the Cooperative Advanced Malignant Melanoma Chemoimmunotherapy Group (ACIMM). Br J Cancer 2002;86:179–84.

214 Keilholz U, Goey SH, Punt CJ, et al. Interferon alfa-2a and interleukin-2 with or without cisplatin in metastatic melanoma: a randomized trial of the European Organization for Research and Treatment of Cancer Melanoma Cooperative Group. J Clin Oncol 1997;15:2579–88.

215 Keilholz U, Punt CJ, Gore M, et al. Dacarbazine, cisplatin, and interferon-alfa-2b with or without interleukin-2 in metastatic melanoma: a randomized phase III trial (18951) of the European Organisation for Research and Treatment of Cancer Melanoma Group. J Clin Oncol 2005;23:6747–55.

216 Mita MM, Rowinsky EK, Forero L, et al. A phase II, pharmacokinetic, and biologic study of semaxanib and thalidomide in patients with metastatic melanoma. Cancer Chemother Pharmacol 2007;59:165–74.

217 Alexander HR Jr, Fraker DL, Bartlett DL. Isolated limb perfusion for malignant melanoma. Semin Surg Oncol 1996;12:416–28.

218 Vrouenraets BC, Nieweg OE, Kroon BB. Thirty-five years of isolated limb perfusion for melanoma: indications and results. Br J Surg 1996;83:1319–28.

219 Noorda EM, Vrouenraets BC, Nieweg OE, et al. Isolated limb perfusion for unresectable melanoma of the extremities. Arch Surg 2004;139:1237–42.

220 Lienard D, Ewalenko P, Delmotte JJ, et al. High-dose recombinant tumor necrosis factor alpha in combination with interferon gamma and melphalan in isolation perfusion of the limbs for melanoma and sarcoma. J Clin Oncol 1992;10:52–60.

221 Takkenberg RB, Vrouenraets BC, van Geel AN, et al. Palliative isolated limb perfusion for advanced limb disease in stage IV melanoma patients. J Surg Oncol 2005;91:107–11.

222 Klein E, Holtermann OA, Helm F, et al. Immunologic approaches to the management of primary and secondary tumors involving the skin and soft tissues: review of a ten-year program. Transplant Proc 1975;7:297–315.

223 Klein E, Schwartz RA, Case RW, et al. Accessible tumors. In: LoBuglio AF, editor. Clinical immunotherapy. New York: Marcel Dekker; 1980. p. 31–71.

224 Morton DL, Eilber FR, Holmes EC, et al. BCG immunotherapy of malignant melanoma: summary of a seven-year experience. Ann Surg 1974;180:635–43.

225 Mastrangelo MJ, Bellet RE, Berkelhammer J, et al. Regression of pulmonary metastatic disease associated with intralesional BCG therapy of intracutaneous melanoma metastases. Cancer 1975;36:1305–8.

226 Wack C, Kirst A, Becker JC, et al. Chemoimmunotherapy for melanoma with dacarbazine and 2,4-dinitrochlorobenzene elicits a specific T cell–dependent immune response. Cancer Immunol Immunother 2002;51:431–9.

227 Radny P, Caroli UM, Bauer J, et al. Phase II trial of intralesional therapy with interleukin-2 in soft-tissue melanoma metastases. Br J Cancer 2003;89:1620–6.

228 King DM, Albertini MR, Schalch H, et al. Phase I clinical trial of the immunocytokine EMD 273063 in melanoma patients. J Clin Oncol 2004;22:4463–73.

229 Scott AM, Lee FT, Hopkins W, et al. Specific targeting, biodistribution, and lack of immunogenicity of chimeric anti-GD3 monoclonal antibody KM871 in patients with metastatic melanoma: results of a phase I trial. J Clin Oncol 2001;19:3976–87.

230 Hsueh EC, Essner R, Foshag LJ, et al. Prolonged survival after complete resection of disseminated melanoma and active immunotherapy with a therapeutic cancer vaccine. J Clin Oncol 2002;20:4549–54.

231 Berd D, Sato T, Cohn H, et al. Treatment of metastatic melanoma with autologous, hapten-modified melanoma vaccine: regression of pulmonary metastases. Int J Cancer 2001;94:531–9.

232 Belli F, Testori A, Rivoltini L, et al. Vaccination of metastatic melanoma patients with autologous tumor-derived heat shock protein gp96-peptide complexes: clinical and immunologic findings. J Clin Oncol 2002;20:4169–80.

233 Lee P, Wang F, Kuniyoshi J, et al. Effects of interleukin-12 on the immune response to a multipeptide vaccine for resected metastatic melanoma. J Clin Oncol 2001;19:3836–47.

234 Slingluff CL Jr, Petroni GR, Yamshchikov GV, et al. Immunologic and clinical outcomes of vaccination with a multiepitope melanoma peptide vaccine plus low-dose interleukin-2 administered either concurrently or on a delayed schedule. J Clin Oncol 2004;22:4474–85.

235 Parmiani G, Castelli C, Dalerba P, et al. Cancer immunotherapy with peptide-based vaccines: what have we achieved? Where are we going? J Natl Cancer Inst 2002;94:805–18.

236 Trefzer U, Herberth G, Wohlan K, et al. Vaccination with hybrids of tumor and dendritic cells induces tumor-specific T-cell and clinical responses in melanoma stage III and IV patients. Int J Cancer 2004;110:730–40.

237 Hersey P, Menzies SW, Halliday GM, et al. Phase I/II study of treatment with dendritic cell vaccines in patients with disseminated melanoma. Cancer Immunol Immunother 2004;53:125–34.

238 Hawkins WG, Gold JS, Blachere NE, et al. Xenogeneic DNA immunization in melanoma models for minimal residual disease. J Surg Res 2002;102:137–43.

239 Essner R. Surgical treatment of malignant melanoma. Surg Clin North Am 2003;83:109–56.

240 Wood TF, DiFronzo LA, Rose DM, et al. Does complete resection of melanoma metastatic to solid intra-abdominal organs improve survival? Ann Surg Oncol 2001;8:658–62.

241 Skibber JM, Soong SJ, Austin L, et al. Cranial irradiation after surgical excision of brain metastases in melanoma patients. Ann Surg Oncol 1996;3:118–23.

242 Fife KM, Colman MH, Stevens GN, et al. Determinants of outcome in melanoma patients with cerebral metastases. J Clin Oncol 2004;22:1293–300.

243 Petersen RP, Hanish SI, Haney JC, et al. Improved survival with pulmonary metastasectomy: an analysis of 1720 patients with pulmonary metastatic melanoma. J Thorac Cardiovasc Surg 2007;133:104–10.

244 Herman P, Machado MA, Montagnini AL, et al. Selected patients with metastatic melanoma may benefit from liver resection. World J Surg 2007;31:171–4.

245 Attia P, Phan GQ, Maker AV, et al. Autoimmunity correlates with tumor regression in patients with metastatic melanoma treated with anti-cytotoxic T-lymphocyte antigen-4. J Clin Oncol 2005;23:6043–53.

246 Phan GQ, Yang JC, Sherry RM, et al. Cancer regression and autoimmunity induced by cytotoxic T lymphocyte-associated antigen 4 blockade in patients with metastatic melanoma. Proc Natl Acad Sci U S A 2003;100:8372–7.

247 Eisen T, Ahmad T, Flaherty KT, et al. Sorafenib in advanced melanoma: a phase II randomised discontinuation trial analysis. Br J Cancer 2006;95:581–6.

248 Becker JC, Kirkwood JM, Agarwala SS, et al. Molecularly targeted therapy for melanoma: current reality and future options. Cancer 2006;107:2317–27.

249 Markovic SN, Geyer SM, Dawkins F, et al. A phase II study of bortezomib in the treatment of metastatic malignant melanoma. Cancer 2005;103:2584–9.

250 Margolin K, Longmate J, Baratta T, et al. CCI-779 in metastatic melanoma: a phase II trial of the California Cancer Consortium. Cancer 2005;104:1045–8.

251 Ryan QC, Headlee D, Acharya M, et al. Phase I and pharmacokinetic study of MS-275, a histone deacetylase inhibitor, in patients with advanced and refractory solid tumors or lymphoma. J Clin Oncol 2005;23:3912–22.

252 Stevens G, McKay MJ. Dispelling the myths surrounding radiotherapy for treatment of cutaneous melanoma. Lancet Oncol 2006;7:575–83.

253 Harwood AR. Conventional fractionated radiotherapy for 51 patients with lentigo maligna and lentigo maligna melanoma. Int J Radiat Oncol Biol Phys 1983;9:1019–21.

254 Farshad A, Burg G, Panizzon R, et al. A retrospective study of 150 patients with lentigo maligna and lentigo maligna melanoma and the efficacy of radiotherapy using Grenz or soft X-rays. Br J Dermatol 2002;146:1042–6.

255 Schmid-Wendtner MH, Brunner B, Konz B, et al. Fractionated radiotherapy of lentigo maligna and lentigo maligna melanoma in 64 patients. J Am Acad Dermatol 2000;43:477–82.

256 Sause WT, Cooper JS, Rush S, et al. Fraction size in external beam radiation therapy in the treatment of melanoma. Int J Radiat Oncol Biol Phys 1991;20:429–32.

257 Trefzer U, Sterry W. Topical immunotherapy with diphenylcyclopropenone in combination with DTIC and radiation for cutaneous metastases of melanoma. Dermatology 2005;211:370–1.

258 Peacock KH, Lesser GJ. Current therapeutic approaches in patients with brain metastases. Curr Treat Options Oncol 2006;7:479–89.

259 Douglas JG, Margolin K. The treatment of brain metastases from malignant melanoma. Semin Oncol 2002;29:518–24.

260 Schwartz RA. Edmund Klein (1921–1999). J Am Acad Dermatol 2001;44:716–8.

Index